CLASSIC PAPERS IN
HYPERLIPIDAEMIA

CLASSIC PAPERS IN
HYPERLIPIDAEMIA

EDITORS
J R QUINEY
Lecturer
Division of Chemical Pathology and Metabolic Disorders
St Thomas' Hospital
London, UK

G F WATTS
Lecturer
Division of Chemical Pathology and Metabolic Disorders
St Thomas' Hospital
London, UK

FOREWORD
B LEWIS
Professor of Chemical Pathology and Metabolic Disorders
St Thomas' Hospital
London, UK

MSD
MERCK
SHARP &
DOHME

science press

Copyright 1989 by Science Press Limited
6 Lowther Road, Barnes, London SW13 9ND
England

British Library Cataloguing in Publication Data
Classic Papers in Hyperlipidaemia
1. Man. Blood. Hyperlipidaemia
2. Quiney, J (Jeremy) II. Watts G. (Gerald)

616. 3'997

ISBN 1-870026-80-2

Designed by Robin Dodd FCSD
Printed and bound in the United Kingdom by
Dotesios Printers Limited, Trowbridge, Wiltshire

FOREWORD

I t cannot have been easy for the authors to select from the voluminous literature on hyperlipidaemia, atherosclerosis and coronary heart disease. Few conditions can have been the subject of a greater research effort, particularly in the past twenty years; and few, more successfully. Whilst many issues remain to be solved, the history of research on the metabolic bases of coronary disease is one of the triumphs of epidemiology, clinical research and cell biology.

Many disciplines have contributed to our understanding of heart disease, and of the potential for its prevention, and Dr Quiney and Dr Watts demonstrate this clearly in their selection of topics. There has been a particular excitement about this development; for those of us who have followed the literature of the subject for some years it has been intellectually satisfying to see the threads of basic research converge into a new and clinically relevant field of medicine.

The scope of the book is also of value for its balance between the early and the current literature. The investigator immersed in the overwhelming task of keeping up with new advances often pays inadequate attention to the earlier classic papers. Moreover, the pattern of coronary disease research and its evolution, with its emphasis on nutritional and other behavioural causes, is, I believe, instructive to those studying other major chronic diseases. There is much to learn from the success story outlined in this volume.

B. Lewis
Professor of Chemical Pathology and
Metabolic Disorders
St Thomas' Hospital
London, UK

INTRODUCTION

Coronary heart disease is the major clinical consequence of atherosclerosis and is the commonest cause of morbidity and mortality in western populations. In the United States, for example, over half a million people die every year from this cause with its attendant colossal medical and financial burdens. A wealth of evidence has now identified hyperlipidaemia, in particular that associated with high cholesterol levels, as intimately involved in atherosclerosis and, hence, a major risk factor for coronary heart disease. The purpose of this book is to present the major milestones which have led to our present state of knowledge about the relationship between hypercholesterolaemia, atherosclerosis and coronary heart disease.

HISTORICAL BACKGROUND

It was probably Leonardo da Vinci (*1452-1519, quoted by Keele, 1952*) who first recognized the macroscopic changes of what we now know as atherosclerosis. When he illustrated the arterial lesions in an elderly man at autopsy, he suggested that the thickening of the vessel wall was due to 'excessive nourishment' from the blood. However, it was Marchand (*circa 1860, quoted by Aschoff, 1924*) who coined the term 'atherosclerosis' to emphasize the pathological findings of atheroma (gruel-like) and sclerosis (hardening) seen in the intimal layer of the aorta and other major arteries.

Early researchers in the field of cardiovascular disease concentrated on the morphology of the atheromatous lesion. Virchow (*1856*) proposed the 'response to injury' theory, in which he gave the first accurate histological account of the process of atherosclerosis. He considered that the first changes involved a 'certain loosening of the connective tissue ground substance' of the intima, and postulated that the swelling of this ground substance was due to 'increased imbibition of fluid elements from the passing blood stream'. As this occurred the connective tissue cells enlarged, divided and formed a localized thickening of the intima; when thickening advanced to a critical degree, fatty metamorphosis took place. Virchow concluded that a mechanical aetiology was most likely.

Virchow's response to injury theory was not without its opponents. Around the same time, von Rokitansky (*1804-1878*) published a parallel view of the pathogenesis of atherosclerosis, the 'thrombogenic' theory. Although there was much contemporary debate as to which was correct, both theories recognized that lipid accumulation was involved in the process of atherosclerosis and they eventually proved not to be mutually exclusive.

Although Vogel had described cholesterol in atheromatous tissue as early as 1847, it was not until the beginning of the twentieth century that the association between elevated serum cholesterol and atheroma was described. Ignatowski (*1908*) reported that the feeding of high protein diets to rabbits led to ostensible atherosclerosis, an observation that was soon to fuel the work of Anitschkow. In 1913, Bacmeister and Henes (*page 26*) described the association of raised serum cholesterol with certain diseases, but they were uncertain as to whether this was a primary or secondary phenomenon. They noted that the serum cholesterol concentrations were increased in patients with chronic renal failure and in those with diabetes mellitus; more significantly, they also reported that a raised serum cholesterol was associated with post-mortem evidence of atherosclerosis, and that the consumption of a low cholesterol diet could reduce the serum cholesterol in living subjects. These observations were developed further by Schmidt (*1914*), who described a new method for measuring cholesterol and used it to investigate xanthomata of the skin. He concluded that the cause of these lesions, previously described as being familial by Fagge (*1837*), was an increase in cholesterol content of the blood and that inheritance played a key role.

Contemporary with these findings was the seminal work of Anitschkow (*page 1*), which involved the feeding of cholesterol to rabbits. He noted that increased serum cholesterol, accelerated the infiltration of fat into the walls of the major arteries. He concluded that experimental atherosclerosis of the artery wall was a primary infiltrative process with re-active secondary changes. The importance of this animal model was the similarity of the morphology and microchemistry of the lesion to those of human atherosclerosis. By pos-tulating that an increase in serum cholesterol caused atheroma, Anitschkow propounded the 'lipid hypothesis'.

One of the strongest pieces of evidence in support of the lipid hypothesis was obtained from clinical observations in patients with inherited disorders of lipoprotein metabolism, especially familial hypercholesterolaemia. Müller (*page 29*) described tendon xanthomata, angina pectoris and hypercholesterolaemia in six patients, three of whom had a strong fam-ily history of similar findings. He pointed out that whilst some patients died suddenly at a relatively young age, the majority developed angina pectoris later in life. The following year Müller emphasized that there was a link between early coronary heart disease and fa-milial hypercholesterolaemia; he described familial hypercholesterolaemia as a genetic disor-der of cholesterol metabolism. Müller's clinical observations were independently confirmed by Adlersberg (*1951*), by Leys (*1951*), and by Slack (*1969*).

THE CONNEXION WITH DIET

Following Anitschkow's work, few systematic experimental studies were conducted, and later Weiss and Minot (*1933*) concluded that there was no convincing evidence that nutri-tion and atherosclerosis were linked. However, after the end of the Second World War, there was renewed interest in the relationship between diet, cholesterol, and atherosclero-sis. Although research initially followed epidemiological lines, it was soon supplanted by several fundamental ward studies on metabolism.

In 1957, Keys (*page 51*) published the first of a series of articles which culminated in the Seven Countries Study. Pointing out the striking variation in the frequency of coronary heart disease between countries, he postulated that this was due to a difference in the dietary intake of fat. Kinsell (*page 46*) showed that the type of fat ingested was important in deter-mining the serum cholesterol: whereas a diet rich in vegetable oils resulted in a pronounced fall in serum cholesterol, rising to base-line levels on resuming a mixed diet, a diet rich in dairy fat had no cholesterol-lowering effect. He also noted that increased consumption of cholesterol did not counterbalance the hypocholesterolaemic effect of diets rich in vegetable oils.

This association between dietary fat and serum cholesterol was emphasized by further population analyses in the Seven Countries Study. During the next few years, Keys (*page 139*) was able to study the effects of mixed diets of various fatty acid compositions in long-term schizophrenics in a Minnesota mental hospital. From these metabolic ward studies, he deduced simple equations for estimating the changes in serum cholesterol from changes in dietary intake of saturated and polyunsaturated fats and of cholesterol.

In order to establish that diet and not racial factors was responsible for the wide variation in coronary heart disease between different populations, Keys (*page 59*) undertook a study of Japanese people living in Japan, Hawaii and the continental USA. Whilst coronary heart disease was rare in Japan and common in Hawaiian Japanese, its incidence was highest in Japanese migrants living in California; the relationship between dietary fat intake and the serum cholesterol concentration was strikingly positive. Although the evidence was by no means conclusive, Keys observed that his findings were largely consistent with the hypothesis that dietary fat was a major determinant of coronary heart disease.

THE CLASSIFICATION OF THE HYPERLIPIDAEMIAS

As the clinical importance of the hyperlipidaemias became evident, the need for a system of nomenclature arose. The classification of the hyperlipidaemias has undergone several metamorphoses over the years. The early literature drew a clear distinction between 'secondary' hyperlipidaemia (such as that associated with diabetes mellitus) and 'essential' or 'primary' hyperlipidaemia. Thannhauser (*1950*) proposed that essential hyperlipidaemia be subdivided into 'juvenile' and 'adult' forms, but this did not prove to be clinically useful. Then Ahrens (*1961*) distinguished between 'fat-induced' and 'carbohydrate-induced' hypertriglyceridaemia, and later a third group of 'mixed' hyperlipidaemias was also recognized. This clinical heterogeneity caused much confusion and engendered a need for a practicable method of identification. This demand was met when Fredrickson, Levy and Lees (*page 82*) published a series of articles in the *New England Journal of Medicine* which provided a comprehensive description and classification of the major hyperlipidaemias. Fundamental to this work was the demonstration by Gofman (*page 39*) that plasma cholesterol and triglycerides were associated with proteins to form water-soluble complexes, the lipoproteins, and the development by Lees and Hatch (*1963*) of a simple method for separating lipoproteins using paper electrophoresis. Although this could also be achieved by ultracentrifugation, only available in research centres, the technique of Lees and Hatch allowed hospital laboratories to undertake the diagnosis of the hyperlipidaemias.

Fredrickson and colleagues were thus able to describe five electrophoretic patterns or phenotypes of hyperlipidaemia and hyperlipoproteinaemia. These were later popularized as the *Fredrickson classification*.

Type I was that of hyperchylomicronaemia alone.

Type II was characterized by a raised beta–band on electrophoresis and corresponded to a raised low density lipoprotein (LDL) concentration alone.

Type III described a combined hyperlipidaemia with a broad beta–band on electrophoresis caused by the accumulation of remnant lipoproteins in plasma. Although the clinical syndrome had been described earlier by Lever (*1954*) and by Adlersberg (*1955*), it was considered to be a variant of type II. It was some years before Utermann (*page 260*) was to describe the underlying abnormality of apoprotein E in these patients.

Type IV arose from isolated hypertriglyceridaemia due to increased concentrations of very low density lipoproteins (VLDL), detectable as a pronounced pre–beta band on electrophoresis.

Type V combined the findings of the type I and type IV patterns.

Although the Fredrickson classification was a striking advance which immediately established the hyperlipidaemias on a practical clinical footing, it did have certain important limitations. The first was pointed out by a World Health Organisation committee headed by Beaumont (*1970*). It was felt that the so-called Type II pattern embodied two distinct and clinically important groups of patients, and this necessitated the further subdivision of the electrophoretic pattern into types IIa and IIb. However, a more critical shortcoming was that the Fredrickson classification failed to provide an aetiological basis for the hyperlipidaemias. This stimulated subsequent work aimed at uncovering the molecular mechanisms underlying clinical disorders of lipoprotein metabolism.

THE RATIONALE FOR PHARMACOTHERAPY

Whilst it is now evident that the majority of hyperlipidaemias encountered in clinical practice can be successfully treated with dietary modification, a proportion of patients, especially those with monogenic disorders of lipoprotein metabolism, require pharmacotherapy. Some of the most effective drug preparations used to treat diet-refractory hypercholesterolaemia are the bile acid-binding resins. Hashim and van Itallie (*page 77*) published data on a bile acid-sequestering agent, cholestyramine, for the reduction of elevated plasma cholesterol concentrations. Their nine patients achieved a mean fall in serum cholesterol of 20-30%: they noted that the compound produced 'occasional gastrointestinal discomfort' but no systemic side-effects. The efficacy of the bile acid-binding resins in treating hypercholesterolaemia and preventing coronary heart disease was later well-emphasized by the Lipid Research Clinics Coronary Primary Prevention Trial (*page 281*) and the Cholesterol-lowering Atherosclerosis Study (*page 340*).

Clinical drug trials have done much to advance our knowledge of the benefits of cholesterol reduction in humans. By 1960, several cholesterol-lowering drugs were available, thus engendering the need for well-designed therapeutic trials. The Coronary Drug Project (*page 214*) was conceived in that year. Its object was to evaluate the efficacy of the then available lipid lowering drugs in the secondary prevention of coronary heart disease in men aged between 30 and 64, all of whom had electrocardiographic evidence of previous myocardial infarction. The drugs used included equine oestrogens (in two doses), clofibrate, dextrothyroxine and nicotinic acid, as well as a lactose placebo. A total of 8341 men were enrolled at 53 centres in North America. The main study was conducted between 1966 and 1975. The higher dose oestrogen regime was terminated in 1970 (after a mean follow-up of 4.7 years) because of an increase in deaths from malignancy. Three treatment groups – clofibrate, nicotinic acid, and placebo – were continued to the scheduled end of the trial (mean follow-up of 6.2 years). The clofibrate group showed no benefit, either in overall mortality or in non-fatal cardiovascular events, and, whilst nicotinic acid produced a 26% reduction in non-fatal myocardial infarction, there was no reduction in overall mortality. Nine years after the termination of this trial, Canner (*page 323*) undertook a further follow-up: mortality from all causes was similar for each drug, but in the nicotinic acid-treated group there was an 11% reduction in total mortality compared to the placebo group.

CORONARY HEART DISEASE AND THE RISK FACTORS

Around the same time that Keys originated his Seven Countries Study (*page 139*), the Framingham Study (*page 152*) was begun in the town of Framingham, Massachusetts, USA. In this observational cohort study, 5127 subjects (2282 men and 2845 women) aged between 30 and 62, none of whom had ostensible coronary heart disease at entry, were followed up over 14 years. Six individuals had serum cholesterol concentrations greater than 10.4 mmol/l (400 mg/100 ml) and a strong family history of heart disease: all died of coronary heart disease during the follow-up period. More modest elevations of cholesterol, range 6.5 – 9.1 mmol/l (250 – 350 mg/100 ml), were also found to be associated with a two- to six-fold increased risk of coronary heart disease (depending on age and sex) when compared with individuals having cholesterol concentrations of around 5.7 mmol/l (217 mg/100 ml). Elevated serum triglyceride was not seen as an independent cardiovascular risk factor.

Framingham was not the only epidemiological study in progress in the 1960s. It was realized that a very large cohort was needed to establish the relationship between risk factors and coronary heart disease. In keeping with this, the principal investigators of five large observational studies – Albany Civil Servants, Chicago People's Gas Company, Chicago Western Electric Company, Framingham and Tecumseh – agreed to pool their data. The importance of elevated serum cholesterol, raised blood pressure and cigarette smoking, as major independent risk factors for coronary heart disease was confirmed by the vast amount of data from this Pooling Project (1978). It is noteworthy that, although an optimal concentration of serum cholesterol was not propounded, it was felt that it would probably be well under 5.2 mmol/l(200 mg/100ml).

THE ROLE OF INHERITANCE

The importance of genetic factors in coronary heart disease was recognized in the last century by Sir William Osler (1897). Müller's findings (page 29) suggested that, in some families, elevated serum cholesterol was responsible for familial aggregation of coronary heart disease. Although the hereditary nature of what was known as essential familial hypercholesterolaemia had been noted in the first half of the twentieth century, it was Khachadurian (page 71) who first proposed, correctly, autosomal co-dominant inheritance. Because of the high prevalence of familial hypercholesterolaemia in the Lebanon, he was able to study twelve patients and their relatives. He characterized homozygous patients as having very high levels of serum cholesterol, extensive tendon xanthomata in childhood and advanced coronary heart disease at a young age. Heterozygotes had a more moderate elevation of serum cholesterol, tendon xanthomata much later in life, and a pronounced risk of coronary heart disease in middle age.

In the early 1970s, prompted by the impressive evidence linking hyperlipidaemia to coronary heart disease, and in the knowledge that certain forms of hypercholesterolaemia were inherited, Goldstein and colleagues (pages 164, 169, 180 and 205) set about performing a detailed genetic analysis of families with hyperlipidaemia; their primary aims were to obtain insight into the inheritance of atherosclerosis and the mechanism of the underlying biochemical lesions. These workers carried out a detailed genetic analysis of fasting plasma cholesterol and triglyceride levels in 2500 relatives of hyperlipidaemic patients chosen from 500 consecutively studied survivors of myocardial infarction in Seattle, Washington State, USA. Their results were published in three adjacent classical papers in the *Journal of Clinical Investigation* (pages 169, 180 and 205) under the umbrella title of Hyperlipidaemia in Coronary Heart Disease.

Using segregation analysis and referring to the distribution of lipids in first, second, third and fourth degree relatives, Goldstein and co-workers concluded that their data best fitted a genetic classification which distinguished three autosomal dominant (monogenic) disorders: familial hypercholesterolaemia, familial hypertriglyceridaemia, and familial combined hyperlipidaemia; polygenic hypercholesterolaemia and sporadic hypertriglyceridaemia were also recognized.

The authors estimated that among 157 hyperlipidaemic survivors of myocardial infarction, at least 68% had hyperlipidaemia of genetic origin. The over-representation of the familial combined hyperlipidaemia was a striking finding, which was confirmed by the parallel observations of Nikillä and Aro (1973).

The new genetic classification of the hyperlipoproteinaemias revealed that a monogenic disorder such as familial combined hyperlipidaemia could exhibit as many as four different phenotypes (for example Fredrickson IIa, IIb, IV and V), and that monogenic and polygenic disorders could share a common phenotype (for example Fredrickson IIa or IIb). The electrophoretic phenotypes described by Fredrickson (*page 82*) were thus demonstrated to arise from a combination of several genetic disorders of lipoprotein metabolism interacting with the environmental factors, diet, drugs and disease, for instance diabetes mellitus, hypothyroidism and renal failure. Thus, the seminal work of the Seattle group provided the basis for our modern classification of clinical disorders of lipoprotein metabolism. Equally important, it gave birth to a new field of research into the genetics of the hyperlipidaemias.

CHOLESTEROL HOMEOSTASIS AND THE LDL RECEPTORS

Concurrently with the Seattle clinical genetic studies, Goldstein and Brown (*page 164*) began a magnificent programme of experimental research which led to the discovery of the LDL receptor and the consequent characterization of the molecular defect responsible for familial hypercholesterolaemia. The impetus for this research was derived from the earlier finding of Bailey (*1967*) that cholesterol could regulate its own metabolism *in vitro*, and also from the work of Khachadurian (*page 71*). Goldstein and Brown began by studying tissue cultures of fibroblasts from patients with homozygous and heterozygous familial hypercholesterolaemia. Initially they demonstrated that fibroblasts from homozygotes had a greatly increased activity of the rate-limiting enzyme of cholesterol biosynthesis, 3-hydroxy-3-methylglutaryl coenzyme A (HMGCoA) reductase. This enhanced activity was found to be due to the decrease in the intracellular free cholesterol concentration, consequent on a defect in the biosynthesis of the LDL receptor. Extending these observations, Goldstein and Brown proposed the now widely-accepted scheme for cholesterol homeostasis in humans: it appears that the binding of circulating LDL to hepatic LDL receptors leads to an increase in the intracellular free cholesterol with three important consequences:

reduction in the activity of HMGCoA reductase which, in turn, reduces the intracellular biosynthesis of cholesterol;

stimulation of the activity of acyl-cholesterol acyl-transferase (ACAT), which increases the storage of cholesterol in esterified form;

inhibition of the synthesis of the LDL receptor at gene level and, in consequence, regulation of the uptake of circulating plasma cholesterol. This provided the molecular basis for Bailey's findings.

Patients with homozygous familial hypercholesterolaemia were found to have no receptors for LDL and a high rate of intracellular cholesterol biosynthesis. Their plasma cholesterol concentrations were raised five- to tenfold above normal, accounting for their accelerated rate of atherosclerosis, and early death from coronary heart disease.

Patients with the heterozygous form, on the other hand, had half the number of LDL receptors compared to control subjects, and a plasma cholesterol two- to three-fold above normal; their rate of atherosclerosis was accelerated but not to the extent seen in the homozygotes. This model fitted perfectly with the inheritance of familial hypercholesterolaemia that Khachadurian had proposed (*page 71*).

In addition to explaining the molecular basis for familial hypercholesterolaemia, the discovery of the LDL receptor by Goldstein and Brown (*page 164*), richly meriting the Nobel Prize for Medicine in 1985, had several other important ramifications. It provided a valuable model which increased our understanding of diseases arising from inherited dysfunction of receptor activity; it directed research towards the role of modified LDL receptors in the pathogenesis of atherosclerosis (*Mahley et al, page 267*); it afforded a testable mechanism to explain the propensity of certain human populations to nutritionally-induced hypercholesterolaemia.

The reciprocal relationship between HMGCoA reductase activity and LDL receptor function also suggested that therapeutic manoeuvres which led to an increased receptor number, for example, the administration of bile acid-binding resins, would lead to an increase in intracellular synthesis of cholesterol, and thus limit their clinical efficacy in reducing raised serum cholesterol levels. This stimulated the search for a new class of drugs which would inhibit the activity of HMGCoA reductase.

Thus Endo and his collaborators (*page 264*) at the Sankyo Drug Company isolated the prototype of this class of drugs, compactin (ML-236B), a fungal metabolite derived from *Penicillium citrinum*. Since the discovery of this parent compound several more potent preparations have been synthesized. These agents have now been shown to reduce total serum cholesterol by 30-40% and LDL cholesterol by 35-50%, with a modest reduction in serum triglyceride and a modest elevation in HDL cholesterol. Consistent with their mode of action, the HMGCoA reductase inhibitors potentiate the action of the bile acid-binding resin, reductions in serum cholesterol of over 50% being reported.

While Goldstein and Brown established LDL as a positive risk factor for coronary heart disease, another lipoprotein subfraction, high density lipoprotein, was receiving attention as a possible negative risk factor. Although HDL cholesterol had previously been reported as too low in some patients with coronary heart disease, it was Miller and Miller (*page 256*) who focused attention on this and the possible role of HDL in 'reverse transport' of cholesterol. That low HDL cholesterol levels, particularly in association with hypertriglyceridaemia, increase the risk of atherosclerosis, was recently well-emphasized by new data from the Framingham Study (*Castelli, 1986*) and by the Helsinki Heart Study (*page 348*).

THE NEED FOR FURTHER INTERVENTION TRIALS

Following the disappointing outcome of the World Health Organization trial of clofibrate (*Committee of Principal Investigators, 1980*), a need arose for further intervention trials aimed at verifying the lipid hypothesis and the efficacy and safety of the drug treatment of the hyperlipidaemias. The Lipid Research Clinics Coronary Primary Prevention Trial (LRC-CPPT, *page 281*) was a randomized double-blind study of the efficacy of reducing elevated serum cholesterol concentrations in the 'primary prevention' of coronary heart disease. It involved 3806 men enrolled at twelve centres in North America; all had primary hypercholesterolaemia with serum cholesterol concentrations of 6.9 mmol/l (265 mg/100 ml) or greater. All participants received dietary advice, and one-half were also prescribed cholestyramine 24 g/day for 7-10 years (mean 7.4 years). The treatment group achieved an average reduction in total serum cholesterol of 13.4% and in LDL cholesterol of 20.8%. There was a 19% reduction in cardiac end-points (deaths from coronary heart disease and/or, definite non-fatal myocardial infarctions), coronary deaths being reduced by 24%. Reductions in serum cholesterol were consistently related to compliance with the drug. However, despite the large reduction in death from coronary heart disease, treatment reduced overall mortality by only 7%, but this was attributed to an excess of deaths from accidents and violence.

Another major primary prevention trial overlapped with the LRCCPPT and was being carried out in Finland, a country known to have a high prevalence of coronary heart disease. The Helsinki Heart Study (*page 348*) was a placebo-controlled, randomized, double-blind study carried out over five years. The subjects, 4081 men aged between 40 and 55 years, with no evidence of overt coronary heart disease and with non-HDL cholesterol greater than 5.2 mmol/l (200 mg/100 ml), were assigned either to a treatment group (600 mg gemfibrozil twice daily), or to a placebo group; all patients consumed a lipid-lowering diet. Gemfibrozil, a fibric acid derivative, led to a marked increase in HDL cholesterol and simultaneous reductions in total cholesterol and triglycerides. Although there was no difference in total mortality between the groups, the incidence of primary end-points (fatal and non-fatal myocardial infarctions plus cardiac deaths) was significantly reduced in the gemfibrozil-treated group. In contrast to the LRCCPPT, the reduction in non-fatal coronary events was attributed not only to lowering of the serum LDL cholesterol but also to the elevation of the serum HDL cholesterol.

Whilst these intervention studies clearly demonstrated that the lowering of elevated serum cholesterol reduced the clinical manifestations of coronary heart disease, they did not provide a morphological basis for the findings. As techniques of coronary angiography and vascular ultrasonography improved, it became possible to study the coronary arteries more directly, and this gave rise to a series of 'regression trials'. A small but well-designed trial by Duffield et al. (page 277) provided evidence that effective treatment of hyperlipidaemia favourably influenced the natural course of symptomatic peripheral atherosclerosis. This and other trials, (Brensilse, Coronary Intervention Study 1984, and Arntzenius, Leiden Intervention Trial 1985) was overshadowed by the Cholesterol-Lowering Atherosclerosis Study: Blankenhorn and colleagues (page 340) demonstrated the substantial benefits not only in grafts, but also in native coronary arteries, resulting from lowering cholesterol by means of colestipol and niacin over a two-year period in 162 non-smoking, male patients who had undergone coronary artery bypass surgery. The aggressive therapy in this trial, where side-effects of constipation and flushing were common, was used to produce large changes in lipoprotein levels (43% reduction in LDL cholesterol together with 37% elevation in HDL cholesterol) sufficient to achieve arterial changes which could be recognized within the two years of the study.

INTERNATIONAL RECOMMENDATIONS – PREVENTION STRATEGIES

The large body of epidemiological, clinical and experimental evidence provided the impetus for authoritative bodies on both sides of the Atlantic to make firm recommendations for the treatment of hyperlipidaemia, thus reducing the risk of atherosclerosis in individuals and in the community. Central to the recommendations of the National Institute of Health Consensus Development Panel (page 316) and the European Atherosclerosis Society (page 357) was the wealth of prospective epidemiological data, particularly that pertaining to the men screened for entry into the Multiple Risk Factor Interventional Trial in the United States (page 334), and the strategies for the prevention of cardiovascular disease discussed by Rose (page 272). It is hoped that the widespread adoption of the guidelines provided by these expert committees will go a long way towards reducing the excess morbidity and mortality attributed to atherosclerosis in western societies.

This personal selection of classic papers in hyperlipidaemia can, inevitably, include only some of the more important contributions. However, it is hoped that they will give an insight into the great progress made in our understanding of the important role of lipids in the pathobiology of atherosclerosis and coronary heart disease.

Jeremy R. Quiney
Gerald B. Watts
United Medical Schools of
Guy's and St. Thomas' Hospitals
London 1989

REFERENCES

Adlersberg D. Hypercholesterolemia with a predisposition to atherosclerosis: an inborn error of lipid metabolism. *American Journal of Medicine*, 1951; **11**: 600.

Adlersberg D. Inborn errors of lipid metabolism. Clinical, genetic and chemical aspects. *Archives of Pathology*, 1955; **60**: 48.

Ahrens *et al*. Carbohydrate-induced lipidaemia in man. Reduction of lipemia by feeding fat. In: Frazer A C (ed) Biochemical problems of lipids, p.304; 1961; Elsevier Publ. Co.; Amsterdam

Arntzenius AC *et al*. Diet, lipoproteins, and the progression of coronary atherosclerosis. The Leiden Intervention Trial. *New England Journal of Medicine* 1985; **312**: 805-811.

Aschoff L. Lectures on Pathology 1924; Hoeber Inc. New York.

Bailey JM. In: Rothblat GH and Kritcheosky D (eds.) Lipid metabolism in tissue culture cells. Vol.6 p.85. 1967; Wistar Institute Press: Philadelphia.

Beaumont JL *et al*. Classification of hyperlipidaemias and hyperlipoproteinaemias. *Bulletin of the World Health Organization*, 1970; **43**: 891-915.

Brensilse JF *et al*. Effects of therapy with cholestyramine on progression of coronary arteriosclerosis: results of the NHLBI Type II Coronary Intervention Study. *Circulation*, 1984; **69**: 313-324.

Castelli WP. The triglyceride issue: a view from Framingham. *American Heart Journal*, 1986; **112**: 432-437.

Committee of Principal Investigators. Report on a WHO cooperative trial on primary prevention of ischaemic heart disease using clofibrate to lower serum cholesterol – mortality follow up. *Lancet*, 1980; **ii**: 379-385.

Fagge CH. General xanthelasma or ritiligoidea. *Transactions of the Pathological Society (London)*, 1837; **24**: 242.

Ignatowski A. *Isvestiya Imperatorshoi Vorenno Medinsinskoy Akademii, St Petersburg*, 1908; **16**: 154-176.

Keele KD. *Leonardo da Vinci on* Movement of the Heart and Blood 1952; Harvey and Blythe, London.

Lees RS and Hatch FT. Sharper separaton of lipoprotein species by paper electrophoreses in albumin-containing buffer. *Journal of Laboratory and Clinical Medicine*, 1963; **61**: 518.

Lever WF *et al*. Idiopathic hyperlipemic and primary hypercholesterolemic xanthomatosis. 1. Clinical data and analysis of the plasma lipids. *Journal of Investigative Dermatology*, 1954; **22**: 33.

Leys D. Tuberous xanthomatosis. *British Heart Journal*, 1951; **13**: 32-36.

Nikkila E A, and Aro A. Family study of serum lipids and lipoproteins in coronary heart disease. *Lancet*, 1973; **i**: 954.

Osler, Sir W. Lectures on angina pectoris and allied states. Appleton – Century – Crofts, New York 1897.

Pooling Project Research Group: Relationship of blood pressure, serum cholesterol, smoking habit, relative weight, and ECG abnormalities to incidence of major coronary events: Final report of the Pooling Project *Journal of Chronic Disease* 1978; 31: 201-306.

Schmidt E. Über die Bedeutung der Cholesterins für die Xanthombildung. *Dermatologische Zeitschrift*. 1914; **21**: 137.

Slack J. Risks of ischaemic heart disease in familial hyperlipoproteinaemic states. *Lancet*, 1969; **ii**: 1380-1382.

Thannhauser SJ. Lipidoses: diseases of the cellular lipid metabolism 1950; Oxford Press: New York.

Virchow R. Phlogose und Thrombose im Gefassystem. In: *Gesammelte Abhandlungen zur Wissenschaftlichen Medizin*, p.458, 1856; Meidinger Sohn, Frankfurt.

Vogel J. The pathological anatomy of the human body 1847. H. Bailliere, London.

von Rokitansky C. Über einiger der wichtigsten Krankheiten der Arterien. *Denkschriften der K. Akademie der Wissenschaften. Wien*, 1852; **4**: 1-72.

Weiss S and Minot GR. Nutrition in relation to arteriosclerosis. In: Cowdrey EV (ed.), Arteriosclerosis 1933; 233-248, Macmillan. New York.

CONTENTS

CONTENTS

CONTENTS

CONTENTS

XVI.

Über die Veränderungen der Kaninchenaorta bei experimenteller Cholesterinsteatose.

Von

Dr. N. Anitschkow.

Aus dem pathologisch-anatomischen Institut der kaiserlichen medizinischen Militär-Akademie zu St. Petersburg.

Hierzu Tafel IX—XI.

———

Die Anzahl der Methoden, die von verschiedenen Autoren angewandt wurden, um atherosklerotische Aortenveränderungen an Kaninchen zu erzielen, ist zurzeit dermaßen angewachsen, daß es eine schwere Aufgabe wäre, alle diese Methoden auch in Kürze wiederzugeben. Wenn wir aber die bei der Anwendung verschiedener Methoden hervorgerufenen Gefäßveränderungen lediglich vom morphologischen Standpunkte aus betrachten, so überzeugen wir uns darin, daß die Mehrzahl der bisher experimentell erzeugten arteriosklerotischen Prozesse der Aortenwandungen sehr nah zueinander steht und sozusagen einen gemeinsamen pathologischen Typus darstellt. Als Hauptrepräsentanten dieses Typus sind bekanntlich jene Veränderungen zu nennen, die man nach wiederholten intravenösen Adrenalininjektionen hervorruft und die in einer Medianekrose mit nachfolgender Verkalkung nekrotischer Massen, mit reaktiven Bindegewebswucherungen, bisweilen auch mit Knorpel- und Knochenbildung bestehen. Alle diese Prozesse scheinen nicht mit denen identisch zu sein, die für die gewöhnliche menschliche Atherosklerose charakteristisch sind.

In den letzten Jahren ist es aber gelungen einen neuen Typus von Veränderungen an Kaninchenaorta zu erzeugen, die sich scharf von denen des erwähnten „adrenalinischen" Typus unterscheiden, und sich nach den Angaben der Autoren teilweise in hypertrophischen, teilweise

Editorial Note: A synopsis of this paper, in English, appears on page 25. The figures which originally appeared at the end of the paper have been omitted.

380   Anitschkow,

in degenerativen Erscheinungen (fettige Metamorphose) der inneren
Schichten der Aortenwandungen äußern. Diese Erscheinungen, die der
menschlichen Atherosklerose nahe stehen, gelang es bisher am deut-
lichsten mit folgenden zwei Methoden hervorzurufen: mittels Ein-
spritzung von Staphylokokkenkulturen (SALTYKOW) und mittels einer
dauernden Fütterung der Tiere mit animalischen Nahrungsmitteln
(IGNATOWSKI, STAROKADOMSKI, STUCKEY, WESSELKIN).

Ich werde an dieser Stelle in die Besprechung der mit der ersten
Methode erzielten Veränderungen nicht eingehen und möchte nur bemerken, daß diese Methode bei Kontrollversuchen, die von einigen Autoren vorgenommen wurden (STAROKADOMSKI (20), REDDINGIUS (16), HERX-
HEIMER (9)) vollkommen negative Resultate gab. Dieser Umstand beweist
schon an und für sich, daß es überhaupt nicht beständig gelingt, die
uns hier interessierenden Veränderungen mittels der genannten Methode
hervorzurufen. Es existieren wahrscheinlich noch einige uns vollkommen
unbekannte und deshalb außer unserer Gewalt liegende Bedingungen,
die für den positiven Erfolg dieser Versuche von Wichtigkeit sind.
Einige von diesen Bedingungen möchte ich noch in den späteren Ausführungen erörtern.

Viel erfolgreicher scheint dagegen die zweite, hauptsächlich im
pathologisch - anatomischen Institute der Petersburger medizinischen
Militärakademie erforschte Methode zu sein, die darin besteht, daß
Kaninchen lange Zeit (2—5 Monate) mit einigen, gegenwärtig schon
genau festgestellten Sorten von Nahrungsmitteln gefüttert werden, wobei
die Tiere gleichzeitig auch die gewöhnliche pflanzliche Nahrung in beliebiger Quantität erhalten. Aus allen hierzu gehörenden Versuchen
erwies es sich, daß bei richtiger Wahl der Nahrungsmaterialien immer
ein und dasselbe Resultat erzielt wird. Es kommen nämlich dabei in
der Wand der Aorta außerordentlich charakteristische hyperplastische und
infiltrative Veränderungen zur Beobachtung, die sich anfangs ausschließlich in der Intima und den inneren Mediaschichten lokalisieren und
nach ihrem morphologischen Bild der menschlichen Atherosklerose
nahestehen.

Dank diesen interessanten Versuchen wurde allmählich eine neue
Gruppe experimenteller Gefäßveränderungen aufgestellt, die man als
„diätetische Atherosklerose" bezeichnen könnte und deren morphologische Hauptmerkmale in den oben zitierten Arbeiten von IGNA-
TOWSKI (10, 11, 12), STUCKEY (21), STAROKADOMSKI (20) u. A. angeführt sind.

An dieser Stelle möchte ich noch darauf hinweisen, daß die von
den genannten Autoren erzielten Gefäßveränderungen gar keine Ähnlichkeit mit denen besitzen, die im Laboratorium von LUBARSCH (14) an
Kaninchen bei Nebennieren- und Lebersubstanzfütterung hervorgerufen
sind. Wie aus der Beschreibung von LUBARSCH klar hervorgeht, be-

Veränderungen der Kaninchenaorta bei experiment. Cholesterinsteatose. 381

standen die von ihm beobachteten Veränderungen in einer Nekrose und Verkalkung der Wandung kleinerer Arterien; die Aortenwandungen blieben dabei aber frei von ausgesprochenen pathologischen Erscheinungen, was gerade das Entgegengesetzte der Versuchsresultate oben zitierter russischer Autoren darstellt.

Gegenwärtig ist somit das allgemeine pathologische Bild der uns interessierenden Aortenveränderungen schon ziemlich genau aufgestellt und die dabei auftretenden Prozesse von denen unterschieden, welche bei anderen Versuchsanordnungen vorkommen. Es bleiben aber auf diesem Gebiete noch Fragen übrig, die für das Verstehen der in Rede stehenden pathologischen Form ein besonderes Interesse darstellen, die aber in den früheren Arbeiten nur wenig berücksichtigt sind.

Eine der wichtigsten dieser Fragen ist gewiß die über die nächste Ursache, die in unserem Falle die Aortenveränderungen hervorruft. Wie ich es schon erwähnt habe, gibt es nur bestimmte Nahrungsmaterialien, welche in Kaninchenorganismus eingeführt, schwere Aortenveränderungen verursachen. IGNATOWSKI (10, 11, 12), der als erster solche Veränderungen notiert hat, glaubte die Entstehung derselben durch die schädliche Wirkung des tierischen Eiweißes erklären zu können. Die nachfolgenden Versuche anderer Autoren schienen aber diese Meinung nicht zu bestätigen. Wie es z. B. aus den Experimenten STUCKEY's (21) hervorgeht, werden mit an Eiweiß besonders reichlichen Stoffen (Hühnereiweiß, Fleischsaft) viel geringere und weit nicht so charakteristische Aortenveränderungen, als bei einer Fütterung mit den Nahrungsmitteln erzielt, die große Mengen verschiedener Fettsubstanzen enthalten. Bei einer sorgfältigen Nachprüfung verschiedener Nährsubstrate erwies es sich dabei, daß es besonders das Eigelb und die Gehirnsubstanz sind, die die stärksten Aortenveränderungen hervorrufen.

Weitere von STUCKEY (22) vorgenommene Fütterungsversuche mit verschiedenen Sorten von reinen Neutralfetten tierischer und pflanzlicher Herkunft haben erwiesen, daß diese Substanzen an und für sich keine Veränderungen der Aortenwandungen verursachen. Fast ebenso negativ fielen auch die Versuche WESSELKIN's (23) mit reinem Lecithin („Agfa") aus. Unter den Fettsubstanzen des Eigelbes blieben somit hauptsächlich nur das Cholesterin bzw. seine Verbindungen übrig, die noch für Ursache der in Rede stehenden Aortenveränderungen gelten könnten.

Diese Voraussetzung wurde namentlich nach den Untersuchungen CHALATOW's (4, 5) über die Leberveränderungen bei Eigelb- und Gehirnsubstanzfütterung besonders wahrscheinlich. Es gelang nämlich CHALATOW zu beweisen, daß bei diesen Fütterungsversuchen eine enorme Ablagerung von kristallinischen Lipoiden in der Leber stattfand und da diese Substanzen nach den Untersuchungen ASCHOFF's (2) u. A. größtenteils aus Cholesterinverbindungen bestehen, so lag es nahe, die Hauptrolle bei

382   A n i t s c h k o w ,

der Entstehung solcher Ablagerungen im Organismus gerade den Cholesterinverbindungen der zum Versuch gebrauchten Nahrungsmittel zuzuschreiben.   Ebensolche Ablagerungen doppeltbrechender flüssig-kristallinischer Cholesterinverbindungen wurden von WESSELKIN (23) auch in
den Aortenwandungen von Kaninchen bei Eigelbfütterung notiert.

Auf diese Weise kamen wir schon in einer früheren Arbeit (1) zum
Schluß, daß es die Cholesterinverbindungen des Eigelbes und Gehirns
sind, die, in den Kaninchenorganismus eingeführt, die von IGNATOWSKI,
STUCKEY u. A. beschriebenen Veränderungen der Aortenwandungen verursachen.

Um die Richtigkeit dieser Meinung außer Zweifel zu stellen, unternahm ich gemeinsam mit Herrn Dr. CHALATOW eine neue Reihe von
Untersuchungen, die darin bestanden, daß Kaninchen täglich im Laufe
von 1—4 Monaten reines Cholesterin (MERCK) in Sonnenblumenöl gelöst
durch eine Magensonde bei einer Temperatur von 35—40 ^{0} C eingeführt
wurde.   Bei dieser Temperatur ist die von uns angewandte Lösung von
0,2—0,8 g Cholesterin (MERCK) in 10—12 ccm Öl längere Zeit haltbar.
Außer Cholesterin und Öl erhielten die Tiere auch ihre gewöhnliche
pflanzliche Nahrung (Heu, Hafer) in beliebiger Quantität.   Als Lösungsmittel für das Cholesterin wurde das Sonnenblumenöl deshalb gewählt,
da es an und für sich sogar bei einer langen Zeit dauernden Fütterung
der Kaninchen mit demselben keine Aortenveränderungen hervorruft.

In dieser Hinsicht dienten uns 2 Kaninchen aus den Experimenten
STUCKEY's als Kontrolle.   Das erste dieser Kaninchen bekam 2 monatelang 25 g Öl täglich, das zweite wurde 4 monatelang mit denselben
Ölmengen (je 25 g täglich) gefüttert.   Wie es aus der Beschreibung
STUCKEY's (22) hervorgeht, konnte er bei diesen Tieren keine mit unbe-
waffnetem Auge bemerkbaren Veränderungen der Aortenwandungen konstatieren.   Dank der Liebenswürdigkeit des genannten Autors hatte ich
die Gelegenheit dieselben Aorten auch mikroskopisch zu untersuchen,
konnte aber dabei auch keine Veränderungen weder in der Intima noch
in der Media der Aortenwandungen finden.

Auf diese Weise wurde festgestellt, daß das Sonnenblumenöl
allein, sogar in reichlichen Mengen in Kaninchenorganismus eingeführt,
nicht imstande ist die Entstehung etwaiger pathologischer Prozesse der
Aortenwandungen zu verursachen und somit als bequemes Lösungsmittel
für das Cholesterin bei Fütterungsversuchen dienen kann.

Die Resultate der Fütterungsversuche an Kaninchen mit reinem
Cholesterin, die schon kurz in unserer früheren Arbeit (ANITSCHKOW
und CHALATOW (1)) erwähnt sind, sind, was die Aortenveränderungen anbetrifft, aus folgender Tabelle zu ersehen.   (Siehe Tabelle I.)

(Tabelle 1 siehe p. 384—385.)

Veränderungen der Kaninchenaorta bei experiment. Cholesterinsteatose. 383

Aus der vorliegenden Tabelle sehen wir, daß es uns in allen Fällen gelungen ist, bei einer dauernden Fütterung der Versuchstiere mit reinem Cholesterin Veränderungen der Aortenwandungen zu erzeugen, die hauptsächlich in einer Ablagerung von doppeltbrechenden Fettsubstanzen in den inneren Schichten der Aortenwandungen und Hyperplasie derselben bestanden.

Wenn wir das Gesamtbild dieser Veränderungen mit denen vergleichen, die von STUCKEY, STAROKADOMSKI und WESSELKIN bei Kaninchenfütterung mit Eigelb erzielt worden sind, so werden wir davon überzeugt, daß diese letzteren vollkommen identisch mit denen sind, die wir mit reinem Cholesterin hervorgerufen haben. Fassen wir dabei noch ins Auge, daß man bei Fütterung mit anderen Lipoiden (Lecithin) und Neutralfetten selbst nach 4—5 monatlicher Fütterung der Kaninchen mit diesen Substanzen gar keine Veränderungen erzeugt (siehe die Untersuchungen von STUCKEY und WESSELKIN), so kommen wir zum folgenden Schlusse: Die sog. diätetische Form der Kaninchenatherosklerose wird augenscheinlich durch das sich in den Nahrungsmitteln befindende Cholesterin bzw. seine Verbindungen verursacht. Somit werden die atherosklerotischen Veränderungen des genannten Typus deshalb bei einer Fütterung mit Eigelb und Gehirnsubstanz beobachtet, weil diese Nahrungmittel eine besonders reichliche Quantität von Cholesterin enthalten.

Aus unseren Untersuchungen geht auch hervor, daß die mit Cholesterin erzielten Veränderungen in ihrer Intensität den eingeführten Cholesterinmengen direkt proportional sind. Diese Tatsache, ebenso wie der Vergleich unserer Versuchsresultate mit denen anderer oben zitierter Autoren schließt in unseren Fällen jede Möglichkeit des Vorhandenseins zufälliger bei Kaninchen spontan vorkommenden Aortenveränderungen aus. Außerdem trifft man bei Kaninchen, soviel mir bekannt, spontane Veränderungen des von uns beobachteten Typus überhaupt nicht, da alle bisher beschriebenen, in der Aorta dieser Tiere spontan auftretenden pathologischen Prozesse ausschließlich der Gruppe der sog. „adrenalinischen" Sklerose angehören, die, wie oben erwähnt, keine Ähnlichkeit mit der uns interessierenden „diätetischen" Gruppe der Aortenveränderungen besitzt. Nur in einem Falle habe ich bei den vorliegenden Versuchen neben den typischen Verfettungsprozessen der inneren Aortenschichten auch Veränderungen des adrenalinischen Typus konstatiert (Versuch Nr. 6), die in einer ausgedehnten Nekrose und Verkalkung der Media bestanden. Da in allen anderen Fällen solche Veränderungen selbst bei längeren Versuchen von mir nie beobachtet wurden, so liegt es nahe, dieselben für spontan entstandene zu halten. Diese Voraussetzung gewinnt um so mehr an Wahrscheinlichkeit, da auch andere Autoren, die sich mit der „diätetischen" Form der Kaninchenatherosklerose beschäftigt haben, nur in ganz seltenen Fällen Mediaveränderungen des „adrenalinischen" Typus

Ta

Nr. der Versuche	Dauer der Versuche Tage	Die tägliche Cholesterindose g	Die Gesamtmenge des eingeführten Cholesterins g	Körpergewicht der Versuchstiere	
				am Anfang des Versuchs g	am Ende des Versuchs g
1	10	0,2—0,5	3,1	1770	1700
2	25	0,2—0,5	10,6	2270	2070
3	26	0,5—0,6	14,2	1050	750
4	55	0,2—0,5—0,7	30,6	1640	1450
5	79	0,2—0,5—0,7 —0,8	57,1	2240	1760
6	81	0,2—0,5—0,7 —0,8	50,75	1370	1130
7	81	0,2—0,5—0,7 —0,8	49,0	1850	1710
8	139	0,2—0,5—0,6 —0,7—0,8	82,7	2240	2150

Veränderungen der Kaninchenaorta bei experiment. Cholesterinsteatose. 385

belle I.

Makroskopische	Mikroskopische
Veränderungen der Aortenwandungen	
Keine Veränderungen	Keine Veränderungen
Keine Veränderungen	Keine Veränderungen
Keine makroskopisch wahrnehmbare Veränderungen	Sehr kleine umschriebene Intimaverdickungen hauptsächlich durch eine Anhäufung von Fettsubstanzen gebildet
Sehr kleine gelbliche Flecke hauptsächlich an den Abgangsstellen der Intercostalarterien lokalisiert	Entsprechend den makroskopisch sichtbaren Flecken Intimaverdickungen mit Fettinfiltration. Anfangsstadien einer Infiltration der Intima mit phagocytierenden Elementen und einer Wucherung der elastischen und Muskelfasern
Gut sichtbare gelbliche Flecke an den Abgangsstellen der Arterien	Dieselben Veränderungen wie im vorigen Falle nur etwas stärker ausgeprägt
Dieselben Veränderungen und daneben eine bedeutende Verdünnung und Derbheit der Aortenwand	Dieselben Veränderungen und außerdem stark ausgeprägte Nekrose- und Verkalkungserscheinungen in der Media
Gelbliche stellenweise miteinander konfluierende Flecke im Arcus und an den Abgangsstellen der Arterien	Bedeutende Verdickung der inneren Aortenschichten mit Fettinfiltration und Wucherung zelliger und faseriger Elemente. Fettablagerungen längs den elastischen Fasern der inneren Mediaschichten
Diffuse Verdickung der Aortenwand im Arcus; die innere Oberfläche verdickter Partien sieht uneben aus und hat eine gelblich-weiße Farbe. Zahlreiche prominente gelbliche Flecke an anderen Stellen der inneren Aortenoberfläche	Außerordentlich starke Intimaverdickung, wobei diese Schicht stellenweise dieselbe Breite wie die Media erreicht. Reichliche Fettsubstanzablagerung in der Intima und in den inneren Mediaschichten. In den veränderten Partien ist eine Wucherung zelliger und faseriger Elemente mit Zerfall derselben scharf ausgeprägt

386   A n i t s c h k o w ,

notierten und deshalb müssen die genannten Veränderungen lediglich als uncharakteristische Nebenerscheinungen der betreffenden Form der Atherosklerose betrachtet werden.

Die vollkommene Identität der bei Cholesterinfütterung beobachteten Aortenveränderungen mit denen, die bei einer Fütterung mit chol-esterinhaltiger Nahrung erzeugt werden, konnte ich selbst an Kaninchenaorten konstatieren. Das zum Vergleich genommene Material wurde mir in liebenswürdiger Weise von Dr. STUCKEY zur mikro-skopischen Untersuchung übergeben und stammte von Kaninchen her, die lange Zeit mit Gehirnsubstanz gefüttert wurden. Die Resultate dieser Untersuchungen ebenso wie die Versuchsanordnung sind aus folgender Tabelle zu ersehen (siehe Tabelle II).

Tabelle II.

Nr. der Versuche	Dauer der Versuche	Menge der täglich ein-geführten Ochsenhirn-substanz	Makroskopische	Mikroskopische
			Veränderungen der Aortenwand	
9	2 Monate	40 g	Kleine weißlich - gelb-liche prominente Flecke an den Abgangsstellen der Arterien und im Arcus	Verdickung der Intima; Ablagerung von Fett-substanzen in derselben und in den inneren Medianschichten
10	3 Monate	40—50 g	Dieselben Verände-rungen, aber stärker ausgeprägt	Stark ausgeprägte In-filtration der inneren Aortenwandschichten mit fettähnlichen Sub-stanzen. Wucherung der zelligen und Zerfaserung der elastischen Elemente in den infiltrierten Aortenpartien

Wenn wir die in der angeführten Tabelle wiedergegebenen Resultate mit denen vergleichen, die wir an mit reinem Cholesterin gefütterten Kaninchen beobachtet haben, so wird uns die vollkommene Ähnlichkeit der in diesen beiden Versuchsreihen gefundenen Aortenveränderungen außer Zweifel. Im weiteren werden wir noch sehen, daß diese Analogie sich auch in den feineren morphologischen und mikrochemischen Be-funden erkennen läßt.

Bevor ich zu dieser Seite der in Rede stehenden Frage übergehen werde, möchte ich noch die Resultate einer anderen Gruppe von Fütterungsversuchen mitteilen, die ich (gemeinsam mit CHALATOW) an

Veränderungen der Kaninchenaorta bei experiment. Cholesterinsteatose. 387

weißen Ratten durchgeführt habe (siehe Tabelle III). Der Zweck dieser Versuche war der, nachzuprüfen, ob auch an anderen Tierarten, außer den Kaninchen Ablagerungen lipoider Substanzen in den Aortenwandungen auf experimentellem Wege hervorzurufen seien. Bei diesen Versuchen wurden Ratten eine lange Zeit mit Eigelb (mit Kuhmilch verrührt) gefüttert, wobei sie auch ihre gewöhnliche Nahrung in beliebiger Menge bekamen. Über die negativen Befunde an Lebern dieser Tiere hat schon CHALATOW in einer seiner Arbeiten (5) ausführlich mitgeteilt. In den Aortenwandungen konnte ich ebenfalls im Gegensatz zu den oben angeführten Resultaten an Kaninchen keine nennenswerten Veränderungen konstatieren.

Tabelle III.

Nr. der Versuche	Anzahl der zum Versuch gebrauchten Ratten	Dauer der Versuche	Anzahl der eingespeicherten Eigelber	Resultate der Experimente
11	5	7 Tage	Alle Ratten bekamen täglich je 1 Eigelb in Kuhmilch zerrieben	Weder makro- noch mikroskopisch wurden etwaige Veränderungen der Aortenwandungen konstatiert
12	4	1 Monat		
13	3	2 Monate		
14	4	3 Monate		
15	2	4 Monate		
16	2	5 Monate		

Die angeführten negativen Ergebnisse der an Ratten angestellten Versuche kann man gewiß durch verschiedene Momente erklären. Die bei diesen Versuchen aufgestellte Tatsache, daß man bei Ratten im Gegensatz zu den Kaninchen in keinem Organe Ablagerungen doppeltbrechender Lipoide erzeugen kann, hängt entweder davon ab, daß die Cholesterinverbindungen bei den Ratten nicht resorbierbar sind, oder sie im Rattenorganismus in einer anderen Form als bei Kaninchen zirkulieren und sich in den Organen nicht ablagern. Die Entscheidung dieser Frage muß man zukünftigen, teilweise von CHALATOW schon in Angriff genommenen, Untersuchungen überlassen. Es sei hier nur der Schluß gezogen, daß für den günstigen Erfolg der Fütterungsversuche mit cholesterinhaltigem Material nicht nur die chemische Konstitution desselben, sondern auch die Art der Versuchstiere von Wichtigkeit ist.

Indem ich die schädliche Wirkung der Cholesterinverbindungen auf die Kaninchenaorta bei einer Kombination derselben mit anderen giftigen Substanzen studieren wollte, unternahm ich schließlich die Untersuchung einer Reihe von Aorten, die von mit Eigelb in Kombination mit Alkohol

388 Anitschkow,

gefütterten Kaninchen herstammten. Das sämtliche Untersuchungsmaterial wurde mir dabei in liebenswürdiger Weise vom Herrn Dr. Schaffir übergeben, der an denselben Tieren die Wirkung genannter Substanzen auf die Leber untersucht hat. In allen diesen Versuchen gelang es stark ausgesprochene Aortenveränderungen desselben Typus zu konstatieren, die für die „diätetische" Form der Kaninchenatherosklerose charakteristisch sind. Weder im Grade ihrer Entwicklung, noch in morphologischen Besonderheiten unterschieden sich die genannten Veränderungen wesentlich von denen die Stuckey bei seinen Fütterungsversuchen mit Eigelb allein erzielt hat. In den von mir untersuchten Aorten wurden nur Mediaverkalkungen häufiger gefunden, als es gewöhnlich bei Fütterungsatherosklerose vorzukommen pflegt, und dieser Umstand konnte sich vielleicht in der Wirkung des den betreffenden Tieren eingeführten Alkohols eine plausible Erklärung finden.

Die Versuchsresultate der letzten Gruppe sind in folgender Tabelle zusammengestellt (siehe Tabelle IV p. 389).

Wenn ich jetzt zur genaueren Beschreibung der bei Cholesterinfütterung an Kaninchen erzielten Aortenveränderungen übergehe, so muß ich in erster Linie einen schon makroskopisch gut erkennbaren Befund, nämlich die Lokalisation der veränderten Teile der Aorta hervorheben. Man trifft dieselben in den nicht allzuschwer veränderten Aorten nur im Arcus und an den Abgangsstellen der aus der Aorta herstammenden Arterien. Die an diesen Stellen vorkommenden Veränderungen bestehen in einer Intimaverdickung in der Form von einzelnen gelblichen Plättchen und Streifen, die in Versuchen von kurzer Dauer nur ganz geringe Dimensionen haben. Bei länger dauernden Versuchen findet man Plättchen und Streifen, die größere Dimensionen erreichen; sie umgeben die Abgangsstellen kleinerer Arterien in der Form von prominenten weißlichen oder gelblichen Ringen und werden dabei auch an anderen Stellen der inneren Oberfläche der Aorta unabhängig von den Abgangsstellen der Arterien gefunden. Bei den länger dauernden Versuchen sieht man schließlich eine diffuse Verdickung der Aortenwandungen, die besonders stark im Arcus aortae ausgeprägt ist. Das Aortenlumen ist dabei erweitert, die Oberfläche der verdickten Aortenwand sieht uneben aus.

Bei mikroskopischer Untersuchung der am wenigsten veränderten Teile der Aortenwandungen, sieht man in der Intima eine Anhäufung kleiner fettähnlichen Tröpfchen (Taf. IX Fig. 1). Dieselbe scheint dicker, als gewöhnlich, zu sein, wobei die Verdickung in den ersten Stadien nicht auf Kosten einer Hyperplasie oder Hypertrophie etwaiger Strukturelemente der Intima selbst vor sich geht. Die verdickten Stellen bestehen nur aus einer relativ schmalen subenthothelialen Schicht, die ein homogenes, teilweise auch feinkörniges Aussehen hat und die oben erwähnten fettähnlichen Tropfen enthält. Es ist schwer, genau zu präzisieren, mit welchen histologischen Elementen die Ablagerung dieser

Veränderungen der Kaninchenaorta bei experiment. Cholesterinsteatose. 389

Tabelle IV.

Nr. der Versuche	Dauer der Versuche	Gesamtmenge des eingeführten 40%igen Alkohols (in ccm)	Anzahl der eingespeicherten Hühnereigelber	Körpergew. am Anfang des Versuchs	Körpergew. am Ende des Versuchs	Veränderungen der Aortenwandungen	
						Makroskopische	Mikroskopische
17	64 Tage	556,4	86	1150	1600	Ziemlich zahlreiche gelbliche Flecke an den Abgangsstellen der Arterien und im Arcus	Entsprechend den makroskopisch veränderten Partien, Aufquellung der Intima und Ablagerung in derselben von fettähnlichen Substanzen
18	80 Tage	690,5	86	1240	1580	Dieselben Veränderungen, aber schwächer ausgeprägt und daneben starke Verdünnung der Aortenwand und Verdichtung derselben im Arcus und im Brustteil	Unbedeutende Aufquellung und Fettinfiltration der Intima. Stark ausgeprägte Mediaveränderungen des adrenalinischen Typus
19	86 Tage	821,0	92	1270	1270	Gut sichtbare gelbliche Flecke an der inneren Aortenoberfläche, daneben Verdünnung und Derbheit der Aortenwandungen	Stark ausgeprägte Verdickung der Intima und Infiltration derselben ebenso wie der inneren Mediaschichten mit Fettsubstanzen. Mediaveränderungen des adrenalinischen Typus
20	87 Tage	873,9	91	1120	1930	Scharf hervortretende prominente Flecken und Streifen an der inneren Aortenoberfläche, besonders an den Abgangsstellen der Arterien ausgeprägt	Dieselben Veränderungen der Intima wie im vorigen Falle. Dagegen die Mediaveränderungen (des adrenalinischen Typus) viel schwächer ausgeprägt
21	107 Tage	1209,6	112	1600	1920	Zahlreiche gelbliche Flecke an der inneren Oberfläche der Aorta, wobei sie im Arcus miteinander konfluieren	Stark ausgeprägte Fettinfiltration der inneren Aortenwandschichten mit einer reichlichen Wucherung des zelligen und faserigen Elemente derselben. Veränderungen des adrenalinischen Typus nicht konstatiert
22	127 Tage	1407,9	132	1030	2370	Diffuse Verdickung der inneren Aortenwandschichten im Arcus. Zahlreiche gelbliche Flecke an anderen Stellen der inneren Aortenoberfläche	Dieselben Veränderungen, aber noch stärker ausgeprägt. Mediaveränderungen des adrenalinischen Typus fehlen

390   A n i t s c h k o w ,

Tropfen verknüpft ist. Jedenfalls sammeln sich die genannten Tropfen
anfangs nicht im Innern etwaiger Zellelemente. In den Endothelzellen
der Aorta sind sie auch nicht zu sehen. Da sie sich aber oft in der
Form einer schmalen Schicht längs den elastischen Fasern (Taf. IX Fig. 2),
besonders auf der Lamina elast. interna, zwischen derselben und der ober-
flächlichen Endothelschicht, konzentrieren, so kann man annehmen, daß
die elastischen Fasern sozusagen Anhaltspunkte darstellen, auf welchen
die Ablagerung fettähnlicher Substanzen vor sich geht. Wie wir es noch
im weiteren sehen werden tritt dabei gleichzeitig auch eine Vermehrung
der elastischen Fasern selbst zum Vorschein. In den frühesten Stadien
des beschriebenen Prozesses weisen aber die elastischen Fasern gar keine
Veränderungen auf.

Die meisten der erwähnten fettähnlichen Tropfen, welche sich in
der Intima ausscheiden, weisen im polarisierten Lichte doppeltbrechende
Eigenschaften auf, wobei sie glänzende Kreuzfiguren bilden (Taf. XI
Mikrophot. 1, 3, 4). Bei leichter Erwärmung verschwinden die anisotropen Eigenschaften der in Rede stehenden Tropfen vollkommen, treten
aber beim Abkühlen wiederum hervor.

Die angeführten Merkmale erlauben schon an und für sich diese
Tropfen hauptsächlich als aus Cholesterinesteren bestehend anzuerkennen.
Aus der weiteren Beschreibung werden wir sehen, daß dieser Schluß
auch in den färberischen Reaktionen dieser Tropfen eine Bestätigung
finden kann.

An einigen Stellen der verdickten Intima gelingt es außer fettähnlichen Tropfen auch einzelne Zellelemente mit rundem dunkeln Kern
und schmalem basophilen Protoplasmasaum zu konstatieren, welche vollkommen den kleinen Blutlymphocyten ähneln (Taf. X Fig. 5 Plb). An
anderen Stellen der Intima findet man noch einige Zellformen, die ein
besonders charakteristisches Aussehen besitzen. Das sind große Zellen
mit breitem schaumartigen Protoplasmaleib und blassem, meist rundem
Kerne (Taf. X Fig. 6, 8 Chol. Ph.). Die Zellkonturen sind entweder
polygonal oder mehr unregelmäßig, wobei sie an kleineren Formen besser,
als an größeren sichtbar sind. Das Protoplasma ist sehr zart und enthält
zahlreiche kleine Vakuolen, die im frischen Zustande einen besonders
starken leicht gelblichen Glanz aufweisen. Im polarisierten Lichte weisen
diese Tropfen doppeltbrechende Eigenschaften auf, wobei die größeren
von ihnen schöne Kreuzfiguren bilden. Auf diese Weise bekommen die
in Rede stehenden Zellen im polarisiertem Lichte ein ganz originelles
Aussehen, indem sie in der Form kugeliger Gebilde erscheinen, die mit
feinsten staubförmigen stark glänzenden tropfigen Einschlüssen erfüllt
sind (Taf. XI Mikroph. 3).

Die beschriebenen anisotropen Substanzen, die man nach ihren Eigenschaften den Cholesterinverbindungen zuzählen kann, nehmen den ganzen
Protoplasmaleib der Intimazellen ein, wobei nur eine sehr schmale peri-

Veränderungen der Kaninchenaorta bei experiment. Cholesterinsteatose. 391

pherische Schicht frei von ihnen ist. Diese Schicht ist vom homogenen Protoplasma gebildet, was besonders an Zellen kleinerer Dimensionen gut zu sehen ist. Die dem Zellkerne am nächsten liegenden Protoplasmateile enthalten die anisotropen Einschlüsse ebenfalls nicht und bestehen aus einem fein retikulierten, basophilen Protoplasma. In diesem perinukleären Protoplasmasaume gelingt es bisweilen eine hellere Zone — wahrscheinlich eine Attraktionssphäre — zu konstatieren.

Die Kerne der in Rede stehenden Zellen sind in den kleineren Elementen klein, dunkel und rund, so daß sie den Lymphocytenkernen nahe stehen. Bisweilen trifft man auch mehr ovale und nierenförmige Kerne. Einige Zellen enthalten 2—3 Kerne. Bei den größeren Intimazellen ist der Kern größer und blasser, wobei er oft an der Peripherie der Zelle liegt. Die Form solcher Kerne ist manchmal unregelmäßig, eckig, die Kerne sehen geschrumpft, pyknotisch aus.

Was die Entstehungsweise der geschilderten Intimazellen anbetrifft, so ist diese Frage außerordentlich schwer zu lösen. Um möglichst viele dieser Elemente in ihren früheren Entwicklungsstadien beobachten zu können, fertigte ich schräge oder der Oberfläche parallel verlaufende Zelloidinschnitte aus den wenig veränderten Aortenwandungen an, wobei die Schnitte nach den von MAXIMOW empfohlenen Methoden bearbeitet wurden. Nur dank dieser Methodik gelang es mir die nötigen Übergangsformen und Merkmale aufzustellen, welche die Natur der in Rede stehenden Zellen und einiger anderen Zellformen der veränderten Aortenschichten aufklären konnten.

Die Endothelzellen können bei der Entscheidung dieser Frage nicht in Betracht gezogen werden, da sie sich vollkommen passiv bei der Bildung der großen Intimazellen verhalten. Sie liegen auf der Oberfläche der verdickten Intima und bilden hier eine scharf abgegrenzte Schicht schmaler, langgezogener Elemente (Taf. X Fig. 5, 7, 8 End.), die keine morphologische Ähnlichkeit mit den in der Intima vorhandenen großen Zellen besitzen.

Viel wahrscheinlicher sind die letzteren von lymphoiden Elementen (Polyblasten) abzuleiten. Wie oben erwähnt, trifft man in der verdickten Intima immer einzelne kleine Lymphocyten, die manchmal eine breitere Protoplasmaschicht als gewöhnlich und größere Kerne aufweisen (Taf. X Fig. 5 Plb). Weiter haben nicht alle, anisotrope Einschlüsse enthaltenden Zellen eine und dieselbe Größe. Die kleineren von ihnen besitzen dabei dunkle, runde Kerne und einen noch nicht so breiten und zarten Protoplasmaleib, der für die größeren Intimazellen charakteristisch ist. Auf diese Weise sieht man in den veränderten Aortenwandungen alle allmählichen Übergangsformen von den kleinen lymphoiden Elementen zu den großen Intimazellen (Taf. X Fig. 7 Plb$_1$ Plb). Diese Befunde gestatten die Entstehungsquelle der oben beschriebenen großen Zellen in den Lymphocyten (Polyblasten) der verdickten Intima zu ersehen. Woraus aber die in der Intima vorkommenden Lymphocyten herstammen ist

392   Anitschkow,

vollkommen unklar. Jedenfalls können sie nur aus folgenden zwei Zellarten entstehen: entweder aus etwaigen schon in der normalen Intima
vorhandenen fixen Zellen (z. B. aus sog. LANHAN'schen Zellen) oder aus
den gewöhnlichen, aus der Blutbahn emigrierten Lymphocyten.

Wie dem auch sei, die großen Intimazellen müssen als typische mit
anisotropen Einschlüssen überladene Phagocyten, Makrophagen oder Polyblasten betrachtet werden. Ebensolche Zellen haben in der Aortenintima
auch die Autoren konstatiert, welche Kaninchen mit cholesterinreichem
Material lange Zeit gefüttert haben (STUCKEY, STAROKADOMSKI). Da ich
dieselben Zellelemente in zahlreicher Quantität auch bei Fütterungsversuchen mit reinem Cholesterin gefunden habe, so unterliegt es keinem
Zweifel, daß es gerade das Cholesterin bzw. seine Verbindungen sind,
mit denen die genannten Makrophagen infiltriert sind. Dafür sprechen
auch die physikalischen und färberischen Reaktionen der in diesen Zellen
vorhandenen anisotropen Einschlüsse, was noch aus weiteren Auslegungen
hervorgehen wird.

An dieser Stelle sei noch darauf hingewiesen, daß ebensolche Zellen
in starker Anhäufung auch in der Intima der menschlichen Aorta bei
Atherosklerose beschrieben wurden. Wenn man die morphologischen
Eigenschaften dieser Elemente, wie sie z. B. RIBBERT (17) geschildert hat,
mit den von uns beschriebenen Intimazellen der Kaninchenaorta ver-
gleicht, so fällt die vollkommene Identität dieser beiden Zellarten sofort
ins Auge. In der Kaninchenaorta hat die großen Intimazellen auch
SALTYKOW (19) bei experimenteller Atherosklerose nach Staphylokokken-
injektionen konstatieren können.

Beiläufig sei es hier erwähnt, daß ähnliche Zellen in reichlicher
Menge auch in anderen Organen des Kaninchens bei Cholesterinfütterungs-
versuchen von mir gefunden sind und daß sie überall zahlreiche anisotrope tropfige Einschlüsse enthalten. Aus diesem Befunde kann man
den Schluß ziehen, daß bei experimenteller Cholesterinsteatose besondere
Zellen, Makrophagen, im Organismus gebildet werden, die die Cholesterinverbindungen aufspeichern. Deshalb liegt es nahe solche Elemente, zu
denen auch die großen Intimazellen gehören, als „Cholesterinesterphagocyten" zu bezeichnen.

Außer den beschriebenen Phagocyten trifft man in der verdickten
Intima der Kaninchenaorta noch andere Zellformen und faserige Bestandteile, die hauptsächlich aus der Media der Aorta herstammen. Es ist
hier notwendig zu bemerken, daß schon in früheren Entwicklungsstadien
des in Rede stehenden Prozesses die Grenze zwischen Intima und Media
verschwindet. Die Lamina elastica interna zerfällt in zahlreiche feinere
Fasern, die in der Richtung der verdickten Intima verlaufen und sozusagen ein Skelett derselben bilden (Taf. X Fig. 9). In den Maschen
des von elastischen Fasern gebildeten Gerüstes liegen die großen Intimaphagocyten (Taf. X Fig. 8 Chol. Ph.) und fein granulierte Massen des bei

Veränderungen der Kaninchenaorta bei experiment. Cholesterinsteatose. 393

Fixierung geronnenen Plasmas, ebenso wie Tropfen fettähnlicher Substanzen.

Nachdem die Lamina elastica interna verschwunden ist, greift der Verfettungsprozeß mit Bildung großer Phagocyten allmählich auch die inneren Schichten der Media an. Hier treffen wir längs der elastischen Fasern auch anisotrope tropfige Ablagerungen (Taf. IX Fig. 2) und eine Zerfaserung der elastischen Lamellen, wobei in den Maschen des elastischen Gerüstes neugebildete phagocytäre Zellformen des oben beschriebenen Typus liegen.

Außer diesen Formen trifft man hier immer noch kleinere lymphoide Wanderzellen, mit rundlichen oder nierenförmigen Kernen und basophilem gut entwickeltem Protoplasma. Die Kerne dieser Zellen sind dunkel, scharf konturiert und enthalten ziemlich grobe Chromatinpartikelchen. Das Protoplasma bildet zahlreiche Pseudopodien und weist eine retikulierte Struktur auf. Neben dem Kerne ist oft ein heller Hof, wahrscheinlich eine Attraktionsphäre, zu sehen.

Einige der in Rede stehenden Zellen besitzen noch kein so scharf entwickeltes Protoplasma, wie die soeben beschriebenen Elemente. Sie haben kleine, runde, sich dunkel färbende Kerne, einen engen basophilen Protoplasmasaum und sind deshalb nach ihren morphologischen Eigenschaften mit den gewöhnlichen kleinen Lymphocyten identisch.

Andererseits besteht zweifellos auch eine nahe morphologische Verwandtschaft zwischen den geschilderten lymphoiden Zellen mit gut entwickeltem Protoplasma und den großen anisotrope Einschlüsse enthaltenden Zellformen. Man trifft nämlich lymphoide Zellen, die neben einem dunklen „lymphoiden" Kern ein verdünntes, vakuolisiertes Protoplasma vom Typus der Intimaphagocyten besitzen. Bei solchen Zellen bemerkt man keine Pseudopodien und sie sehen oft polygonal aus. Mit einem Worte nähern sie sich vollkommen in ihren morphologischen Eigenschaften den oben beschriebenen typischen „Cholesterinesterphagocyten".

Auf diese Weise besitzen wir auch in den späteren Entwicklungsstadien des pathologischen Prozesses morphologische Merkmale, welche für die Entstehung der großen Intimaphagocyten aus den lymphoiden Wanderzellen sprechen. Die beschriebenen Phagocyten sind aber nicht die einzigen Zellelemente, die man in den veränderten Intima- und Mediateilen findet. Außer ihnen kommen hier, besonders in den späteren Entwicklungsstadien des Prozesses, noch andere aus der Media herstammende Zellformen vor. Wie oben erwähnt, greift allmählich der pathologische Prozeß auch die inneren Schichten der Media an, wobei die elastischen Lamellen sich in eine Unmenge feiner elastischer Fasern umwandeln, die die großen phagocytierenden Zellen umflechten (Taf. X Fig. 9). Die zwischen den elastischen Lamellen liegenden glatten Muskelfasern treten dabei als wichtige Bestandteile der veränderten Partien

394   A n i t s c h k o w ,

ein und bilden hier eine besondere Art von Zellen, die überall zwischen
den Phagocyten zu sehen sind.

Wenn man die inneren Schichten der Media besonders an parallel
zur inneren Oberfläche der Aorta gerichteten Schnitten untersucht, so
findet man hier viele Muskelzellen, die auffallende Veränderungen aufweisen. Sie verlieren ihre regelmäßige Verteilung und verlaufen in verschiedensten Richtungen. Einzelne Muskelfasern werden dabei weit von-
einander getrennt und ändern ihre äußere Form stark. Sie werden nämlich
breiter, quellen bedeutend auf und weisen an den Rändern zahlreiche
zackige Ausläufer auf (Taf. X Fig. 10). Das Protoplasma solcher Zellen
ist gut entwickelt und stark basophil. Es enthält oft einzelne ziemlich
große, runde Vakuolen (Taf. X Fig. 12) und ist fein faserig. Der Kern
behält noch seine längliche Form, kann aber auch breiter, als gewöhnlich,
werden.

Die beschriebenen Muskelzellen liegen überall in den Maschen der
aufgequollenen und zerfaserten Mediaschichten. Im Innern dieser Maschen
befinden sich die großen Phagocyten, die geronnenen körnigen Plasmamassen und Tröpfchen fettähnlicher Substanzen. Die Muskelzellen liegen
dabei oft den Phagocyten dicht an, wobei sie dieselben in der Form von
Halbringen umspinnen. Sie bekommen dabei zahlreiche feine und zier-
liche, wurzelförmige Ausläufer, die nebst den elastischen Fasern ein
eigenartiges Netz oder Reticulum bilden, in dessen Maschen sich die
soeben genannten Bestandteile befinden (Taf. X Fig. 11).

Die eigentümlich verästelte Form, die bei diesem Prozesse die
Muskelfasern der Media annehmen, soll nicht als vollkommen ungewöhnlich
für die genannten Elemente betrachtet werden. Wie es z. B. aus der
Beschreibung v. EBNERs (8) hervorgeht, kommen in den inneren Mediaschichten auch unter normalen Bedingungen verästelte glatte Muskelfasern vor.

Außer den großen Phagocyten, lymphoiden Wanderelementen und
Muskelzellen sind in den veränderten Intima- und Mediapartien noch
andere Zellformen zu sehen, die aber in viel geringerer Anzahl als die
übrigen Zellelemente vorkommen. Das sind teilweise die gewöhnlichen
Blutleukocyten und zwar hauptsächlich die eosinophilen, teilweise ebenfalls
eosinophile Granula enthaltende Elemente, die aber einen viel größeren
und regelmäßigeren Kern, als die Leukocyten besitzen. Wahrscheinlich
stellen diese Zellen unreife Formen eosinophiler bzw. pseudoeosinophiler
Leukocyten dar. Was die Entstehungsweise solcher unreifen Formen
betrifft, so konnte ich diese Frage infolge der geringen Anzahl derselben in den veränderten Aortenpartien nicht lösen.

Allmählich dringen die geschilderten pathologischen Prozesse in die
Tiefe der Aortenwandungen ein, obwohl sie nie die ganze Media an-
greifen und sich hauptsächlich nur in den oberflächlichsten Partien derselben lokalisieren (Taf. IX Fig. 3). Dabei wiederholen sich überall eben-

Veränderungen der Kaninchenaorta bei experiment. Cholesterinsteatose. 395

dieselben Vorgänge, die wir schon oben erwähnt haben. In den weniger affizierten Partien trifft man nur eine Ablagerung fettähnlicher Substanzen an den elastischen Fasern und eine Aufquellung des interstitiellen Grundgewebes der Aortenwandungen an. Daneben bemerkt man das Auftreten lymphoider Wanderzellen, wobei gleichzeitig auch die Bildung eines feinen Gerüstes aus zerfaserten elastischen Lamellen und auseinandergeschobenen Muskelelementen vor sich geht. In den Maschen des genannten Gerüstes befinden sich die großen Phagocyten, welche aus den lymphoiden Wanderzellen (Polyblasten) herstammen, ebenso wie fein granulierte oder homogene Infiltrationsmassen und fettähnliche doppeltbrechende Tropfen.

Die großen phagocytierenden Zellen oder „Cholesterinesterphagocyten" weisen oft Zeichen einer allmählichen Degeneration auf, was stellenweise besonders an den stark veränderten Partien der Aortenwandungen zu sehen ist. Die Kerne solcher Zellen werden pyknotisch oder lösen sich allmählich auf und verschwinden. Das Protoplasma verliert seine Konturen und verwandelt sich in eine feinkörnige, zahlreiche tropfige, Fettsubstanzen enthaltende, unförmige Masse. An vielen Stellen treffen wir degenerative Erscheinungen auch in den zwischen den großen Phagocyten liegenden Muskelfasern und auf diese Weise entstehen vereinzelte kleine Atheromherde.

Die direkten Folgen der geschilderten Aortenveränderungen liegen vor der Hand: dank der reichlichen Infiltration mit neugebildeten Zellelementen und Fettsubstanzen werden die Aortenwandungen dicker. Zugleich verlieren sie aber teilweise ihre Festigkeit, da eine bedeutende Quantität der in den inneren Mediaschichten vorhandenen elastischen Lamellen zerstört wird. Diese Veränderungen führen natürlich zu einer Erweiterung des Gefäßes, was in der Tat in den betreffenden Fällen stets einzutreten pflegt. Über die späteren Stadien der Entwicklung geschilderter atheromatösen Prozesse konnte ich auf Grund meiner Präparate kein positives Urteil gewinnen. Nach den Angaben von STUCKEY (21) tritt in diesen Stadien eine reichliche Produktion von fibrösem Gewebe in den veränderten Aortenwandungen ein, das die weitere Zerstörung derselben verhindert. Da aber in meinen Versuchen relativ frühere Entwicklungsstadien des atheromatösen Prozesses verfolgt wurden, so gelang es mir nicht, die genannte fibröse Umwandlung veränderter Aortenpartien zu konstatieren.

Nachdem in vorliegenden Ausführungen die morphologischen Merkmale und die Entstehung der Aortenveränderungen bei experimentell hervorgerufener Cholesterinsteatose angeführt wurden, gehe ich zur Besprechung mikrochemischer und färberischer Reaktionen der fettähnlichen Substanzen über, die bei unseren Experimenten in reichlicher

396   Anitschkow,

Quantität die Aortenwandungen infiltrierten. Nach ihrer Lage könnte man diese Substanzen in intra- und extracelluläre einteilen, da aber diese beiden Gruppen keine wesentliche mikrochemische, bzw. färberische Differenz untereinander aufwiesen, so hielt ich diese Einteilung für unzweckmäßig. In Anbetracht unserer Aufgabe wäre es richtiger die in Rede stehenden Substanzen nach ihren physikalischen Eigenschaften zu klassifizieren und zwar dieselben in kristallinische anisotrope und amorphe isotrope einzuteilen.

Die anisotropen Substanzen befanden sich in Form flüssiger Sphärokristalle und komplizierter myelinähnlichen Figuren teilweise im Inneren der großen Makrophagen, wo sie eine Unmenge kleiner tropfiger Protoplasmaeinschlüsse bildeten (Taf. XI Mikroph. 3), teilweise außerhalb der Zellen, längs der elastischen Fasern, wobei sie in einer Mischung mit anderen Fettsubstanzen als erste Spuren einer beginnenden Infiltration der Aortenwandungen mit fettähnlichen Substanzen erschienen. Nach dem Zerfall der großen Makrophagen werden die in ihrem Protoplasma vorhandenen anisotropen Tropfen frei und befinden sich jetzt in der Grundsubstanz der veränderten Aortenwandungen zwischen den amorphen isotropen Massen. Die Mehrzahl fettähnlicher Tropfen wies im polarisierten Lichte schöne Kreuzfiguren auf, die beim Erwärmen verschwanden und nach Abkühlen wiederum hervortraten. Bei Formolfixierung verwandeln sich die in Rede stehenden anisotropen Substanzen in nadelförmige feste Kristalle, die bei 54° C schmelzen und nach Abkühlen wiederum die flüssig-kristallinische Form annehmen.

Ich habe keine Absicht verschiedene, im polarisierten Lichte bei experimenteller Verfettung der Aortenwandungen erscheinende Formen doppeltbrechender Substanzen, zu beschreiben, da der Besprechung dieser Formen, die auch in anderen Organen der betreffenden Tiere in reichlicher Quantität vorhanden sind, eine spezielle Arbeit CHALATOW's (6) gewidmet ist.

Wenn ich nun zur Besprechung der mikrochemischen Reaktionen flüssig-kristallinischer und amorpher Fettsubstanzen der Aortenwandungen übergehe, so muß ich zu allererst die Lösbarkeit derselben im Äther, Alkohol abs., Aceton und Xylol erwähnen. Die kristallinischen Formen sind dabei schwieriger, als die amorphen lösbar. Es genügt nämlich eine ¹/₂—1 Minute lange Wirkung des absoluten Alkohols, damit sich die amorphen Substanzen lösen, wobei sie bei nachfolgenden speziellen Färbungen schon nicht nachweisbar sind. Die kristallinischen Formen bleiben aber dabei noch gut erhalten und erst nach einer längeren Wirkung des Alkohols abs. verschwinden auch diese vollkommen.

Die für Cholesterin charakteristischen Reaktionen mit Schwefelsäure und Jod, ebenso wie die GOLODETZ'sche Reaktion, ergaben nur undeutliche, eher negative Resultate. Bei der Färbung mit Sudan III wurden die flüssig-kristallinischen Tropfen ebenso wie die amorphe Sub-

Veränderungen der Kaninchenaorta bei experiment. Cholesterinsteatose. 397

stanz gelblich-rot gefärbt. Einige Tropfen wiesen aber dabei eine intensiv rote Färbung auf, was für ihren Bestand aus Neutralfetten sprach. Bei Betrachtung ungefärbter Schnitte gelang es in der Tat zwischen anisotropen Tropfen auch solche zu konstatieren, die keine doppeltbrechenden Eigenschaften besaßen. Diese Tropfen trifft man in späteren Entwicklungsstadien des pathologischen Prozesses in besonders reichlicher Menge an und auf Grund ihrer Isotropie und der roten Färbung wahrscheinlich ebenderselben Tropfen mit Sudan III, ist man berechtigt sie als Neutralfette zu betrachten.

Die Nilblausulfatfärbung wies in den veränderten Aortenpartien verschiedenste Nuancen auf. Die kristallinischen Substanzen wurden violett und rosa, die amorphen bläulich und schmutzig-violett gefärbt. Nach $^{1}/_{2}$—1 Minute langer Wirkung von Alkohol abs. und nachfolgender Färbung mit Nilblau blieben die amorphen Substanzen ungefärbt, die kristallinischen behielten dagegen ihre Färbung und doppeltbrechende Eigenschaft bei.

Die LORRAIN-SMITH-DIETRICH'sche Methode fiel in allen Fällen positiv aus. Wie die amorphen Substanzen, so die Mehrzahl der kristallinischen Tropfen, auch wurde dabei schwarz gefärbt. Nach einer $^{1}/_{2}$—1 Minute langer Wirkung von absolutem Alkohol wurden die amorphen Substanzen aufgelöst und wiesen keine Färbung mehr nach der betreffenden Methode auf. Die kristallinischen Formen, die dabei unaufgelöst blieben, wiesen bei nachfolgender Färbung nach der DIETRICH'schen Methode ebenfalls keine positive Reaktion auf. Dieser Befund stimmt vollkommen mit den Angaben KAWAMURA's (13) überein, daß die flüssig-kristallinischen Formen fettähnlicher Substanzen, die aus Cholesterinester bestehen, sich negativ zur DIETRICH'schen Methode verhalten. Den positiven Ausfall der Reaktion, die ohne vorhergehende Bearbeitung der Schnitte im Alkohol vorgenommen wurde, kann man ebenso wie in den Fällen KAWAMURA's durch das Vorhandensein anderer lipoider Substanzen und zwar der Fettsäuren und Seifen erklären. Da letztere eine innige Mischung mit den Cholesterinestern und sogar Hüllen um die anisotropen Tropfen herum bilden, so liegt es nahe, daß sich das positiv erscheinende Resultat der DIETRICH'schen Reaktion der Cholesterinester in dieser Tatsache eine plausible Erklärung findet.

Die Methode von CIACCIO wurde von mir nur in einem Falle angewandt, wobei es gelungen ist, eine schwach rötliche Färbung der körnigen amorphen Massen, die die Aortenwandungen infiltrierten, zu erzeugen. Die anisotropen Tropfen blieben dabei ungefärbt.

Die FISCHLER'sche Methode ergab mir nur ein schwach positives Resultat, das in einer schwärzlichen Färbung der veränderten Aortenpartien bestand. Der schwarze Farbenton schien dabei am stärksten in der Umgebung einzelner anisotropen Tropfen ausgeprägt zu sein, wobei die Tropfen selbst keine positive Reaktion aufwiesen. Somit hing dieses

398   A n i t s c h k o w ,

Resultat vom schwach positiven Verhalten der amorphen Massen, die
die Aortenwandung infiltrierten, zur erwähnten Reaktion ab.

Da mich einige Reaktionen z. B. die von FISCHLER das Vorhandensein von Seifen als Bestandteile dieser amorphen Massen voraussetzen
ließen, habe ich an Gefrierschnitten von veränderten Aortenwandungen
auch Reaktionen auf Kalkseifen und anderen Kalkverbindungen ausgeführt. Die KOSSA'sche und RIEHL'sche Methode, die für kohlen- bzw.
phosphorsauren Kalk empfohlen wurden, fielen dabei, ebenso wie die
Salzsäure- und Schwefelsäurereaktion (Bildung von CO_2-Bläschen und
von Gipskristallen), vollkommen negativ aus. Es sei hier erwähnt, daß
dieselben Reaktionen, an nekrotischen Mediapartien bei dem adrenalinischen Typus von Sklerose angewandt, mir stets positive Resultate ergaben. Man muß also annehmen, daß die Kalkverbindungen, die einer-
seits in der Media bei Adrenalinsklerose, andererseits in der Intima und
inneren Mediapartien bei Cholesterinverfettung abgelagert werden — wenn
es sich überhaupt im letzteren Falle um Kalkablagerungen handelt —,
eine verschiedene chemische Struktur besitzen.

Die Frage über die chemische Natur dieser Verbindungen wurde
von mir auf Grund ihrer Lösbarkeit in verschiedenen Reagentien gelöst.
Bei der Färbung mit BÖHMER'schem Hämatoxylin werden die amorphen
Massen der Aortenwandungen blau gefärbt. Da diese Färbung nicht
ausschließlich von Kalkseifen, sondern auch von Schleim und Eisen-
verbindungen abhängig sein kann, so wurde der erste mittels spezifischer
Reaktionen (Thionin, Mucikarmin) und die zweiten durch die Bearbeitung
der Schnitte in Oxalsäurelösung ausgeschlossen.

Nach 10 minutiger Behandlung in 3—5 % iger Salzsäure verlieren
die betreffenden Partien der Aortenwandungen die Fähigkeit nicht, mit
Hämatoxylin positive Reaktion aufzuweisen. Es genügt aber eine kurze
(3—5 minutige) Wirkung von Alkohol abs. oder von einem Gemische
von Alkohol mit Äther, damit diese Fähigkeit vollkommen verloren
gehe. Dieser Umstand beweist, daß die von mir in den veränderten
Aortenpartien konstatierten vermutlichen Kalkablagerungen aus im Äther
und Alkohol leicht löslichen Kalkverbindungen bestehen, d. h. daß sie
wahrscheinlich zum fettsauren Kalk gehören.

Auf diese Weise konnte ich auf Grund angeführter mikrochemischer
Reaktionen 2 Hauptsorten chemischer Verbindungen konstatieren, die in
beträchtlicher Menge die veränderten Aortenwandungen bei experimenteller Cholesterinsteatose infiltrieren. Die einen sind doppeltbrechend
und geben alle Reaktionen, die nach KAWAMURA für Cholesterinester
charakteristisch sind. Die anderen kommen in einer isotropen, amorphen,
z. T. körnigen Form vor und sind auf Grund entsprechender Reaktionen
wahrscheinlich den Kalkseifen zuzuzählen. Bemerkenswert ist, daß eben
dieselben chemischen Komponenten die Hauptbestandteile der sich auch
bei menschlicher Atherosklerose in der Aortenintima befindenden lipoiden

Veränderungen der Kaninchenaorta bei experiment. Cholesterinsteatose. 399

Substanzen bilden (KAWAMURA). Was den Mechanismus der Ablagerung dieser Substanzen bei Kaninchenversuchen anbetrifft, so scheint auch in diesem Falle die von RIBBERT (17) und ASCHOFF (3) angegebene Erklärung vollkommen zu genügen. Wie es oben beschrieben wurde, geht der pathologische Prozeß in der Kaninchenaorta auf die Weise vor sich, daß anfangs eine Aufquellung der betreffenden Partien der Aortenwandungen und eine Infiltration derselben mit amorphen, körnigen Plasmamassen eintritt, die auch zahlreiche doppeltbrechende Tropfen fettähnlicher Substanzen enthalten. Dieses Bild entspricht vollkommen jenen Anfangsstadien der Aortenveränderungen, die von RIBBERT beschrieben sind und kann freilich vom Standpunkte eines primären Plasmaeinpressens in die oberflächlichsten Schichten der Aortenwandungen beurteilt werden. In den eingepreßten Plasmamassen kommen nun weitere chemische Vorgänge zum Vorschein, die eine Ausscheidung flüssig-kristallinischer Cholesterinester und wahrscheinlich des fettsauren Kalks verursachen. Da wir in Blutpräparaten der betreffenden Versuchstiere keine Cholesterinester in flüssig-kristallinischer Form konstatiert haben, so muß man annehmen, daß diese Formen in den Aortenwandungen selbst gebildet werden.

Was die Entstehung der Kalkablagerungen anbetrifft, so ist in unseren Fällen die Erklärung ASCHOFF's (3) in demselben Grade, wie bei der menschlichen Atherosklerose, passend. Wenn bei partieller Zerstörung von Cholesterinestern freie Fettsäuren gebildet werden, so können dieselben natürlich in eine Verbindung mit dem Kalk des Blutplasmas eintreten und somit Kalkablagerungen der veränderten Aortenwandungen bilden.

––––––––

Die Bestätigung am experimentellen Material der Ansichten, die für die Enstehung atherosklerotischer Aortenveränderungen beim Menschen ausgesprochen wurden, scheint mir deshalb von Interesse zu sein, da es einen der besten Beweise für die Identität beider Prozesse bietet.

Die oben beschriebenen experimentellen Angaben weisen uns darauf hin, daß es sich bei den experimentellen atherosklerotischen Prozessen hauptsächlich um eine Infiltration der Aortenwandungen mit fettähnlichen Substanzen, keineswegs aber um eine primäre fettige Degeneration etwaiger Bestandteile der Wandungen handelt. In den ersten Entwicklungsstadien des atherosklerotischen Prozesses werden die Fettsubstanzen in vollkommen unveränderten, teilweise nur aufgequollenen Wandschichten der Aorta abgelagert und erst viel später, wenn diese Substanzen in zahlreicher Quantität durch die Phagocyten aufgespeichert werden, kommen in den letzteren, ebenso wie in den faserigen Bestandteilen der Aortenwand, degenerative Erscheinungen vor.

400   Anitschkow,

Der Umstand, daß die von mir geschilderten atherosklerotischen Aortenveränderungen eine rein infiltrative Natur besitzen, findet noch in folgender Tatsache Bestätigung. Bei unseren Experimenten wurden nämlich direkte, toxische Momente, die etwaige degenerative Veränderungen der Aortenwandungen hervorrufen, ausgeschlossen. Infolge einer Fütterung mit relativ kleinen Mengen von reinem Cholesterin haben wir nur eine dauernde Erhöhung der Gesamtmenge von Cholesterinverbindungen im Organismus erzielt und dies führte stets zu einer Ausscheidung von Cholesterinestern in verschiedenen Organen. Wir haben also einen rein infiltrativen Prozeß hervorgerufen, der durch eine Erhöhung des Cholesteringehalts im Organismus bedingt wurde.

Man muß annehmen, daß unter normalen Bedingungen ein gewisser Mechanismus existiert, dank dem das mit Speise eingespeicherte Cholesterin nirgends im Organismus in bedeutender Menge abgelagert wird. Wir haben in unseren Versuchen an Kaninchen experimentell diesen Mechanismus zerstört, indem wir in den Kaninchenorganismus erhöhte Mengen Cholesterins, bzw. seiner Verbindungen einführten, die der Organismus nicht zu eliminieren imstande war. Deshalb trat eine Ablagerung des genannten Stoffes in verschiedenen Organen in der Form von flüssig-kristallinischen Fettsäureesteren ein — ein Vorgang, der gewiß rein infiltrativer Natur ist.

Es sei hier auch hervorgehoben, daß bei weitem nicht alle Organe als Ablagerungsstätten der anisotropen Fettsubstanzen erscheinen. Es gelang uns z. B. solche Ablagerungen hauptsächlich in der Leber, Nebennieren, Aortenwandungen und blutbildenden Organen hervorzurufen.

Was den Grund für diese Empfindlichkeit der betreffenden Organe zu den Cholesterinverbindungen anbelangt, so können wir diesen zurzeit nicht angeben. Bezüglich der Aortenwandungen wissen wir, daß sie auch beim Menschen eine Prädilektionsstelle für die Ablagerung doppeltbrechender Cholesterinestern bilden. Auf Grund der am menschlichen Material gemachten Beobachtungen konnte man sich aber bisher noch keine klare Vorstellung über den Zusammenhang zwischen der in Rede stehenden Ablagerung der Cholesterinester in den Aortenwandungen und der Entwicklung atherosklerotischer Veränderungen derselben gewinnen. Viele Autoren sind sogar geneigt, das Vorhandensein doppeltbrechender Lipoide in den veränderten Aortenschichten für einen sekundären z. T. degenerativen Prozeß zu halten, der sich an die primären hyperplastischen Intimaveränderungen anschließt. Auf Grund der in dieser Arbeit angeführten Beobachtungen, muß aber diese Vorstellung über den Entwicklungsprozeß atherosklerotischer Aortenveränderungen, wenigstens für die experimentelle Atherosklerose vom „diätetischen" Typus abgelehnt werden. In der Tat werden die fettähnlichen Substanzen anfangs in ganz morphologisch unveränderten Aortenwandungen

Veränderungen der Kaninchenaorta bei experiment. Cholesterinsteatose. 401

abgelagert. Die sich später allmählich entwickelnden pathologischen Prozesse können dabei leicht nur als sekundär betrachtet werden. Sie stellen sozusagen eine spezifische Reaktion der Aortenwandungen auf die Ablagerung fettähnlicher Substanzen dar und nach ihren morphologischen Eigenschaften können sie ohne Schwierigkeit von diesem Standpunkte aus beurteilt werden.

Auf diese Weise kommen wir zum Schluß, daß die von uns experimentell hervorgerufenen atherosklerotischen Prozesse der Aortenwandungen einen primär infiltrativen Prozeß mit nachfolgenden reaktiven Erscheinungen darstellen. Da in unseren Versuchen auch in anderen Organen eine enorme Ablagerung doppeltbrechender fettähnlicher Substanzen stattfand, so sind wir schließlich berechtigt, die Aortenveränderungen bei unseren Tieren nur als eine der Teilerscheinungen einer allgemeinen Cholesterinsteatose zu betrachten.

Gewiß stellt der Reichtum der Organismussäfte an Cholesterinverbindungen nicht den einzigen Moment dar, welcher bei der Entstehung atherosklerotischer Veränderungen von Bedeutung ist. Vielleicht gibt es noch Substanzen, welche die Bildung von Cholesterinablagerungen in den Aortenwandungen begünstigen und sogar bei normalem Cholesteringehalt im Blute die Entwicklung dieser Ablagerungen zu verursachen vermögen. Von diesem Standpunkte aus können vielleicht auch die von SALTYKOW (18) erzielten Versuchsresultate beurteilt werden. Wenn dieser Autor mit Hilfe von Staphylokokkeneinspritzungen Atherosklerose bei Kaninchen hervorgerufen hat, so steht noch die Frage offen, ob die Staphylokokkentoxine an und für sich auf eine direkte Weise die Aortenveränderungen verursacht haben, oder letztere erst sekundär infolge einer Zerstörung des Cholesterinstoffwechsels dank der angewandten Intoxikation entstanden sind. Diese Intoxikation hat vielleicht auch eine morphologisch nicht nachweisbare Wirkung auf die Gefäßwandungen, dank der die Entwicklung der Cholesterinablagerungen in denselben erfolgen kann.

Alle diese Fragen sind gewiß zurzeit noch nicht zu entscheiden und bedürfen zu ihrer Beantwortung neuerer ausführlicher Experimente.

Wie es oben erwähnt wurde, steht der von uns an Kaninchen erzielte atherosklerotische Prozeß der menschlichen Atherosklerose sehr nahe und diese Ähnlichkeit tritt nicht nur in morphologischen, sondern auch in mikrochemischen Besonderheiten der beiden Prozesse zum Vorschein. Es scheint aber, daß man zwischen diesen Prozessen auch im pathogenetischen Sinne eine gewisse Parallele ziehen dürfte. Wie es aus den chemischen Blutuntersuchungen CHAUFFARD's (7) und PRIBRAM's (15) hervorgeht, ist bei Atherosklerotikern der Cholesteringehalt des Blutes stets erhöht und somit sind bei ihnen die Bedingungen für die Entstehung von Cholesterinablagerungen in verschiedenen Organen günstig.

402   A n i t s c h k o w ,

Dank dem erhöhten Cholesteringehalt des Organismus sind gerade solche
Kranken für die Entstehung der Ablagerungen von Cholesterinverbindungen besonders prädisponiert und da die Aortenwandungen ein
Organ darstellen, wo am öftesten diese Ablagerungen stattfinden, so liegt
die Voraussetzung nahe auch beim Menschen, in analoger Weise wie
bei unseren Versuchen, die beiden Erscheinungen — den erhöhten Cholesteringehalt des Organismus und die Entstehung atherosklerotischer Aortenveränderungen — in eine ursächliche Beziehung miteinander zu stellen.
Es besteht also zwischen dem Resultate der hier angeführten Experimente
und den Angaben der menschlichen Pathologie nicht nur im morphologischen und mikrochemischen, sondern wahrscheinlich auch im ätio-
logischen Sinne eine gewisse Verwandtschaft.

Literaturverzeichnis.

1) ANITSCHKOW u. CHALATOW, Über experim. Cholesterinsteatose, Zentralbl. f. allg.
    Pathol. u. pathol. Anat. Bd. 24 1913.
2) ASCHOFF, L., Zur Morphologie der lipoiden Substanzen, Ziegler's Beiträge Bd. 47
    1910.
3) —, Diskussionsbemerkung zu SALTYKOW, Verhandlg. d. deutsch. pathol. Gesellsch.
    14. Tag. 1910.
4) CHALATOW, Über die Veränderungen von Kaninchenleber unter dem Einfluß
    einer reichlichen animal. Nahrung, Ber. d. Russ. pathol. Gesellsch. Bd. 2
    1910/11.
5) —, Über das Verhalten der Leber gegenüber den verschiedenen Arten von
    Speisefett, Virchow's Archiv Bd. 207 1912.
6) — Über die flüssigen Kristalle im Organismus, erscheint in Frankf. Zeitschr. f.
    Pathologie 1913.
7) CHAUFFARD, Les depôts locaux de la choléstérine, Rev. de med. Oct. 1911.
8) v. EBNER, Koelliker's Handb. d. Gewebelehre d. Menschen Bd. III 1902.
9) HERXHEIMER, zit. n. SALTYKOW (19).
10) IGNATOWSKI, Über den Einfluß der animal. Nahrung auf den Kaninchenorganis-
    mus, Ber. d. K. mil.-med. Akad. zu St. Petersburg Bd. 16 1908.
11) —, Über die Veränderungen d. parench. Organe unter dem Einflusse des animal.
    Eiweißes, ebenda Bd. 17 1908.
12) —, Über die Wirkung des tierischen Eiweißes auf die Aorta, Virchow's Archiv
    Bd. 192 1909.
13) KAWAMURA, Cholesterinestervorfettung, Jena 1911.
14) LUBARSCH, Über alimentäre Schlagaderverkalkung, Münch. med. Wochenschr.
    Nr. 30 1910.
15) PRIBRAM, Über den Cholesteringehalt des Blutes, Prag. med. Wochenschr. Nr. 17
    1912.
16) REDDINGIUS, zit. n. SALTYKOW (19).
17) RIBBERT, Über die Genese der arterioskl. Veränderungen, Verhandlg. d. deutsch.
    pathol. Gesellsch. 8. Tag. 1904.
18) SALTYKOW, Atherosklerose bei Kaninchen nach wiederholt. Staphylokokkeninjekt.,
    Ziegler's Beiträge Bd. 43 1908.
19) —, Weitere Untersuch. über die Staphylokokken-Atherosklerose, Verhandlg. d.
    deutsch. pathol. Gesellsch. 14. Tag. 1910.
20) STAROKADOMSKI, Zur Frage über die experim. Arteriosklerose, I.-D., St. Peters-
    burg 1909.
21) STUCKEY, Über die Veränderungen d. Kaninchenaorta unter dem Einflusse einer
    reichl. animal. Nahrung, I.-D., St. Petersburg 1910.
22) STUCKEY, Über die Aortenveränderungen unter dem Einfluß verschiedener Arten
    von Fetten, Zentralbl. f. allg. Pathol. u. pathol. Anat. Nr. 21 1912.
23) WESSELKIN, Über die Ablagerungen fettähnlicher Substanzen in den inneren
    Organen. Russki Wratsch Nr. 21 1912.

A synopsis of
Changes in rabbit aorta due to experimentally induced cholesterolsteatosis
by Dr N Anitshkow

Pathological-Medical Institute of the Imperial Military Academy,
St. Petersburg. 1913
Prepared by Madeleine Kinsella B.A., M. Litt.,
University of Marburg, W. Germany

In their research into the causes of hypercholesterolaemia, the author, with other colleagues at the Imperial Military Academy of St. Petersburg, experimented with rabbits in order to reproduce in them a form of arteriosclerosis as similar as possible to that found in man. They were able to establish a new group of vascular changes which they termed "dietetic arteriosclerosis". They discovered that these severe changes in the rabbit aorta could only be induced by feeding them certain food-stuffs. Stuckey *et al.* fed the rabbits egg yolk, while Anitschkow and Cholatow used pure cholesterol dissolved in sunflower oil. Anitschkow pointed out that his experimental animals, and those fed by Stuckey with egg yolk, all showed exactly the same changes in the aorta and that the common factor was cholesterol. He also found that the intensity of these changes was directly proportional to the amount of cholesterol ingested by the animals. He discounted the possibility of spontaneous changes in the rabbit aorta on a scale sufficiently large to distort the experiments. The results of these experiments are supported by detailed tables of the doses given to the animals and are correlated to the findings of the macroscopic and microscopic examinations. Anitschkow also carried out similar experiments on rats but failed to produce similar results. No changes of any consequence were to be found in the rats. He concluded that not only the chemical content of the cholesterol but also the type of animal used was of importance.

The author then described the specific changes he observed in the rabbit aorta. After detailing the morphological characteristics and the genesis of changes in the aorta caused by experimentally induced hypercholesteraemia, he then proceeded to discuss the microchemical and colour reaction of the fat-like substances that had penetrated the aortic walls of the rabbits in substantial quantities. These were the subject of an exhaustive series of experiments using several different methods.

Anitschkow summarized his results by stating that the experimental material at the disposal of himself and his colleagues enabled the theories about the origins of arteriosclerotic changes in human aorta to be tested and confirmed. However, the reasons for the sensitivity of the aortic walls, liver and adrenal glands to cholesterol compounds were not yet understood.

In conclusion he expressed his conviction that a definite connection existed, not only on a morphological and microchemical level, but also on an aetiological level, between the results of these experiments and the information available from human pathology.

Aus der Medizinischen Klinik in Freiburg i. Br.
(Direktor: Prof. de la Camp.)

Untersuchungen über den Cholesteringehalt des menschlichen Blutes bei verschiedenen inneren Erkrankungen.[2])

Von Priv.-Doz. Dr. Bacmeister und Dr. Henes (New York).

In der letzten Zeit hat die Vervollkommnung chemischer Methoden uns die Möglichkeit gebracht, unsere Kenntnis über das Vorkommen und den Stoffwechsel des Cholesterins im menschlichen und tierischen Organismus zu vertiefen und zu erweitern. Wir haben gelernt, daß gewisse Krankheiten mit einer Vermehrung, andere mit einer Verminderung des Cholesterinspiegels im Blute einhergehen, und es erhebt sich die Frage, ob diesen Schwankungen bestimmte, für die Krankheit charakteristische Vorgänge im Organismus entsprechen. Es scheint, daß der Cholesteringehalt für gewisse immunisatorische Prozesse im Körper von Bedeutung ist, daß die Abwehrmaßregeln des Organismus für die verschiedensten pathologischen Vorgänge und der innere und äußere Cholesterinstoffwechsel in gewissen Beziehungen stehen. Wir haben in letzter Zeit in unserer Klinik ein großes Material der verschiedensten Krankheitszustände (über 100 Fälle) auf den Cholesteringehalt des Blutes geprüft, und im folgenden soll in aller Kürze über die Hauptergebnisse referiert werden. Wir versagen es uns, an dieser Stelle auf die Resultate anderer Arbeiten einzugehen und die ganze einschlägige Literatur zu bringen.

Die genaueren Resultate wird einer von uns (Dr. Henes, der die technischen Bestimmungen ausführte) mit genauer Angabe der Technik unter Berücksichtigung der Literatur ausführlich an anderer Stelle veröffentlichen.

Wir bedienten uns des Extraktionsverfahrens, wie es von Weston und Kent angegeben wurde. Für die kolorimetrische Bestimmung haben wir nach kurzer Zeit das Verfahren dieser Autoren aufgegeben, weil wir damit keine hinreichend konstanten Resultate erhielten. Wir haben dann das Extraktionsverfahren von Weston und Kent mit der kolorimetrischen Methode von Grigaut verbunden und in dieser Weise die Untersuchungen ausgeführt. Wir haben uns nicht davon überzeugen können, daß nach der Verseifung eine Ansäuerung notwendig ist — wie Bürger und Beumer verlangen —, um das Cholesterin zu extrahieren, sondern haben gefunden, daß bei genügend langem, unter Schütteln fortgesetztem Extrahieren diese Fehlerquelle praktisch ausgeschaltet werden kann. Herr Prof. Autenrieth und Herr Dr. Funk von der Medizinischen Abteilung des hiesigen Chemischen Institutes hatten die Liebenswürdigkeit, mit anderen Methoden, die Herr Prof. Autenrieth in nächster Zeit der Veröffentlichung übergeben wird, dieselben Blutmengen derselben Fälle mehrfach zu untersuchen, und sie erzielten übereinstimmende Werte mit uns. Ebenso ergab die Digitoninmethode, die verschiedentlich zur Kontrolle mit herangezogen wurde, die Richtigkeit unserer Werte.

In 9 Fällen fanden wir bei normalen, gesunden Menschen Werte, die zwischen 1,10 und 1,80 g pro 1000 ccm schwankten, mit einem Durchschnitt von 1,48. Uebereinstimmend mit vielen anderen Autoren fanden wir, daß der Cholesteringehalt des Blutes von der Diät beeinflußt wird, daß eine geringe Vermehrung des Gesamtcholesterins im Blute bei cholesterinreicher Nahrung auftritt. Wir versuchten festzustellen, wie die Verteilung des Cholesterins auf die einzelnen Blutbestandteile sich vollzieht und ob die Verhältniszahl des Cholesteringehaltes zwischen Serum und roten Blutkörperchen bei physiologischen und pathologischen Zuständen sich ändert. Dr. Henes, der auch diese Untersuchungen ausführte, fand, daß das Serum bei normalen Fällen allein durchschnittlich 55,6%, die roten Blutkörperchen 44,4 % des Gesamtcholesterins enthielten. Nach einer physiologischen Vermehrung des Cholesterins im Blute (entsprechende Mahlzeit), waren die Verhältniswerte 54,5 % und 45,5, und ebensowenig fand eine stärkere Verschiebung bei pathologischer Zunahme statt. Das prozentuale Verhältnis des Cholesteringehaltes der einzelnen Blutbestandteile scheint sich nach diesen Untersuchungen bei der Hypercholesterinämie nicht zu ändern, und dasselbe darf man wohl

auch von der pathologischen Hypercholesterinämie annehmen. Demnach bleibt es sich praktisch gleich, ob man vollständiges Blut oder Serum allein bei der quantitativen Bestimmung benutzt.

Wir haben dann 14 Fälle von chronischen Nierenerkrankungen untersucht. Je schwerer der Allgemeinzustand durch die Erkrankung beeinträchtigt war, umso höher war der Cholesteringehalt des Blutes; einen hohen Wert erhielten wir bei der chronischen Urämie (2,2). Unabhängig war die Vermehrung des Cholesterins im Blut von der Eiweißausscheidung im Urin. Wir erhielten normale Werte bei hohem Albumengehalt, wenn der Allgemeinzustand gut war, stark erhöhte Werte bei geringerer Eiweißausscheidung bei schwer geschädigtem Allgemeinstatus. Interessant war, daß in einem Fall von Urämie der Cholesterinwert des Blutes kurz vor dem Tode erheblich sank (0,9).

Bei 13 Fällen von Atherosklerose konnten wir immer dann eine Vermehrung des Cholesterinspiegels im Blute feststellen, wenn klinisch der Prozeß noch in der Entwicklung begriffen war. Bei ausgebildeten Fällen mit hohem Blutdruck (nicht kompliziert durch Schrumpfnieren) waren die Werte meist normal oder nur gering erhöht. Bei zwei Fällen von Apoplexie bei alten Leuten auf atherosklerotischer Grundlage war eine Vermehrung des Blutcholesterins nicht nachweisbar, beide Fälle hatten keine Nierenkomplikationen.

Fast regelmäßig wurde eine Hypercholesterinämie beim Diabetes mellitus gefunden (6 Fälle); ob hier die Vermehrung mit der wachsenden Zuckerausscheidung steigt, konnten wir nicht feststellen, da nur leichtere Fälle zur Beobachtung kamen. Einmal konnten wir im Coma diabeticum kurz vor dem Tode untersuchen und fanden hier den hohen Wert von 3,0. In 4 Fällen von Fettsucht wurde dreimal eine erhebliche Vermehrung nachgewiesen 1,9—2,2. Ein Fall von chronischer Gicht zeigte keine Abweichung von der Norm, während beim Diabetes insipidus der Wert von 2,0 gefunden wurde.

Interessant war das Verhalten des Cholesterins im Blut bei Infektionskrankheiten. Als Regel können wir sagen, daß bei jedem höheren Fieber der Cholesteringehalt sofort heruntergeht, das haben wir in gleicher Weise gefunden bei Typhus, Scharlach, Pneumonie, Erysipel, Sepsis etc. Je höher das Fieber, desto geringer der Cholesterinspiegel im Blut. Mit der Abnahme der Temperatur steigt der Cholesterinwert wieder an, langsam oder schnell entsprechend der Temperatur. Diese Abnahme während des Fiebers scheint eine direkte Funktion der erhöhten Temperatur und ihrer Folgen zu sein, denn in 2 Fällen ziemlich schwerer Gesichtsrose, bei die Temperatur nicht über 36,8° war, konnten wir keine größere Verminderung feststellen (1,3 und 1,8). Dauert das Fieber nur wenige Tage, so geht der Cholesteringehalt des Blutes nach unseren Untersuchungen zur Norm zurück; so fanden wir in 6 Scharlachfällen, bei denen nur wenige Tage ein allerdings meist hohes Fieber bestanden hatte, mit Abklingen des Fiebers ziemlich normale Werte. Wenn aber das Fieber längere Zeit angehalten hatte, so erhob sich der Cholesterinspiegel längere Zeit über die Norm, so bei der Pneumonie und vor allem beim Typhus, bei dem in 3 Fällen die Hypercholesterinämie noch wochenlang zu beobachten war und bis zur Entlassung der Fälle anhielt. Bei der Lungentuberkulose scheint der allgemeine Zustand den wichtigsten Faktor für den Cholesteringehalt des Blutes abzugeben; bei dieser Krankheit haben wir trotz hoher Temperaturen normale, ja sogar erhöhte Werte gefunden, wenn der allgemeine Ernährungszustand gut, tiefe Werte selbst bei nur geringem Fieber, wenn die Auszehrung vorgeschritten war.

Aehnliche Resultate wie bei der chronischen Tuberkulose erhielten wir bei malignen Tumoren; auch hier gingen die Werte herab, wenn die Kachexie einsetzte, während in der ersten Entwicklungsperiode der Geschwülste fast regelmäßig eine leichte Steigerung — eine Hypercholesterinämie — nachzuweisen war. Bei nicht komplizierten kompensierten Herzfehlern und bei einigen Systemerkrankungen des Rückenmarks waren keine besonderen Abweichungen von der Norm zu finden.

Die genauen Tabellen und Werte werden in nächster Zeit von Dr. Henes publiziert werden.

---

[1]) Essai d'une conception nouvelle de la Parasyphilis etc. Presse médicale 1911, Nr. 100, S. 1035

[2]) Nach einem Vortrag in der Freiburger medizinischen Gesellschaft am 18. Februar 1913.

Editorial Note: A synopsis of this paper, in English, appears on page 28.

Zusammenfassung. Aus unseren Untersuchungen geht hervor, daß cholesterinarme Diät, Alter, Abzehrung, schlechter Allgemeinzustand und vor allem Temperaturerhöhung vermindernd auf den Cholesteringehalt des Blutes wirken.

Bei cholesterinreicher Kost, bei allen schweren Stoffwechselerkrankungen, Diabetes, Fettsucht, Nephritis, frischer Atherosklerose, fanden wir eine ausgesprochene Hypercholesterinämie. Ob beim Typhus, der von allen anderen Infektionskrankheiten eine Sonderstellung einnimmt, die Hypercholesterinämie, die mit Beginn der Rekonvaleszenz einsetzt und Wochen hindurch dauern kann, das Resultat eines lange dauernden Fiebers mit seinen Folgen ist, oder durch spezifische Vorgänge im Körper ausgelöst wird, wollen wir nicht entscheiden. Auf die Rekonvaleszentennahrung ist sie, wie der Vergleich mit anderen Infektionskrankheiten zeigt, sicher nicht allein zu schieben.

Wir stehen noch ganz im Beginn unserer Kenntnisse über die Verbreitung und die Bedeutung des Cholesterins im menschlichen Organismus.

Aus den Arbeiten von Dorée und Gardner, Fraser und Ellis geht wohl mit Sicherheit hervor, daß das Cholesterin in den Körper mit der Nahrung eingeführt und nicht von diesem gebildet wird. Die Flintsche Theorie, daß das Cholesterin ein Produkt der Zersetzung des Nervengewebes sei, ist von Grigaut und Laroche widerlegt.

Wir wissen jetzt aber auch, daß das Cholesterin ein stetiger Bestandteil der tierischen Zellen ist und in allen Körperflüssigkeiten erscheint. Wir haben gelernt, daß in fast gesetzmäßiger Weise bei bestimmten Krankheiten das Cholesterin im Blut angehäuft wird, bei anderen pathologischen Vorgängen regelmäßig vermindert erscheint. Noch wissen wir nicht, ob es sich hier um sekundäre Stoffwechselvorgänge handelt, oder ob dem Cholesterin irgendeine aktive Rolle im Kampfe des Organismus gegen die Krankheit zuzuschreiben ist. Noch gilt es, die einzelnen Bausteine zusammenzutragen und unsere Erfahrungen, die wir auf Grund vervollkommneter Methode erworben haben, zu mehren. Ehe wir nicht die Bedeutung des Cholesterinstoffwechsels im normalen und kranken Organismus erkannt haben, sind alle therapeutischen Versuche mit dem Cholesterin, wie sie von verschiedenen Seiten ausgeführt wurden, verfrüht und ein Arbeiten im Dunkeln.

A synopsis of
Investigations into the cholesterol content of human blood in various internal diseases
by Dr. Bacmeister and Dr. Henes
prepared by Madeleine Kinsella, B.A., M.Litt.,
University of Marburg, W. Germany

The authors collected and examined blood samples, to determine the cholesterol content, from over 100 cases representing a wide range of illnesses, in order to determine the blood cholesterol content. This article is a report of the main results obtained. The extraction process used was that devised by Weston and Kent. Blood samples from the same patients were also tested by Authenrieth and Funk, using a different method, and their results agreed with those of the authors.

14 cases of chronic renal disease were examined. It was found that the weaker the patient's general state of health, the higher the blood cholesterol content. A high value was also present in cases of chronic uraemia.

In 13 cases of arteriosclerosis an increase in the blood cholesterol level was always present in the developing stages of the disease. In fully developed cases with high blood pressure but no renal atrophy, the values were mainly normal, or only slightly raised. Hypercholesterolaemia was found in most of the six cases of diabetes mellitus and the four cases of obesity showed a considerable increase in cholesterol.

One of the most interesting results, in the opinion of the authors, was the reaction of blood cholesterol in infectious diseases. As a general rule, a high temperature depressed the cholesterol content of the blood. This phenomenon was observed in, for instance, typhus, scarlet fever and pneumonia. The higher the fever, the lower the cholesterol level in the blood. If the fever lasted only a couple of days, then the cholesterol content returned to normal, but in the case of pneumonia or typhus where the temperature remains high for a prolonged period, then the cholesterol content rose above normal levels and hypercholesterolaemia could be observed in the patients for several weeks.

In pulmonary tuberculosis the patients general state of health was the most important factor influencing blood content of cholesterol. If it was good, normal to raised levels were found in spite of a high temperature. If bad, due to the disease being in advanced stages, then the levels remained low. Similar results were also observed in cases of malign tumours.

The authors then summarized the results as follows: The study showed that a low cholesterol diet, age, emaciation, poor state of health and, in particular, high temperature were factors which had a lowering effect on the cholesterol content of the blood. A diet high in cholesterol, all serious metabolic disorders, diabetes, obesity, nephritis, and arteriosclerosis in its initial stages were all factors in the development of hypercholesterolaemia. The reasons for hypercholesterolaemia in typhus still had to be researched more thoroughly. The authors emphasized that much remained to be discovered about the role of cholesterol in the body and its function in the body's fight against disease. Premature attempts to use it in therapy would have little chance of success.

8. **Carl Müller,** Oslo:

Xanthomata, Hypercholesterolemia, Angina Pectoris.

Since FR. HARBITZ, in 1925, mentioned xanthomata this question has been later on touched upon in the Norwegian literature by himself as well as by several other authors (JOHN HALD, G. RAEDER). In all, eight to ten cases of this kind have been mentioned in the literature of our country, rather as curiosities.

Of especial interest in regard to these patients is the circumstance that five of them *died suddenly* and unexpectedly, apparently with symptoms of paralysis of the heart. In those cases where necropsy was undertaken the cause of death proved to be vessel changes, viz. deposits of xanthomatous masses in the aorta, on the aortic valves, and in the coronary arteries. — This condition attracted attention owing to the fact that it was evidently *hereditary*. It is inherited as a pronounced dominant quality, either as a clinically provable xanthomatosis, or as a hypercholesterolemia. Report on similar cases have appeared in other countries also.

Xanthomata are generally interpreted as a symptom indicating a constitutional anomaly in the metabolism, a *lipoidosis*. Hypercholesterolemia does not seem to be always present in these patients. It is certain that such a change in the blood may be at hand without provable xanthomata. The cause of this anomaly in the metabolism is unknown. The lipoids, circulating in the blood, are presumably not deposited exclusively under the skin at fixed points in the form of nodules, but also in the mucous membranes, e. g. in those of the mouth and the biliary ducts and above all in the arteries where changes are thus evoked which may not be distinguished in any way either microscopically or macroscopically from those observed in an ordinary arteriosclerosis.

There is no occasion in this lecture to refer to other clinical types of lipoidosis nor to the presence of hypercholesterolemia as a symptom in several diseases.

76

Reports of cases.

I came across my first case by the middle of April 1937.

Patient No. 1: male, aged 45, observed non-dolorous nodules on the dorsal side of several fingers when 30 years old. About the same time he noticed deposits on the elbows, below the ligamentum patellae and the achilles tendons. (Se figures 1, 2, and 3). The localization of these nodules is almost symmetrical and they have grown very slowly during all these years and only troubled him from the cosmetic point of view. They are of varying consistence being in most places almost like infiltrated glandular tissue and almost bony hard under ligamentum patellae. The deposits do not adhere to the skin, which is not discoloured, but they are adherent to

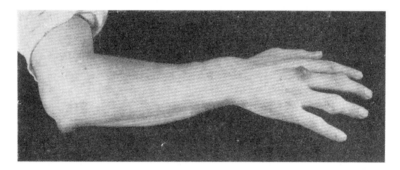

Fig. 1.

the underlying tissues, tendons and capsular ligaments or fascia. In March 1932, a nodule was extirpated on the dorsal side of the ring-finger. Partial extirpation of the tendon infiltrated by the nodule was also necessary. Under the microscope the tumor was found to consist of *xanthomatous tissue.* The patient was admitted to hospital on April 14th 1937 on account of cardiac symptoms. He has been suffering from dyspnea in connection with excertion for 10 years and during the last two or three years from typical angina pectoris. The pain disappears when he rests. After an exercise test the electrocardiogram showed signs of myocardial involvement. A blood cholesterole examination made in 1932 showed occurrence of 331 mgs. per cent; in April 1937 the cholesterol content was 560 mgs. per cent; R.R. 125/75 mm. Hg.; Wassermann reaction —. The family history of the patient: *both his father and mother died of angina pectoris at the age of 77 and 66 years. His mother had nodules on her hands. One of the patients sisters has the same cardiac symptoms as the patient, nodules on the hands and hypercholesterolemia (in 1932).* Two children in the same family are well and have no visible nodules. Their blood has not been examined.

77

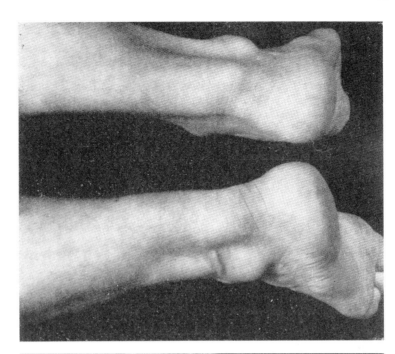

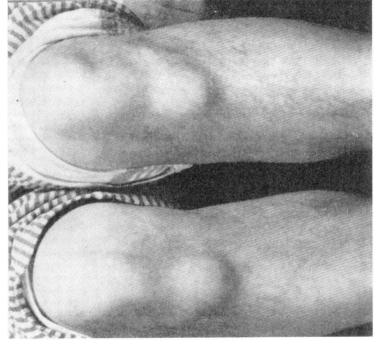

Fig. 2 and 3.

78

Patient No. 2: I came across a few days later: male aged 76. In 1935 I treated him for angina pectoris, from which he had suffered increasingly for 16 years. But I did not at the time connect his xanthomata with the heart-disease. He saw me now because he was almost unable to walk owing to angina pectoris. The electrocardiogram showed signs of myocardial involvement. R.R. — 140/95 mm. Hg. — The blood cholesterol was 304 mgs. per cent. He died at home on the 2nd June 1937 of angina pectoris. — This patient had had xanthomata for 40 years. Their growth was exceedingly slow from year to year and they did not trouble him. The localization was much the same as in the previous case. See figures 4, 5, and 6).

Patient No. 3: a brother of the above patient, aged 73. He has had angina pectoris during the last 6 years. Examination of the heart (by electrocardiogram and x-rays) revealed nothing abnormal. R.R. 150/100; the blood cholesterol was 440 mgs. per cent. On fingers, knnees and heels nodules similar to those in the two previous cases but less obvious. (See figure 7.) He has had these nodules for about 30 years.

Patient No. 4: daughter of Patient No. 2 and niece of Patient No. 3, aged 37. She is well, especially no signs of cardiac disease but nodules on the dorsal side of both the middle-fingers and on each side of the tuberositas tibia. R.R. 120/85 mm. Hg. The blood cholesterol was 350 mgs. per cent. It may be further mentioned about this family that the father of the above two brothers (thus the grandfather of this patient) had very marked nodules on the hands and died of angina pectoris at the age of 58. *Xanthomata thus occurred in three generations in this family.*

These two family histories have reminded me of a number of previously observed patients. A follow-up examination of these patients and their families gave the following results.

Patient No. 5: A married woman, aged 55, saw me on account of angina pectoris in the years 1928—1930. I remember having observed xanthomata on all the four eye-lids. The angina pectoris commenced in February 1928, the xanthomata were noticed by her in 1922. The Physician in Chief, OLAF RØMCKE, M. D., Drammen, who treats her at present, has kindly placed at my disposal the following data concerning her: Now the xanthomata encircle both her eyes like rings. The angina pectoris, which is alleviated by nitroglycerine, seems to have remained unchanged ever since 1928. The electrocardiogram now also shows signs of myocardial involvement. R.R. (during the period 1928—30 and now) about 150 mm. Hg. Wassermann reaction (in 1928) —. The family history of the patient is as follows: Her mother is said to have died from "a tumor on a blood vessel", ascertained at the post-mortem examination. She was treated for heart-disease and had xanthomata in the face. One of the patient's sisters has similar xanthomata and heart-disease, one of her brothers has heart disease too, but no xanthomata. The patient has two healthy children 27 and 29 years of age.

79

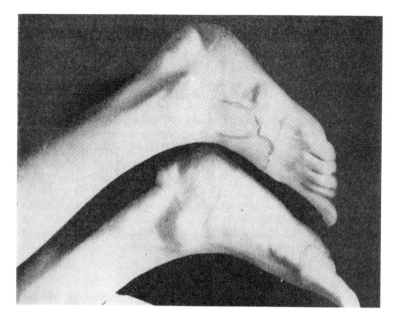

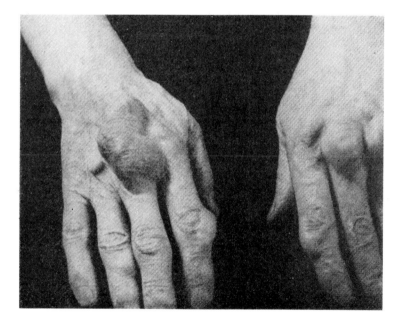

Fig. 4 and 5.

80

Patient No. 6: female, aged 68, was treated by me during many years for angina pectoris. She saw me again 3 weeks ago as her trouble had increased considerably. I now observed that she had xanthomata on the upper left eye-lid, which had previously escaped my notice. She had had it for at least 30 years and a similar nodule had been removed from her upper right eye-lid about 25 years ago. On the middle and basal joint of both her middle-fingers I found small nodules, hardly visible but easily palpated, which the patient herself had not noticed. The electrocardio-gram showed signs of an old coronary thrombosis. R.R. 140/95 mm. Hg. The blood cholesterol was 234 mgs. per cent. The family history of the patient: Her grandfather, on the father's side, and her father both died of angina pectoris at a fairly advanced age. A sister and a brother also died of the same disease, both over 60 years old. The patient's sister,

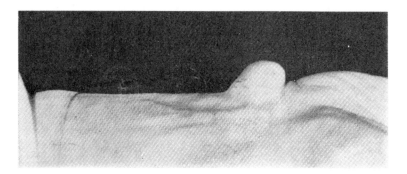

Fig. 6.

whom I treated until her death, had for many years suffered from slight anginal troubles, when coronary thrombosis rapidly ended her days. Some years ago I had the opportunity to examine the son of this patient also. He was at that time about 40 years old and had angina pectoris. This patient has not suffered from rheumatic fever or syphilis (Wassermann reaction —); blood-pressure normal. At the age of 42 this man suddenly died from angina pectoris. It is now too late to find out whether any one of the deceased in this family had had xanthomata, but xanthomatosis and hypercholesterolemia having been ascertained in one of the members unquestionably throws a new light on this family history.

Finally, I have during the last 3 months seen three cases of typical coronary thrombosis (two men and one woman), who all had xanthomata on the eye-lids. The family history was either negative in these cases or there was no available history.

The first three family histories confirm the previous experiences according to which multiple xanthomata are a hereditary disease

81

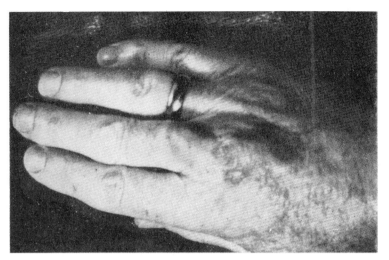

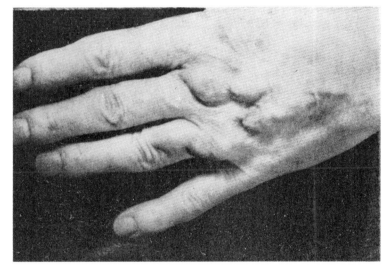

Fig. 7.

6

82

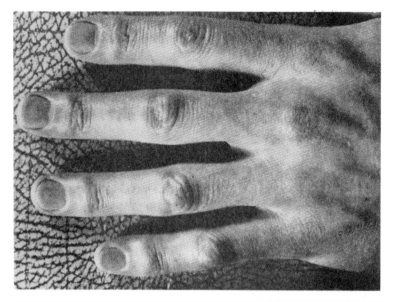

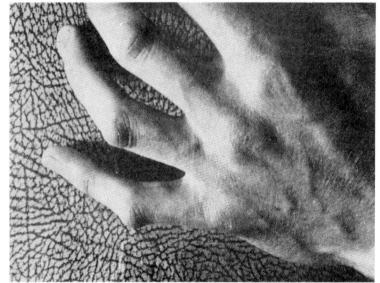

Fig. 8.

83

causing pronounced predisposition for cardiac diseases. The same hereditary predisposition was probably present in the fourth family also.

While the majority of cases, at any rate those so far published in Norway, had a fatal issue, i. e. the patients died suddenly of heart failure when still young or comparatively young, it appears that the members of the families mentioned above can show the same clinical picture of angina pectoris and that they have reached the age at which this disease usually appears. We have heard also that those who died of this disease were no longer young. These experiences seem thus to show that xanthomata and the lipoidosis connected with them should interest clinicians not only because they may cause sudden death by heart-disease in young people but also because angina pectoris of the common type may be evoked thereby at an advanced age. It is too early to express an opinion as to how often this cause of angina pectoris asserts itself. The fact that we have been able to collect so many cases in such a short time seems anyway to indicate that we have here to do with a causal factor of practical importance. Especially it seems that our attention should be turned in this direction in the case of families where heart-diseases are common and whorse etiology cannot apparently be traced back to the common causes, hypertension, rheumatic infection, and syphilis. If we want to widen our experiences on this subject it is necessary to pay the greatest possible attention to the family history in heart diseases. As hypertension is considered a hereditary cause of arteriosclerosis and angina pectoris, it should be emphasized that the blood-pressure was not particularly high in any of the examined patients.

It is generally easy to diagnose xanthomata when we have to do with the symmetrically placed and plainly visible nodules and also with the xanthomata (»xanthelasms») on the eye-lids. But the nodules may easily be overlooked if they are small (as in Case No. 4). It is to be observed that the nodules were not yellowish in colour in any of my cases. These nodules may be hardly mistaken for HEBERDEN's nodes or deposits of uric acid, but easily for GARROD's pads, localized on the upper side of the joint between the 1st and 2nd finger phalanx. These pads seem to occur very frequently. While searching for nodules I was able to ascertain that three of the younger physicians at the hospital

84

had them (Figure 8); and all three were able to tell me that such nodules occurred also in other members of the family, being thus presumably *hereditary*. Six of GARROD's twelve patients had at the same time DUPYTREN's contraction also. These pads consist of fibrous tissue and have nothing to do with xanthomata.

References.

GARROD, A. E.: St. Barthol. Hosp. Reports. 1893, vol. XXIX p. 157.
—»— British Med. Journ. July 2. 1904, p. 8.
HARBITZ, FR.: Svulster inneholdende xanthomvæv, Norsk Magasin for Lægevidenskapen. 1925, p. 321, No. 4.
—»— Xanthomatose og plutselig død. Ibid. 1936, p. 695, No. 7.
—»— Ibid. 1936, p. 1317.
WHITE HALE, W.: On pads on finger-joints. Quarterly journ. of med. 1907—09, vol. I, p. 479.
RAEDER, I. G.: Om stoffskifteforholdene ved lipoidose. Norsk magasin for lægevidenskapen. 1936, p. 113, No. 2.

Discussion.

BING: Expresses his thanks for the interesting report and demonstrates sciopticon pictures (see Figure) showing the deposits of fat in the aorta of a man aged 30, in whom was at several examinations stated hyperlipemia with about 1.5 per cent total fat and 400 mg. per cent cholesterol. The

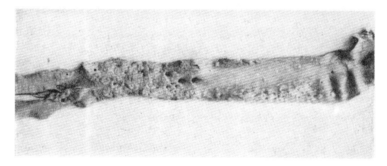

deposits were situated in the same manner as in atherosclerosis. Yellow fat deposits were also observed in the coronary arteries. Sciopticon pictures are besides shown of the same patient's kidneys, which were small, yellowish-white, with numerous granules of fat and protein in the tubuli.

SALVESEN: Described a case of chronic lipoid-nephrosis in which lipemia developed simultaneously with general xanthomatosis. Treatment with diet poor in fats caused disappearance both of the lipemia and the cutaneous xanthomata.

ULTRACENTRIFUGAL STUDIES OF LIPOPROTEINS OF HUMAN SERUM

By JOHN W. GOFMAN, FRANK T. LINDGREN, AND HAROLD ELLIOTT

(*From the Division of Medical Physics, Donner Laboratory, University of California, Berkeley*)

(Received for publication, January 21, 1949)

In spite of several extensive ultracentrifugal studies of human sera by Mutzenbecher, McFarlane, and Pedersen, the interpretation of the patterns observed has remained in doubt. Specifically, the greatest difficulties encountered by previous workers have arisen in their efforts to study undiluted human sera. McFarlane (1) referred to marked distortions in the pattern observed with undiluted human serum and suggested a trial and error dilution of the serum with salt solution to minimize such distortions. Pedersen (2) recommended diluting sera with various salt or buffer solutions to 40 per cent of the initial concentration, since under these conditions "adequate" resolution of the albumin and so called "X protein" peaks in the sedimentation diagram could be made. Both these workers found the apparent concentration of the X protein to vary considerably with respect to both over-all protein and salt concentration. The variations in concentration ranged from a value of X protein constituting up to 30 per cent of the serum proteins when studied in concentrated serum to an immeasurably small value when the serum was greatly diluted. Pedersen has explained this variation in X protein concentration by assuming this molecule to be a labile complex of albumin, globulin, and lipides which dissociates with increasing dilution of the serum.

On the basis of ultracentrifugal studies of human sera by the present authors, a wholly different interpretation of the ultracentrifugal patterns observed is given herewith. This interpretation indicates that the X protein concentration in human sera is vastly smaller than reported by Pedersen or McFarlane, but more consistent with electrophoretic data for the low density B_1 lipoproteins. Further, the ultracentrifugal pattern observed for human serum with increasing dilution can be explained without assuming that any dissociation of X protein occurs.

EXPERIMENTAL

An electrically driven ultracentrifuge designed by E. G. Pickels was employed, the Thovert-Philpot-Svensson cylindrical lens-refractive index method for the observation of migrating boundaries being utilized (3). All runs were made between 25 and 30° at rotor speeds of 59,780 R.P.M.,

974 LIPOPROTEINS IN HUMAN SERUM

giving centrifugal fields between 240,000g and 300,000g, at the meniscus and base, respectively. Blood was obtained from presumably normal individuals in the postabsorptive state.

A large number of undiluted sera were studied ultracentrifugally. Typical patterns obtained approximately 2 hours after reaching full speed are shown in Fig. 1. The vertical bar seen in Fig. 1, *b*, *c*, and *d* in the albumin complex represents a region of refractive index gradient in the cell so great that an entering light beam is completely thrown out of the optical system. We have determined that this bar has no bearing on the symmetry or asymmetry of the albumin peak. Of great interest is the "dip" below the base-line characteristically associated with the asymmetric boundary of the albumin complex. Pedersen accounted for albumin boundary asymmetry as being due to the presence of a density-sensitive lipoprotein (*X* protein), the $S_{20,w}$ value of which is very close to that of albumin. However, a two-component resolution, assuming a protein of this nature, even if present in the high concentration which Pedersen described,

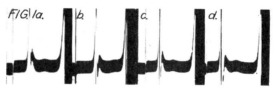

FIG. 1. Ultracentrifugal patterns of normal undiluted human sera obtained approximately 2 hours after the rotor attained full speed.

could not conceivably give rise to the "dip" phenomenon which we have observed. An explanation is possible if we assume that the asymmetry and "dip" result from a piling up of the lipoprotein along the albumin concentration gradient at the sedimenting albumin boundary. Fig. 2, *a* gives the concentration diagram for a lipoprotein which for any reason has completely piled up in the region of the albumin gradient. The theory of the diagonal bar-cylindrical lens method of recording refractive index boundaries reveals that such a pile up must give rise to a *biphasic* curve (Fig. 2, *b*). In Fig. 2, *c* is given the concentration diagram for lipoprotein, in process of piling up, and for albumin, and in Fig. 2, *d*, the separate corresponding optical patterns expected. Fig. 2, *e* shows the albumin and lipoprotein pile up patterns in a single composite picture, which is the net result observed with the ultracentrifuge. A comparison of Fig. 2, *e* with the experimental observations of Fig. 1 demonstrates the plausibility of our hypothesis of the origin of the "dip" phenomenon.

It is of interest to consider how the observed ultracentrifugal pattern will vary with *slight* displacement of the lipoprotein pile up relative to the position of the albumin concentration gradient. Fig. 3, a shows the separate albumin and lipoprotein patterns with such relative displacements. Fig. 3, b shows the corresponding composite patterns. All these types of distortions of the albumin boundary complex have been observed by altering serum density (see Fig. 3, c). Sucrose, sodium chloride, or magnesium sulfate added in quantities sufficient to give equivalent density increments produces the same type of pattern distortion.

The basis for the pile up phenomenon is the difference in sedimentation rates of the lipoprotein on either side of the albumin boundary gradient. A related type of anomaly occurring in mixtures of proteins, without a pile up but due to the same fundamental cause, has been previously described and mathematically treated by Johnston and Ogston (4). Two main factors contribute to this change: The viscosity of the albumin-containing solution is higher than the viscosity of its own supernatant so-

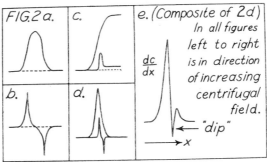

FIG. 2. Pile up analysis and the resulting "dip" phenomenon that is observed ultracentrifugally (see the text for a complete explanation).

lution, and the effective buoyant force on sedimenting molecules is not the same in the albumin solution as in the supernatant solution, since the density difference between sedimenting particle and sedimenting medium is not the same in the two solutions. This is particularly important for the lipoprotein, the density of which is very close to that of the serum itself.

Two major types of situations can in general result in the pile up of lipoprotein: (a) The lipoprotein sediments in the same direction as the albumin. Here buoyancy difference and viscosity difference are additive in slowing lipoprotein sedimentation in the albumin solution relative to that in supernatant solution. Now, if lipoprotein has a sedimentation rate in supernatant solution greater than the albumin sedimentation rate, whereas the lipoprotein in albumin solution sediments more slowly than albumin itself, then the effect will be to produce a progressive pile up of lipoprotein somewhere in the albumin concentration gradient. Since in

976   LIPOPROTEINS IN HUMAN SERUM

this instance the lipoprotein sediments with the albumin boundary, it cannot be seen as an independently sedimenting component.

(b) The lipoprotein sediments toward the albumin boundary from both sides. This is mandatory if the lipoprotein density falls between the density of albumin solution and that of the supernatant solution. Here, if the lipoprotein sediments more rapidly in supernatant solution than does albumin, an appreciable pile up will be expected. It is this situation which, we believe, usually exists in undiluted serum. Further, small density increments produced by salt or sucrose addition to serum may be expected to shift the pile up along the albumin concentration gradient and thus give rise to a variety of bizarre patterns described in Fig. 3.

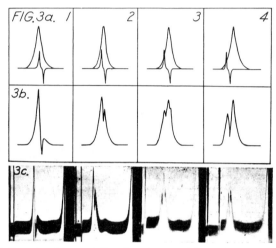

FIG. 3. Variations in ultracentrifugal patterns with variations in the location of the lipoprotein pile up on the albumin concentration gradient.

In the situation described in section b, a lipoprotein boundary migrating toward the center of rotation may or may not be observed. If the migration is slow, the boundary may be poor or may be lost entirely, due to the factors usually operative in producing diffuseness of boundaries.

A third situation may arise when the density of the solution is raised to the point where lipoprotein migrates in the direction opposite to albumin both above and below the albumin boundary. In this case, the analysis of Johnston and Ogston applies and predicts the possibility of some distortion of the albumin boundary. However, no pile up phenomenon will be expected along the albumin concentration gradient. It is to be noted here that, for lipoprotein, the viscosity and buoyancy effects operate in opposite directions, so that distortions will tend to be minimized.

It is thus evident that the classical method of boundary resolution applied to the albumin boundary is not applicable. Determinations such as those of Pedersen and McFarlane measure, therefore, some function of the concentration of lipoprotein that has piled up in the albumin boundary, but by no means the true serum lipoprotein content.

In view of the low density of the lipoprotein (specific volume 0.97), a method capable of measuring its concentration in human serum is available; namely, flotation. The necessary requirement that the density of the serum be greater than that of the lipoprotein may readily be achieved by the addition of small quantities of sodium chloride. Once the lipoprotein has moved a small distance away from the base of the cell in flotation, it then moves in an essentially homogeneous medium. Fortunately, the rate of flotation can be made sufficiently rapid so that the lipoprotein concentration measurements can be made before its boundary is obscured by meeting the sedimenting protein components. Fig. 4, a, b, and c shows the progressive flotation of the low density lipoprotein, as studied in serum

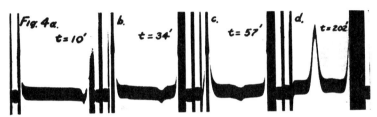

FIG. 4. Progressive flotation of lipoprotein in a serum containing 7.8 per cent added NaCl.

containing 7.8 per cent of added sodium chloride. The lipoprotein appears as an "inverse" peak, which is fully expected from the theory of the optical system. Since the specific refractive increment of the lipoproteins is very close to that for other proteins (5), the area under this peak is a measure of the concentration of the lipoprotein. At the density chosen for these studies, the albumin peak is essentially symmetrical (Fig. 4, d). A comparison of the area under the lipoprotein peak with that under the albumin peak gives a measure of the abundance of low density lipoprotein relative to those substances measured ultracentrifugally as albumin.

Ten sera from normal male and female young adults were studied by the method of flotation. The results tabulated in Table I indicate the lipoprotein concentration to be of the order of 5 per cent of total serum proteins, an abundance far lower than that quoted in the literature on the basis of previous interpretation of sedimentation diagrams.

The X protein has been suggested by Pedersen to be a labile complex of albumin, globulin, and lipides on the basis of changes in the apparent concentration of this component with changes in the serum protein and

978   LIPOPROTEINS IN HUMAN SERUM

salt concentrations. The pile up theory presented here could readily explain the apparent changes in concentration of lipoprotein observed by Pedersen without invoking any dissociation of the molecule. In Table II is given the concentration of lipoprotein at various total protein and salt concentrations for a single serum. Within the experimental

TABLE I

Low Density Lipoprotein Content of Ten Normal Human Sera

Serum No.	Sp. gr. of serum	Total protein	Lipoprotein	Lipoprotein
		gm. per 100 ml.	*gm. per 100 ml.*	*per cent of total*
1	1.0305	8.10	0.20	2.5
2	1.0310	8.26	0.23	2.8
3	1.0276	7.08	0.40	5.6
4	1.0298	7.86	0.35	4.4
5	1.0314	8.40	0.24	2.9
6	1.0288	7.50	0.23	3.0
7	1.0294	7.70	0.45	5.8
8	1.0278	7.14	0.43	6.0
9	1.0244	5.96	0.33	5.7
10	1.0240	5.82	0.20	3.4

TABLE II

Low Density Lipoprotein Content of a Single Human Serum Sample Obtained from Different Salt and Total Protein Concentrations

Preparation of serum sample	Cell used	Resultant sp. gr.	Lipoprotein	Lipoprotein
	ml.		*gm. per 100 ml.*	*per cent of total protein*
3.0% NaCl added	0.3	1.048	0.33	4.6
4.7% " "	0.3	1.060	0.33	4.7
6.1% " "	0.3	1.069	0.42	6.0
7.8% " "	0.3	1.081	0.40	5.6
9.4% " "	0.3	1.093	0.41	5.8
1 volume serum + 1 volume 8% NaCl	0.8	1.042	0.40	5.6
1 " " + 3 volumes 8% NaCl	0.8	1.048	0.46	6.5

error of measuring small areas, the data indicate no significant variation of lipoprotein content and hence the stability of this molecule, in accord with the report of Edsall (6) on the relative stability of the low density B_1 lipoprotein to such manipulations as precipitation and resolution.

It has been further stated that a density-sensitive component is present only in the sera of humans (7). Ultracentrifugal studies reported elsewhere[1]

[1]Lindgren, F. T., Elliott, H. A., and Gofman, J. W., in preparation.

have demonstrated the presence of such a component in about 60 per cent of rabbit sera.

SUMMARY

1. The difficulties which have prevented a satisfactory interpretation of the ultracentrifugal pattern of human serum, both diluted and undiluted, have been reviewed.

2. The observation of a "dip" in the ultracentrifugal pattern of undiluted human sera has led the present authors to explain the major peculiarities of albumin boundary asymmetry as being due to a pile up of lipoprotein (X protein) on the albumin concentration gradient. The existence of the pile up phenomenon renders classical two-component resolution of asymmetrical albumin boundaries completely erroneous both in the calculation of sedimentation rates and concentration of lipoprotein.

3. A method for measuring the concentration of low density lipoproteins by flotation has been described and applied. The results of analysis of lipoprotein concentrations by this method are in much better agreement with electrophoretic and fractionation data concerning this lipoprotein than are the data in the literature up to the present. The data obtained in the present work render unnecessary the postulation of a great degree of lability of lipoprotein with variation in salt and protein concentration.

BIBLIOGRAPHY

1. McFarlane, A. S., *Biochem. J.*, **29**, 660 (1935).
2. Pedersen, K. O., Ultracentrifugal studies on serum and serum fractions, Upsala, **33** (1945).
3. Pickels, E. G., *Chem. Rev.*, **30**, 341 (1942).
4. Johnston, J. P., and Ogston, A. G., *Tr. Faraday Soc.*, **42**, 789 (1946).
5. Edsall, J. T., *Advances in Protein Chem.*, **3**, 393 (1947).
6. Edsall, J. T., *Advances in Protein Chem.*, **3**, 459 (1947).
7. Pedersen, K. O., *J. Phys. and Colloid Chem.*, **51**, 156 (1947).

DIETARY MODIFICATION OF SERUM CHOLES-
TEROL AND PHOSPHOLIPID LEVELS*

To the Editor:

For more than a generation the matter of relationship between diet and serum lipids, as well as the relationship between diet and the development of clinical atherosclerosis has been a disputed subject. It has been stated and denied that diets high in cholesterol result in significant elevation of the serum cholesterol level in human subjects (1). Recently it has been reported that diets high in fat, even though they may be low in cholesterol, under some circumstances will result in significant elevation of serum cholesterol (2, 3).

In this institution over the past two years, as part of studies in various aspects of lipid metabolism, patients have been maintained on chemically constant formula diets over prolonged periods of time. Some of these diets have been extremely high in fat content. Others have been relatively high in carbohydrate. In some instances, the fat has been derived from vegetable sources; in others, from dairy fat; and in others, from egg yolk. Under the conditions of these studies, the following results have been obtained:

1 All patients receiving carbohydrate-free diets containing large amounts of vegetable fat, usually in conjunction with protein (calcium caseinate), had a major and maintained fall in the concentrations of serum cholesterol and phospholipids, which continued throughout the period of diet administration. A prompt rise to base-line levels occurred when the patient resumed a "usual" mixed diet (Fig. 1). The magnitude of the fall averaged nearly 100 mg./100 cc. for total cholesterol, and approximately 5 mg./100 cc. for serum lipid phosphorus (equivalent to a fall of 125 mg. of lecithin per 100 cc.). Most of the fall in cholesterol is referable to a decrease in the amount of esterified cholesterol. Twelve such patients have been studied in this manner. The study shown in Figure 1 is representative of the group.

2. The addition of as much as 60 grams of cholesterol daily to the diet high in vegetable fat did not result in significant elevation of the serum cholesterol level (Fig. 2). It is possible that the time factor may have been insufficient.

* This work has been supported in part by grants from the National Institutes of Health and from the Armour Laboratories.

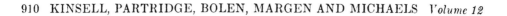

910 KINSELL, PARTRIDGE, BOLEN, MARGEN AND MICHAELS *Volume 12*

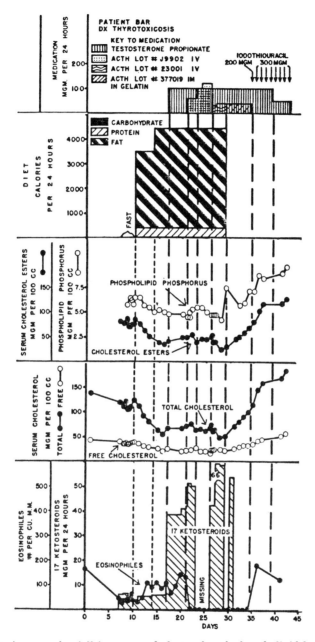

FIG. 1. Showing a major fall in serum cholesterol and phospholipid levels during ingestion of a diet containing very large amounts of vegetable fat. A prompt rise occurred when an average mixed diet was resumed. On the basis of other studies, the hormonal therapy played little or no role in the fall in serum lipids under these experimental conditions.

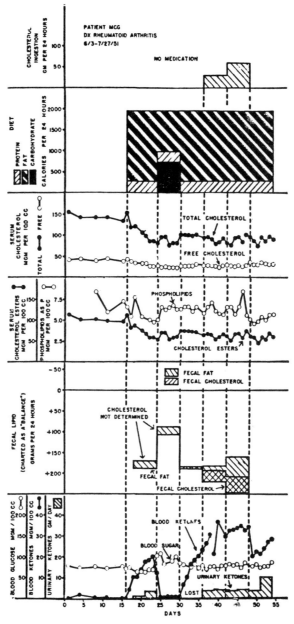

FIG. 2. Despite absorption of large amounts of administered cholesterol, no significant elevation of the serum cholesterol level ensued.

912 KINSELL, PARTRIDGE, BOLEN, MARGEN AND MICHAELS *Volume 12*

3. Patients maintained on formula diets containing fat of dairy origin or derived from egg yolk, the amount of fat being equal to that administered as vegetable fat, had levels of serum cholesterol and phospholipids essentially identical with those observed in the same patients on an average mixed diet (Fig. 3). The cholesterol content of the egg yolk diet (equivalent to 36 egg yolks) was 9.6 grams per day.

4. Patients maintained on diets containing constant amounts of pro-

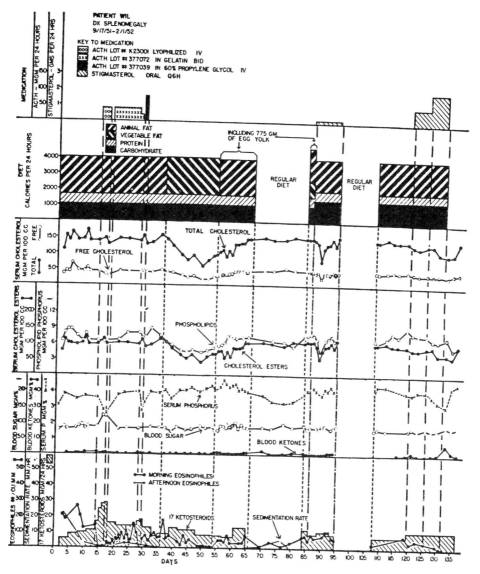

Fig. 3. Relationship of fat of animal and of vegetable origin to the concentration of serum lipids. The changes during stigmasterol administration may be of significance.

tein, but varying proportions of carbohydrate and fat, showed some variability in the levels of serum lipids. These data will be reported later.

From the foregoing observations, it would appear that the ingestion of synthetic diets containing large amounts of vegetable fat consistently results in an impressive fall in the level of serum cholesterol and of phospholipids. Whether this is the result of a positive effect of some material present in the vegetable fat, or attributable to lack of dietary cholesterol, is not yet clearly established. The findings of Peterson *et al.* in chicks (4), and the fall in the serum cholesterol level in one patient during the administration of stigmasterol (Fig. 3), might suggest that the former mechanism was responsible. This is being investigated.

The relationship of the above findings to normal and abnormal cholesterol metabolism in human subjects is unknown at the present time.

Acknowledgment

Grateful acknowledgment is made to Dr. Warren Cox, Mead Johnson and Company, for supplies of Casec; to Dr. Edward Hays and Dr. Grosvenor Bissell of the Armour Laboratories for cerebroside (which was used interchangeably with "Tween 80" as an emulsifying agent) and for supplies of stigmasterol; to Mr. C. D. Pratt for supplies of the emuslifying agent used, namely, polyoxyethylene (20) sorbitan mono-oleate, manufactured and sold by Atlas Powder Company under the trade mark "Tween 80."

Institute for Metabolic Research,
Highland Alameda County Hospital,
Oakland, California.

LAURANCE W. KINSELL, M.D.
JOHN PARTRIDGE, M.D.†
LENORE BOLING, M.D.
SHELDON MARGEN, M.D.‡
GEORGE MICHAELS, PH.D.

with the technical assistance of
Florence Olson, Sadie Smyrl,
and Nancy Dawson.

REFERENCES

1. WEINHOUSE, S.: The blood cholesterol, *Arch. Path.* **35**: 438–500, 1943.
2. KEYS, A.; MICHELSON, O.; MILLER, E. V. O., and CHAPMAN, C. B.: The relation in man between cholesterol levels in the diet and in the blood, *Science* **112**: 79–81, 1950.
3. GOFMAN, J. W.: Personal communication.
4. PETERSON, D. W.: Effect of soybean sterols in the diet on plasma and liver cholesterol in chicks, *Proc. Soc. Exper. Biol. & Med.* **78**: 143–147, 1951.

† Schering Research Fellow in Endocrinology, 1950–52.
‡ Damon Runyon Clinical Research Fellow, 1949–51.

THE LANCET]   ORIGINAL ARTICLES   [NOV. 16, 1957

PREDICTION OF SERUM-CHOLESTEROL RESPONSES OF MAN TO CHANGES IN FATS IN THE DIET *

ANCEL KEYS

M.A., Ph.D. California, Ph.D. Cantab.

JOSEPH T. ANDERSON

Ph.D. Rochester

FRANCISCO GRANDE

M.D. Madrid

From the Laboratory of Physiological Hygiene of the University of Minnesota, Minneapolis, and Hastings State Hospital, Minnesota

A SHARP decrease in the amount of ordinary fats in the usual American or Western European diet, without any change in the amount of calories or vitamins, lowers the serum-cholesterol level. The fall is rapid in the first few days, but after a few weeks there is an approach to a new plateau (Keys et al. 1950, Mellinkoff et al. 1950, Groen et al. 1952, Keys 1952, Keys et al. 1955). Such low-fat diets usually contain less cholesterol and animal proteins, but the change in the serum-cholesterol level in man does not depend on this fact (Keys et al. 1956b, Keys and Anderson 1957). The responsible agent is clearly either in the quality of the fats or in the ratio of fat to carbohydrate calories.

The most striking difference between an ordinary American diet and a low-fat diet is in the amount of animal fat. The usual diets of 119 Minnesota businessmen were measured with great care in 1953–54 by a team headed by Miss Sadye Adelson from the U.S. Department of Agriculture Research Service ; they showed an average intake of 115 g. of fat, of which 85 g. was animal fat. Diets containing very little fat may provide less than 5 g. of animal fat (a decrease of 94%), whereas the vegetable fat in such diets may amount to 15–20 g. (a decrease of 40–50%). A moderately low-fat diet for such men would contain something like 50 g. of total fat, half from animal sources, making a decrease of 5 g. of vegetable fat and 70 g. of animal fat. Such a change in diet quickly lowers the serum-cholesterol level.

It is tempting, then, to ascribe the effect of low-fat diets to the decrease in animal fat, especially since some vegetable oils given in large amounts in synthetic concoctions may depress the serum-cholesterol level (Kinsell et al. 1952, Ahrens et al. 1954, Bronte-Stewart et al. 1956, Beveridge et al. 1956). However, the free use of vegetable fat in otherwise low-fat diets may raise the serum-cholesterol level (Keys et al. 1950). Clearly the analysis of the effects of dietary fats on the serum-cholesterol should be made in terms of chemical composition rather than of origin.

Accordingly for the past six years we have conducted controlled dietary experiments in the metabolic research unit of the Hastings State Hospital, using diets with fixed adequate amounts of calories, proteins, and vitamins but with different amounts and kinds of fats (Anderson et al. 1957). Most of the dietary comparisons were made from both forward and backward dietary changes—i.e., changing from diet X to diet Y and vice versa. Standard periods on each diet were from two to nine weeks, usually four weeks. In all the experiments the experimental diets were preceded by at least four weeks' standardisation on fixed "normal" diets. In each series of experiments 12–27 men were studied on each of two to six diets. In addition we have the data

from three experiments in Shime, Japan, on Japanese coalminers (Keys et al. 1957b).

We report here the serum-cholesterol responses to different amounts of dietary glycerides of saturated (S), monoethenoid (M), and polyethenoid (P) fatty acids producing 9–44% of calories derived from fats. Besides normal " house diets " and low-fat diets, the experiments involved commercial grades of butter-fat, olive oil, cotton-seed oil, corn oil, sunflower-seed oil, hydrogenated coconut oil (' Hydrol '), sardine oil, safflower oil, several varieties of margarine, and the mixed fats of ordinary American diets.

Diets

Our aim was to obtain information about the effects of the fatty acids in the presence of ordinary foods in mixed diets ; so formula and synthetic diets were not used. Calorie equilibrium was maintained at all times. The calorie requirements of the individual men at Hastings were estimated by measuring the intakes of food at constant body-weight during a control period of four weeks before each of the series of experiments. In the Shime experiments (Keys et al. 1957b) the change in the diet was an isocaloric substitution of fat (butter-fat or one of two kinds of margarine) for 450 calories of rice carbohydrate, the regular diet of the men otherwise being continued throughout ; there was no significant change in body-weight.

The diets in the Hastings experiments conformed to the general pattern of menus in the United States, 37–42% of calories being from fats and 13–15% from proteins, and the day's calories being apportioned roughly as 25%, 35%, and 40% for breakfast, luncheon, and dinner respectively. Seven rotating " house-diet " menus were devised so that the individual calorie requirements were easily supplied by altering the allowances of jam, sugar, potatoes, and bread. Similarly seven menus of " low-fat-base " diet were devised to resemble the house diet except that the fats and the corresponding calories were much decreased, the whole being arranged so that either an experimental fat or carbohydrates (jam, sugar, potatoes, and bread) could be added to bring the total amount of calories to that needed for equilibrium. These house and low-fat-base diets varied slightly from one set of experiments to another, but the nutrient contents are exemplified in table I as computed from average values for the nutrients in each of the food items in each day's menu.

The low-fat-base diet provided an average of about 400 mg. less cholesterol daily than did the corresponding house diet, but variations of twice this amount of cholesterol are without effect on the serum-cholesterol level (Keys et al. 1956b). The low-fat-base diet also tended to average 5–10 mg. lower in the daily tocopherol content than did the house diet, but in unpublished experiments we have found that even the addition of 100 mg. of α-tocopherol to the daily diet has no effect on the serum-cholesterol level.

The house and low-fat-base diets at Hastings were closely matched in total proteins, and there was no major difference in the proportions of proteins from animal and vegetable sources in the two kinds of diets. This agreement was assured by the use of casein, egg-white, and skim-milk in the low-fat-base diets. In any case, large differences in the amount of animal protein (± 10% of calories in the form of casein) in such diets have no significant influence on the serum-cholesterol level of man (Keys and Anderson 1957).

Measurements of body-weight and of the foods eaten by each man during the preliminary control periods at Hastings were used in estimating the calorie requirements to maintain equilibrium during the experimental periods. These individual allowances were adjusted weekly, if

* The data cited here were obtained with the help of research grants from the National Dairy Council, Chicago ; the Minnesota Heart Association ; the Nutrition Foundation, New York ; the American Heart Association ; the Schweppe Foundation, Chicago ; the Winton Companies Fund ; and Mr. David Winton, of Minneapolis.

960 THE LANCET]   ORIGINAL ARTICLES   [NOV. 16, 1957

TABLE I—NUTRIENT CONTENTS OF REPRESENTATIVE HOUSE AND LOW-FAT-BASE DIETS IN THE HASTINGS EXPERIMENTS

Diet	Day	Cal.	Prot. (g.)	Total fat (g.)	Vit. A I.U.	Aneurine (mg.)	Riboflavine (mg.)	Nicotinic acid (mg.)	Pyridoxine (mg.)	Ascorbic acid (mg.)	Tocopherol (mg.)	Phytosterol (mg.)	Cholesterol (mg.)	Iron (mg.)
House	1	3159	101	138	4600	2·1	2·4	23	1·9	71	56	91	1110	15
,,	2	3217	98	136	10,600	1·8	2·2	20	2·4	158	9	57	680	16
,,	3	3183	98	139	5000	3·3	2·1	13	1·1	68	8	75	730	13
,,	4	3173	102	140	3300	2·7	2·4	20	1·3	136	7	64	510	16
,,	5	3208	99	138	17,100	1·6	2·4	17	1·8	71	8	60	870	16
,,	6	3219	94	136	22,800	1·3	2·2	19	1·8	97	11	94	690	20
,,	7	3195	103	137	8100	1·7	2·1	23	2·5	128	7	80	610	17
,,	Mean	3183	99	138	10,200	2·1	2·2	19	1·8	104	15	74	740	16
Low-fat-base	1	2290	99	39	17,900	1·8	3·0	18	1·8	128	6	49	340	18
,,	2	2290	99	38	8800	1·3	2·9	23	1·8	162	7	70	280	21
,,	3	2330	101	39	17,100	1·8	2·9	19	1·7	84	8	83	280	17
,,	4	2290	97	37	3400	1·7	2·8	17	1·8	106	4	41	280	17
,,	5	2320	102	37	2000	1·8	3·1	20	2·1	101	5	75	300	16
,,	6	2340	100	40	3700	1·7	2·9	19	1·9	148	5	59	310	16
,,	7	2320	102	41	3600	1·6	2·8	18	2·1	105	5	66	300	19
,,	Mean	2311	100	39	8100	1·8	2·9	19	1·9	118	6	63	300	18
Experimental fat	..	900	..	100	..	..	..	..	..	..	..	..	..	..
,, ,, + L.F.B.	..	3211	∴	139	..	..	..	..	..	..	..	..	..	..

needed, during the experimental periods according to the indications from the weekly (nude) body-weights. These calorie adjustments were made by changing the allowances of sugar, jam, potatoes, and bread. A change of 3 kg. or more in body-weight over an entire experiment was considered to indicate failure to maintain calorie equilibrium.

At Hastings the men were under surveillance by special attendants for 24 hours daily both in the quarters where they spent most of the time and during their standardised outdoor recreation. Fixed recipes were followed, all food servings were measured, and plate waste and extra portions were recorded for each man. All experimental fats were purchased in large lots and stored in full sealed containers at −20°C until used. Other staple foods were similarly bought in large lots and stored. Bread was baked on the premises. Fresh milk and eggs were procured from a constant local source. The meals were prepared and served in a special diet kitchen, used for no other purpose, within the metabolic research unit. In the Shime series the butter and margarines used were single lots, of which sealed samples were sent by air to the United States for analysis.

Analytical Methods

Serum-cholesterol was determined in duplicate on samples of venous blood drawn with the patient at rest, in most cases on two occasions, a day or two apart, at the end of each dietary period. These samples were analysed in duplicate, and the average of the four results was

TABLE II—ANALYTICAL VALUES OBTAINED ON FATS USED IN DIETARY EXPERIMENTS

Fat	Iodine value	Glycerides of fatty acids (%) Saturated	Mono-ethenoid	Poly-ethenoid
Butterfat 1	32	57	39	4
,, 2	35	56	39	5
Coconut oil (hydrol)	3	97	3	0
Corn oil 1	120	12	37	51
,, 2	128	16	26	58
Cotton-seed oil	108	25	25	50
Olive oil 1	85	12	80	8
,, 2	86	13	75	12
,, 3	85	15	72	12
Margarine A	39	65	25	10
,, B (all veg.)	37	64	30	6
Safflower oil 1	144	12	10	78
,, ,, 2	144	14	8	78
,, 3	146	10	12	78
Sardine oil *	188	23	23	54
Sunflower-seed oil	131	10	28	62

* Fatty acid composition from Brocklesby and Harding (1938) and Hilditch (1956) for *Sardinops cœrulea* oil of same iodine value.

taken to be the best estimate of the true value. The method was that of Abell et al. (1952) modified by Anderson and Keys (1956). β-lipoprotein cholesterol was also measured in most of the experiments by the method of Anderson and Keys (1956) but the results are not reported here.

The fat analyses were made by the methods recommended by the American Oil Chemists' Society (1950). For the experimental fats and oils values were obtained for unconjugated dienes, trienes, tetraenes, monoenes, saturated fatty acids, conjugated dienes, non-saponifiable lipid, and the percentage of trans acids. Such detailed analysis of the " sardine " oil (from *Sardinops cærulea*) was not attempted, but the iodine and saponification values of the oil used agreed well with samples of the same oil analysed in detail by Brocklesby and Harding (1938).

Subjects

The men at Hastings were " stabilised " schizophrenics judged, on the basis of extensive examinations and tests, to be physically and metabolically normal.† Men who became ill or otherwise deviated, as well as those whose body-weight changed as much as 3 kg. in an experiment, were excluded. 66 men served successfully as subjects. They were aged 32–56, except 1 man in one experiment who was aged 62. None of them was unusually thin or fat, but on the average they were about 10% lighter in weight than the average of Minnesota businessmen of the same age and height (Anderson et al. 1957). Their average height was 173·5 cm. (5 ft. 8 in.) and average weight (nude) 69·8 kg. (10 st. 13¹/₂ lb.).

At Shime the subjects were 18 Japanese men, aged 22–54 (average 39·8), working at their regular occupations as coalminers (Keys et al. 1957b). All were judged clinically healthy on the basis of physical examinations and blood analyses. None was unusually thin or fat. Initially there were 21 Japanese, but 3 were discarded : 1 developed a cold with fever, 1 developed persistent diarrhœa ascribed to the unaccustomed fat in the diet, and 1 lost 2 kg. of weight.

Fatty-acid Composition of Experimental Fats

The iodine and saponification values of the experimental fats and oils were measured in this laboratory, and estimates of fatty-acid composition were obtained from Bailey (1951), Eckey (1954), and Hilditch (1956) for

† Permission for each subject to participate in these trials was obtained in writing from his nearest relative. The trials were conducted under careful and continuous medical supervision, and the patients were at all times friendly and cooperative.

THE LANCET]   ORIGINAL ARTICLES   [NOV. 16, 1957   961

samples of the same fats having iodine values matching the samples used here. These values were used in devising the diets.

Detailed analyses of the fats were made on samples of fats and oils sent to the Research and Development Department, Miami Valley (Ohio) Laboratories of the Procter and Gamble Co.; Dr. J. C. Cowan at the Northern Utilisation Research Branch (Peoria, Illinois) of the Agricultural Research Service, U.S. Department of Agriculture; and Dr. Raymond Paschke, Research Laboratories of General Mills, Inc. (Minneapolis). Dr. Ralph Holman, of the Hormel Research Institute, Austin, Minnesota, measured the percentages of polyethenoids independently in four kinds of fats.

Table II summarises the analyses of the experimental fats and oils expressed as percentages of the glycerides in the form of saturated (S), monoethenoid (M), and polyethenoid (P) fatty acids. The last-named grouping was adopted because of uncertainties of analysis and identification within the polyethenoids and because, as will appear later, a more elaborate classification of the polyethenoids seems to be unnecessary for the present purpose. These analytical results are in good agreement with those previously published for the same fats and oils with similar iodine values. Trans acids were negligible except in the margarines.

Fatty-acid Composition of Diets

From data published by Bailey (1951), Eckey (1954), and Hilditch (1956) and from a few special analyses of foods used here a table was compiled for the average fatty-acid composition (S, M, and P) of about 96% of the fats in the foods used in the Hastings and Minneapolis experiments.

The remaining 4% of the dietary fat was in low-fat vegetables and fruits for which it was impracticable to estimate fatty acids for every item separately. The average for this latter group of items was estimated to be 10% saturated, 30% monoethenoid, and 60% polyethenoid fatty acids, and these figures were applied in the computations. Since only 4% of the total fat was involved, at worst no more than trivial errors could result.

In most of the diets used at Hastings the comparisons were between the effects of different test fats added to a constant low-fat-base diet; hence the only variable was

TABLE III—COMPARISON OF ESTIMATED AND ANALYSED PER-CENTAGES OF FATTY-ACID GLYCERIDES OF SATURATED MONOETHENOID, AND POLYETHENOID FATTY ACIDS IN DIETS USED AT HASTINGS

No.	Diet code	Fat (g. daily)	Diet type	Source of data	Fat (%) S	M	P
1	1KH	138·2	House, as served	Estimate	47·2	45·1	7·7
	,,	,,	,, ,, ,,	Analysis	53·3	39·4	7·3
2	4KH	137·4	House, as served	Estimate	48·6	44·6	6·8
	,,	,,	,, ,, ,,	Analysis	47·5	45·3	7·2
3	2MB	38·3	Low fat base M	Estimate	46·0	43·3	10·7
	,,	,,	,, ,, ,, ,,	Analysis	43·3	46·2	10·5
4	2M18C	138·3	M18C as served	Estimate	51·5	43·1	5·4
	,,	,,	,, ,, ,,	Analysis	50·8	43·9	5·3
5	2M12C	138·3	M12C as served	Estimate	52·1	42·7	5·2
	,,	,,	,, ,, ,,	Analysis	51·3	43·4	5·3
6	3N	37·8	Low fat base N	Estimate	46·0	43·1	10·9
	,,	,,	,, ,, ,, ,,	Analysis	42·1	49·5	8·4
7	3NCr	137·8	NCr as served	Estimate	21·6	31·5	46·9
	,,	,,	,, ,, ,,	Analysis	20·6	33·2	46·2
8	3NSa	137·8	NSa as served	Estimate	21·3	19·9	58·8
	,,	,,	,, ,, ,,	Analysis	20·2	20·8	59·0

Pure estimates versus direct analysis are shown for items 1, 2, 3 and 6. For items 4, 5, 7, and 8 analytical data on experimental fats were used in both "Estimate" and "Analysis" values for diets as served.

TABLE IV—INTRA-INDIVIDUAL VARIABILITY OF SERUM-CHOL-ESTEROL LEVEL (MG. PER 100 ML.) INDICATED BY VALUES OBTAINED 1 OR 2 WEEKS APART IN MEN SUBSISTING IN CALORIE EQUILIBRIUM ON RIGIDLY CONTROLLED DIET

—	—	Hastings men	U.S. army soldiers
1	N	834	38
2	$\Sigma\Delta^2/2N = (S.E.M.)^2$	132	144
3	S.E.M.	±11·52	±12·00
4	S.E. of S.E.M.	±0·28	±1·38
5	Grand mean cholesterol	228·2	209·7
6	100 × line 3/line 5	±5·04 %	±5·72 %

the 70–75% of the total dietary fat represented by the experimental fat for which detailed analyses were available.

Direct analyses were made of the entire combined foods of representative weeks of house and low-fat-base diets. The procedure was to set a dummy place at each meal for a week and to serve this dummy the specified amounts of each item in the menu for that day. Each meal was mixed and ground immediately after the food items had been measured out, and the mixture was stored at −20°C until the week's collection was completed. At the end of the week the entire collection of twenty-one meals was thawed, mixed, and passed through a meat-grinder, a measured amount of water being added to facilitate mixing. Checks of beginning and end weights showed an average of 99·5% of food weight accounted for. Weighed portions of this diluted mixture were mixed in a Waring blender. Portions of this final slurry were frozen on the walls of wide-mouthed short flasks and dried in vacuo from the frozen state. The dried residue was saponified, acidified, and extracted with ethyl ether. After evaporation of the solvent in vacuo the lipid was dissolved in petroleum ether and kept at −20° until analysed.

Table III gives the analytical results obtained in this way from two weeks of house diets and from two weeks of low-fat-base diets, together with the corresponding composition computed by adding the estimated average values for each of the foodstuffs. Table III also shows the analyses of four experimental fat diets as served and, for comparison, the corresponding values obtained by adding the known values for the (analysed) test fats to the estimates for the low-fat-base diets.

The estimated and analytical values agree very well, particularly for the polyethenoids (P in table III). For the low-fat-base diets plus added test fats—i.e., experimental diets as actually served (items 4, 5, 7, 8 in table III)—no discrepancy larger than 1% was observed. With the house diets the estimates tended to be slightly too low for saturated fats (average −2·2%) and slightly too high for monoethenoids (average +2·5%); these differences approach the limits of analytical and sampling error for fatty acids in such mixed fats.

Variability in Serum-cholesterol Levels

Consideration of the reliability of estimates of serum-cholesterol levels and of intra- and inter-individual variability is essential for analysing the results of dietary experiments. For this purpose we have 3336 cholesterol analyses comprising 834 sets of measurements on 66 men at Hastings, each set consisting of analyses in duplicate on each of two samples of blood drawn one or two weeks apart from 1 man subsisting on a controlled fixed diet maintained for at least three weeks before drawing the first sample. Table IV summarises this material. The standard error of measurement (S.E.M.) in the 1668 pairs of duplicate analyses in this series is ±3·64 mg. of cholesterol per 100 ml. of serum, calculated from the sum of the differences between duplicates (Δ), without regard to sign, as $(S.E.M.)^2 = \Sigma\Delta^2/2N$. This is a measure of analytical error. The variability of the men is indicated by calculating the S.E.M. in the same way

962   THE LANCET)   ORIGINAL ARTICLES   [NOV. 16, 1957

TABLE V—SERUM-CHOLESTEROL LEVELS * AT HASTINGS ON HOUSE DIET ON TWO OCCASIONS 1 WEEK APART AND CHANGES DURING SUCCESSIVE WEEKS ON LOW-FAT DIET

Case no.	House diet		Δ on low-fat diet for weeks				
	31 Jan.	7 Feb.	1	2	3, 4	5, 6	7, 8, 9
1	206	209	−15	−33	−28	−37	−24
2	224	236	−9	−22	−6	+3	−52
3	174	167	−23	−23	−36	−33	−25
4	160	184	−26	−17	−19	−7	−22
5	184	196	−30	−22	−17	−30	−33
6	301	291	−29	−63	−63	−66	−50
7	240	238	−50	−75	−66	−61	−36
8	281	264	−49	−74	−73	−87	−94
9	228	240	−22	−54	−28	−39	−39
10	172	166	−13	−33	−16	−26	−24
11	227	236	−39	−38	−31	−37	−33
12	201	173	+1	+2	−4	+6	−15
13	284	251	−24	−42	−52	−51	−37
14	240	230	−17	−25	+11	−8	−18
Mean S.E.	223·0 ±11·7	220·1 ±10·3	−24·6 ± 3·8	−37·1 ± 6·0	−30·6 ± 6·7	−33·8 ± 7·2	−35·9 ± 5·3

* Mg. per 100 ml.

but using for Δ the difference between the means of the values recorded for the first and second occasions; this gave S.E.M. = ±11·52 mg. per 100 ml., or ±5·04% of the grand mean cholesterol level.

For comparison we have data from 38 American soldiers maintained in the laboratory for a month on a constant ration with rigidly standardised conditions of exercise and rest. The intra-individual variability does not significantly differ from that of the men at Hastings.

The variability between individuals is still greater, of course, even when we are concerned only with clinically healthy men of the same age, engaged in the same activity, and eating precisely the same diet. The inter-individual variability in the Hastings experiments is indicated by the standard deviations of the mean values at the ends of the experimental periods, these means being computed from the averages for each man, for whom two samples were analysed, each in duplicate. The grand average of these standard deviations was ±33·58 mg. per 100 ml., or ±14·7% of the grand mean serum-cholesterol level.

Table V illustrates the intra- and inter-individual variability as well as the variability in the serum-cholesterol response to a change in dietary fat. This experiment was selected for illustration because the variability is about as large as is ever encountered in these experiments, and because the experiment lasted long enough to show the characteristic time course of the response. A highly significant change in the serum-cholesterol level takes place within a week after a change in diet fat; by the end of the second week a relative plateau is reached, and no further significant change can be observed within the next month or two.

Experimental Data and their Analysis

The experimental data are summarised in table VI. The fats in the diets are expressed as percentages of the total calories contributed by glycerides of saturated (S), monoethenoid (M), and polyethenoid (P) fatty acids. Table VI gives the means (and standard errors) of serum-cholesterol levels for the groups of men at the end of each dietary period. The problem then is to discover whether the differences between the serum-cholesterol levels on these diets are systematically related to these dietary variables, and how such a relationship is best expressed.

For a given group of men the average serum-cholesterol level in calorie equilibrium on a given diet may be related to the diet composition:

$$(1) \qquad Chol._1 = a + bS_1 + cM_1 + dP_1$$

where Chol. is the serum-cholesterol level in mg. per 100 ml., a is a characteristic of the particular group of men, independent of the diet fat, and b, c, and d are multiplying coefficients that express the influence of S, M, and P respectively per unit of those dietary factors. On a different diet, everything else being the same, it would follow that:

$$Chol._2 = a + bS_2 + cM_2 + dP_2;$$

so the change in the serum-cholesterol level is indicated by subtraction:

$$(2) \qquad \Delta\,Chol._{1,2} = b(S_1 - S_2) + c(M_1 - M_2) + d(P_1 - P_2).$$

Table VII gives the 64 sets of such differences available for the solution of equation 2. For the initial analysis the data marked with asterisks were omitted because (1) the effects of corn oil may not be fully explained in terms of fatty-acid composition (Keys et al. 1957a); (2) the polyethenoids in fish oils may not be comparable with those in other foods; (3) the men in Japan may not be comparable with the men in Minnesota; and (4) preliminary analysis has suggested that hydrol may require special consideration.

There were, then, 41 sets of comparisons available for the initial analysis, 10 being in a single series, JWX. Least-squares solutions of equation 2 were obtained by the method of matrices for these JWX data and, separately, for the 31 other sets of data. Statistical tests showed that the regressions and the component variances

TABLE VI—AVERAGE PERCENTAGES OF TOTAL CALORIES FROM GLYCERIDES OF S, M, AND P FATTY ACIDS FOR EACH DIETARY PERIOD AND MEAN (AND STANDARD ERROR) TOTAL SERUM-CHOLESTEROL LEVELS AT END OF EACH DIETARY PERIOD

Expt. no.	Diet type	No. of men	Calories from fats (%)				Serum-chol. (mg. per 100 ml.)
			Total	S	M	P	
C	Low-fat	16	8·5	3·7	3·5	1·3	198·2 ± 7·0
,,	Olive oil	,,	25·2	5·6	17·4	2·2	213·6 ± 9·1
,,	Cotton-seed oil	,,	25·1	7·8	7·7	9·4	208·8 ±10·2
D	House	12	37·7	17·2	17·1	3·4	225·2 ±10·7
,,	Low-fat	,,	15·9	7·0	7·2	1·7	198·1 ± 9·1
,,	Butter-fat	,,	39·5	18·3	15·2	6·0	231·9 ± 9·2
,,	Cotton-seed oil + marg.	,,	38·4	14·9	16·5	7·0	211·9 ± 9·4
F	House	18	40·0	18·8	17·8	3·4	231·8 ±11·1
,,	Butter-fat	,,	37·8	20·4	15·0	2·4	234·8 ± 8·5
,,	Low-fat	,,	11·4	5·2	4·8	1·4	203·0 ± 7·9
,,	Cotton-seed oil	,,	37·7	11·9	11·2	14·6	204·4 ±11·3
G	House	27	36·7	16·4	16·2	4·1	222·3 ± 7·3
,,	Lard	,,	37·8	15·7	18·0	4·1	221·4 ± 9·5
,,	Butter-fat	,,	37·8	20·6	14·5	2·7	240·9 ± 8·0
HWX	House	13	40·8	18·7	19·4	2·7	221·3 ±11·7
,,	Low-fat	,,	11·4	4·7	5·2	1·5	186·3 ± 9·3
,,	Cotton-seed oil	,,	37·0	10·9	11·3	14·8	179·5 ±10·1
,,	Corn oil	,,	37·4	7·5	13·6	16·3	160·2 ± 9·0
HYZ	House	12	41·1	18·9	19·2	3·0	213·3 ± 8·2
,,	Low-fat	,,	11·8	4·8	5·4	1·6	181·0 ± 7·2
,,	Cotton-seed oil	,,	37·5	11·1	11·6	14·8	178·2 ± 8·8
JWX	House	14	40·8	18·7	19·2	2·9	219·9 ±11·0
,,	Butter-fat	,,	36·8	19·3	15·6	1·9	223·5 ± 9·1
,,	Low-fat	,,	11·3	5·1	5·4	0·8	184·7 ± 5·8
,,	Olive oil	,,	37·4	7·9	26·7	2·8	187·9 ± 8·4
,,	Sunflower-seed oil	,,	37·0	7·4	12·7	16·9	170·0 ± 9·0
,,	Corn oil	,,	37·6	7·6	14·6	15·4	160·7 ± 9·2
JYZ	House	12	41·9	19·6	19·7	2·9	220·1 ±10·1
,,	Butter-fat	,,	38·8	21·0	16·0	1·8	219·2 ± 9·4
,,	Cotton-seed oil	,,	39·2	12·0	12·0	15·2	183·7 ± 7·3
,,	Olive oil	,,	39·3	8·1	28·3	2·9	189·9 ± 6·4
,,	Sardine oil	,,	39·2	11·4	11·9	15·9	179·8 ± 5·2
,,	Corn oil	,,	39·0	7·8	14·6	16·6	159·7 ± 9·0
KWY	House	13	36·6	17·9	16·6	2·1	206·1 ± 6·9
,,	Safflower oil	,,	44·4	18·9	17·3	8·2	196·5 ± 6·8
Shime (A)	Control	7	10·3	2·3	4·0	4·0	145·4 ±14·4
,,	Butter-fat	,,	22·6	9·7	8·4	4·5	163·0
(B)	Control	6	10·3	2·3	4·0	4·0	135·7 ±11·0
,,	Margarine 1	,,	22·6	10·3	7·1	5·2	154·7
(C)	Control	5	10·3	2·3	4·0	4·0	163·2 ±16·6
,,	Margarine 2	,,	22·6	10·1	7·7	4·8	177·4
HYZ	Hydrol	12	37·6	30·6	5·9	0·9	224·3 ± 8·4
,,	,,	,,	,,	23·8*	5·9	0·9	,, ,,

* Only fatty acids with 12 or more carbons in the chain counted.

THE LANCET]   ORIGINAL ARTICLES   [NOV. 16, 1957   963

were not significantly different ; so it was concluded that pooling of the entire 41 sets of data would be legitimate, and the following solution was obtained for the combined data :

$$\text{(2a)} \qquad \Delta \text{ Chol.} = -1 \cdot 68 + 2 \cdot 76 \Delta S + 0 \cdot 05 \Delta M - 1 \cdot 35 \Delta P,$$

where Δ Chol. is in mg. per 100 ml.

On testing the significance of the contributions of the several coefficients it is found that, expressing these as t values, we have for a, $t = 0 \cdot 98$; for b, $t = 15 \cdot 15$; for c, $t = 0 \cdot 36$; and for d, $t = 7 \cdot 19$. Since we have 37 degrees of freedom (41–3–1), both b and d make very highly significant contributions to the prediction, but neither a nor c is significant. Accordingly, the third-order equation (2) may be replaced by a second-order equation ;

and, further, since the constant a is insignificant, we may stipulate that the final regression equation should pass through the zero-zero origin. New least-squares solutions were then obtained for the equation :

$$\text{(3)} \qquad \Delta \text{ Chol.} = b \Delta S + d \Delta P,$$

for the JWX series, the remaining 8 series, and, since the regressions and variances indicate homogeneity, the combined 41 sets of data. The results of these calculations are given in table VIII.

The final result is :

$$\text{(3a)} \qquad \Delta \text{ Chol.} = 2 \cdot 74 \Delta S - 1 \cdot 31 \Delta P.$$

The application of equation 3a to these 41 sets of data yields the results shown in the accompanying figure.

TABLE VII—MEAN DIFFERENCES IN PERCENTAGES OF CALORIES IN DIETS PROVIDED BY GLYCERIDES OF (S), (M), AND (P) FATTY ACIDS, TOGETHER WITH CORRESPONDING MEAN ($\pm$ STANDARD ERROR) DIFFERENCES IN SERUM-CHOLESTEROL AT ENDS OF DIETARY PERIODS

Expt. no.	Diet comparison			Δ Diet fats, % cal.			Δ Chol. (mg. per 100 ml.)	
				S	M	P	Mean	S.E. of mean
C	Low-fat	minus	olive oil	− 1·9	−13·9	− 0·9	−15·4	± 5·8
,,	,,	,,	cotton-seed oil	− 4·1	− 4·2	− 8·1	−10·6	± 6·4
,,	Olive oil	,,	,, ,,	− 2·2	9·7	− 7·2	4·8	± 5·3
D	House	minus	low-fat	10·2	9·9	1·7	27·1	± 4·2
,,	,,	,,	butter-fat	− 1·1	1·9	− 2·6	− 6·7	± 4·7
,,	,,	,,	cotton. + marg.	2·3	0·6	− 3·6	13·3	± 4·4
,,	Low-fat	,,	butter-fat	−11·3	− 8·0	− 4·3	−33·8	± 3·7
,,	,,	,,	cotton. + marg.	− 7·9	− 9·3	− 5·3	−13·8	± 5·3
,,	Butter-fat	,,	,, ,,	3·4	− 1·3	− 1·0	20·0	± 5·1
F	House	minus	butter-fat	− 1·6	2·8	1·0	−12·4	± 4·7
,,	,,	,,	low-fat	13·6	13·0	2·0	28·8	± 4·8
,,	,,	,,	cotton-seed oil	6·9	6·6	−11·2	28·4	± 3·7
,,	Butter-fat	,,	low-fat	15·2	10·2	1·0	42·4	± 4·2
,,	,,	,,	cotton-seed oil	8·5	3·8	−12·2	42·0	± 4·9
,,	Low-fat	,,	,, ,,	− 6·7	− 6·4	−13·2	− 0·4	± 4·2
G	House	minus	lard	0·7	− 1·8	0·0	0·9	± 3·3
,,	,,	,,	butter-fat	− 4·2	1·7	1·4	−18·6	± 3·6
,,	Lard	,,	,,	− 4·9	3·5	1·4	−19·5	± 3·9
HWX	House	minus	low-fat	14·0	14·2	1·2	35·0	± 5·1
,,	,,	,,	cotton-seed oil	7·8	8·1	−12·1	41·8	± 4·7
,,	,,	,,	corn oil *	11·2	5·8	−13·6	61·1	± 5·4
,,	Low-fat	,,	cotton-seed oil	− 6·2	− 6·1	−13·3	6·8	± 4·4
,,	,,	,,	corn oil *	− 2·8	− 8·4	−14·8	26·1	± 3·9
,,	Cotton-seed oil	,,	,, ,, *	3·4	− 2·3	− 1·5	19·3	± 4·2
HYZ	House	minus	low-fat	14·1	13·8	1·4	32·3	± 5·2
,,	,,	,,	cotton-seed oil	7·8	7·6	−11·8	35·1	± 5·0
,,	,,	,,	hydrol *	−11·7	13·1	1·8	−11·0	± 2·8
,,	Low-fat	,,	cotton-seed oil	− 6·3	− 6·2	−13·2	2·8	± 4·5
,,	,,	,,	hydrol *	−25·8	− 0·7	0·4	−43·3	± 7·4
,,	Cotton-seed oil	,,	,, *	−19·5	5·5	13·6	−46·1	± 6·8
JWX	House	minus	butter-fat	− 0·6	3·6	1·0	− 3·6	± 3·8
,,	,,	,,	low-fat	13·6	13·8	2·1	35·2	± 6·0
,,	,,	,,	olive oil	10·8	− 7·5	0·1	32·0	± 6·2
,,	,,	,,	sunflower-seed oil	11·3	6·5	−14·0	49·2	± 6·1
,,	,,	,,	corn oil *	11·1	4·6	−12·5	59·2	± 6·0
,,	Butter-fat	,,	low-fat	14·2	10·2	1·1	38·8	± 6·1
,,	,,	,,	olive oil	11·4	−11·1	− 0·9	35·6	± 4·7
,,	,,	,,	sunflower-seed oil	11·9	2·9	−15·0	53·5	± 7·4
,,	,,	,,	corn oil *	11·7	1·0	−13·5	62·8	± 3·5
,,	Low-fat	,,	olive oil	− 2·8	−21·3	− 2·0	− 3·2	± 5·4
,,	,,	,,	sunflower-seed oil	− 2·3	− 7·3	−16·1	14·7	± 6·3
,,	,,	,,	corn oil *	− 2·5	− 9·2	−14·6	24·0	± 6·1
,,	Olive oil	minus	sunflower-seed oil	0·5	14·0	−14·1	17·9	± 5·1
,,	,,	,,	corn oil *	0·3	12·1	−12·6	27·2	± 3·6
,,	Sunflower-seed oil	,,	,, ,, *	− 0·2	− 1·9	1·5	9·3	± 2·8
JYZ	House	minus	butter-fat	− 1·4	3·7	1·1	0·9	± 4·4
,,	,,	,,	cotton-seed oil	7·6	7·7	−12·3	36·4	± 5·1
,,	,,	,,	olive oil	11·5	− 8·6	0·0	30·2	± 4·6
,,	,,	,,	sardine oil *	8·2	7·8	−13·0	40·3	± 5·3
,,	,,	,,	corn oil *	11·8	5·1	−13·7	60·4	± 5·6
,,	Butter-fat	,,	cotton-seed oil	9·0	4·0	−13·4	35·5	± 5·4
,,	,,	,,	olive oil	12·9	−12·3	− 1·1	29·3	± 4·3
,,	,,	,,	sardine oil *	9·6	4·1	−14·1	39·4	± 5·6
,,	,,	,,	corn oil *	13·2	1·4	−14·8	59·5	± 5·7
,,	Cotton-seed oil	,,	olive oil	3·9	−16·3	12·3	− 6·2	± 5·2
,,	,, ,,	,,	sardine oil *	0·6	0·1	− 0·7	3·9	± 5·2
,,	,,	,,	corn oil *	4·2	− 2·6	− 1·4	24·0	± 5·6
,,	Olive oil	,,	sardine oil *	− 3·3	16·4	−13·0	10·1	± 4·6
,,	,,	,,	corn oil *	0·3	13·7	−13·7	30·2	± 4·8
,,	Sardine oil	,,	,, ,, *	3·6	− 2·7	− 0·7	20·1	± 3·8
KWY	House	minus	safflower oil	− 1·0	− 0·7	− 5·9	9·6	± 4·4
Shime (A)	Control	minus	butter-fat *	− 7·4	− 4·4	− 0·5	−17·6	± 5·2
(B)	,,	,,	margarine 1 *	− 8·0	− 3·1	− 1·2	−19·0	± 8·0
(C)	,,	,,	,, 2 *	− 7·8	− 3·7	− 0·8	−14·2	± 6·9

* See text.

TABLE VIII—VALUES OF COEFFICIENTS FOUND FOR EQUATION : Δ CHOL. $= b\Delta s + c\Delta M + d\Delta P$ AND FOR THIS EQUATION OMITTING TERM FOR ΔM (I.E., c = 0)

Line no.	Data used	No. of comparisons	b	c	d
1	Series JWX ..	10	2·91	−0.11	−1·28
2	Total of 9 series..	41	2·73	0·01	−1·31
3	Series JWX ..	10	2·87	0	−1·27
4	8 Other series ..	31	2·68	0	−1·31
5	Total of 9 series..	41	2·74	0	−1·31

Note that, for the construction of the figure, the direction of dietary comparison in each case was chosen so as to provide positive values for observed Δ Chol. Subtracting the diets in the opposite direction would yield a corresponding figure running down into the lower left-hand quadrant of the X-Y plot.

The figure also shows, as barred circles, the application of equation 3a to the 3 sets of data from the Shime experiment and, as solid circles, the 4 comparisons of " sardine " oil with other fats and oils (excluding corn oil). The results of these 7 comparisons are all satisfactorily predicted from equation 3a.

However, test with 12 comparisons involving corn oil shows that equation 3a consistently overestimates the cholesterol values on the corn-oil diet by an average value of 11·0 mg. per 100 ml. (s.e. = ±0·89). The least-squares regression equation for estimating the observed Δ Chol. in a corn-oil diet comparison from the predicted value from equation 3a is :

Observed Δ Chol. = 11·53 + 0·97 (predicted Δ Chol.)

In other words, the average fall in serum-cholesterol level in changing from butter-fat, house, low-fat, olive oil, cotton-seed oil, or sunflower-seed oil to corn oil can be estimated by calculating the predicted value from equation 3a, multiplying by 0·97, and adding 11·53 mg. per 100 ml. The observed serum-cholesterol values are highly correlated with the (uncorrected) values predicted from equation 4, the coefficient of correlation for the 12 comparisons being r = 0·978. It appears that the correction is a simple additive factor uncorrelated with the size of the observed Δ Chol. ; in this series of 12 observations the mean Δ Chol. range is 9·3–62·8 mg. per 100 ml.

In the hydrol comparisons (HYZ series) equation 3a overestimates Δ Chol. by an average of 26 mg. per 100 ml. This discrepancy might be related to the trans acids in this hydrogenated fat, or perhaps the short-chain fatty acids in coconut oil (about 18% of the total being in 8- and 10-carbon chains) are responsible. If it is taken

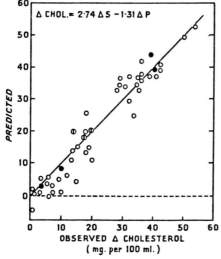

Δ Chol. observed vs. predicted from equation 3a: *open circles, data used in developing equation 3a; barred circles,* Japanese coalminers; *solid circles,* sardine oil.

that the term " saturated acids " for the present purpose refers to fatty acids with chain lengths of 12 or more carbon atoms, the value for S in hydrol is decreased, as indicated at the bottom of table VI, and computations on this basis with equation 3a gives good agreement. In the 3 hydrol comparisons (HYZ in table VII) the observed values for Δ Chol. are −11·0, −43·3, and −46·1, and the predicted values from equation 3a, only fatty acids of 12 or more carbons being considered, are −9·8, −46·5, and −46·6 respectively. Applying the same convention regarding chain length to all the comparisons in table VII does not change any of the other results appreciably.

Prediction from only Total Fat and Iodine Values

In many situations it is easier to obtain information about the total fat content of diets and the average iodine value than to estimate the amounts of the several classes of fatty acids. Can this more limited information serve for prediction of Δ Chol. ? It is obvious that diets containing large amounts of fish oils would not fit in any such scheme because the higher degrees of unsaturation of the fish oils beyond the dienes does not seem to be reflected in the serum-cholesterol level (Keys et al.

TABLE IX—RELIABILITY OF PREDICTION OF SERUM-CHOLESTEROL RESPONSE (Δ CHOL.) TO CHANGE IN DIET FATS INDICATED BY AVERAGE OF DISCREPANCIES (DISREGARDING SIGN) BETWEEN OBSERVED Δ CHOL. AND Δ CHOL. PREDICTED FROM S AND P FATTY ACIDS

(3A) Δ Chol. = 2·74Δs − 1·31ΔP, and Δ Chol. predicted from total fat (F) and iodine value (J)

(5) Δ Chol. = 73·6($F_1/J_1 - F_2/J_2$).
All values in mg. of Cholesterol per 100 ml.

Prediction from	Average discrepancy	S.D.	S.E.
1. Equation 5	9·84	±6·80	±1·06
2. Equation 3a	3·65	±2·94	±0·46
3. Difference line 1–line 2 ..	6·19	..	±1·16

1957a). But for other ordinary food fats the iodine value of a mixture is related to the proportions of saturated, monoethenoid, and polyethenoid fatty acids in a fairly uniform way. If the average chain lengths of the groups of fatty acids is 18 carbons, and if the polyethenoid fatty acids are dienes (linoleic acid), we have the formula :

(4)   Iodine value = 86 M′ + 173 P′,

where M′ and P′ refer to the proportions of these acids (as glycerides) in the total fat. With most ordinary diets, including low-fat diets and diets with added ordinary food fats, equation 4 is a good approximation. We have found good agreement between the iodine value computed in this way and that measured directly on the mixed fats extracted from an ordinary house diet. Accordingly it may be suggested that, as a simple approximation, the serum-cholesterol level should tend to be directly proportional to the amount of dietary fat and its average degree of saturation (or inversely related to the degree of unsaturation). And when the diet is changed, we might have :

(5) Δ Chol. = $k(F_1/J_1 - F_2/J_2)$,

where F is the amount of total fat, J the iodine value of that fat, and k a constant. For convenience we can express F as the percentage of total calories provided by fats.

To test this equation we have obtained the value for k for the same 41 sets of dietary differences and observed Δ Chol. values we used in obtaining equation 3a. The mean value of k was 73·60, with a standard error of ±7·38. When this value is substituted in equation 5 and the equation is applied to the 41 sets of experimental data, the mean discrepancy between observed and predicted values for Δ Chol. proves to be almost three times as large as found in the application of equation 3a to the same data. The computations are summarised in table IX.

The iodine value and total fat, expressed in equation 5, however, do have predictive value, as shown by the coefficient of correlation between Δ Chol. predicted from it and Δ Chol. observed : $r = 0.899$. The corresponding correlation involving Δ Chol. predicted from equation 3a is $r = 0.978$.

The reason for the limited reliability of the computation using iodine values is clear if we consider the coefficients in equations 2b and 3a. If we have two diets with total fats providing 40% of all calories in both cases but the fats are made up of 10%, 80%, and 10% of S, M, and P acids respectively in one case and 40%, 20%, and 40% respectively in the other, the iodine values will be the same. But from equation 2b we would predict that the serum-cholesterol level would be higher on the second diet by 17.2 mg. per 100 ml., since $S_1 = 4$, $S_2 = 16$, $P_1 = 4$, $P_2 = 16$, so Δ Chol.$_{1-2} = 2.71 (12) - 1.31 (12) = 17.2$.

Discussion

The prediction equations developed here apply only to the conditions of these experiments—namely, adult men aged 30–55, in calorie equilibrium, and with a constant rate of energy expenditure, who are consuming diets containing 10–40% of calories from fats, with periods on each diet of about two to four weeks. Moreover we are concerned with " control " serum-cholesterol levels less than 300 mg. per 100 ml. on ordinary diets of the type where S is about 18% and P about 4% of total calories. Finally, these predictions are for group averages; the reliability of individual prediction is low because of the intra- and inter-variability noted above and because the magnitude of Δ Chol. for a given dietary change tends to be related to the characteristic serum-cholesterol level of the individual. Larger values for Δ Chol. are found in men with idiopathic hypercholesterolæmia. The magnitude of Δ Chol. from a given change in dietary fat tends to be directly related to the intrinsic serum-cholesterol level on a reference diet—e.g., one in which $S = 18\%$ and $P = 4\%$ of calories.

It cannot be stated how well the numerical data which have been developed here, including the values of the coefficients in equations 3a and 5, will apply to other groups of men and in other conditions. There are no published data from experiments elsewhere that conform precisely to the conditions of the present study. After this work was finished the papers of Ahrens et al. (1957) and Malmros and Wigand (1957) appeared. Though the data published in these papers do not allow exact comparison, they seem to be at least in fair agreement with the present results and with equation 3a.

The slightly aberrant results obtained with corn oil merit comment. In experiments on animals Jones et al. (1956) report a cholesterol-depressing factor in corn oil not explained by its fatty-acid composition, and from experiments on 57 men. Beveridge et al. (1957) conclude that at least part of the effect of corn oil in the diet must result from something other than fatty acids. It is significant that Ahrens et al. (1957) could not produce a greater effect with safflower-seed oil on the serum-cholesterol level than with corn oil. Very recently we compared corn oil with safflower-seed oil in 141 university students and found a slightly greater cholesterol depression on the corn-oil diet. Perhaps the sterol content of the corn oil is responsible, as suggested by Beveridge et al. (1957).

The total cholesterol responses to the diet reported here are wholly explained by changes in the β-lipoprotein fraction, and this fraction alone is primarily

responsible for the differences observed in comparing populations subsisting on different diets (Anderson and Keys 1956, Keys et al. 1956a, Anderson et al. 1957, Keys et al. 1957b).

As regards population comparisons, the question arises whether the observed differences in mean serum-cholesterol levels can be predicted by applying equation 3a to the dietary data. Most of these dietary data provide only very rough estimates of the proportions of the several classes of fatty acids, but it is clear that the observed Δ Chol. is usually considerably larger than would be predicted from equation 3a. The signs and relative values of Δ Chol. are in general agreement, but the magnitude is something like twice what would be predicted from these experiments. The most reasonable explanation is that maintenance for many years on a diet produces larger effects than result in a few weeks or months.

The experiments reported here clearly indicate that the saturated fatty acids, at least those of chain length longer than 10 carbons, have about twice as much effect in raising the serum-cholesterol level as the cholesterol depressing effect of an equal amount of polyethenoids or linoleic acid. This being so, it is not surprising that it is indicated that monoethenoids (oleic acid) have relatively little effect on the serum-cholesterol level. But that oleic acid has absolutely no effect, as indicated in the derivation of equation 3a, cannot be concluded with certainty, because in most of the diets the variation in oleic acid is correlated to some extent with variations in the saturated fatty acid. Experiments are now in progress that should settle the oleic-acid question.

In any case it appears that the speculation that hypercholesterolæmia is simply a manifestation of a deficiency of " essential " fatty-acids (Sinclair 1956) cannot be supported. An excess of saturated fatty acids in the diet seems to explain the high serum-cholesterol levels in populations subsisting on luxurious American and European diets. To lower the serum-cholesterol level adequately a decrease in the intake of saturated fats seems to be more important than an increase in linoleic or other polyethenoids. The mere addition to the diet of small amounts of fats very rich in linoleic acid can have very little effect, and the addition of amounts adequate to have a real effect means an undesirable increase in calories. Fortunately, substitution of one type of fat for the other is both effective and acceptable for dietetic practice.

Summary

Groups of 12 to 27 men at a time were studied in calorie balance in dietary experiments controlled so that each man was maintained for 4 weeks of standardisation and then for 2–9 weeks on each of 2–6 diets differing in fat content, covering the range of 9–44% of calories from fats, with an experimental fat usually representing about three-fourths of the total fat. Fats studied included butter-fat, hydrogenated coconut oil (hydrol), olive oil, cotton-seed oil, corn oil, sunflower-seed oil, safflower oil, fish oil (Sardinops cœrulea), and the mixed food fats of ordinary American diets. The intakes of fats, as percentages of total calories provided from glycerides of saturated (S), monoethenoid (M), and polyethenoid (P) fatty acids, were estimated for each man on each diet.

Statistical analysis of the serum-cholesterol levels at the end of each dietary period yielded the least-squares multiple regression equation for the averages of groups of subjects :

$$\Delta \text{ Chol.} = 2.74 \Delta S - 1.31 \Delta P,$$

where Δ Chol. is the average change in mg. of total cholesterol per 100 ml. of serum predicted from the changes in the diet in S and in P, for all fats save corn oil and hydrol. The equation overestimates by an average of 11 mg. per 100 ml. the serum-cholesterol level on diets providing 20–30% of calories from corn oil. The equation is satisfactory in hydrol comparisons if S is interpreted to mean only fatty acids with more than 10 carbons..

Prediction of Δ Chol. can also be made, but with less accuracy, from :

$$\Delta \text{ Chol.} = 73 \cdot 6(F_1 J_1 - F_2/J_2),$$

where F is the percentage of total calories from all fats and J is the mean iodine value of those fats. With the group averages from 41 sets of dietary comparisons the average discrepancy between Δ Chol. observed and that predicted from this equation was $9 \cdot 84 \pm 1 \cdot 06$ mg. per 100 ml. The corresponding averaging discrepancy in S and P was $3 \cdot 65 \pm 0 \cdot 46$ mg. per 100 ml.

These equations are much more reliable for groups of men than for individuals because of spontaneous inter- and intra-individual variability.

These experiments and their analysis offer no support for the suggestion that a deficiency of essential fatty acids produces the high serum-cholesterol levels characteristic of populations subsisting on luxurious American and Western European diets. Effective correction of these high serum-cholesterol levels involves a decrease in the most common fats in such diets and the secondary substitution of fats high in polyethenoid fatty acids.

We are grateful for assistance in the statistical analysis to Mr. Norris Schulz and Mr. Malempati Rao and in fat analysis to the Research Division of Procter and Gamble Co., Cincinnati (Dr. Lloyd Beck, Dr. F. H. Mattson, and Dr. P. W. Ifland) ; to Dr. J. C. Cowan, of the U.S. Department of Agriculture laboratories at Peoria, Illinois ; Dr. Raymond Paschke, Research Laboratories, General Mills, Inc., Minneapolis ; and Dr. Ralph Holman, Hormel Research Institute, Austin, Minnesota. Mrs. Nedra Foster supervised the technicians who did the cholesterol analyses and collaborated with Mrs. Helen Williams in devising recipes and menus and in the dietary analyses.

REFERENCES

Abell, L. L., Levy, B. B., Brodie, B. B., Kendall, F. E. (1952) J. biol. Chem. 195, 357.

Ahrens, E. H. Jr., Blankenhorn, D. M., Tsaltas, T. T. (1954) Proc. Soc. exp. Biol., N.Y. 86, 872.

— Hirsch, J., Insull, W. Jr., Tsaltas, T. T., Blomstrand, R., Peterson, M. L. (1957) Lancet, i, 943.

American Oil Chemists' Society (1956) Official and Tentative Methods. 2nd ed., Chicago.

Anderson, J. T., Keys, A. (1956) Clin. Chem. 2, 145.

— — Grande, F. (1957) J. Nutr. 62, 421.

Bailey, A. E. (1951) Industrial Oil and Fat Products. 2nd ed., New York.

Beveridge, J. M. R., Connell, W. F., Mayer, G. A. (1956) Canad. J. Biochem. Physiol. 34, 441.

— — — (1957) Fed. Proc. 16, 11.

Brocklesby, H. N., Harding, K. F. (1938) J. Fish Res. Bd Can. 4, 55.

Bronte-Stewart, B., Antonis, A., Eales, L., Brock, J. F. (1956) Lancet, i, 521.

Eckey, E. W. (1954) Vegetable Fats and Oils. New York.

Groen, J., Tjiong, B. K., Kamminga, C. E., Willebrands, A. F. (1952) Voeding, 13, 556.

Hilditch, T. P. (1956) The Chemical Constitution of Natural Fats. 3rd ed., New York.

Jones, R. J., Reiss, O. K., Huffman, S. (1956) Proc. Soc. exp. Biol., N.Y. 93, 88.

Keys, A. (1952) Circulation, 5, 115.

— Anderson, J. T. (1957) Amer. J. clin. Nutr. 5, 29.

— — Aresu, M., Biörck, G., Brock, J. F., Bronte-Stewart, B., Fidanza, F., Keys, M. H., Malmros, H., Poppi, A., Posteli, T., Swahn, B., del Vecchio, A. (1956a) J. clin. Invest. 35, 1173.

— — Fidanza, F., Keys, M. H., Swahn, B. (1955) Clin. Chem. 1, 34.

— — Grande, F. (1957a) Lancet, i, 66.

— — Mickelsen, O., Adelson, S. F., Fidanza, F. (1956b) J. Nutr. 59, 39.

— Kimura, N., Kusukawa, A., Yoshitomi, M. (1957b) Amer. J. clin. Nutr. 5, 245.

— Mickelsen, O., Miller, E. v. O., Chapman, C. B. (1950) Science, 112, 79.

Kinsell, L. W., Partridge, J., Boling, L., Margen, S., Michaels, G. (1952) J. clin. Endocrin. 12, 909.

Malmros, H., Wigand, G. (1957) Lancet, ii, 1.

Mellinkoff, S. M., Machella, T. E., Reinhold, J. G. (1950) Amer. J. med. Sci. 220, 203.

Sinclair, H. M. (1956) Lancet, i, 381.

LESSONS FROM SERUM CHOLESTEROL STUDIES IN JAPAN, HAWAII AND LOS ANGELES *†

By Ancel Keys, Ph.D., *Minneapolis, Minnesota,* Noboru Kimura, M.D.,
Kyushu, Japan, Akira Kusukawa, M.D., *Fukuoka, Japan,*
B. Bronte-Stewart, M.D., *Oxford, England,*
Nils Larsen, M.D., F.A.C.P., *Honolulu, Hawaii,*
and Margaret Haney Keys, B.Sc.,
Minneapolis, Minnesota

Two years ago, at the meeting of the College in Philadelphia, we reported some of our findings in South Africa. These data were in conformity with the hypothesis that dietary fat is an important element in the remarkable differences between populations in the frequency of coronary heart disease.[1,2]

It is now possible to report related findings in Japan and on Japanese in Hawaii and in Los Angeles.

The basic question under investigation is this: What causes the striking differences in the frequency of coronary heart disease in different populations? Research on this question, and related studies on the cholesterol lipoprotein system in the blood in controlled dietary experiments on man, have led to a hypothesis about the influence of dietary fats on the development of coronary heart disease. The hypothesis may be stated as follows:

1. The etiology of coronary heart disease is multiple, but the development of the majority of cases in our society is dominated by the long-time effect of a rich fatty diet and an endless succession of fat-loading meals.

2. One effect of our kind of high fat diet is hypercholesterolemia, and this is so universal among us that our so-called cholesterol norms are simply standards for preclinical coronary disease. Hypercholesterolemia promotes atherosclerosis.

3. Fatty meals induce changes in the coagulability and other characteristics of the blood that favor thrombosis and inhibit fibrinolysis.[3,4,5]

4. Food fats differ in their effect on the blood cholesterol, but those fats most favored and abundant in our own diet are more powerful in promoting hypercholesterolemia than are those food oils that have a neutral or oppos-

* From the Symposium on the Pathogenesis of Coronary Heart Disease, presented at the Thirty-eighth Annual Session of The American College of Physicians, Boston, Massachusetts, April 10, 1957.

From the Laboratory of Physiological Hygiene, University of Minnesota, Minneapolis, and the First Medical Clinic, University of Kyushu Medical School, Fukuoka, Japan.

† The research reported here was made possible by grants from the American Heart Association, New York, the National Dairy Council, Chicago, the Tobacco Research Committee, New York, Mr. David Winton and the Winton Companies Fund, Minneapolis, and local sources in Japan.

Requests for reprints should be addressed to Laboratory of Physiological Hygiene, University of Minnesota, Stadium, Gate 27, Minneapolis 14, Minnesota.

ing effect. It takes about 2 gm. of linoleic acid to offset the effect of 1 gm. of palmitic or stearic acid.[6]

5. The thrombus-inducing factor or factors in food fats and oils cannot be attributed to the fatty acids as such, and corn oil is no better than beef fat in this respect.[5]

TABLE 1

Mortality Rates, per 100,000 of Given Age, for Men Aged 50 to 54 in 1953–54 (From Official Vital Statistics)

Cause	U.S.A.	Japan
1. All causes	1,189	1,163
2. Infective and parasitic diseases	39	177
3. All neoplasms	206	236
4. Coronary (Internat. List Nos. 420, 422)	445	33
5. Hypertension plus Cerebrovascular Lesions	115	251
6. All violence	124	112
7. Ill defined and not known	13	35

6. Obesity, physical inactivity and economic privilege do not, of themselves, necessarily lead to the development of coronary heart disease.[7, 8, 9] But the rich man's table is apt to offer only a choice among rich foods. In America now we are all economically privileged, we are protected from exercise, the fat of the land is ours, and we try to fight obesity by cutting out bread and potatoes. So almost all Americans now eat high fat diets; we are pleased to be able to afford the most expensive fats, that is, the most highly

TABLE 2

Comparison between Mortality Rates from Vital Statistics and Calculated from a Nationwide Morbidity Survey with Follow-Up on Lethality (Data from Kusukawa, 1956)

Cause	Lethal Rate per 100 Cases	Death Rate From Morbidity +Lethality	Death Rate From Vital Statistics
All morbidity	0.7	758	970
I. Infective and parasitic	1.2	115	147
VII. Circulatory diseases	2.9	58	64
XVII. All violence	0.5	29	34

saturated fats. Our situation is at the opposite extreme from that in Japan, where the diet is remarkably low in fats. Table 1 summarizes some vital statistics.

Of all large countries with detailed vital statistics, Japan reports the lowest mortality rate from coronary heart disease. Mortality rates from tuberculosis, cancer and cerebrovascular lesions are known to be high, yet the total mortality of middle aged men is somewhat less than our own. This lends credibility to the remarkable discrepancy in coronary mortality shown here.

TABLE 3

Experience with Japanese Patients of Three Private Clinics in Japan and Three in
Hawaii during the Month of March, 1956 (Data collected by
Dr. B. Bronte-Stewart)

Place	Total	Number of Patients Seen Hypertensive	Coronary
Honolulu	433	50	34
Fukuoka	381	38	1

Moreover, as table 2 shows, a large scale morbidity survey in Japan, with follow-up to find lethality, yielded reasonable agreement on the mortality rate for International List (1948), Category VII, Circulatory Diseases.[10] In spite of much rheumatic and hypertensive heart disease in Japan, the total mortality from circulatory diseases is low.

Such facts called for an extensive research program on the Japanese in Japan, in Hawaii and in California. Table 3 summarizes findings in private medical practice on Japanese in Fukuoka, Japan, and in Honolulu. This experience of the private practitioners in Hawaii and in Japan is no different from that in the big public hospitals. Dr. Paul White and other internists who checked these hospitals will testify that coronary heart disease is fairly common among Japanese in Hawaii but very rare in Japan. Hypertension is common in both regions.

Figure 1 summarizes findings on the frequency of severe atherosclerosis in consecutive autopsies, deaths from all causes. We checked the compara-

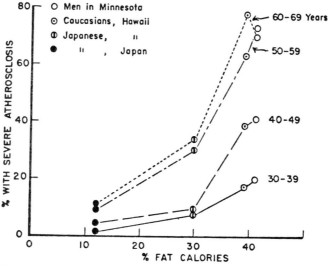

FIG. 1. Percentage of consecutive autopsies, deaths from all causes, showing severe (Mayo Clinic grades 3 and 4) coronary atherosclerosis among men aged 30 to 69 years, in Minnesota (400 autopsies), in Hawaii (141 Japanese, 270 Caucasians), and in Fukuoka, Japan (400 autopsies). The average percentage of calories provided by fats in the diet for these populations is given on the abscissa.

bility of methods and grading.   Minnesotans and Caucasians in Hawaii are almost identical, but the incidence of severe atherosclerosis in Japanese men in Kyushu is only a tenth as great.   Japanese men in Hawaii are intermediate.   We lack comparable data for Japanese in California, but at least it is known that coronary heart disease is their leading cause of death, and the representation of the disease at the Los Angeles Japanese Hospital and in private practice there is much the same as for the Caucasians in California. According to vital statistics, Japanese in California appear to be no different from other Californians; coronary heart disease is their leading cause of death.

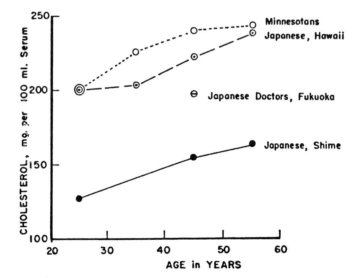

Fig. 2.   Mean serum total cholesterol concentrations for clinically healthy men engaged in sedentary and light activity occupations.   N = 153 for Shime (49, 54, and 50 men in third, fifth and sixth decades, respectively), N = 122 for Japanese in Hawaii (34, 27, 33, and 28 men in third, fourth, fifth and sixth decades, respectively), N = 52 for Fukuoka doctors (ages 40 to 49), and N = 940 for Minnesotans (163, 186, 234, and 357 men in third, fourth, fifth and sixth decades, respectively).

Obviously something happens to Japanese when they move to Hawaii and begin to adopt American customs.   And when they become fully Americanized in California, this includes conformity with our American pattern of excessive coronary heart disease.

Figure 2 summarizes total serum cholesterol findings in clinically healthy men engaged in sedentary and light activity occupations, all studied in 1956 with the same methods and by the same analysts.   The values for the 110 Japanese men in Hawaii average 76 mg.% higher than those for their 153 counterparts in Kyushu, while those for the 831 Minnesotans are higher still.

These 1956 measurements probably represent the situation during a number of preceding years among Minnesotans and men in Japan, but there is some question about the former dietary situation in Hawaii, where Ameri-

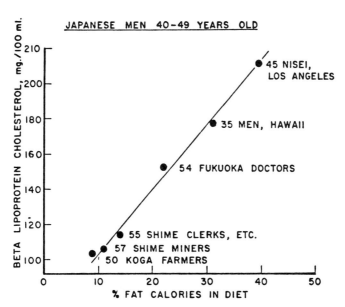

FIG. 3. Mean percentage of calories provided by all fats in the diet and concentration of beta lipoprotein-cholesterol in the serum of Japanese men aged 40 to 49 in Japan, in Hawaii, and in Los Angeles.

canization of the resident Japanese has progressed rapidly in the last few years, especially among the younger men. Note the high value for the youngest group in Hawaii; these young men are now just as addicted to hamburgers and ice cream as are the local Caucasians.

Figure 3 summarizes cholesterol and dietary data for men aged 40 through 49. It was possible to make dietary studies on all subjects. The same chief dietitian, Mrs. S. Miyamoto, supervised the work in Hawaii and Los Angeles, while in Kyushu a team of 10 dietitians conducted the household inventory and purchase surveys. Fats provided less than 10% of total calories for the farmers at Koga, and the highest fat intake in Kyushu was that of the 54 physicians, who got an average of 22% of their calories from fats. In Hawaii the Japanese men of this age averaged a little over 30% fat calories, and in Los Angeles the average was almost 40%. Serum cholesterol was linearly related.

TABLE 4

Mean Alpha and Beta Lipoprotein-Cholesterol Concentrations in the Blood Serum of Sedentary Japanese Men, aged 40 to 49, Matched as to Relative Fatness; Also Average Percentage of Calories Provided by Fats in the Diets of These Same Men

Place	% Fat Calories	Cholesterol, mg.%	
		α	β
Shime	13	40.3	120.3
Honolulu	32	40.4	183.0
Los Angeles	40	35.2	212.7

This relationship is not dependent upon differences in total calories or obesity. Table 4 compares 40-to-49 year old Japanese men matched in relative obesity by measurements of the subcutaneous fat thickness with skinfold calipers. This table also shows that the total cholesterol differences are fully accounted for by differences in the concentration of beta lipoprotein choles-

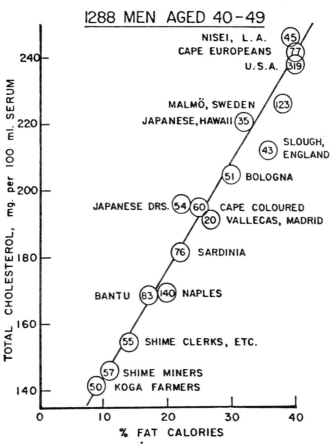

FIG. 4. Mean percentage of calories provided by all fats in the diet and concentration of total cholesterol in the serum of 1,288 clinically healthy men aged 40 to 49 in gainful employ in the United States, (Minnesota railroad clerks, switchmen, dispatchers, Minneapolis firemen, Los Angeles Caucasians), Malmö, Sweden (shipyard workers, firemen, clerks, engineers, foremen), Bologna (policemen, factory workers, businessmen), Sardinia (policemen, firemen, coal miners), Naples (firemen, steelworkers, clerks), and in other groups as indicated. Numbers within the circles show the number of men in each group.

terol. The lipoproteins were separated by paper electrophoresis, and cholesterol was measured in separate fractions. As in our other population studies, alpha lipoprotein cholesterol does not vary beyond the range of about 35 to 45 mg. per 100 ml.

These findings on Japanese are, as shown in figure 4, in conformity with the data on other racial groups. The dietary and cholesterol data suggest no peculiarity of Japanese or Bantu or Americans or Italians, and so on. They all conform to the same pattern. Further, this graph shows no peculiarity of men doing heavy manual labor as contrasted with men in sedentary and light work. Heavy labor here is represented by the Japanese farmers at Koga and the miners at Shime, Bantu at Cape Town, the steel workers at Ilva near Naples, coal miners at Bacu Abis, Sardinia, and shipbuilders at Malmö, Sweden.

In Japan we were able to make a small dietary experiment, summarized in figure 5, on 18 Japanese coal miners.[11] Fifty grams of butter or margarine were isocalorically substituted for rice in their customary diet. In

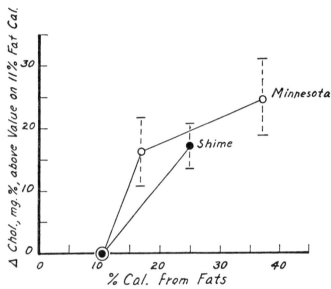

FIG. 5. Mean change in serum total cholesterol of Japanese coal miners at Shime and of Minnesota Hastings State Hospital men in response to isocaloric substitution of butterfat or margarine for carbohydrate in a low fat diet. Vertical broken lines show standard errors.

11 days there was a significant rise in the serum cholesterol, and this corresponded in magnitude to the results of similar experiments made on Minnesota men at the Hastings State Hospital. We conclude that the low cholesterol values of the Japanese in Japan is fully explained by the fat, or lack of it, in the diet.

There is, however, the question as to the kind of fat in the Japanese and the American diets. Table 5 summarizes fat calories according to source for the Japanese studied in Shime, Honolulu and Los Angeles, and for the Caucasian controls studied in parallel in Honolulu and in Los Angeles. Except in Los Angeles, the Japanese get a larger proportion of their calories from fish and marine invertebrates than do the Caucasians. All groups except the Japanese at Shime get most of their diet fats from meat, eggs, and dairy products, that is from relatively saturated fats.

In controlled dietary experiments we have found that fish oil, in spite of its extreme degree of unsaturation, does not have any remarkable cholesterol-lowering effect; it is about equivalent to cottonseed oil in this respect.[12] Calculations indicate, in fact, that more than the two double bonds in linoleic are without further effect on the blood cholesterol.

TABLE 5

Percentages of Total Calories in the Diet from Fats Classified as to Source; Clinically Healthy Men Studied in 1956

Source	Japanese			Caucasians	
	Shime	Honolulu	Los Angeles	Honolulu	Los Angeles
Meat, eggs and dairy products	3.3	20.2	28.1	33.7	28.0
Fish and other marine animals	5.9	1.4	0.8	0.8	0.5
Vegetable sources	2.8	10.2	10.2	6.7	13.9
Total	12.0	31.8	39.1	41.2	42.4

Table 6 summarizes the average fatty acid contributions to the diet in Kyushu and in Minnesota and Los Angeles. The fatty acids, as the glycerides, are expressed as percentages of the total calories. This is the result of summing up the fatty acid contents of each of the food items in the recorded food consumption. It is apparent that the diet in the United States differs from the Japanese diet primarily in the much larger content of saturated and mono-ethenoid (one double bond) fatty acids. Our diet contains much more linoleic acid than does the Japanese, and even the total of polyethenoid fatty acids is greater in our diet than in the Japanese diet.

TABLE 6

Percentages of Total Dietary Calories from Fatty Acids, as Glycerides, in Diets of Men Studied in Minnesota and Los Angeles and in Kyushu, Japan

Fatty Acids	U.S.A.	Kyushu
Saturated	17.6%	2.6%
Mono-ethenoid	17.3	4.7
Linoleic	4.6	2.6
Other poly-ethenoid	0.5	2.1
Total	40.0%	12.0%

This is, in fact, the general pattern of diets in most populations. As populations increase their fat consumption, they do so mainly by increasing their use of meat and dairy fats, but their intake of linoleic or so-called essential fatty acids also rises somewhat. The resulting rise in serum cholesterol is attributable to an increased intake of saturated fats and not to a decreased intake of unsaturated fats.

The relative influence of different fats on the serum cholesterol-lipoprotein system of man has been the subject of a major research program in

Minnesota for the last six years. Over 20,000 subject-days of controlled dietary experiments on man have recently been analyzed. The result is to show that 1 gm. of saturated fat requires about 2 gm. of linoleic acid to counter the effect on the serum cholesterol. This agrees with our population studies and the conclusion that in natural human diets the content of saturated fatty acids is dominant. Frying the hamburger steak in sunflower seed oil does not seem to be the solution.[12]

CONCLUSION

The low incidence of atherosclerosis and coronary heart disease in Japan is clearly established. Among Japanese, as among other peoples, the incidence of coronary heart disease is directly related to the average level of serum cholesterol, and it is unnecessary to invoke racial or other factors in explanation.

The serum cholesterol level in Japanese men is directly related to the percentage of calories provided by fats in the diet. The effect of the fats is dominated by the saturated fats of meats and dairy products. Among Japanese, as in most of the world's populations, when the diet is increased in fats, this increase is mainly accounted for by increasing consumption of the more saturated types of fats, as represented in beef, pork and dairy products.

These findings do not constitute proof of the hypothesis that dietary fat is a major factor in the development of coronary heart disease. But the findings are consistent, in detail, with the theory.

The theory is consistent not only with our findings in comparing Japan with the United States—it is consistent also with the results of our studies in North and South Italy, in South Africa, in England, in Spain, in Sweden and, most recently, in Finland. It is consistent with the findings of others in Guatemala, in Israel, in India, in Nigeria and in West Germany. So far, all investigations on populations subsisting on low-fat diets show such populations to be characterized by a low incidence of atherosclerosis and coronary heart disease and a low average level of cholesterol in the blood in comparison with populations who subsist on high fat diets. All populations known to have an incidence of the disease comparable to that in the United States or in Great Britain obtain at least a third of their calories in the form of fats in which fats from meats and dairy products make a large contribution.

Two exceptions to these rules have been claimed—the Eskimo and the Navajo Indian. On investigation, however, these "exceptions" prove to be based on faulty or absent information, and failure to realize that in both of these small populations the number of men of an age appropriate to the exhibition of coronary heart disease is extraordinarily small. The majority of Eskimos in modern times eat a diet considerably lower in fats than do contemporary Americans, and the few primitive Eskimos who do eat a high fat diet (only slightly higher in fat calories than the diet in the United States) consume very little of the common meat and dairy fats characteristic of the United States and other regions where coronary heart disease is common. In any case, practically nothing is known about the frequency of coronary atherosclerosis and heart disease among Eskimos.

Study of the Navajo Indians does not support the suggestion that the Navajos eat the high fat diet typical of most Americans today, yet suffer no coronary heart disease. Navajo diets are not high in total fats and are very low in dairy fats. The average age of the Navajo population is far lower than that of the United States as a whole (about half of them are 15 years old or younger), and there are no reliable data on the frequency of atherosclerosis or coronary heart disease among them. Arteriosclerotic heart disease and myocardial infarction are not vanishingly rare, and the incidence seems to be roughly what would be expected with a diet of around 25% fat calories, including little or no butterfat. In other words, the Navajos apparently resemble the inhabitants of Sardinia or the Cape colored people of South Africa in these respects.

Summary

1. Studies on the diet, the serum cholesterol and the frequency of atherosclerosis and coronary heart disease have been made in Japanese in Japan, where coronary heart disease is rare, in Hawaii, where it is fairly common but less so than among local Caucasians, and in California, where the local Japanese are similar to the local Caucasians in regard to the frequency of the disease. In middle age, coronary heart disease is at least 10 times as common in the United States as in Japan.

2. In 475 Japanese the serum cholesterol concentration showed a linear relationship to the percentage of calories provided by fats in the diet from a low among farmers at Koga, and a slightly higher average among miners at Shime, Japan, to a high among Nisei in Los Angeles, who were not significantly different from local Caucasians in this respect. These differences (averaging 96 mg. per 100 ml. comparing 40-to-49 year old Koga farmers, eating less than 10% fat calories, with Los Angeles Nisei of the same age, eating 39% fat calories) were accounted for by beta lipoprotein cholesterol, the alpha fraction showing no significant variation. These differences are not accounted for by differences in climate, relative obesity, physical activity, the use of alcohol and tobacco, the concentration of protein in the diet or the intake of "essential" fatty acids.

3. The findings on the Japanese are consistent with the theory that an important factor in producing differences in the frequency of coronary heart disease in populations is the proportion of calories in the diet provided by fats, particularly the common saturated fats.

ACKNOWLEDGMENT

The results reported here could not have been obtained without able and generous assistance and coöperation. *In Japan:* Dr. Masakazu Yoshitomi, Dr. Nobuki Endo, Dr. Y. Noda, Dr. R. Kikuno, Dr. G. Hashimoto, Mr. S. Miwa, Mr. P. Ishida, Mrs. M. Yasutake, Miss T. Oka, Mrs. T. Tsutsumi, Mrs. T. Takimoto, and the Staff of the 1st Medical Clinic of Kyushu University and of the Shime Hospital. *In Hawaii:* Mr. and Mrs. Steve Chinen, Mr. K. Goto. *In Los Angeles:* Dr. John Denny, Dr. T. Watanabe, Dr. Ben Kondo, Dr. Ed Phillips, Dr. George Matsumo, Dr. Robert Stivelman, Mrs. Nedra Foster. Mrs. Shizuko H. Miyamoto supervised the dietary work both in Los Angeles and in Hawaii. Dr. Joseph T. Anderson supervised the cholesterol measurements in Minneapolis on serum samples sent from Japan, Hawaii and Los Angeles.

SUMMARIO IN INTERLINGUA

Esseva studiate le dieta, le cholesterol seral, e le frequentia de atherosclerose e morbo coronari in subjectos japonese (1) in Japon, ubi morbo cardiac coronari es rar, (2) in Hawai, ubi illo es satis commun inter le japoneses sed minus commun que inter le residente caucasianos, e (3) in California, ubi le residente japoneses es simile al residente caucasianos con respecto al frequentià del morbo. Inter individuos de etate medie, morbo cardiac coronari es al minus 10 vices plus commun in le Statos Unite que in Japon.

Determinationes del cholesterol seral in 475 masculos japonese de etates de inter 40 e 49 annos monstrava un relation linear inter le cholesterol seral e le procentage del calorias providite per grassias in le dieta. Tanto le nivello de cholesterol como etiam le procentage del calorias representate per grassias in le dieta esseva plus basse inter le fermeros de Koga, levemente plus alte inter le mineros de Shime, e le plus alte inter le nisei de Los Angeles (qui non differeva significativemente ab le caucasianos local in iste respecto). Iste differentias amontava a un valor medie de 96 mg de cholesterol per 100 ml quando fermeros de Koga, de etates de inter 40 e 49 annos e alimentate con dietas in que minus que 10 pro cento del calorias esseva fornite per grassias, esseva comparate con le nisei de Los Angeles, del mesme gruppo de etate sed con dietas in que 39 pro cento del calorias esseva fornite per grassia. Le differentias se concentrava in le fraction lipoproteinic beta. Le fraction alpha non monstrava un variation significative. Le differentias del cholesterol non se explica per differentias de climate, del obesitate relative, del activitate physic, del uso de alcohol e tabaco, del concentration de proteina in le dieta, o del ingestion de acidos grasse "essential."

Iste constatationes in subjectos japonese es de accordo con le theoria que un importante factor in le production del differentias del numero de casos de morbo cardiac coronari in varie populationes es le proportion de calorias dietari providite per grassias, specialmente le commun grassias saturate.

Le constatationes es de accordo con le resultatos de nostre previe studios in Nord- e Sud-Italia, in Sud-Africa, in Anglaterra, in Espania, in Sveda, e, le plus recentemente, in Finlandia.

BIBLIOGRAPHY

1. (a) Keys, A.: The cholesterol problem, Voeding (Amsterdam) **13**: 539–555, 1952.
   (b) Keys, A.: Human atherosclerosis and the diet, Circulation **5**: 115–118, 1952.
   (c) Keys, A.: Atherosclerosis: a problem in newer public health, J. Mt. Sinai Hosp. **20**: 118–139, 1953–54.
   (d) Keys, A.: Prediction and possible prevention of coronary disease, Am. J. Pub. Health **43**: 1399–1407, 1953.
2. Keys, A.: The diet and the development of coronary heart disease, J. Chron. Dis. **4**: 364–380, 1956.

94   KEYS ET AL.   January 1958

3. Buzina, R., and Keys, A.: Blood coagulation after a fat meal, Circulation **14**: 854–858, 1956.
4. Keys, A., Buzina, R., Grande, F., and Anderson, J. T.: Effects of meals of different fats on blood coagulation, Circulation **15**: 274–279, 1957.
5. Greig, H. B. W.: Inhibition of fibrinolysis by alimentary lipaemia, Lancet **2**: 16–18 (July 7) 1956.
6. Keys, A., Anderson, J. T., and Grande, F.: "Essential" fatty acids, degree of unsaturation, and the effect of corn (maize) oil on the serum-cholesterol level in man, Lancet **1**: 66–68 (Jan. 12) 1957.
7. Keys, A.: Obesity and degenerative heart disease, Am. J. Pub. Health **44**: 864–871, 1954.
8. Brozek, J., and Keys, A.: Overweight, obesity, and coronary heart disease, Geriatrics **12**: 79–87, 1957.
9. Keys, A., Anderson, J. T., Aresu, M., Biörck, G., Brock, J. F., Bronte-Stewart, B., Fidanza, F., Keys, M. H., Malmros, H., Poppi, A., Posteli, T., Swahn, B., and del Vecchio, A.: Physical activity and the diet in populations differing in serum-cholesterol, J. Clin. Investigation **35**: 1173–1181, 1956.
10. Kusukawa, A.: Statistical findings on the incidence of coronary heart disease in Japan, *in* World trends in cardiology, edited by A. Keys and P. D. White, 1956, Hoeber-Harper, New York, pp. 159–163.
11. Keys, A., Kimura, N., Kusukawa, A., and Yoshitomi, M.: Serum cholesterol in Japanese coal miners: a dietary experiment, Am. J. Clin. Nutrition **5**: 245–250, 1957.
12. Keys, A., Anderson, J. T., and Grande, F.: Serum-cholesterol response to dietary fat, Lancet **1**: 787 (Apr. 13) 1957.

The Inheritance of Essential Familial Hypercholesterolemia*

Avedis K. Khachadurian, M.D.

Beirut, Lebanon

Essential familial hypercholesterolemia (EFH) is a hereditary disorder characterized by elevation of the serum cholesterol and phospholipid levels in the presence of normal serum triglyceride levels, the development of cutaneous and tendinous xanthomas, corneal arcus and, most important of all, a tendency to early atherosclerosis which may result in death from coronary occlusion. In patients presenting the full syndrome the differential diagnosis from other causes of hypercholesterolemia and xanthomatosis presents little difficulty.

Although the familial nature of the condition was recognized at the beginning of this century, and numerous pedigrees have been reported and analyzed since, there is still controversy about the mode of inheritance of the disorder. In 1949 Stecher and Hersh [1] analyzed thirty-seven pedigrees previously reported by Boas, Parets and Adlersberg [2] and concluded that hypercholesterolemia was transmitted as a Mendelian dominant gene. This analysis supported the previous report of Müller [3]. Wilkinson, Hand and Fliegelman [4] were the first to emphasize the variations in the severity of the disease and from the study of a very large kindred they concluded that the disease was transmitted as an autosomal, incompletely dominant gene; xanthoma tuberosum or tendinosum representing the homozygous state, and hypercholesterolemia with or without xanthelasma representing the heterozygous state. This theory acquired many supporters, among others Adlersberg [5].

Objections were soon raised to this theory following the discovery that persons with xanthomatosis, and therefore presumably homozygotes, did not invariably have two abnormal parents nor were all their children hypercholesterolemic. Thus Leonard [6] described eleven families with twenty-nine cases of hypercholesterolemia and four cases of xanthomatosis and concluded that the condition was probably inherited as a dominant trait. Harris-Jones, Jones and Wells [7], who had previously agreed with Wilkinson's incompletely dominant theory of transmission, concluded from an analysis of three additional families "that there is no evidence that xanthomatosis represents the homozygous state" for the condition. Piper and Orrild [8], from a follow-up study of fifty persons, concluded that xanthomatosis depends largely on the level of serum cholesterol and the duration of hypercholesterolemia and that the condition is transmitted as a dominant trait. Wheeler [9] reported on twelve patients with the "full syndrome" of hypercholesterolemia, clear serum and tendon xanthomas and concluded that the condition was transmitted as a dominant gene. However, he could not rule out the possibility that the homozygous state could produce a more severe form of the disorder. In 1959 Hirschhorn and Wilkinson [10] reported on three additional families and concluded that in the majority of the kindreds reported the mode of inheritance conforms to that of an incompletely dominant gene, but they also entertained the possibility that there could be two forms of inheritance. In the same year Adlersberg and Schaefer [11] concluded from their studies that the condition is transmitted by "a dominant gene with incomplete penetrance . . . the penetrance of the gene increasing with age." Epstein and his co-workers [12] noted that the mating of two hypercholesterolemic, nonxanthomatous persons has not been described a sufficient number of times to determine if 25 per cent of their children had xanthomatosis. From the analysis of the data in a family with

* From the Departments of Biochemistry and Internal Medicine, American University of Beirut, School of Medicine, Beirut, Lebanon. This study was supported in part by National Institutes of Health Grant AM 04270. Manuscript received September 3, 1963.

Inheritance of Essential Familial Hypercholesterolemia—*Khachadurian*   403

TABLE I

CLINICAL AND LABORATORY FINDINGS IN TEN FAMILIES WITH ESSENTIAL
FAMILIAL HYPERCHOLESTEROLEMIA

Case	Relation to Propositus	Age at Last Visit (yr.)	Serum			Xanthoma		Heart Disease		Remarks
			Choles-terol (mg. %)	Phospho-lipid Phos-phorus (mg. %)	Total Lipid Esters (mEq. %)	Degree	Age at Onset (yr.)	Degree	Age at Onset (yr.)	
A1	Father	55	486	—	—	0		+		Related to wife; dyspnea on exertion
A2	Mother	45	472	—	—	0		0		Four other children with no skin lesions
A3	Propositus female	20	600–942	—	—	++++	8	++++		History of "rheumatic fever" with migra-tory polyarthritis; angina pectoris aortic stenosis; died at age 21 of myocardial infarction
B1	Father	45	372	—	—	0		0		
B2	Mother	35	327	—	—	0		0		
B3	Propositus male	14	884	—	—	++++	3	++++	13	Severe angina and dyspnea on exertion
C1	Father	30	—	—	—	0		0		Second cousin of wife
C2	Mother	30	—	—	—	0		0		Two other children have no skin lesions
C3	Propositus female	8	965	—	—	++++	3	++	8	Aortic stenosis; left ventricular hyper-trophy, no symptoms
D1	Father	28	—	—	—	0		0		First cousin of wife
D2	Mother	25	—	—	—	0		0		Two other children with no skin lesions
D3	Propositus female	5	1,132	—	—	++++	3	+	5	Grade 1 aortic systolic murmur
E1	Father	45	—	—	—	0		+		From same village as wife; died at age 45 from "heart attack"
E2	Mother	40	—	—	—	0		0		Two other children with no skin lesions
E3	Propositus female	29	550–1,200	19	—	++++	7	++++	16	History suggestive of rheumatic poly-arthritis; hematuria; aortic stenosis, angina—lost to follow up; believed to have died at age 29
F1	Father	—	—	—	—	++++	—	++++	—	From same village as wife; died at age 30 suddenly; one brother died young from heart attack, had xanthomas; father died of heart attack, from same village as mother
F2	Mother	35	305	—	—	0		0		
F3	Brother	22	319	—	—	0		0		
F4	Sister	—	—	—	—	++++	—	++++	—	Died of heart attack
F5	Propositus male	19	896	21	2.9	++++	Birth	++++	15	Aortic stenosis and regurgitation
G1	Father	40	391	12	1.6	0		0		Originates from same village as wife
G2	Mother	29	291	10	1.4	0		0		
G3	Brother	12	135	6.5	0.74	0		0		
G4	Propositus male	9	746	16.7	2.1	++++	3	++	8	Aortic stenosis; no symptoms
G5	Brother	5	157	6.5	0.86	0		0		
H1	Father	45	—	—	—	0		0	—	Originates from same village as wife
H2	Mother	40	—	—	—	0		0	—	
H3	Propositus male	18	651	14.6	1.7	+++	14	0		No murmurs
H4	Brother	6	240	7.8	0.97	0		0		
H5	Brother	4	215	7.6	0.92	0		0		
H6	Sister	3	746	17.7	2.2	+	2	0		
H7	Sister	2	124	6.2	0.79	0		0		
I1	Paternal grand-father	—	—	—	—	0		0		Died of old age
I2	Paternal grand-mother	70	501	13.6	1.9	+	65	0		
I3	Father	50	405	10.8	1.3	0	0	0	0	From same village as wife
I4	Mother	40	325	8.9	1.2	0	0	0	0	
I5	Propositus male	22	470	11.5	1.4	++++	7	++++	20	History of polyarthritis at age 15; aortic stenosis, severe angina; died at age 22 suddenly
I6	Brother	18	645	16	2.0	++++	6	0		
I'1	Paternal uncle	45	541	14.5	1.8	+	40	0		Brother of I3; xanthelasma, 1 by 1 cm. nodules over both elbows
I'2	Wife of uncle	34	165	6.9	1.1	0		0		
I'3	Nephew	4	158	6.6	0.93	0		0		
I'4	Niece	3	158	6.3	0.74	0		0		
I'5	Niece	1½	—	—	—	0		0		

(Continued)

404   Inheritance of Essential Familial Hypercholesterolemia—*Khachadurian*

TABLE I (*Continued*)

CLINICAL AND LABORATORY FINDINGS IN TEN FAMILIES WITH ESSENTIAL
FAMILIAL HYPERCHOLESTEROLEMIA

Case	Relation to Propositus	Age at Last Visit (yr.)	Serum			Xanthoma		Heart Disease		Remarks
			Choles-terol (mg. %)	Phospho-lipid Phos-phorus (mg. %)	Total Lipid Esters (mEq. %)	Degree	Age at Onset (yr.)	Degree	Age at Onset (yr.)	
J1	Father	54	318	12.7	1.33	+	50	0		Second cousin of wife; thick xanthelasma, bilateral
J2	Mother	50	319	13.9	1.78	0		0		
J3	Brother	31	190	10.2	1.15	0		0		
J4	Sister	30	289	13.9	1.49	0		0		
J5	Sister	27	300	13.6	1.28	0		0		
J6	Propositus male	23	618	20.5	1.78	++++	7	+++		History of "rheumatic fever" and poly-arthritis; aortic stenosis; dyspnea and angina on exertion
J7	Brother	21	205	9.6	1.04	0		0		
J8	Brother	16	296	12.1	1.1	0		0		
J9	Sister	14	730	19.5	1.74	++++	7	++	13	History of "rheumatic fever" and poly-arthritis; aortic stenosis; mild angina on exertion
J10	Brother	13	281	11.1	1.06	0		0		
J11	Sister	7	160	8.1	0.71	0		0		

268 members previously reported by Wilkinson et al. [4] and the data available in the literature they concluded that there was no firm basis for attributing xanthomatosis to a single gene or to the coexistence of two abnormal alleles. In 1960 Fredrickson [13] reached a similar conclusion after a comprehensive review of the literature.

The present paper reports twelve cases of extensive xanthomatosis in ten Arab sibships. A definite inheritance pattern for essential familial hypercholesterolemia emerging from the study of these sibships is presented.

MATERIALS AND METHODS

All the index cases reported in this paper were studied at the Hospital or the Outpatient Department of the American University of Beirut. The diagnostic criteria for essential familial hypercholesterolemia consisted of hypercholesterolemia with a clear serum, xanthomatosis and the apparent absence of causes of secondary hyperlipemia. The clinical and laboratory data pertinent to this study are reported in Table I. Members of the families whose age is mentioned in column 3 of Table I were interviewed and examined. Information about the other members was obtained from relatives. Families A, B, E, F, G, H, I, I' and J were studied by me, the last six families being seen during a period of eighteen months. Serum cholesterol levels for families A, F, G, H, I, I' and J were determined in my laboratory using a modification [14] of the Lieberman-Burchard reaction. The cholesterol determinations for the other families were carried out

in the clinical laboratory of the Hospital where the Liebermann-Burchard reaction and the method of Zak et al. [15] were used at various periods. Serum phospholipids were determined by the method of Stewart and Hendry [16] and the total lipid esters by the method of Stern and Shapiro [17].

COMMENTS

In the ten index cases of xanthomatosis recorded in Table I marked hypercholesterolemia was present and extensive xanthomatosis (Fig. 1) developed before the age of fifteen (in one case the lesions were reported to be present at birth); in eight there is definite evidence of heart disease. In all instances in which the serum cholesterol was determined in the parents, values were found to be definitely above normal. There is consanguinity in five families, in four other families the parents originate from the same village and stated that they could not rule out consanguinity. These findings leave little doubt that the ten propositi reported on herein represent the homozygous state for familial hypercholesterolemic xanthomatosis.

The difficulties in establishing the mode of inheritance of essential familial hypercholesterolemia have arisen mainly from lack of agreement as to the criteria for the diagnosis of the heterozygote. Thus, the presence of xanthomas has been taken by some workers as evidence for homozygosity while others have presented data

Inheritance of Essential Familial Hypercholesterolemia—*Khachadurian*   405

to indicate that xanthomatosis can develop in heterozygotes. Our data indicate that xanthomas can develop in heterozygotes. However, in these subjects the lesions develop late in life and are small in size and few in number. To illustrate this point the grandmother (Case I2) and the uncle (Case I'1) of the propositus in family I have been included in this report. (Fig. 2.) In the grandmother xanthelasma and a small xanthoma developed at the age of sixty-five. One of her children has a normal serum cholesterol level and four of five of her children aged forty and above have no skin lesions. In the uncle xanthomas developed at the age of forty, the nodules are limited to his elbows and are 1 cm. in diameter. Two of his children have normal serum cholesterol levels. During the past year I have studied three additional patients in their fifth and sixth decades who have coronary heart disease, small cutaneous and tendinous xanthomas of recent onset and moderate hypercholesterolemia. They had a total of twelve children aged four to thirty, all

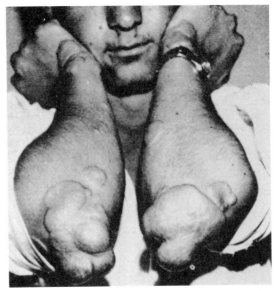

FIG. 1. Xanthomatosis in a homozygote (Patient F5, age nineteen).

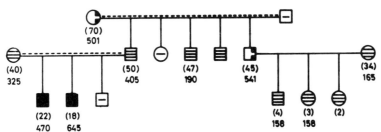

FIG. 2. Pedigree of Family I illustrating the presence of xanthomas in heterozygotes.

were free of xanthomatous lesions and the serum cholesterol level was below 200 mg. per cent in three of them. Hypercholesterolemia being an invariable finding in patients heterozygous for essential familial hypercholesterolemia, these five persons with xanthomatosis could not be homozygotes since some of their children are normocholesterolemic.

The severity of the atherosclerotic lesions parallels that of the xanthomatous lesions in this series. Thus while definite cardiac lesions developed in childhood or adolescence, in eight of the ten propositi, only one of the parents that I examined had findings suggestive of heart involvement.

In these patients the level of serum cholesterol follows a bimodal distribution distinguishing the homozygotes from the heterozygotes, especially within individual families. That an overlap of

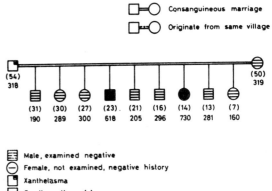

FIG. 3. Pedigree of Family J illustrating Mendelian ratios of autosomal recessive inheritance.

406 Inheritance of Essential Familial Hypercholesterolemia—*Khachadurian*

values between the two groups can occur is illustrated by the findings in family I in which the propositus had a single serum cholesterol determination of 470 mg. per cent while his heterozygous uncle and grandmother had levels of 541 and 501 mg. per cent, respectively. The wide fluctuations in the serum cholesterol level reported by many investigators and illustrated in patients A3 and E3 could be responsible for this observation. However, when all three cardinal manifestations of the disease are taken together, there is little difficulty in differentiating the heterozygotes from the homozygotes. The Mendelian ratio of 1:2:1 for homozygous normal, heterozygote and homozygous abnormal is obtained in this series and illustrated in Figure 3.

Recognition that xanthomatosis can occur both in the heterozygote as well as in the homozygote will resolve the controversy now prevalent in the literature by explaining the fact that persons with xanthomatosis can have normocholesterolemic children as well as the finding that the number of hypercholesterolemic children born to this group is substantially greater than the number of their normocholesterolemic children [15].

At its lower margin the serum level of cholesterol in the heterozygote can merge with values obtained for the "normal" population. In this study the dividing line between normal and abnormal was set at 250 mg. per cent. However, one patient (Case H5, a four year old boy with a serum level of 215 mg. per cent) probably represents a heterozygote in view of a cholesterol level of 124 mg. per cent in his two year old sister. Since the metabolic defect responsible for essential familial hypercholesterolemia is not known at present, the heterozygote without xanthomatosis can be diagnosed with certainty only if he comes from a family with a positive history for essential familial hypercholesterolemia. It is therefore impossible to know what proportion of the population with moderate hypercholesterolemia carries the abnormal gene.

During the last two decades extensive studies have been carried out to determine the environmental factors regulating serum cholesterol level. The enthusiasm created by these studies may have diverted attention from the hereditary factors determining the level of the serum cholesterol and the degree of atherosclerosis [11]. That genetic factors may be important in certain populations is illustrated by the study of the cases presented by Boas et al. [2] and analyzed by Stecher et al. [1]. In this study, in which patients were selected because of coronary artery disease starting before the age of fifty, hypercholesterolemia was transmitted as a Mendelian dominant gene and most probably represented the heterozygous state for essential familial hypercholesterolemia.

SUMMARY

Twelve patients with marked hypercholesterolemia and extensive xanthomatosis, representing ten sibships, are described. The presence of hypercholesterolemia in all the parents tested and the high incidence of consanguinity in these sibships leaves little doubt that these patients are homozygotes.

The inheritance pattern in these sibships conforms to that of an incompletely dominant gene. Persons homozygous for the condition have high levels of serum cholesterol, extensive xanthomas starting in childhood, and frequently advanced heart disease in youth. Heterozygous persons have moderate elevation of the serum cholesterol and xanthomatosis to a small extent may develop late in life. The occurrence of xanthomatosis in the heterozygote as well as in the homozygote reconciles the opposing theories for the inheritance of the disorder.

Acknowledgment: I wish to thank H. Chaglassian, M.D., A. Kurban, M.D., F. Farah, M.D., S. Najjar, M.D., G. Rubeiz, M.D. and A. Tuma, M.D. for referring patients and collaborating in their study. Thanks are also due to J. L. Wilson, M.D. for suggestions in the preparation of the manuscript. Mr. Apkar Mirakian gave able technical assistance.

REFERENCES

1. STECHER, R. M. and HERSH, A. H. Note on genetics of hypercholesterolemia. *Science*, 109: 61, 1949.
2. BOAS, E. P., PARETS, A. D. and ADLERSBERG, D. Hereditary disturbance of cholesterol metabolism. A factor in the genesis of atherosclerosis. *Am. Heart J.*, 35: 611, 1948.
3. MÜLLER, C. Xanthomata, hypercholesterolemia, angina pectoris. *Acta med. scandinav.*, 89 (supp.): 75, 1938.
4. WILKINSON, C. F., JR., HAND, E. A. and FLIEGELMAN, M. F. Essential familial hypercholesterolemia. *Ann. Int. Med.*, 29: 671, 1948.
5. ADLERSBERG, D. Hypercholesterolemia with predisposition to atherosclerosis. *Am. J. Med.*, 11: 600, 1951.
6. LEONARD, J. C. Hereditary hypercholesterolemic xanthomatosis. *Lancet*, 2: 1239, 1956.
7. HARRIS-JONES, J. N., JONES, E. G. and WELLS, P. G.

Inheritance of Essential Familial Hypercholesterolemia—*Khachadurian*   407

Xanthomatosis and essential hypercholesterolemia. *Lancet*, 1: 855, 1957.

8. PIPER, J. and ORRILD, L. Essential familial hypercholesterolemia and xanthomatosis. *Am. J. Med.*, 21: 34, 1956.

9. WHEELER, E. O. The genetic aspects of atherosclerosis. *Am. J. Med.*, 23: 653, 1957.

10. HIRSCHHORN, K. and WILKINSON, C. F. The mode of inheritance in essential familial hypercholesterolemia. *Am. J. Med.*, 26: 60, 1959.

11. ADLERSBERG, D. and SCHAEFER, L. E. The interplay of heredity and environment in the regulation of circulating lipids in atherogenesis. *Am. J. Med.*, 26: 1, 1959.

12. EPSTEIN, F. H., BLOCK, W. D., HAND, E. A. and FRANCIS, T. F., JR. Familial hypercholesterolemia, xanthomatosis and coronary heart disease. *Am. J. Med.*, 26: 39, 1959.

13. FREDRICKSON, D. S. Essential familial hyperlipidemia. In: The Metabolic Basis of Inherited Disease. Edited by Stanbury, J. B., Wyngaarden, J. B. and Fredrickson, D. S. New York, 1960. McGraw-Hill Book Co.

14. ABELL, L. L., LEVY, B. B., BRODIE, B. B. and KENDALL, F. E. A simplified method for the estimation of total cholesterol in serum and demonstration of its specificity. *J. Biol. Chem.*, 195: 357, 1952.

15. ZAK, B., DICKENMAN, R. C., WHITE, E. G., BURNETT, H. H. and CHERNEY, P. J. Rapid estimation of free and total cholesterol. *Am. J. Clin. Path.*, 24: 1307, 1954.

16. STEWART, C. P. and HENDRY, E. B. The phospholipins of blood. *Biochem. J.*, 29: 1683, 1935.

17. STERN, I. and SHAPIRO, B. A rapid and simple method for the determination of esterified fatty acids and for total fatty acids in blood. *J. Clin. Path.*, 6: 158, 1953.

289

Cholestyramine Resin Therapy for Hypercholesteremia

Clinical and Metabolic Studies

Sami A. Hashim, MD, and Theodore B. Van Itallie, MD

Cholestyramine resin, a bile-acid-sequestering agent, was administered to nine hypercholesteremic patients for periods of one month to four years. By promoting fecal excretion of bile acids, the resin appears to induce an increase in the rate of cholesterol conversion to bile acids in the liver, often resulting in a diminution of plasma cholesterol levels. During daily treatment with 13.3 gm of cholestyramine, eight of the subjects achieved mean serum total cholesterol levels that ranged from 80% to 50% of the average control values. The decreases were sustained for the duration of treatment. Two patients and one normal subject exhibited marked increases in fecal bile-acid excretion during resin administration, but neutral sterol output did not change consistently. The preparation produced occasional gastrointestinal discomfort; however, systemic side effects were not encountered.

Cholestyramine is a quaternary ammonium anion exchange resin with a polystyrene polymer skeleton. As the chloride salt, it binds bile acids both in vitro and in vivo, exchanging chloride for bile acid.[1] When the resin is administered to certain animals used for experimental purposes and to man, it sequesters bile acids in the gut, preventing their reabsorption and thereby promoting their excretion in the feces.[1,2] Because of its insolubility in water and high molecular weight (over 1 million), the resin presumably is not absorbed from the intestine.

Cholestyramine has been shown to lower serum cholesterol in the dog,[1] the cockerel,[1] and man.[3,4] It also is effective in the treatment of pruritus associated with incomplete biliary obstruction.[2,5-7]

The present report describes clinical and biochemical observations on nine patients with "primary" hypercholesteremia treated with cholestyramine for periods up to four years.

From the Department of Medicine, St. Luke's Hospital, and the Institute of Nutrition Sciences, Columbia University, New York.

Read in part before the annual meeting of the American Society for Clinical Nutrition, Atlantic City, May 2, 1964.

Reprint requests to Amsterdam Ave and 113th St, New York 10025 (Dr. Van Itallie).

Materials and Methods

The nine patients treated with cholestyramine are identified and their diagnoses shown in Table 1. All remained ambulatory during the study. Three were consuming diets rich in polyunsaturated fatty acids; the remainder ate a regular diet. None of the patients was given supplementary vitamins. At least three control determinations of serum total cholesterol and cholesterol esters were performed on each patient over a span of two to three weeks before cholestyramine administration was begun. The method of Sperry and Brand[8] was used to measure cholesterol and its esters in serum. All patients received 13.3 gm of cholestyramine resin per day in four equally divided doses. The medication was taken after each meal and at bedtime. Throughout, blood samples were obtained for lipid analyses at weekly or, occasionally, biweekly intervals. (In patient 8 blood lipid measurements were made less frequently, the average interval being 40 days.) In seven patients the cholestyramine was given without interruption; in two individuals, treatment was discontinued and started again (once in patient 8 and three times in patient 7) to establish the reproducibility of the cholesterol-lowering effect.

At various intervals following initiation of treatment, the following additional studies were performed: prothrombin activity, serum level of chloride, plasma carbon dioxide content, serum glutamic oxalacetic transaminase (SGOT) and alkaline phosphatase activities, serum thymol turbidity, serum albumin and globulin concentrations and serum bilirubin. Because of the report[9] that cholestyramine administration may enhance calcium absorption, serum calcium also was measured. Because of Schaffner's[10] suggestion that cholestyramine administration might have been responsible for inducing biliary calcification in three cases of biliary cirrhosis, the livers of all nine patients were x-rayed.

Fecal output of bile acids and neutral sterols was determined by analysis of individual 24-hour fecal samples. The stools were collected in 95% ethanol

Table 1.—Studies of Hypercholesteremic Patients During Treatment With Cholestyramine Resin

Patient No. Sex/Age	Other Lesions	Diet	Duration of Treatment, Days	Studies During Cholestyramine Treatment (Days of Treatment Prior to Test Shown in Parentheses)								
				Serum Ca, Mg/100Cc	Serum Cl, mEq/L	Alkaline Phosphatase, King-Armstrong Units	SGOT,* Units	Prothrombin Activity, % of Normal	Albumin/ Globulin, Gm/100Cc	CO₂ Content, mEq/L	X-ray of Liver†
1 M/37	....	Regular	271	10.0 (127)	100 (127)	4.9 (127)	18 (127)	100 (55) 100 (127)	4.2/ 2.4 (127)	25	Negative (120)
2 F/54	Xanthomatosis	Regular	414	9.9 (414)	100 (414)	6.2 (414)	18 (414)	100 (414)	4.8/ 3.2 (414)	27	Negative (414)
3 M/52	Xanthomatosis	Regular	365	10.0 (365)	105 (365)	8.1 (365)	29 (365)	100 (365)	4.8/ 2.5 (365)	24	Negative (365)
4 F/27	Xanthelasma	PUFA-‡ rich	30	10.4 (30)	101 (30)	6.4 (30)	12 (30)	100 (30)	4.7/ 2.8 (30)	....	Negative (30)
5 M/39	....	Regular	170	9.7 (150)	106 (150)	4.6 (150)	17 (150)	100 (150)	4.8/ 2.2 (150)	....	Negative (170)
6 F/62	....	Regular	90	10.1 (60)	103 (60)	6.2 (60)	18 (60)	100 (60)	4.8/ 2.8 (60)	....	Negative (90)
7 F/54	....	Regular	154	10.0 (154)	102 (154)	5.0 (154)	16 (154)	100 (154)	4.1/ 2.6 (154)	26 (154)	
			110	9.9 (110)	100 (110)	6.0 (110)	12 (110)	100 (110)		25 (110)	Negative (110)
8 F/32	Xanthomatosis, CHD§	PUFA- rich	1,460	9.1 (1,460)	103 (1,460)	12.0 (1,460)	30 (1,460)	100 (1,460)	4.5/ 2.4 (1,460)	26 (1,460)	Negative (1,460)
9 F/25	Xanthomatosis, CHD	PUFA- rich	579	9.7 (523)	100 (523)	10.1 (523)	20 (523)	100 (523)	4.6/ 3.3 (523)	24 (523)	Negative (579)

*Serum glutamic oxaloacetic transaminase.
†For calcification.
‡Polyunsaturated fatty acid.
§Coronary heart disease.

and the contents thoroughly homogenized. The analyses were performed on aliquot samples of the clear supernatant, obtained after the solids had settled. While the subjects were being administered cholestyramine, a saturated solution of ammonium carbonate was added to the fecal samples to free the bile acids from the resin. The bile acids and neutral sterols were then separated from the other constituents by ion exchange column chromatography as described by Kuron and Tennent.[11] The eluates obtained from the columns were clear and, from these, the dihydroxy and trihydroxy bile acids were measured spectrophotometrically,[12,13] and lithocholic acid by glass paper chromatography.[14] The neutral sterols were also measured by glass paper chromatography.[14,15]

Results

Serum Total and Esterified Cholesterol.—The effect of cholestyramine on serum total and esterified cholesterol levels in the nine patients is summarized in Table 2. Eight of the patients exhibited appreciable decreases in serum cholesterol during cholestyramine treatment. The mean serum total cholesterol levels during treatment were calculated from consecutive determinations performed during the latter portion of the treatment period, after the values had stabilized. These means varied from 80% to 50% of the average control values.

The pattern of response of patient 7 to intermittent treatment with cholestyramine over a 600-day period is shown graphically in Fig 1. In four treatment periods, each following a control period, there

was a rapid and striking decrease in serum total cholesterol values. Cholesterol esters followed a parallel course. The reduced cholesterol levels were maintained as long as treatment was continued. Individual treatment periods ranged up to 154 days. Also, a prompt cholesterol rise occurred each time cholestyramine was discontinued.

Fecal Bile Acids and Neutral Sterols.—The effect of cholestyramine administration on fecal excretion of bile acids and neutral sterols in two female patients with hypercholesteremia, one with marked xanthelasma and the other with extensive xanthomatosis, is shown in Table 3. For comparison, the response of a normal male subject, on a regular diet, to similar doses of cholestyramine also is shown. Neither he nor the two patients changed their diets while the fecal sterol studies were being carried out. The normal subject had a fivefold increase in fecal bile acids during the six-day period of cholestyramine treatment. The bile acid excretion rate returned promptly to pretreatment values upon cessation of cholestyramine administration. One hypercholesteremic subject, patient 9, exhibited an eightfold increase in bile acid excretion on 13.3 gm of cholestyramine per day and an elevenfold increase when the dose was changed to 20 gm/day. The other hypercholesteremic patient (No. 4) exhibited a fourfold increase in bile acid output in response to cholestyramine. The normal subject and both patients showed little or no increase in neutral sterol excretion during cholestyramine administration. Although patient 9 exhibited a striking increase in bile acid output in response to cholestyramine, serum

Table 2.—Serum Cholesterol Responses to Cholestyramine Resin (13.3 Gm/Day) in Nine Patients

Patient No. Sex/Age	Serum Cholesterol,* Mg/100 Ml						Duration of Treatment Days	% Decrease From Control in Mean Serum Cholesterol Values	
	Control			During Cholestyramine Treatment					
	Total	Ester	N†	Total	Ester	N†		Total	Ester
1 M/37	341 ± 27	249 ± 25	13	264 ± 29	206 ± 33	10	271	23	17
2 F/54	419 ± 5	310 ± 7	5	337 ± 24	251 ± 21	25	414	20	19
3 M/52	438 ± 37	338 ± 33	9	326 ± 23	246 ± 26	20	365	25	27
4 F/27	578 ± 40	412 ± 24	6	291 ± 7	213 ± 7	5	30	50	48
5 M/39	376 ± 14	291 ± 15	5	234 ± 11	183 ± 10	7	170	38	37
6 F/62	337 ± 11	262 ± 12	4	210 ± 6	141 ± 12	9	90	38	46
7 F/54	428 ± 16	329 ± 13	6	211 ± 14	147 ± 7	4	70	50	55
	426 ± 26	329 ± 23	7	232 ± 11	172 ± 10	7	64	45	48
	340 − 386‡	254 − 279‡	2	223 ± 15	173 ± 15	6	154	38	35
	376 ± 18	269 ± 37	6	220 − 208‡	127 − 125‡	3	28	42	52
8 F/32	756 ± 46	535 ± 61	4	533 ± 38	398 ± 27	4	174	29	26
	836 ± 69	606 ± 94	3	659 ± 67	480 ± 60	25	1,460	21	21
9 F/25	620 ± 39	447 ± 21	4	652 ± 51	477 ± 40	26	579	+5	+7

*Means and standard deviations.
†Number of consecutive determinations during latter portion of treatment period.
‡Ranges.

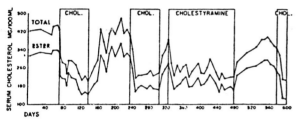

1. Effect of cholestyramine on serum cholesterol in a 54-year-old woman with hypercholesteremia.

total cholesterol and cholesterol ester levels remained virtually unchanged. In contrast, patient 4 had a marked decrease in serum cholesterol concurrently with the augmentation of her fecal bile acid excretion rate. The normal subject also showed a drop in serum cholesterol values at the time his fecal output of bile acids increased. In all three subjects studied from the standpoint of fecal bile acid output, excretion rates remained elevated as long as resin treatment was continued.

Clinical Observations and Laboratory Tests.—In general the cholestyramine was well tolerated. Because of the sandy consistency of the resin, the patients often preferred to mix the powder with a variety of foods such as fruit juices and applesauce. Some patients took the material in capsule form. Once ingested, the preparation produced occasional gastrointestinal discomfort, ranging from slight distension to manifest peptic distress. Such symptoms, more frequent during early treatment, tended to disappear after the first few weeks of resin therapy. It should be emphasized that the patients had volunteered for treatment and were well motivated toward the study. Several patients complained of constipation, which was usually controllable by adjustment of the fibre content of the diet. Systemic side effects were not encountered.

Four patients had generalized xanthomatosis and one xanthelasma at the time cholestyramine administration was begun. After prolonged treatment with the resin, all the patients with xanthomas showed some softening and diminution in size of plain and tuberous lesions; however, the changes were not quantified. One patient had several large xanthomas excised from the elbows after 30 months of treatment with cholestyramine. After 18 more months of treatment with the resin, there was no evidence of recurrence of the lesions. On previous occasions, without hypocholesteremic therapy, xanthomas removed by surgery had reappeared within six months. During a 30-day treatment period the patient with xanthelasma showed no change in palpebral deposits.

A variety of blood values was obtained in all nine subjects after cholestyramine had been administered for varying periods. The results summarized in Table 1 show that serum calcium, chloride, and carbon dioxide values were normal, as were the serum alkaline phosphatase, SGOT, prothrombin activity, and serum proteins. X-ray films of the liver of all nine patients failed to disclose evidence of enlargement or abnormal calcification.

Comment

The mechanism by which cholestyramine appears to lower the serum cholesterol level is outlined in Fig 2. By interfering with bile acid reabsorption from the intestine, cholestyramine reduces sharply the traffic of bile acids returning to the liver via the portal vein. The rate at which hepatic cholesterol is converted to bile acids is controlled in part by the concentration of bile acids reaching the liver at any given time.[16,17] Thus, cholestyramine administration would be expected to promote cholesterol oxidation to bile acids by virtue of its interference with the enterohepatic bile acid cycle.

Since the plasma cholesterol is in equilibrium

Table 3.—Effect of Cholestyramine (13.3 Gm/Day) on Fecal Sterol Excretion in
Two Hypercholesteremic Patients and Normal Subject

Patient No. Sex/Age	Fecal Bile Acids, Mg/Day* (Days of Periods)			Fecal Neutral Sterols, Mg/Day*,		
	Control (I)	During Cholestyramine Treatment	Control (II)	Control (I)	During Cholestyramine Treatment	Control (II)
4 F/27	289 ± 73 (4)	1,506 ± 503 (10)	309 ± 72 (2)	1,186 ± 183	1,090 ± 248	950 ± 110
9 F/25	150 ± 119 (5)	1,243 ± 592 (31) 1,685 ± 732† (14)	....	792 ± 426	439 ± 106 619 ± 204	....
Normal M/32	233 ± 124 (7)	1,298 ± 528 (6)	317 ± 64 (7)	798 ± 350	1,098 ± 453	1,050 ± 247

*Means and standard deviations are given.
†Dose of cholestyramine increased to 20 gm/day.

with liver cholesterol, it is not surprising that bile acid sequestration can lower the concentration of circulating cholesterol by diverting more liver cholesterol to bile acid synthesis.

Normally, the bile acids that escape reabsorption from the intestine and are lost in the feces are replaced by new bile acids produced in the liver. This and other homeostatic mechanisms favor the maintenance of a stable plasma cholesterol level for a given individual. Since resin administration is associated with plasma cholesterol lowering, it must be presumed that, until a new steady state is achieved, the rate of fecal sterol loss during cholestyramine administration is more rapid than the rate of new cholesterol synthesis.

The two patients with hypercholesteremia and xanthomatous manifestations readily increased their fecal output of bile acids in response to cholestyramine administration (Table 3). This result suggests that the "metabolic lesion" in such patients does not entail blockade of cholesterol oxidation. The lack of response of the serum cholesterol to cholestyramine administration in patient 9 may have been due to (1) an enhanced capacity of the liver to synthesize new cholesterol to replace that lost in the feces (in contrast with the other subjects studied) or (2) mobilization of cholesterol from massive tissue deposits into the plasma at a rate approximately equal to that at which cholesterol was being removed by the liver. The fact that there was a gradual reduction in the size of the xanthomas in this patient over a 19-month period of cholestyramine treatment gave some support to the latter possibility.

There is evidence that large doses of cholestyramine resin (30 gm/day) can induce mild to moderate malabsorption in normal human subjects.[1] For this reason, the effect of prolonged cholestyramine resin treatment (13.3 gm/day) on vitamin K absorption (as indicated by prothrombin activity) was determined in each patient. Prothrombin activity remained normal in all of the patients despite the fact that supplementary vitamin K was not given. It should be pointed out that none of the subjects in this series had evidence of impaired liver function or disease affecting intestinal absorption.

Values of serum calcium, alkaline phosphatase, SGOT, albumin, and globulin remained normal dur-

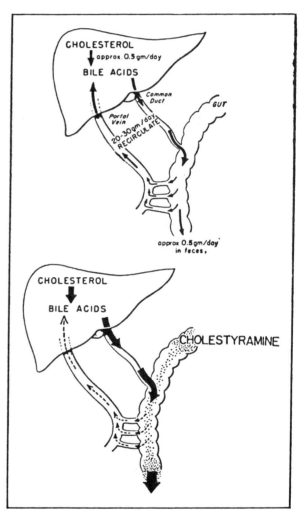

2. Postulated effect of cholestyramine on enterohepatic cycle of bile acids. Top, Enterohepatic cycle of bile acids. Bottom, Effect of bile acid sequestrant on cycle.

ing cholestyramine treatment. Because the resin was administered as the chloride salt, serum chlorides and carbon dioxide content were measured to determine whether the calculated chloride load (up to 40 mEq/day) had altered the blood electrolytes adversely. No such abnormalities were found after prolonged cholestyramine administration; however, the data do not provide information concerning possible acute effects of cholestyramine on carbon dioxide content. X-ray studies of the liver of the nine patients disclosed no evidence of abnormal calcification (Table 1). It should be emphasized that the patients referred to by Schaffner[10] had advanced liver disease, while the subjects in the present series exhibited normal hepatic function.

Since cholestyramine promotes excretion of the steroid nucleus in the feces and, presumably, is not absorbed from the intestinal lumen, it has advantages as a cholesterol-lowering drug. It is noteworthy that the resin appears to act by accelerating the major mechanism by which cholesterol and its products normally leave the body. Thus, despite its physical consistency and the relatively large dose that must be ingested to induce appreciable lowering of the serum cholesterol, cholestyramine must be considered a promising hypocholesteremic agent, combining effectiveness with safety.

This investigation was supported in part by Public Health Service research grant AM-08107.

The cholestyramine resin used in this investigation was supplied as Cuemid by Merck Sharp & Dohme Research Laboratories, West Point, Pa, and as Questran by Mead Johnson & Co., Evansville, Ind.

References

1. Tennent, D.M., et al: Plasma Cholesterol Lowering Action of Bile Acid Binding Polymers in Experimental Animals, *J Lipid Res* 1:469-473 (Oct) 1960.

2. Carey, J.B., Jr., and Williams, G.: Relief of Pruritus of Jaundice With Bile Acid Sequestering Resin, *JAMA* 176:432-435 (May 6) 1961.

3. Bergen, S.S., Jr., et al: Effect of Anion Exchange Resin on Serum Cholesterol in Man, *Proc Soc Exp Biol Med* 102:676-679 (Oct) 1959.

4. Horan, J.M.; DiLuzio, N.R.; and Etteldorf, J.N.: Use of Anion Exchange Resin in Treatment of Two Siblings With Familial Hypercholesteremia, *Pediatrics* 64:201-209 (Jan) 1964.

5. Hashim, S.A., and Van Itallie, T.B.: Use of Bile Acid Sequestrant in Treatment of Pruritus Associated With Biliary Cirrhosis, *J Invest Derm* 35:253-254 (Nov) 1960.

6. Van Itallie, T.B., et al: Treatment of Pruritus and Hypercholesteremia of Primary Biliary Cirrhosis With Cholestyramine, *New Eng J Med* 265:469-474 (Sept 7) 1961.

7. Keczkes, K.; Goldberg, D.M.; and Fergusson, A.G.: Xanthomatous Biliary Cirrhosis Treated With Cholestyramine, *Arch Intern Med* 114:321-328 (Sept) 1964.

8. Sperry, W.M., and Brand, F.C.: Colorimetric Determination of Cholesterol, *J Biol Chem* 150:312-324 (July) 1943.

9. Briscoe, A.M., and Ragan, C.; Enhancement of Calcium Absorption in Man by Bile Acid Sequestrant. *Amer J Clin Nutr* 13: 277-284 (Nov) 1963.

10. Schaffner, F.: Cholestyramine, Boon to Some Who Itch, editorial, *Gastroenterol* 46:67-70 (Jan) 1964.

11. Kuron, G.W., and Tennent, D.M.: Ion-Exchange Procedure for Separating Bile Acids From Feces and Serum, *Fed Proc* 20: 268, (March) 1961.

12. Mosbach, E.H., et al: Determination of Deoxycholic and Cholic Acids in Bile, *Arch Biochem* 51:402-410 (Aug) 1954.

13. Irvin, J.L.; Johnston, D.G.; and Kopala, J.: Photometric Method for Determination of Cholates in Bile and Blood, *J Biol Chem* 153:439-457 (Jan) 1944.

14. Swartwout, J.R., et al: Quantitative Glass Paper Chromatography: Micro-determination of Plasma Cholesterol, *J Lipid Res* 1:281-285 (July) 1960.

15. Intengen, C.L.: Studies on Coconut Oil, thesis, Columbia University, New York, 1961.

16. Bergström, S.: Metabolism of Bile Acids, *Fed Proc* 21 (suppl 11 [pt 2]):28-32 (July-Aug) 1962.

17. Van Itallie, T.B., and Hashim, S.A.: Clinical and Experimental Aspects of Bile Acid Metabolism, *Med Clin N Amer* 47: 629-648 (May) 1963.

18. Hashim, S.A., and Van Itallie, T.B.: Experimental Steatorrhea Induced in Man by Bile Acid Sequestrant, *Proc Soc Exp Biol Med* 106:173-175 (Jan) 1961.

MEDICAL PROGRESS

FAT TRANSPORT IN LIPOPROTEINS — AN INTEGRATED APPROACH TO MECHANISMS AND DISORDERS*

Donald S. Fredrickson, M.D.,† Robert I. Levy, M.D.,‡ and Robert S. Lees, M.D.§

BETHESDA, MARYLAND

THE subjects of this review are the plasma lipoproteins, their structure and functions and the ways in which they are disordered in certain diseases. The intent is not to discuss lipoproteins for their own sake, however, but to exploit their potential for illuminating the common and often frustrating clinical problem of hyperlipidemia. The finding of an abnormal concentration in plasma of cholesterol, glycerides or a given class of the lipoproteins often raises questions of cause and relief that have no certain answer. These will not necessarily be forthcoming in this report. What will be attempted is the reduction of current information about fat transport and metabolism to the minimum terms needed by a physician to obtain a rational approach to the patient with hyperlipidemia and to keep abreast of new developments in this rapidly expanding field.

The integration of information and concepts about normal mechanisms and clinical disorders will proceed from more theoretical to more practical grounds. The first part of the review will outline the normal tasks of fat transport and describe how the several plasma lipids and certain proteins interact in their performances. The proteins that have evolved mainly to participate in transport of esterified lipids and the lipoproteins that they form will be closely examined. This will include analysis of several inheritable diseases in which one of these proteins is deficient to gain perspective on the functions that they apparently serve.

A detailed discussion of hyperlipidemia will follow. This will be based on an approach developed primarily for the study of genetically determined abnormalities, but acquired or nonfamilial disorders, including changes in lipid concentrations secondary to other known disease, will be dealt with as well. All these disorders are translated into *hyperlipoproteinemia* on the premise — for which supporting evidence will be presented — that lipoprotein patterns offer necessary information not provided by analyses of plasma lipids alone. Some simple new nomenclature is offered since the older terminology

*From the Laboratory of Molecular Diseases, National Heart Institute.

†Director and chief, Laboratory of Molecular Diseases, National Heart Institute.

‡Head, Section on Lipoproteins, Laboratory of Molecular Diseases, National Heart Institute.

§Assistant professor and associate physician, Rockefeller University.

obscures the heterogeneity that has recently been discovered. Attention will also be paid to practical steps to diagnosis and conservative therapy suitable for the great majority of patients with hyperlipoproteinemia.

It will be necessary to cover the enormous literature in the area of this report in a selective rather than a comprehensive fashion. Whenever possible general references will be introduced with major topics and the number of specific citations held to a minimum.

THE NORMAL FAT-TRANSPORT TASKS[1-4]

It seems wisest to begin by considering the kinds and amounts of lipids that move through the extracellular waterways. Most of the lipid in plasma at any one time is usually not in rapid transit from one tissue to another. Cholesterol and phospholipids, which represent about two thirds of the plasma lipid, have a much slower turnover than fatty acids. In quantitative terms the major fat-transport tasks are movement of free fatty acids and fatty acid esters of glycerol (glycerides). The lipoprotein concentrations in plasma are directly and indirectly influenced by this traffic, which in turn depends on many factors, an important one of which is the state of carbohydrate metabolism.

FREE FATTY ACIDS

By far the greatest amount of fat transported through the plasma compartment is in the form of free fatty acids. This is despite their relatively insignificant contribution to the total plasma lipid concentration. In the fasting subject, there are from 0.3 to 0.7 mEq. per liter of plasma, about 8 to 20 mg. of the total lipid concentration of 400 to 800 mg. per 100 ml. The content of individual free fatty acids is similar but not identical to that of adipose-tissue triglycerides, from which they mainly originate. These fatty acids do not actually circulate in the "free" state but bound to albumin. The free-fatty-acid-albumin complex is formed immediately when fatty acids are released into the bloodstream and the complex releases its fatty acid at sites of utilization, which include liver, muscle, heart and many other tissues. This process is under sensitive metabolic control that is rapidly adjusted to meet the body's ever-changing need for metabolic fuel. Release of free fatty acids depends acutely on the availability of insulin, but is further adjusted by the sympathetic nervous system and by circulating catecholamines; adrenocortical hormones, thyroid hormone, glucagon and several anterior pituitary hormones also have permissive or secondary roles in mobilization of free fatty acids.

In the postabsorptive state from 50 to 90 per cent of the body's total energy needs are met by free fatty acids delivered from the adipose tissue. More than 25 gm. per hour may be transported through plasma during the day although much of this is re-esterified rather than oxidized immediately. The major direct contribution of the free fatty acids to plasma lipid concentrations is their conversion in the liver to glycerides. When flux of free fatty acids to the liver is unusually high, in considerable excess of the ability of that organ to burn them, the outpouring of such glyceride can be great, leading to a form of "endogenous hyperlipemia." Although the importance of free fatty acid transport cannot be overemphasized it would be tangential to our purposes to attempt to cover many details available in a number of reviews.[1-4] Free fatty acids will be mentioned further only when directly pertinent to lipoprotein metabolism and disorders thereof.

Glyceride Transport

Exogenous. From the first days of life a second major task must be performed, the disposal of glycerides that are ingested in the amount of 1 to 2 gm. per kilogram of body weight daily. These are hydrolyzed in the intestinal lumen and taken up along with smaller amounts of other lipids and lipid-soluble substances. In the mucosal cells glycerides are reformed and collected into particles. (The term particle is conventionally applied to circulating lipid-protein complexes large enough to be seen in the light microscope — that is, about 0.1 μ or larger.[5]) The chylomicrons or "exogenous particles" formed in the intestinal cells during fat absorption are released into intestinal lymphatics and enter the bloodstream through the thoracic duct. Either at the capillary surface or immediately on entering cells in adipose tissue, liver, heart and other organs, the chylomicron glycerides are hydrolyzed, and the constituent fatty acids reformed into other esters within the cell.

Endogenous. The plasma of normal fasting subjects contains glyceride in concentrations of 10 to 190 mg. per 100 ml. This glyceride, which appears for the most part to be synthesized in the liver, is in the form of very-low-density lipoproteins that will be called pre-β in this review. If the concentration of such glyceride is abnormally increased the pre-β lipoproteins become larger or particulate in size. Such "endogenous particles" differ from chylomicrons not only in their origin but also in their physical properties and their content of cholesterol, phospholipid and glyceride.[6,7]

The turnover of glycerides in pre-β lipoproteins seems to be slower than that in chylomicrons. This is more probably due to their smaller average size[6,7] than to any chemical differences, since it has been suggested that the clearing rate of particles is proportional to size.[8] At ordinary plasma concentrations the rate of removal has been calculated to be about 2 gm. per hour.[9] This estimate is subject to a number of qualifications and possibly much variation, but its relatively low order of magnitude implies that factors that accelerate synthesis and secretion of these lipoproteins may rapidly produce endogenous hyperlipemia.

36   THE NEW ENGLAND JOURNAL OF MEDICINE   Jan. 5, 1967

MINOR TRANSPORT TASKS

Cholesterol Transport[10][14]

In contrast to the large amounts of free fatty acids and glyceride that must be transported through the plasma compartment each day, the net movement of cholesterol between tissues appears to be small indeed. From 100 to 500 mg. of cholesterol per day is usually absorbed from the diet, to which is added roughly another gram of sterol resorbed from the intestinal lumen upon its secretion from bile or intestinal mucosa. Most tissues are capable of cholesterol synthesis, and none has been known to require that cholesterol be transported to it via the plasma to meet its demands, although this may be occurring, for example, in organs using cholesterol as a precursor for hormone synthesis.

An unknown amount of cholesterol must be re-transported to the liver to take advantage of this organ's unique capability to degrade sterol to bile acids, which may then be excreted. The circulating red blood cells, for example, represent a total pool of about 4 gm. of cholesterol. With the replacement of 1 per cent of this mass per day about 40 mg. of cholesterol must be transferred from sites where red cells are broken down to where they are made, or the cholesterol must be catabolized. The total of all such anabolic and catabolic processes is a daily body turnover of cholesterol approximating 1 gm.[10,11]

Cholesterol coming in from the intestine does so in association with chylomicrons, and much of this seems to disembark in the liver. From this point the exogenous cholesterol, like that which is made endogenously, is usually carried from tissue to tissue in the form of α and β lipoproteins. There is rapid exchange of free cholesterol between the various transport forms and many tissues, most swiftly between plasma, liver and red blood cells; the resultant randomization of molecules makes any calculation of net transport from tracer studies most difficult. For present purposes, the important conclusion to be drawn is that most of the cholesterol in plasma is not earmarked as cargo but is there for another purpose, as a structural component of lipoproteins, vehicles for transport of other lipid.

Phospholipid Transport

The phospholipids, which in plasma are mostly phosphatidyl choline and sphingomyelin,[15] exceed all other lipid classes in their contribution to the total mass of lipids. If these molecules have a role in carrying specific fatty acids between tissues it has thus far been a silent one. The total plasma phospholipid pool is estimated to turn over about every three days in man.[16] It is possible to reach erroneous conclusions about the turnover of phospholipids if they are considered as a single pool, for many molecular species, differing in fatty acid content, are represented. One cannot escape the intuitive conclusion, however, that the phospholipids, always predictable in their composition and varying only sluggishly in concentration, are mainly in plasma to function as "biologic detergents." Their high surface activity promotes stability at the oil-water interfaces represented by the lipoproteins and their interactions with plasma.

Carotenoids and Fat-Soluble Vitamins[17-21]

The diet contains several milligrams of various carotenoids per day. These pigments are of importance to man because some of them are convertible in the intestine into vitamin A. This essential fat-soluble vitamin is present in the diet in only microgram quantities. During digestion, vitamin A alcohol (retinol) and ester, formed in the gut from β carotene, are transported along with unchanged carotene into the bloodstream in association with lymph chylomicrons. In the postabsorptive state the carotenes are found mainly in the β lipoproteins whereas vitamin A (retinol) is associated with still unidentified proteins of density greater than the lipoproteins (more than 1.21).

Vitamin E is also transported from the intestine in the chylomicron lipids, and carried in the blood predominantly with the β lipoproteins. Little is known about the transport of vitamins D and K, but these too are probably adsorbed to the chylomicrons and carried on the β lipoproteins in the postprandial state.

To summarize the known demands for lipid transport in man and quite likely many other species, the movement of fatty acids for maintenance of "caloric homeostasis" far overshadows all other requirements. Food intake gives rise to several tidal waves of exogenous glyceride. As the last of these ebbs, and the delivery of dietary glucose declines as well, an increase in movement of free fatty acids out from the adipose tissues occurs. Some of these fatty acids and carbohydrates are converted to endogenous glycerides. The ones that the liver cannot store are sent back to the adipose tissue. The interactions of these several transport circuits and their responses to changing demands will crop up frequently as this discussion proceeds, for they are the basis for several forms of hyperlipoproteinemia.

In considering the manner in which lipids combine with proteins to serve the major transport tasks, we shall, again, only mention the important transport pathway for free fatty acids. Albumin is uniquely involved, and the protein-lipid complex formed is neither considered a lipoprotein nor measured in the usual quantification of lipids or lipoproteins. When albumin is deficient or free fatty acid concentrations are unusually high free fatty acids may travel with lipoproteins and affect the lipoprotein patterns, but these are special cases rarely encountered. The lipoproteins, on the other hand, are the keys to a more rational approach to hyperlipidemia, and the proteins involved and their various combinations with lipids will now be examined in some detail.

THE PLASMA LIPOPROTEINS[1,5,22-24]

None of the plasma lipids are sufficiently polar to circulate free in solution. They depend upon interactions with protein, and the resulting "macromolecules" or "micromicelles" are referred to by the generic term of lipoproteins. There is a tendency to restrict the term "lipoprotein" to the soluble complexes and to use the name "particle" for those that scatter light and approach a 2-phase distribution of lipid and plasma as they get large. For purposes of simplification the concept will be adopted here that there are 2 basic kinds of lipoproteins, the α and the β, and that these act to solubilize varying amounts of glyceride. Followed to its logical conclusion, this means that particles therefore contain lipoproteins. The advantages of this point of view, which has not been strictly proved to be true, will emerge presently.

There is much uncertainty about the structural relations of the lipid to the proteins in these macromolecules. It remains to be proved for any of the lipoprotein forms whether the protein serves as a film over the surface of all the lipid, exists as a central core or is sandwiched between alternate lipid moieties. The nature of the bonds between lipid and protein in the lipoproteins is also speculative. Few are covalent.[25] They are strong enough to resist dissociation during the physical processes used to isolate the lipoproteins; yet they allow for the exchange of lipid between plasma lipoproteins themselves and between tissue and plasma lipoproteins.

Isolation[1,26,27]

There are many methods for isolating and characterizing lipoproteins. These take advantage of the fact that the lipoproteins behave as euglobulins but have physical properties that are determined by their content of both protein and lipids and permit separation by methods as diverse as salting out, ethanol-salt fractionation,[28] precipitation by antibodies and nonspecific polyanions,[29] electrophoresis,[30-32] ultracentrifugation[33,34] and chromatography.[35-38]

Lipoproteins isolated by other technics are invariably equated with lipoproteins prepared by the 2 most widely used methods, ultracentrifugation and electrophoresis, which have the greatest range and adaptability. The analytical ultracentrifuge, which can quantitatively determine an almost limitless number of subgroups (S_f classes) of lipoproteins varying by small increments of differences in their densities, has capabilities beyond the current requirements of many experimental or clinical studies.[39]

The groups of lipoproteins important in clinical work are 4: high-density or α lipoproteins; low-density or β lipoproteins; very-low-density or pre-β- (also called α_2-) lipoproteins; and chylomicrons. Although everyone agrees with this subdivision as far as it goes there is not complete accord over how these groups of lipoproteins are related to each other or whether they contain subgroups that also have independent metabolic behavior.

This uncertainty is moving toward resolution through wider employment of immunochemical standards for comparing the content and measuring the purity of lipoproteins isolated by different procedures. The lipoproteins are good antigens. Their specificity devolves from the protein moiety, the lipids contributing in only a minor way as haptenes. The search for immunochemical determinants has exposed the presence of several different proteins and greatly enhanced the understanding of lipoproteins in general.

The Lipoprotein Apoproteins

Two different proteins are consistently isolated from plasma lipoproteins. A third has been found in 1 group of lipoproteins. These proteins, which some favor calling apoproteins in the lipid-free state, are generally designated as A (or α), B (or β) and C proteins. They differ in their terminal residues, total amino acid content and immunochemical behavior. The presence of 1 or both of the A and B proteins, combined with lipid, accounts for the known functions and chemical properties of all the plasma lipoproteins with one exception. This is the frequent demonstration of aminoterminal serine and threonine in proteins obtained from very-low-density lipoproteins, attributed by some to the C protein.

Normally, the A protein is the only protein found in the α_1-migrating (high-density) lipoproteins and the B protein in the β-migrating (low-density) lipoproteins. In some diseases the normal distribution of either protein is distorted. For example, A protein appears in the low-density lipoproteins in obstructive liver disease and in the rare disease, abetalipoproteinemia. At times the B protein appears in the high-density lipoproteins; most commonly this implies that the manipulations involved in lipoprotein isolation have been too severe. Both proteins can be isolated in the very-low-density lipoproteins and chylomicrons.

The appearance of A and B proteins individually in the 2 soluble lipoproteins and together in the larger glyceride-rich particles is the basis for the major simplification of lipoprotein metabolism adopted for this review (Fig. 1). This concept[40] is simplistic and vulnerable to a number of possible contradictions as knowledge of lipoproteins unfolds. In brief, it assumes that A and B proteins are the primary components of the lipoproteins. In plasma they usually occur with predictable complements of lipid that feature differing proportions of cholesterol and phospholipids. When glycerides appear in quantity these 2 lipoproteins become involved with its transport. Glyceride (Fig. 1) thus becomes the third and most dynamic factor in determining the nature of the lipoprotein distribution in plasma.

ALPHA LIPOPROTEIN

A crude α lipoprotein was isolated from horse serum in 1929 by Macheboeuf,[41] who used salt precipitation in a way somewhat similar to the later

38   THE NEW ENGLAND JOURNAL OF MEDICINE   Jan. 5, 1967

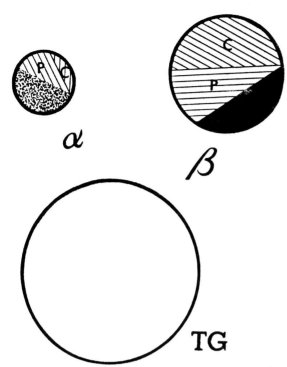

FIGURE 1. *Symbols for the 3 Most Important Factors in the Simplest Concept of Fat Transport by Lipoproteins* — α = *Alpha Lipoprotein,* β = *Beta Lipoprotein; TG = Triglyceride; the Phospholipid (P), Cholesterol (C) and Protein (Stippled for A Apoprotein and Solid for B Apoprotein)* — *Allotted Areas in the Symbols Comparable to Their Contribution by Weight to the Lipoproteins. In all subsequent figures the protein moiety only will be shown in the circular lipoprotein symbols.*

Cohn fractionation method.[28] The Cohn fraction IV-I contains lipoproteins that have α_1 mobility on either free, starch or paper electrophoresis and correspond to the "high-density" lipoproteins isolated in the ultracentrifuge between the densities of 1.063 and 1.21. Alpha lipoproteins are normally not precipitated by polyanions like heparin that aggregate all the low-density lipoproteins and are thus the only lipoproteins remaining in the supernatant after such treatment of plasma. They have the highest content of phospholipids and protein of all the lipoproteins. They are relatively stable and can be delipidated with solvents to yield a water-soluble A protein containing only a little phospholipid. The physical and chemical properties of the α lipoproteins are better known than are those of the lower-density lipoproteins. The metabolism of the latter has been far better studied, however, owing in part to the interest generated by their frequent indictment for complicity in causing atherosclerosis.

Inferences from what little is known of the comparative biochemistry of lipoproteins suggests that on the evolutionary scale the α lipoproteins may be the older of the 2 major soluble lipoproteins. In many mammals (when not hibernating) the bulk of the lipid content in the postabsorptive plasma is present in α lipoproteins.[34] In man and other primates the total weight and lipid content of the β lipoproteins is greater. Nevertheless, in human

plasma there is still much more A protein than B (approximately 140 mg. of the former as compared to 80 mg. of the latter per 100 ml.).

Neither Cohn fractionation, electrophoresis nor polyanion precipitation alone provides α lipoproteins uncontaminated by other serum proteins. Preparative ultracentrifugation must be employed when it is desired to isolate a large quantity of material as nearly pure as possible. In our experience, the highest yields are obtained by ultracentrifugation of plasma that has been brought to a density of 1.21 by the addition of salt. The supernatant is washed free of nonlipoprotein material by ultracentrifugation repeated once or, at most, twice. All the low-density lipoproteins are then precipitated with heparin and manganese.[42] Alpha lipoproteins isolated in this way ideally should contain only A protein. As determined immunochemically, however, traces of B protein are not uncommonly present.

The A Protein[22,27]

Pure α lipoproteins can be extracted to obtain the A protein. Several stages of delipidation are possible. Exposure of the lipoproteins to cold ether alone extracts only some of the cholesterol and fails to remove any of the phospholipids. Pretreatment of the lipoproteins with trypsin, chymotrypsin, or phospholipases increases the amount of lipids extracted by ether. Delipidation of lyophilized α lipoproteins in the presence of starch granules[43] removes all the neutral lipids and leaves a phospholipid protein that is quite stable and may represent an important structural unit or stage in lipoprotein formation. The best method to date for obtaining A protein that is water soluble is prolonged treatment of α lipoproteins with ethanol and ether in the cold. The product still contains a small amount of tightly bound phospholipids.

The essentially lipid-free A protein obtained by ethanol-ether extraction still contains over 3 per cent carbohydrate by weight.[44,45] The B protein isolated from β lipoproteins similarly contains carbohydrates.[46] The total amount of carbohydrates present in the lipoproteins before delipidation, their exact chemical form and whatever function they are serving remain to be determined.

The A protein obtained in this fashion seems to be a polymer or aggregate whose components readily separate and recombine in response to changes in pH, ionic strength and the presence or absence of urea or detergents like sodium dodecyl sulfate.[27,47,48] The protein may consist of identical subunits whose molecular weight has been estimated to be between 23,000 and 36,000.[48,49] Upon exposure of the A protein to depolymerizing agents, the polymer of $S_{20w}4.5$ yields several units of $S_{20w}2.3$. These units reaggregate rapidly in solution. It is believed that the A protein in native α lipoprotein represents a polymer of 2 to 6 units.

These subunits contain aminoterminal aspartic

acid and carboxyterminal threonine. In the amino acid analyzer their composition is indistinguishable. They have large amounts of glutamic acid and leucine and small amounts (1 or 2 moles per mole of protein) of isoleucine, methionine and cystine.[49,50]

Upon electrophoresis in either agar or agarose the A protein migrates more slowly than the native α lipoprotein. On starch or Pevikon this difference is reversed. The A protein appears to have a high degree of helical structural organization whether lipid is present or not, suggesting that the tertiary structure of the protein is independent of its interactions with lipid.[51]

The A protein reacts with antiserums against α lipoproteins. When ^{131}I-labeled A protein is introduced into plasma, it disappears at the same rate as α lipoprotein.[27,52] The A protein has great avidity for lipid. Whenever it is exposed to lipid suspensions in vitro or to other lipoproteins nearly all of it is recovered with the lipid or lipoproteins.

Alpha Lipoproteins[53-55]

There has not yet been convincing proof that A protein is present in plasma except as α lipoprotein. When plasma is ultracentrifuged at density 1.21 the lipoprotein-poor infranate usually yields a small amount of immunoprecipitate with anti-α-lipoprotein serum. There is no certainty that this represents α lipoprotein or A protein that was present in the native state because the process of ultracentrifugation delipidates some α lipoproteins and the products of this transformation also sediment at density 1.21.[50] Recently, an "apoprotein" capable of recombining with lipid has been described in similar preparations (density greater than 1.21 infranatant fractions) from rat plasma.[56] This protein has not yet been shown to be A (or B) protein.

The lipid and protein sedimenting at density greater than 1.21, sometimes collectively called "very-high-density lipoproteins," still remain uncertainly related to the rest of the plasma lipoproteins. This fraction accounts for about 8 per cent of the plasma phospholipids and includes trace amounts of neutral lipid. Most of the phospholipids are lysolecithins.[57] It has been proposed these may be the product of a plasma enzyme transferring a fatty acid molecule from lecithin to esterify cholesterol.[58] The lysolecithin may be complexed with albumin,[59] but further experimental confirmation is needed.

Normally most of the α lipoproteins can be isolated from plasma between the densities of 1.063 and 1.21. This is a rather broad density band, which can be further subdivided in the ultracentrifuge.[33] The heavier α-lipoprotein fractions contain relatively more A protein and phospholipid and less cholesterol than the lighter ones. The "average" α lipoproteins are composed (in dry weight) of 45 to 55 per cent protein, about 30 per cent phospholipid and about 18 per cent cholesterol. Five sixths of the latter is esterified. Small amounts of glyceride are also found in most preparations. The hydrated lipoproteins contain about 15 per cent water. Estimates of molecular weight vary from 165,000 to 400,000.[27,49,60] As determined by light-scattering and viscometry the lipoprotein seems to be a prolate ellipsoid about 300 × 50 Å.[60,61]

Compared to the β lipoproteins, the α lipoproteins contain relatively more esterified cholesterol and phospholipids. The fatty acid patterns of the different lipid moieties are similar in the 2 lipoproteins.[62] The ratio (by weight) of sphingomyelin to lecithin in α lipoproteins is about 0.2.[63]

Immunochemistry[50]

The immunochemistry of the plasma lipoproteins is summarized in Figure 2. The α lipoproteins and their A protein are less antigenic than the larger and more lipid-rich β lipoproteins. When the latter are present even in trace amounts they stimulate the production of a potent anti-β-lipoprotein serum. This is a persistent problem in preparation of antiserums to α lipoproteins. As previously indicated, antiserum prepared to either the A protein or the α lipoprotein usually crossreact. Only 1 immunologic form of α lipoprotein is usually detectable in fresh plasma. At least 1 other antigenic form becomes readily detectable after ultracentrifugation, freeze thawing or brief storage at room temperature. These 2 α lipoprotein antigens are only partially crossreactive with most antiserums. We have designated the native α lipoprotein as "αLP$_A$." This is represented by the forward migrating α-precipitation line in Figure 2. The slower migrating antigen (αLP$_B$) is partially delipidated α lipoprotein believed to contain a smaller polymer of the basic subunit of A protein. Only αLP$_A$ is present in the high-density lipoproteins isolated between density 1.063 and 1.12 (called the HDL$_2$ subclass when it is quantified in the analytical ultracentrifuge).[33] Both αLP$_A$ and αLP$_B$ are present in the subclass separated in the ultracentrifuge between densities 1.12 and 1.21 (called HDL$_3$ in the analytical ultracentrifuge). Since αLP$_B$ is formed during ultracentrifugation it has been suggested that the relative concentrations of HDL$_2$ and HDL$_3$ may represent the degree to which native α lipoproteins are dissociated in the ultracentrifuge.[50] The plasma concentrations of these 2 "forms" of α lipoproteins vary greatly with certain metabolic disorders as they are measured in the analytical ultracentrifuge.[64] It is possible that this is a function not only of the degree of dissociability of the lipoproteins but also of other factors still unappreciated that may control the amount of lipid associated with the A protein or its state of polymerization. Other small peaks have been seen in the analytical ultracentrifuge besides the HDL$_2$ and HDL$_3$ fractions.[65] The possibility that these are technical artifacts has been raised.[66]

BETA LIPOPROTEINS

The Lipoprotein

The β lipoproteins represent a second homoge-

40 THE NEW ENGLAND JOURNAL OF MEDICINE Jan. 5, 1967

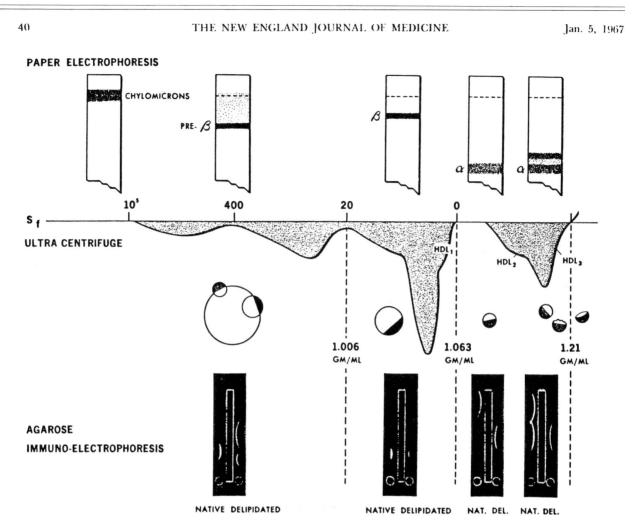

FIGURE 2. *Schematic Representation of the Major Portions of the Lipoprotein Spectrum as Defined by Paper Electrophoresis, the Ultracentrifuge and by Immunoelectrophoresis Using Antiserums Reacting with Both α and β Lipoproteins. The protein content is also depicted as in Figure 1.*

ous component of the plasma lipoproteins. In the newborn infant practically all the plasma lipid not present in α lipoproteins is found in β lipoproteins.[67] This perhaps "ideal" condition also holds in most healthy, actively growing young human beings in the postabsorptive state. As the members of most populations grow older, however, there is a progressive departure from this simple picture of plasma lipoproteins.

Beta lipoproteins migrate with sharp boundaries in the β zone on most types of electrophoresis and can be isolated in bulk in the Cohn fraction III-0. In the ultracentrifuge β lipoproteins are isolated between the densities 1.006 and 1.063 and have a mean density of about 1.03.[33] Like the α lipoproteins, β lipoproteins are found at densities less than 1.006 when plasma glyceride concentrations rise. In these cases they do not *usually* have their β mobility but are part of the pre-β lipoproteins and chylomicrons. In the analytical ultracentrifuge, according to the technic of Gofman et al.,[33,64] the pure β lipoproteins normally are in the S_f subclass of 0-20; they have a mean S_f of 6 and are mostly in the subclass S_f 0-12. (S_f refers to Svedberg units of flotation

expressed in 10^{-13} cm. per second per dyne per gram).

In man β lipoproteins are the major cholesterol-bearing lipoproteins. In the dry state a "typical" β lipoprotein consists (by weight) of 20 to 25 per cent protein, 8 per cent free and 35 per cent esterified cholesterol, 22 per cent phospholipid and 10 per cent triglyceride.[68] In its native state it is extensively hydrated. The fatty acid components of its constituent lipids are similar to those found in the total plasma lipids and in α lipoproteins.[53] There is relatively more sphingomyelin in the β lipoproteins than in α, ratio of the sphingomyelin to lecithin being about 0.4.[63]

The molecular weight of representative β lipoproteins has been estimated at anywhere from 1.3 to 3.2×10^6.[61,69] Light-scattering studies indicate that the usual complex is dyssymetric and a prolate ellipsoid of about 150×350 Å.[61]

Mild treatment with cold ether or n-heptane readily removes much of the cholesterol and glycerides from the β lipoproteins.[22,27,43] Attempts to remove the neutral lipids more completely or to strip away phospholipids usually yield a gel-like product that is irreversibly aggregated. Both the state of hydration and the presence of lipid appear to be very important in maintaining the integrity of β lipoproteins. Recently, delipidation in the presence of depolymerizing agents like urea and sodium dodecyl sulfate has shown promise of yielding a lipid-free and soluble protein from β lipoprotein.[70]

The B Protein[71-76]

The difficulties encountered in obtaining lipid-free B protein leave it less well characterized than the A protein. The low-density lipoproteins in egg yolk (lipovitellin) have been suggested as a model for β lipoprotein.[77] When these are delipidated stepwise formation of smaller protein components, each approximately half the size of its immediate precursor, occurs. The total number of polypeptide chains is partially dependent on the total lipid content of the complex. Analogous but less complete experiments with human β lipoproteins suggest that the B protein in the native lipoprotein consists of several identical or at least similar peptide chains. Two identical protein units of molecular weight 380,000 have been reported in lipoproteins having an S_f 7.9 flotation value. Other predictions of protein molecular weight have been as low as 250,000. Recent work suggests a protein on the order of 100,000 molecular weight as a possible repeating subunit.[76] The B protein contains aminoterminal glutamic acid, carboxyterminal serine and a total amino acid pattern that differs from the A protein particularly in the relative contents of isoleucine, leucine, glutamic acid and alanine.[27,50,74]

Immunochemistry[78,79]

Immunochemical studies of β lipoproteins are subject to difficulties not encountered with α owing to interactions with media commonly used for precipitation reactions. Precipitation lines may appear that do not reflect true immunoprecipitation. Purified agar and especially sulfate-free agar (agarose) have made it easier to work with β lipoproteins. In agarose they migrate in the β region and, although they still do not diffuse freely, usually give a sharp immunoprecipitation line with anti-β-lipoprotein serums (Fig. 2).

Most antiserums reacting with β lipoproteins also react with the soluble phospholipid-protein complex obtained by mild ether delipidation. Some antibodies fail to react with the products of more vigorous lipid extraction, suggesting that the neutral lipids of the lipoproteins are important as haptenes. It has not yet been shown that an anti-β-lipoprotein serum will react with a completely lipid-free B protein. This has made it impossible to learn whether B protein circulates in plasma or exists in tissues without appreciable amounts of associated lipid.

Thus far it appears that all β lipoproteins obtained from a given subject are antigenically homogeneous, but it is likely that as methods are improved antigenic forms of β lipoprotein sharing only partial

identity will be detected in the same individual as is the case with α lipoproteins. Several variations (polymorphism) in plasma β lipoproteins have already been reported in man. These fall into 3 categories. In the first place, minor antigenic differences occur between the β lipoproteins in different subjects; these appear to be genetically determined.[80,84] They are usually demonstrable by immunochemical technics using antiserums obtained from patients who have had multiple blood transfusions. Secondly, there are cases in which β lipoproteins differ from the normal in their electrophoretic and ultracentrifugal behavior. A peculiar "broad" β lipoprotein found in Type III hyperlipoproteinemia will later be described in detail. There is also a recently described "double β-lipoprotein" anomaly first detected by starch-gel electrophoresis and restricted thus far to 1 family.[85] Here there appears to be an alteration in the physical state, perhaps in degree of polymerization, of some of the β lipoproteins, giving them greater density and a higher molecular weight than the normal. This intriguing abnormality may provide a means for learning more about what controls the normal structure of the lipoprotein. Finally, the β lipoproteins also contain enzyme activity, especially esterases.[86] It is not yet known whether this is located in the B protein or represents other proteins adsorbed to the β lipoprotein molecules.

STRUCTURE AND INTRACELLULAR METABOLISM OF THE LIPOPROTEINS

No further attempt will be made here to review the fine structure of lipoproteins. The subject must lean heavily upon analogies drawn from colloidal and surface chemistry or study of bimolecular leaflets such as myelin, and little progress beyond the theoretical has been made. Since the plasma lipoproteins provide uniquely accessible models for approaching the structural features of other lipid-protein complexes in cells, knowledge in this area may be expected to increase rapidly.

When certain difficulties encountered in the study of tissue lipoproteins are overcome it will also be possible to learn more about how and where the plasma lipoproteins are synthesized and broken down. It is not easy to apply to tissues the technics presently used with plasma lipoproteins. Frequent contamination of tissues with plasma, lability of the relatively weak lipid-protein bonds and frequent exchange or adherence of labeled precursors to lipoproteins all complicate experiments dealing with cellular lipoproteins.

There is fairly good evidence that the liver is capable of synthesizing lipoproteins identical to those found in plasma. Incorporation of ^{14}C labeled amino acids, and apparently net synthesis of β lipoproteins (density less than 1.063), occurs in rat-liver slices and perfused rat livers.[87-89] The ability of the rat liver to make lipoproteins that correspond in peptide pattern to plasma α lipoproteins has been

42   THE NEW ENGLAND JOURNAL OF MEDICINE   Jan. 5, 1967

similarly demonstrated,[90] and synthesis of lipoproteins has been reported in rat-liver microsomes.[91]

Less conclusive experiments suggest that intestinal-mucosa cells can incorporate labeled amino acids into both α and β lipoproteins.[92-94] This is in keeping with a recent report that the hepatectomized dog can still synthesize plasma lipoprotein,[95] but there yet is no basis for assessing the contribution of the intestine to the plasma lipoprotein pools.

Inhibitors of protein synthesis such as puromycin cause accumulation of lipid in both the intestinal and liver cells and therefore presumably inhibit either the synthesis or the release of plasma lipoproteins.[96,97] In the liver the same effect has been shown for hepatotoxins such as carbon tetrachloride. Orotic acid not only produces a fatty liver but eliminates nearly all the plasma β lipoprotein in rats, a nearly specific effect that is quickly reversed by adenine.[98,99]

Turnover of plasma α lipoproteins has been studied by labeling of the protein with [131]I. The biologic half-life of the protein, either in lipoprotein or as apoprotein is about four days.[27,52,100] A similar half-life has been obtained with β lipoprotein tagged with either ^{131}I or [35]S.[100,101] The plasma lipoprotein proteins thus turn over faster than most other major plasma proteins with the exception of fibrinogen.[101]

Recapitulation

Those who feel no great concern with the minutiae concerning the plasma lipoproteins may find it easiest to consider the essential elements as being 3, all represented symbolically in Figure 1. Two of these are lipoproteins. Each consists of a different protein, the A (or α) and the B (or β), that has unusual affinity for lipids and prefers to circulate in extracellular fluid accompanied by a complement of cholesterol and phospholipid. The lipoproteins that result have densities and electrostatic charges that differ sufficiently to permit their operational definition by several technics. By the most commonly employed methods, electrophoresis and the ultracentrifuge, they are identified as α, or high-density, lipoproteins and β, or low-density, lipoproteins.

The α and β lipoproteins normally account for about 90 per cent of the cholesterol and phospholipid in plasma. The concentrations of those lipids undergo very little tidal change in comparison to that of the other major group of neutral lipids found in plasma, the glycerides. Glycerides are the third element in any discussion of lipoproteins and fat transport (Fig. 1). They are the dynamic factor to which the α and β lipoproteins seem related as vehicles are to cargo. When appreciable glyceride is present in plasma it associates with both α and β lipoproteins in such a way as to decrease their density and alter the net effect of the charges on the lipoproteins. The resultant combinations differ, depending on whether the glycerides are coming in from the diet or are made in the body. This distinction is of great importance when one is in dealing

with hyperlipoproteinemia and merits detailed consideration, which will be given in the next section of this review.

(To be continued)

REFERENCES

1. Fredrickson, D. S., and Gordon, R. S., Jr. Transport of fatty acids. *Physiol. Rev.* **38**:585-630, 1958.
2. Olson, R. E., and Vester, J. W. Nutrition-endocrine interrelationships in control of fat transport in man. *Physiol. Rev.* **40**: 677-733, 1960.
3. Fritz, I. B. Factors influencing rates of long-chain fatty acid oxidation and synthesis in mammalian systems. *Physiol. Rev.* **41**:52-129, 1961.
4. Steinberg, D. Fatty acid mobilization — mechanisms of regulation and metabolic consequences. In *The Control of Lipid Metabolism*. Edited by J. K. Grant. 191 pp. New York: University Press, 1963. (Biochem. Society Symposium 24.) Pp. 111-143.
5. Dole, V. P., and Hamlin, J. T., III. Particulate fat in lymph and blood. *Physiol. Rev.* **42**:674-701, 1962.
6. Bierman, E. L., Porte, D., Jr., O'Hara, D. D., Schwartz, M., and Wood, F. C., Jr. Characterization of fat particles in plasma of hyperlipemic subjects maintained on fat-free high-carbohydrate diets. *J. Clin. Investigation* **44**:261-270, 1965.
7. Lees, R. S., and Fredrickson, D. S. Differentiation of exogenous and endogenous hyperlipemia by paper electrophoresis. *J. Clin. Investigation* **44**:1968-1977, 1965.
8. Quarfordt, S. H., and Goodman, D. S. Heterogeneity in rate of plasma clearance of chylomicrons of different size. *Biochim. et biophys. acta* **116**:382-385, 1966.
9. Reaven, G. M., Hill, D. B., Gross, R. C., and Farquhar, J. E. Kinetics of triglyceride turnover of very low density lipoproteins of human plasma. *J. Clin. Investigation* **44**:1826-1833, 1965.
10. Bergström, S. Metabolism of bile acids. *Federation Proc.* **21** (Supp. 11):28-32, 1962.
11. Danielsson, H. Present status of research on catabolism and excretion of cholesterol. *Advances in Lipid Research* **1**:335-385, 1963.
12. Spritz, N., Ahrens, E. H., Jr., and Grundy, S. Sterol balance in man as plasma cholesterol concentrations are altered by exchanges of dietary fats. *J. Clin. Investigation* **44**:1482-1493, 1965.
13. Wilson, J. D., and Lindsey, C. A., Jr. Studies on influence of dietary cholesterol on cholesterol metabolism in isotopic steady state in man. *J. Clin. Investigation* **44**:1805-1814, 1965.
14. Goodman, D. S. Cholesterol ester metabolism. *Physiol. Rev.* **45**:747-839, 1965.
15. Phillips, G. B. Phospholipid composition of human serum lipoprotein fractions separated by ultracentrifugation. *J. Clin. Investigation* **38**:489-493, 1959.
16. Moser, H. W., and Emerson, K., Jr. Estimation of phospholipid phosphorus turnover time in man: studies in normal individuals, in patients with nephrotic syndrome and in other types of hyperlipemia. *J. Clin. Investigation* **34**:1286-1296, 1955.
17. Deuel, H. J., Jr. Metabolism and nutritional value of carotenoids and vitamins A. In *The Lipids*. Vol. 3. 1065 pp. New York: Interscience, 1957. P 421.
18. Krinsky, N. I., Cornwell, D. G., and Oncley, J. L. Transport of vitamin A and carotenoids in human plasma. *Arch. Biochem.* **73**:233-246, 1958.
19. McCormick, E. C., Cornwell, D. G., and Brown, J. B. Studies on distribution of tocopherol in human serum lipoproteins. *J. Lipid Research* **1**:221-228, 1960.
20. Olson, J. A. Biosynthesis and metabolism of carotenoids and retinol (vitamin A). *J. Lipid Research* **5**:281-299, 1964.
21. Huang, H. S., and Goodman, D. S. Vitamin A and carotenoids. I. Intestinal absorption and metabolism of ^{14}C-labeled vitamin A alcohol and β-carotene in rat. *J. Biol. Chem.* **240**:2839-2844, 1965.
22. Gurd, F. R. N. Some naturally occurring lipoprotein systems. In *Lipide Chemistry*. Edited by D. J. Hanahan. 325 pp. New York: Wiley, 1960. P. 260.
23. Vandenheuvel, F. A. Origin, metabolism, and structure of normal human serum lipoproteins. *Canad. J. Biochem. & Physiol.* **40**:1299-1326, 1962.
24. Salem, L. Role of long-range forces in cohesion of lipoproteins. *Canad. J. Biochem. & Physiol.* **40**:1287-1297, 1962.
25. Fisher, W., and Gurin, S. Structure of lipoproteins: covalently bound fatty acids. *Science* **143**:362, 1964.
26. Lindgren, F. T., and Nichols, A. V. Structure and function of human serum lipoproteins. In *The Plasma Proteins*. Vol. II.

Edited by F. W. Putnam. 518 pp. New York: Academic Press, 1960. P. 1.

27. Scanu, A. M. Factors affecting lipoprotein metabolism. *Advances in Lipid Research* **3**:63-138, 1965.

28. Cohn, E. J., et al. Preparation and properties of serum and plasma proteins. IV. System for separation into fractions of protein and lipoprotein components of biological tissues and fluids. *J. Am. Chem. Soc.* **68**:459-475, 1946.

29. Cornwell, D. G., and Kruger, F. A. Molecular complexes in isolation and characterization of plasma lipoproteins. *J. Lipid Research* **2**:110-134, 1961.

30. Jencks, W. P., Hyatt, M. R., Jetton, M. R., Mattingly, T. W., and Durrum, E. L. Study of serum lipoproteins in normal and atherosclerotic patients by paper electrophoretic techniques. *J. Clin. Investigation* **35**:980-990, 1956.

31. Kunkel, H. G., and Trautman, R. α_2 Lipoproteins of human serum: correlation of ultracentrifugal and electrophoretic properties. *J. Clin. Investigation* **35**:641-648, 1956.

32. Nikkilä, E. Studies on lipid-protein relationships in normal and pathological sera and effect of heparin on serum lipoproteins. *Scandinav. J. Clin. & Lab. Investigation* **5** (Supp. 8):1-101, 1958.

33. de Lalla, O. F., and Gofman, J. W. Ultracentrifugal analysis of serum lipoproteins. In *Methods of Biochemical Analysis*. Edited by D. Glick. 528 pp. New York: Interscience, 1954. P. 459.

34. Havel, R. J., Eder, H. A., and Bragdon, J. H. Distribution and chemical composition of ultracentrifugally separated lipoproteins in human serum. *J. Clin. Investigation* **34**:1345-1353, 1955.

35. Hjertén, S. Calcium phosphate chromatography of normal human serum and of electrophoretically isolated serum proteins. *Biochim. et biophys. acta* **31**:216-235, 1959.

36. Carlson, L. A. Chromatographic separation of serum lipoproteins on glass powder columns: description of method and some applications. *Clin. chim. acta* **5**:528-538, 1960.

37. Cramér, K. Serum β-lipoprotein lipids and protein in normal subjects of different sex and age. *Acta med. Scandinav.* **171**:413-427, 1962.

38. Peeters, H., and Laga, E. Electrochromatography of serum lipoproteins. In *Protides of the Biological Fluids*. Edited by H. Peeters. 476 pp. Amsterdam C: Elsevier, 1963. P. 134.

39. Ewing, A. M., Freeman, N. K., and Lindgren, F. T. Analysis of human serum lipoprotein distributions. *Advances in Lipid Research* **3**:25-61, 1965.

40. Fredrickson, D. S., and Levy, R. I. Functional view of plasma lipoproteins. In *Proceedings of The Mosbach Colloquium of the Society for Physiological Chemistry*. Heidelberg: Springer (in press).

41. Macheboeuf, M. M. A. Recherches sur les phosphoaminolipides et les stérides du sérum et du plasma sanguins. I. Entraînement des phospholipides, des stérols et des stérides par les diverses fractions au cours du fractionnement des protéides du sérum. *Bull. Soc. chim. biol.* **11**:268-293, 1929.

42. Burstein, M., and Samaille, J. Sur un dosage rapide du cholesterol lié aux α- et aux β-lipoprotéines du sérum. *Clin. chim. acta* **5**:609, 1960.

43. Gustafson, A. New method for partial delipidization of serum lipoproteins. *J. Lipid Research* **6**:512-517, 1965.

44. von Schultze, H. E. Über Glykoproteine. *Deutsche med. Wchnschr.* **83**:1742-1752, 1958.

45. Epstein, F. H., and Block, W. D. Glycoprotein content of serum lipoproteins. *Proc. Soc. Exper. Biol. & Med.* **101**:740-742, 1959.

46. Marshall, W. E., and Kummerow, F. A. Carbohydrate constituents of human serum β-lipoprotein: galactose, mannose, glucosamine and sialic acid. *Arch. Biochem.* **98**:271-273, 1962.

47. Sanbar, S. S., and Alaupovic, P. Effect of urea on behavior of protein moiety of human-serum α-lipoproteins in solution. *Biochim. et biophys. acta* **71**:235, 1963.

48. Scanu, A. Forms of human serum high density lipoprotein protein. *J. Lipid Research* **7**:295-306, 1966.

49. Shore, V., and Shore, B. Protein subunit of human serum lipoproteins of density 1.125-1.200 gram/ml. *Biochem & Biophys. Research. Commun.* **9**:455-460, 1962.

50. Levy, R. I., and Fredrickson, D. S. Heterogeneity of plasma high density lipoproteins. *J. Clin. Investigation* **44**:426-441, 1965.

51. Scanu, A. Studies on conformation of human serum high-density lipoproteins HDL$_2$ and HDL$_3$. *Proc. Nat. Acad. Sc.* **54**:1699-1705, 1965.

52. Furman, R. H., Sanbar, S. S., Alaupovic, P., Bradford, R. H., and Howard, R. P. Studies of metabolism of radioiodinated human serum alpha lipoprotein in normal and hyperlipidemic subjects. *J. Lab. & Clin. Med.* **63**:193-204, 1964.

53. Freeman, N. K., Lindgren, F. T., and Nichols, A. V. Chemistry of serum lipoproteins. In *Progress in the Chemistry of Fats and*

Other Lipids. Vol. 6. Edited by R. T. Holman, W. O. Lundberg and T. Malkin. 364 pp. New York: Macmillan, 1963. P. 215.

54. Oncley, J. L. Lipid protein interactions. In *Brain Lipids and Lipoproteins, and the Leucodystrophies*. Edited by J. Folchi-Pi and H. Bauer. 213 pp. Amsterdam C: Elsevier, 1963. P. 1.

55. Fredrickson, D. S. Familial high-density lipoprotein deficiency: Tangier disease. In *The Metabolic Basis of Inherited Disease*. Second edition. Edited by J. B. Stanbury, J. B. Wyngaarden and D. S. Fredrickson. 1434 pp. New York: McGraw-Hill, 1966. P. 486.

56. Roheim, P. S., Miller, L., and Eder, H. A. Formation of plasma lipoproteins from apoprotein in plasma. *J. Biol. Chem.* **240**:2994-3001, 1965.

57. Phillips, G. B. Lipid composition of human serum lipoprotein fraction with density greater than 1.210. *Proc. Soc. Exper. Biol. & Med.* **100**:19-22, 1959.

58. Glomset, J. A. Further studies of mechanism of plasma cholesterol esterification reaction. *Biochim. et biophys. acta* **70**:389-395, 1963.

59. Switzer, S., and Eder, H. A. Transport of lysolecithin by albumin in human and rat plasma. *J. Lipid Research* **6**:506-511, 1965.

60. Hazelwood, R. N. Molecular weights and dimensions of some high-density human serum lipoproteins. *J. Am. Chem. Soc.* **80**:2152-2156, 1958.

61. Björklund, R., and Katz, S. Molecular weights and dimensions of some human serum lipoproteins. *J. Am. Chem. Soc.* **78**:2122-2126, 1956.

62. Lindgren, F. T., Nichols, A. V., and Wills, R. D. Fatty acid distributions in serum lipids and serum lipoproteins. *Am. J. Clin. Nutrition* **9**:13-23, 1961.

63. Nelson, G. J., and Freeman, N. K. Phospholipid and phospholipid fatty acid composition of human serum lipoprotein fractions. *J. Biol. Chem.* **235**:578-583, 1960.

64. Gofman, J. W., et al. Serum lipoprotein transport system in health, metabolic disorders, atherosclerosis and coronary artery disease. *Plasma* **2**:413-484, 1954.

65. Barclay, M., Barclay, R. K., Terebus-Kekish, O., Shah, E. B., and Skipski, V. P. Disclosure and characterization of new high-density lipoproteins in human serum. *Clin. chim. acta* **8**:721-726, 1963.

66. Lindgren, F. T. New high-density lipoproteins in human serum? *Clin. chim. acta* **9**:402-404, 1964.

67. Auerswald, W., Doleschel, W., and Müller-Hartburg, W. Flotationsanalytische Untersuchungen der Lipoproteinverteilung im mütterlichen und im Nabelschnurblut. *Klin. Wchnschr.* **41**:580-584, 1963.

68. Bragdon, J. H., Havel, R. J., and Boyle, E. Human serum lipoproteins. 1. Chemical composition of four fractions. *J. Lab. & Clin. Med.* **48**:36-42, 1956.

69. Oncley, J. L., Scatchard, G., and Brown, A. Physical-chemical characteristics of certain of proteins of normal human plasma. *J. Physiol. Chem.* **51**:184-198, 1947.

70. Granda, J. L., and Scanu, A. Studies on protein moiety of serum low-density lipoproteins (LDL). *Federation Proc.* **24**:224, 1965.

71. Shore, B. C- and N-terminal amino acids of human serum lipoproteins. *Arch. Biochem.* **71**:1-10, 1957.

72. Bernfeld, P., and Kelley, T. F. Proteolysis of human serum β-lipoprotein. *J. Biol. Chem.* **239**:3341-3346, 1964.

73. Banasyak, L. J., and McDonald, H. J. Proteolysis of human serum β-lipoproteins. *Biochemistry* **1**:344-349, 1962.

74. Margolis, S., and Langdon, R. G. Studies on human serum β$_1$-lipoprotein. I. Amino acid composition. *J. Biol. Chem.* **241**:469-476, 1966.

75. Idem. Studies on human serum β$_1$-lipoprotein. II. Chemical modifications. *J. Biol. Chem.* **241**:477-484, 1966.

76. Idem. Studies on human serum β$_1$-lipoprotein. III. Enzymatic modifications. *J. Biol. Chem.* **241**:485-493, 1966.

77. Augustyniak, J., Martin, W. G., and Cook, W. H. Characterization of lipovitellenin components, and their relation to low-density lipoprotein structure. *Biochim. et biophys. acta* **84**:721-728, 1964.

78. Levy, R. I., Lees, R. S., and Fredrickson, D. S. Nature of prebeta (very low density) lipoproteins. *J. Clin. Investigation* **45**:63-77, 1966.

79. Levy, R. I., Fredrickson, D. S., and Laster, L. Lipoproteins and lipid transport in abetalipoproteinemia. *J. Clin. Investigation* **45**:531-541, 1966.

80. Blumberg, B. S., Bernanke, D., and Allison, A. C. Human lipoprotein polymorphism. *J. Clin. Investigation* **41**:1936-1944, 1962.

81. Berg, K. New serum type system: Lp system. *Acta path. et microbiol. Scandinav.* **59**:369-382, 1963.

44   THE NEW ENGLAND JOURNAL OF MEDICINE   Jan. 5, 1967

82. Allison, A. C., and Blumberg, B. S. Serum lipoprotein allotypes in man. In *Progress in Medical Genetics*. Vol. 4. Edited by A. G. Steinberg and A. G. Bearn. 280 pp. New York: Grune, 1965. P. 176.

83. Speiser, P., and Pausch, V. Das erbliche Serum β-lipoprotein System Lp (α, x) *Ann. pardiat.* **205**:193-202, 1965.

84. Berg, K. New serum type system in man — Ld system. *Vox Sang* **10**:513-527, 1965.

85. Seegers, W., Hirschhorn, K., Burnett, L., Robson, E., and Harris, H. Double beta lipoprotein: new genetic variant in man. *Science* **149**:303, 1965.

86. Lawrence, S. H., and Melnick, P. J. Enzymatic activity related to human serum beta-lipoprotein: histochemical, immunoelectrophoretic and quantitative studies. *Proc. Soc. Exper. Biol. & Med.* **107**:998-1001, 1961.

87. Radding, C. M., Bragdon, J. H., and Steinberg, D. Synthesis of low- and high-density lipoproteins by rat liver *in vitro. Biochim. et biophys. acta* **30**:443, 1958.

88. Marsh, J. B., and Whereat, A. F. Synthesis of plasma lipoprotein by rat liver. *J. Biol. Chem.* **234**:3196-3200, 1959.

89. Haft, D. E., Roheim, P. S., White, A., and Eder, H. A. Plasma lipoprotein metabolism in perfused rat livers. 1. Protein synthesis and entry into plasma. *J. Clin. Investigation* **41**:842-849, 1962.

90. Radding, C. M., and Steinberg, D. Studies on synthesis and secretion of serum lipoproteins by rat liver slices. *J. Clin. Investigation* **39**:1560-1569, 1960.

91. de Jong, J. B., and Marsh, J. B. Synthesis of plasma lipoproteins by rat liver ribosomes. *Federation Proc.* **25**:581, 1966.

92. Rodbell, M., Fredrickson, D. S., and Ono, K. Metabolism of chylomicron proteins in dog. *J. Biol. Chem.* **234**:567-571, 1959.

93. Hatch, F. T., Hagopian, L. M., Rubinstein, J. J., and Canellos, G. P. Incorporation of labeled leucine into lipoprotein protein by rat intestinal mucosa. *Circulation* **28**:659, 1963.

94. Isselbacher, K. J., and Budz, D. H. Synthesis of lipoproteins by rat intestinal mucosa. *Nature* (London) **200**:364, 1963.

95. Roheim, P. S., Gidez, L. I., and Eder, H. A. Extrahepatic synthesis of lipoproteins of plasma and chyle: role of intestine. *J. Clin. Investigation* **45**:297-300, 1966.

96. Robinson, D. S., and Seakins, A. Development in rat of fatty livers associated with reduced plasma-lipoprotein synthesis. *Biochim. et biophys. acta* **62**:163-165, 1962.

97. Sabesin, S. M., Drummey, G. D., Budz, D. M., and Isselbacher, K. J. Inhibition of protein synthesis: mechanism for production of impaired fat absorption. *J. Clin. Investigation* **43**:1281, 1964.

98. Windmueller, H. G. Orotic acid-induced, adenine-reversed inhibition of hepatic lipoprotein secretion in rat. *J. Biol. Chem.* **239**:530-537, 1964.

99. Windmueller, H. G., and Levy, R. I. Complete and reversible inhibition of hepatic beta-lipoprotein release in rat by orotic acid. *Circulation* **34**:239, 1966.

100. Gitlin, D., et al. Studies on metabolism of plasma proteins in nephrotic syndrome. II. Lipoproteins. *J. Clin. Investigation* **37**:172-184, 1958.

101. Volwiler, W., et al. Biosynthetic determination with radioactive sulfur of turn-over rates of various plasma proteins in normal and cirrhotic man. *J. Clin. Investigation* **34**:1126-1146, 1955.

MEDICAL PROGRESS

FAT TRANSPORT IN LIPOPROTEINS — AN INTEGRATED APPROACH TO MECHANISMS AND DISORDERS (Continued)*

DONALD S. FREDRICKSON, M.D.,† ROBERT I. LEVY, M.D.,‡ AND ROBERT S. LEES, M.D.§

BETHESDA, MARYLAND

GLYCERIDE TRANSPORT

Two Forms of Plasma Glyceride Transport

In subjects on fat-free diets the plasma lipid concentrations vary little throughout the day and tend to be highest just before breakfast.[102] When the diet contains fat the levels of cholesterol and phospholipids in plasma are still relatively constant, but the glyceride concentration, as already intimated, is quite variable. It is lowest during the early morning hours (when blood samples for analysis are usually taken) and rises sharply, reaching a peak about three hours after breakfast. The concentration is boosted again by the midday meal, and after some decline in the afternoon, again rises after dinner, ebbing during the night.

The form in which glycerides are transported in the plasma depends on whether their immediate source is dietary fat or endogenous synthesis (Fig. 3). In normal subjects before breakfast, and in those on fat-free diets at all times, the plasma glycerides are exclusively of endogenous origin and are carried predominantly on pre-β lipoproteins and particles. Glycerides from dietary fat, on the other hand, are carried on the chylomicrons.

*From the Laboratory of Molecular Diseases, National Heart Institute.

†Director and chief, Laboratory of Molecular Diseases, National Heart Institute.

‡Head, Section on Lipoproteins, Laboratory of Molecular Diseases, National Heart Institute.

§Assistant professor and associate physician, Rockefeller University.

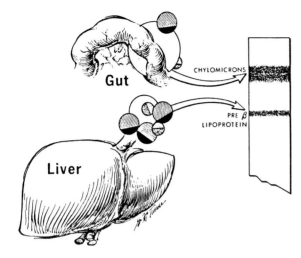

FIGURE 3. *Origins of Plasma Glycerides and the Lipoproteins in Which They Are Found as Separated by Paper Electrophoresis.*

METHODS

Analytical methods for the detection and quantitation of α and β lipoproteins are relatively simple, and the technics employed are generally comparable from one laboratory to another. In the analysis of the glyceride-rich lipoproteins, however, there is no such uniformity. Many different procedures are used, none of them ideal. The ones that are of greatest value at present have one common feature, the ability to provide a qualitative separation of lipoproteins and particles carrying mainly endogenous glycerides from those containing exogenous glycerides. These technics, collated in Table 1, will be considered one by one.

Ultracentrifugation

The preparative ultracentrifuge separates lipoproteins according to their flotation characteristics, which depend upon size and density. It can be used to separate the main chylomicron (exogenous) glyceride mass from the endogenous particles. Such separations are not complete, however, for the flotation rates of chylomicrons and endogenous particles overlap.[6,7,103] Thus, the "chylomicron" fractions prepared by exposure of plasma to centrifugal fields of about 10^5 g. per minute may contain a variable mixture of endogenous as well as exogenous particles. After this fraction has been removed a species of very-low-density lipoproteins can next be isolated

that is generally considered endogenous in origin. It is of S_f 20–400 and identical to the pre-β lipoproteins separated by paper electrophoresis.[104] By manipulation of the diet of subjects serving as lipoprotein sources — for example, fat-free diets, high in carbohydrate, which induce high concentrations of endogenous glycerides, or high-fat diets, which produce transient chylomicronemia — the preparative ultracentrifuge may be used to obtain quantities of pure or nearly pure particles of the two types.[7,78]

Precipitation

Precipitation methods are among the oldest of the technics for preparing lipoproteins and are of great usefulness in the isolation of pure lipoproteins.[29] No reliable way has yet been found to use precipitation alone for precise subfractionation of very-low-density lipoproteins and particles. Dextran sulfate, amylopectin sulfate, heparin or polyvinylpyrrolidone precipitate endogenous and exogenous particles together.[29] The combination of gradient flotation and precipitation by polyvinylpyrrolidone is used to separate chylomicrons into 2 classes, "primary" and "secondary" particles, and these exogenous particles can also be separated from endogenous particles.[6,105] This technic can be employed to distinguish endogenous and exogenous hyperlipemia and is particularly useful for preparative work since the flocculated particles can be recovered for lipid and other analyses.

Electrophoresis

It was noted quite early in the study of plasma by free electrophoresis that the turbidity in lipemic samples obscured underlying protein peaks.[106] Exogenous particles in lymph were shown to migrate with albumin whereas those in plasma moved with β globulin. When the simpler technic of electrophoresis in an inert medium of starch granules was devised, similar turbid peaks were found and the separateness of an α_2 lipoprotein (pre-β lipoproteins on paper electrophoresis) established.[107] More recently it has been demonstrated that exogenous particles in plasma may accumulate in 2 regions on starch blocks.[6,108] Exogenous particles in the α_2 zone are called "primary" because they appear in plasma early after fat ingestion. The other group of exogenous particles appear somewhat later in the β zone and are called "secondary." The primary particles

TABLE 1. *Very-Low-Density Lipoproteins—Composition and Correlations.*

BAND ON PAPER ELECTROPHORESIS	MIGRATION IN STARCH-BLOCK ELECTROPHORESIS	LOCATION IN POLYVINYL-PYRROLIDONE DENSITY GRADIENT	APPROXIMATE S_f BY ULTRACENTRIFUGATION	PROTEIN	LIPID		
					GLYCERIDE	CHOLESTEROL	PHOSPHOLIPID
				% total weight	% total lipid	% total lipid	% total lipid
Chylomicron	α_2 (primary particles)	Top	>400	0.5–2.5	79–95	2–12	3–15
	β (secondary particles)	Bottom	>400				
Pre-β	α_2	Throughout tube	>400	2–10	60–80	10–20	10–20
			20–400	10–13	50–70	10–25	15–25

tend to be superimposed upon endogenous lipoproteins and particles when the latter are present.

Similar separations can be achieved with the simpler technic of paper electrophoresis. It was early noted that with barbital buffer, chylomicrons remain at the origin, as do the larger endogenous particles, whereas the smaller particles and S_f 20-400 lipoproteins form a "pre-β" band.[104,109,110] When albumin is added to buffer to decrease adsorption to the paper sharper separations are obtained.[111,112] The chylomicrons (both "primary" and "secondary" exogenous particles) remain at the point of application; the endogenous glyceride-rich lipoproteins are concentrated in the pre-β position, with trailing of the larger endogenous particles between the origin and pre-β region.[7,112]

Nature of Pre-β Lipoproteins[7R]

The pre-β lipoproteins and endogenous particles cover a wide density spectrum varying from 1.006 to 0.93. Their composition depends on their density. As the density decreases, the relative proportion of glyceride rises, and that of protein falls. The fatty acid pattern of a given subclass is not the same in all subjects; grosser differences may obtain between normal and abnormal subjects. Nevertheless, certain generalizations can be made about the composition of the usual pre-β group of lipoproteins (Table 1). Lipids make up over 85 per cent of the total weight of the complex, protein being 2 to 15 per cent. Glyceride is the major lipid class. When pre-β lipoproteins and particles are isolated under conditions that minimize lipid exchange with other lipoproteins, the glyceride fatty acid composition is that of endogenously synthesized fat, low in linoleic acid and high in palmitic and oleic acids.[6,7]

Proteins in Pre-β Complexes[7R,113]

The protein moiety of pre-β lipoproteins was for a long time considered to be mainly or exclusively the B protein, identical to that in the β lipoproteins.[114] Native pre-β lipoproteins react with anti-β-lipoprotein serums and not with anti-α serums. Certain chemical findings, however, were never explained by the assumption of a single protein. The increased electrophoretic mobility of pre-β lipoproteins over that of β lipoproteins, the higher ratio of phospholipid to cholesterol and a significant content of aminoterminal aspartic acid (the same as in the A protein) in the protein residues, spurred a search for other companions of the B protein in pre-β lipoproteins. Recently, it has been shown that after careful delipidation of pre-β lipoproteins significant amounts of both α and β lipoproteins are immunologically identifiable (Fig. 2). Hydrolysis of pre-β lipoproteins catalyzed by postheparin enzymes also immediately increases the plasma content of α and β lipoproteins. In subjects fed various experimental diets the concentrations of pre-β lipoproteins vary inversely with those of α and β lipoproteins. The evidence is good that both the A and B proteins, probably as their lipoproteins, are normally present in the triglyceride-rich complexes grouped as pre-β (very-low-density) lipoproteins.

C protein.[113] Analyses of the proteins obtained in pre-β lipoproteins and particles usually reveal some aminoterminal residues (threonine and serine) differing from those in the A or B proteins. The amounts have been variable, and the source conjectural.[1] In recent years one series of studies have dealt with the isolation of a third protein, called apoprotein C. This apoprotein has been isolated as a phospholipid-protein complex along with the A and B apoproteins after lyophilization and partial delipidation of very-low-density lipoproteins with heptane. Whether the particle sources of this protein contain glycerides of endogenous or exogenous origin has not been established. The C apoprotein is characterized as a 7S protein with hydrated density of 1.09 (gm. per milliliter) and a molecular weight of about 834,000. Although it appears homogeneous in the analytical ultracentrifuge it migrates as a double band with a prealbumin position on starch-gel electrophoresis and contains both aminoterminal serine and threonine. The C apoprotein fails to react with antiserums to α and β lipoprotein. Peptide fingerprints obtained by trypsin or pepsin digestion have been considered different from those of the A and B apoproteins. The C apoprotein apparently binds phospholipid more avidly than A or B. The bid of C protein for entry into the family of fat-transporting proteins is greeted with great interest. Although its presence in glyceride-rich particles is as indubitable as its separateness from apoproteins A and B, it remains for further work to demonstrate its specificity and its physiologic role. There is not yet sufficient knowledge about it to fit C protein into any of the concepts being developed in this review, and it does not appear in any of the accompanying illustrations.

Metabolism of Endogenous Glyceride[1,3,4,115-117]

Considerable evidence points to the liver as the major site of synthesis of the endogenous triglyceride and presumably elaboration of many if not all of the circulating pre-β lipoproteins. An important source of fatty acid substrate for glyceride synthesis is the plasma free fatty acids. The flux of free fatty acids into liver, heart, skeletal muscle and other tissues is governed by their rate of release from adipose tissue. Any factor that increases lipolysis or decreases glycerol esterification in the adipose tissue causes outpouring of free fatty acids.[118] Much of this free fatty acid is removed by the liver, and the excess beyond what it can use or store is resynthesized into glycerides and resecreted as pre-β lipoproteins since the acids apparently are not returned to adipose tissue as such. A significant "overshoot" in release of free fatty acids, therefore, may temporarily elevate the plasma glyceride concentration. Potential causes of hyper-pre-β lipoproteinemia include a number of abnormal physiologic states that are accompanied by increased release of free fatty acids.

Carbohydrate induction.[119-124] Endogenous hyperlipemia perhaps first became a distinctly recognized phenomenon in 1950, when Watkin and his co-workers[119] noted that fat-free, high-carbohydrate diets increased the glyceride concentration in a group of hypertensive men. Many others have confirmed and extended these observations. The concept of carbohydrate-induced hyperlipemia is an important outgrowth of such studies. Not all carbohydrate induction is abnormal, however, for it is now clear that the response of practically all subjects to very high-carbohydrate feeding is conversion of much of the carbohydrate to fat and its eventual release into the plasma as pre-β lipoproteins. In healthy young subjects the plasma glyceride rises to a peak three to ten days after the beginning of carbohydrate feeding and usually falls slowly thereafter despite continuation of the diet. The response is widely variable; the average rise in glyceride concentration is about 200 mg. per 100 ml. above the initial level, but in a "normal" subject may be as much as 400 mg. per 100 ml.[124] The ease of induction of endogenous hyperlipemia in normal subjects is probably due to the relatively limited rate of removal of such lipid from the plasma. The previously mentioned estimates of a turnover rate of glycerides in pre-β lipoproteins of about 2 gm. per hour in the adult have been obtained in subjects with normal and somewhat elevated glyceride concentrations.[9] The capacity of removal mechanisms to adapt to higher loads has not been established. The question of whether endogenous and exogenous glycerides are removed by an identical mechanism also has not been resolved and is important to the understanding of certain kinds of hyperlipemia.[117] In some experiments tagged glycerides in fatty acids administered in a form comparable to the pre-β lipoproteins have been found predominantly in the liver in the fasting state and in the adipose tissue in the fed state.[116] In others, the role of the liver in removing endogenous glycerides has seemed unimportant.[125]

Particles of Exogenous Glyceride (Chylomicrons)[1,5,108,117]

Definition. The term chylomicron was coined in 1920 for the visible particles that appear in lymph and blood in response to fat feeding and contain the fed triglycerides.[126] For a time all particulate lipid was given this name, but it has become useful to return to the original meaning to provide some easy way of distinguishing dietary particles.[5]

It is easier to define chylomicrons in physiologic than in operational terms (Table 1). They float too rapidly in the ultracentrifuge to be quantified by optical means, and arbitrary centrifugal forces have been adopted for their definition and isolation. Sometimes, all particles having an S_f greater than 400 have been considered chylomicrons. Endogenous particles may also have flotation rates of this order, however, and the ultracentrifuge sometimes cannot

be used to separate chylomicrons from significant quantities of endogenous particles.

In free or starch-block electrophoresis chylomicrons have a wide range of mobility. Those isolated from thoracic-duct lymph migrate with albumin.[5] As already noted, in plasma they may move with α_2 globulin (primary particles) or with β globulin (secondary particles).[108] Endogenous particles likewise have α_2 mobility and cannot always be separated clearly from chylomicrons by this technic. One separation of the 3 types of particles by polyvinylpyrrolidone gradient tubes has already been described.[6]

For clinical purposes the presence of chylomicrons in plasma is most conveniently indicated by paper electrophoresis. In albumin-containing buffer chylomicrons remain as a distinct band at the origin on electrophoresis whereas all other lipoprotein species migrate to some extent (Fig. 3).[7]

Composition (Table 1). In the light or electron microscope the chylomicrons appear to be spheres that vary in diameter from about 0.1 to 5.0 μ. The upper limit may reflect aggregation during isolation, and it is possible that circulating chylomicrons are not larger than about 1 μ. Chylomicrons, like pre-β lipoproteins, are made up mainly of glyceride, with lesser amounts of phospholipid and cholesterol. The proportions depend on the average size of the particles under study. Usually less than half the cholesterol is esterified, as compared to 65 to 75 per cent of esters in other lipoproteins. Patients with severe chylomicronemia may have a low percentage of esterified cholesterol in the plasma without the usual implication of abnormal liver function.

The protein content of chylomicrons is usually between 0.5 and 2.5 per cent of their total weight. Reports of higher protein content are probably due to contamination of the isolates. There is no general agreement about the nature of this protein or whether it is an intrinsic part of the chylomicron.[5,27,127-129] It therefore does not appear in Figure 2. Even in chylomicrons washed many times by ultracentrifugation several different serum proteins, including albumin and gamma globulin, can often be identified immunologically. Amino acid or peptide analyses on such small quantities of protein are subject to errors compounded by the probability that a mixture of proteins is usually present. Aminoterminal aspartic and glutamic acid are often obtained, and the aminoterminal serine and threonine typical of apoprotein C are inconsistently present. Considering all the available evidence, the 2 proteins obtained most consistently after delipidation are the A and B proteins. These can be seen best by immunologic means, but peptide analyses have also demonstrated the A protein on one occasion.[128] It is not known how the chylomicrons are actually stabilized, and some or all of the proteins present could be adsorbed to the surface or dissolved in these complexes without serving a functional purpose. It seems clear that upon entering plasma, chylomicrons take on additional protein, for the protein content is higher than that of similar particles isolated from lymph and, as noted earlier, the electrophoretic mobility also changes.[106] We shall have occasion shortly to examine evidence that the 2 major plasma lipoproteins have more than a casual relation to the chylomicron.

Origin of chylomicrons.[5,130] In the intestinal lumen dietary glycerides are dispersed by the action of bile salts and rendered easily vulnerable to hydrolysis by lipases. The resulting products are micelles containing glycerol, free fatty acids, monoglycerides and diglycerides that are taken up by intestinal epithelial cells and there resynthesized to triglycerides. Cholesterol, phospholipid and probably protein are added, and the resulting chylomicrons are extruded from the mucosal cell into the lymphatic spaces. The precise details of chylomicron formation and movement from the base of the jejunal epithelial cell into the lymphatics are not known. Chylomicrons travel in the intestinal lymph through the regional lymph nodes and the thoracic duct into the venous blood.

Chylomicron removal.[117] Chylomicrons are rapidly removed from the plasma. When chylomicrons containing tagged glycerides are infused into human subjects they disappear with a half-time of five to fifteen minutes.[131] From the distribution of tagged glyceride fatty acids it appears that most organs of the body rapidly receive chylomicron fatty acids. The possibility that some of the glycerides are hydrolyzed very rapidly and the resulting fatty acids distributed as free fatty acids to some tissues has to be considered in the interpretation of experimental studies of glyceride removal. It appears from such studies in several species that after an overnight fast the major site of chylomicron removal may be the liver. In animals allowed access to food most of the chylomicrons may be cleared by adipose tissue. The concept of net hepatic removal of chylomicron glycerides has recently been challenged by experiments in which rat livers were perfused with chylomicrons in the presence and absence of heparin.[132] Without heparin, which may release lipolytic enzymes into the medium, there was no net uptake or metabolism of the particles. When heparin was added to the perfusate, uptake and oxidation began immediately. Other perfusion experiments[133] have not been in agreement, however, and the question of direct participation of the liver in glyceride removal remains unsettled.

The role of lipolysis.[117,134] It is fairly certain that a hydrolytic step must initiate or accompany the removal of chylomicrons from the circulation. The evidence is inferential and of the following nature. Although the endothelium of the hepatic sinusoids may contain spaces that could admit chylomicrons, the capillary walls in other tissues appear continuous. Passage of chylomicrons through the endothelial wall by pinocytosis has not been convincingly demonstrated by the electron microscope. Further-

more, during removal of glycerides, the fatty acids appear quickly in the free fatty acids, perhaps 10 per cent of which represent fatty acids coming in with the glycerides.[135] Tagged fatty acids appearing in liver do not remain in the glycerides in which they were delivered but are rapidly reshuffled, many appearing in phospholipids. The initial hydrolysis of the glycerides entering extrahepatic tissues is believed by some to be catalyzed by lipoprotein lipase concentrated in the capillary wall.[117] Lipoprotein lipase catalyzes the hydrolysis to fatty acid and glycerol of glycerides in chylomicrons and other lipoproteins, and will also split artificial fat emulsions if they are first activated by added serum or plasma. Parenteral administration of heparin and other polyanions causes lipoprotein lipase activity to appear rapidly in plasma. The activity rapidly disappears if liver function is normal. There is evidence that postheparin lipolytic activity is due to more than 1 enzyme, including a phospholipase.[136] The intravascular lipolysis induced by heparin or similar agents is a gross exaggeration of normal chylomicron removal to the extent that the fatty acids cannot all be removed by the immediately adjacent tissues. The free fatty acid content does rise slightly during normal chylomicron clearing. How much lipoprotein lipase is present in the adipose tissue cells themselves as opposed to their capillary epithelium is unclear.[137] It has been detected in hepatic-vein blood[138,139] but never convincingly demonstrated in liver parenchymal cells. The level of lipoprotein lipase in adipose tissue bears a relation to the insulin activity. In rats made diabetic with alloxan the enzyme activity is low and restored to normal by insulin treatment.[140]

Recapitulation. Plasma glycerides are transported by 2 different systems. Dietary fat is carried from the intestine into the bloodstream as large particles (chylomicrons), consisting mainly of glycerides. Phospholipids, cholesterol and a little protein are also present and probably stabilize the particle. The presence of chylomicrons can be established, and the quantity estimated by several technics. One of the simplest and most useful is based on the lack of mobility of chylomicrons on paper electrophoresis. The plasma concentration of chylomicrons is variable and dependent upon the timing of fat ingestion. Only quantities below the limits of detection by paper electrophoresis are normally present after an overnight fast. The disposal of these particles is relatively rapid and depends upon 2 major steps. The first is hydrolysis, which possibly takes place at the capillary wall and is catalyzed by lipoprotein lipase. The second is the ability of tissues beyond the capillary wall to take up the fatty acids released. In the adipose tissue, one of the major sites of disposal, re-esterification depends upon an adequate supply of α glycerolphosphate, which in turn is derived from glucose breakdown. The fate of the other constituents of the chylomicron, which seem to include small amounts of α and β lipoproteins, is not known. It is possible that chylomicrons after removal of some of their glycerides become pre-β lipoproteins. Alpha and β lipoproteins, freed of their mantle of glycerides, may join others of their species in the plasma.

Glycerides synthesized in the liver either from carbohydrate or from re-esterification of circulating free fatty acids are transported from that organ in pre-β lipoproteins and larger endogenous particles. These represent a broad spectrum of density and size from particles large enough to be seen in the light microscope to others merging with the density limits of the soluble β lipoproteins. The endogenous particles have higher protein and cholesterol content than the chylomicrons and different properties. On paper electrophoresis, they migrate in the pre-β range with increasing trailing as particle size increases. Their concentration in plasma changes slowly but can vary widely over the period of a few days, particularly in association with marked changes in the carbohydrate content of the diet. The removal rate of glyceride in the pre-β lipoproteins seems to be slower than that of glyceride in chylomicrons. The large endogenous particles may be cleared at about the same rate as chylomicrons, however, and it has not been shown that glyceride molecules of different origin have different disposal mechanisms.

INHERITED LIPOPROTEIN DEFICIENCY STATES

Several mutations in man have been discovered that have laid to rest all uncertainty that the A and B proteins in lipoproteins have separately evolved to serve different functions. They have also considerably illuminated some of the transport tasks that each lipoprotein seems to serve and illustrated something about the genetic control of their plasma concentrations.

In 2 genetically determined disorders the normal β or α lipoproteins respectively are completely missing from the plasma. These are abeta-lipoproteinemia and familial α-lipoprotein deficiency (Tangier disease). The latter is termed "deficiency" because small amounts of α lipoproteins are present, but they appear to be abnormal judging from available immunochemical evidence. The clinical details of these 2 diseases have been extensively reviewed, and attention can be focused here on the disabilities in fat transport that accompany absence of one or the other class of lipoproteins.

Abeta-lipoproteinemia[141] [143]

In 1950, 2 patients with neurologic abnormalities and "crenated" red blood cells (acanthocytes)[144] became the first of about 30 patients with a singular disorder subsequently reported from America, Britain and Europe. At first the acanthocytosis seemed the most striking finding; a very low concentration of plasma cholesterol was then noted and absence of β lipoproteins was demonstrated in

1960.[145] Other investigators confirmed that several patients had severe deficiency or absence of all the plasma lipoproteins of density less than 1.063, including the absence of any chylomicronemia after the feeding of fat. The name abeta-lipoproteinemia was then suggested[145] and has gained general acceptance on the assumption that this describes the primary inherited defect.

The disease is usually expressed in infancy by retarded growth associated with steatorrhea and abdominal distention. Malabsorption becomes less marked in late childhood and is succeeded by progressively more severe neurologic deficits, including loss of muscle strength and nystagmus and signs of degeneration of the posterolateral columns and cerebellar tracts. Pigmentary retinal degeneration and visual difficulties appear. Life expectancy is limited; at least 1 death has been associated with persistent cardiac arrythmias. Deposition of ceroid pigment in the tissues is a prominent finding. The plasma and tissue phospholipids are unusually low in essential fatty acids. A deficiency of the latter or some other dietary constituent whose intake is dependent upon fat absorption may be the basis of the changes in erythrocyte membranes and nerve-cell structures that seem to underlie the many features of the disease. Sibs can be affected, and sometimes there is parental consanguinity, but vertical transmission has never been observed. The disease appears to be the expression of a double dose of a mutant autosomal allele. In 1 set of parents the β lipoproteins have been low,[145] but at present there is no way to distinguish most of the presumed heterozygotes.

The plasma lipoprotein pattern in abeta-lipoproteinemia is illustrated in Figure 4. The evidence indicates that there is no β lipoprotein in plasma. Immunochemical methods capable of detecting less than 1/10,000 of the β lipoprotein in normal plasma have revealed none in 6 patients from 4 kindreds.[79] The average plasma concentrations of cholesterol

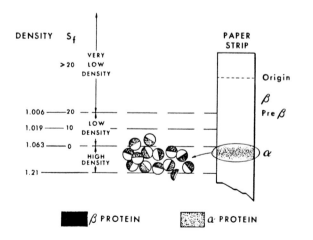

FIGURE 4. *Lipoprotein Pattern in Abeta-lipoproteinemia.*
The key clinical features are hypolipidemia and clear plasma, malabsorption, cerebellar ataxia, peripheral neuropathy, acanthocytosis, retinitis pigmentosa and autosomal recessive inheritance.

100 THE NEW ENGLAND JOURNAL OF MEDICINE Jan. 12, 1967

(20 to 90 mg. per 100 ml.) and of phospholipids (35 to 95 mg. per 100 ml.) are the lowest seen in any human disease. Glyceride concentrations approach the vanishing point — less than 10 to 20 mg. per 100 ml.

As shown in Figure 4 abeta-lipoproteinemia provides one of the rare instances in which α lipoproteins appear in the density region of 1.019 to 1.063 that is usually the exclusive preserve of the β lipoproteins. These α lipoproteins have a mean density that is lower than usual, probably as the result of a large lipid complement carried by the A protein. The A protein seems otherwise to be perfectly normal. The α lipoproteins are immunochemically identical to those in normal subjects, and the A protein has an amino acid composition indistinguishable from the normal.[79]

The omission of all β-lipoprotein-containing complexes (compare Figure 4 with Figure 5) is associated with the abolition of practically all glyceride transport in abeta-lipoproteinemia. The most obvious defect is a total inability to form chylomicrons.

Patients with abeta-lipoproteinemia digest glycerides, absorb the resulting monoglycerides and free fatty acids into the intestinal mucosa cells and reform them into triglycerides, but fail to release chylomicrons. Of great interest is the ability to produce in rats a similar defect in the intestine by abolishing protein synthesis with puromycin.[93,94] As patients with abeta-lipoproteinemia get older, they "learn" to absorb some fat, but must do so through another pathway such as transport of long-chain fatty acids via the portal circulation; they never have chylomicrons in peripheral blood.

When the patients are fed diets high in carbohydrates designed to induce production of endogenous glycerides and release of pre-β lipoprotein, no increase in plasma glycerides occurs and no trace of pre-β lipoproteins appears.[79] Diets that contain more than 20 gm. of carbohydrate per kilogram of body

weight have been used. A liver biopsy has been obtained on 1 patient who was regularly on a relatively high-carbohydrate diet and revealed tissue containing excessive amounts of glyceride.[141] Thus, it appears that, like the intestinal mucosa, the liver in a patient with abeta-lipoproteinemia is able to produce and store glycerides but cannot transfer the lipid into the plasma.

The abnormalities found in the intestine and liver of patients with this disease, along with the nearly complete absence of glyceride in plasma, strongly invite the conclusion that the B protein has a specific function in the transport of both exogenous and endogenous glyceride from cells. This function cannot be adequately assumed by A protein.

Hypobeta-lipoproteinemia

A few patients with familial deficiency of β lipoproteins (as opposed to their absence) have been reported.[146,148] Beta lipoprotein concentrations have been 10 to 50 per cent of normal, with comparable decreases in plasma cholesterol, phospholipids, glycerides and probably in essential fatty acids. Some patients have had abnormally fragile red cells or acanthocytes and progressive neuromuscular difficulties developing in adulthood. In at least 1 of the reported families, the data indicate that the defect could be transmitted as an autosomal dominant; the mutations are probably different from that producing abeta-lipoproteinemia.

Fat absorption and chylomicron formation are not abolished in hypobeta-lipoproteinemia. Presumably, sufficient β lipoprotein is formed to meet these requirements, but it is likely that these patients are operating at minimal levels of B protein and its lipoprotein. For example, in 1 patient with severe hypobeta-lipoproteinemia and acanthocytosis neurologic symptoms developed only after the fourth pregnancy. Presumably, the hyperglyceridemia of pregnancy creates greater demand for glyceride transport and therefore for B protein.

Familial hypobeta-lipoproteinemia must be differentiated from that secondary to acute infections, other severe debilitating illnesses or malabsorption due to different gastrointestinal lesions. Undoubtedly as population surveys increase more patients will be found with similar decreases in β-lipoprotein production or increased catabolism. A spectrum of inherited states with different degrees of β-lipoprotein deficiency may eventually be uncovered.

Familial Alpha-Lipoprotein Deficiency (Tangier Disease)[55]

The analogue of abeta-lipoproteinemia was discovered in 1960 and called Tangier disease after the first 2 examples, in siblings five and six-years-old, from Tangier Island in Chesapeake Bay. Since that time the authors have had the opportunity to study 6 more examples, in 3 pairs of siblings from different families unrelated to the Tangier population.

In Tangier disease the plasma concentrations of cholesterol average 70 mg. per 100 ml. (with a

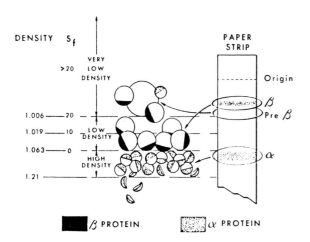

FIGURE 5. Normal Lipoprotein Pattern in a Young Subject after an Overnight Fast.
Pre-β Lipoprotein May Not Be Present.

range of 50 to 130 mg.), and that of phospholipids about 100 mg. (range of 70 to 140 mg.), both similar to those found in abeta-lipoproteinemia. The glyceride concentrations tend to be modestly elevated in the postabsorptive state (range of 120 to 280 mg.). The dramatic abnormality that uniquely characterizes the disease is the great size and peculiar orange color of the tonsils. Even small tags remaining after tonsillectomy have the telltale appearance. These changes are due to a gross deposition of cholesterol esters in reticuloendothelial tissues, sometimes also associated with enlargement of liver, spleen and lymph nodes. All the known clinical manifestations of the disorder appear to be secondary to the deposition of lipid, which is widespread and can also be found in cutaneous lesions and the cornea, blood vessels and reticuloendothelial cells in the rectal mucosa. One adult patient had pancytopenia corrected by removal of an enlarged spleen. His affected sibling died at the age of forty-eight years with a probable myocardial infarction.

Alpha-lipoprotein deficiency seems certain to be the primary inheritable defect, and extensive study of the pedigrees has revealed the expression in a clear genetic mode. The presence of a single abnormal autosomal gene results in abnormally low plasma concentrations of α lipoprotein (in terms of lipoprotein cholesterol, below 32 mg. per 100 ml. in males and 35 mg. per 100 ml. in females) but no significant tissue lipid deposition.[149] The homozygous abnormal genotype is expressed by near absence of all plasma high-density or α lipoproteins and tissue accumulation of cholesterol esters.

The plasma of the homozygote usually appears to be completely devoid of α lipoproteins after paper electrophoresis or ordinary immunophoresis. With appropriate antiserums and concentration of the plasma, however, a small amount of α lipoprotein can be detected. This lipoprotein can be isolated between the densities of D 1.063 and 1.21 in the ultracentrifuge and concentrated in a manner similar to that of normal α lipoprotein. It contains cholesterol and phospholipid and has an α_1 mobility like that of α lipoprotein. It also reacts with anti-α-lipoprotein serum, and when used as an antigen, provokes antibodies to itself as well as normal α lipoproteins. Despite these similarities to native α lipoprotein, however, further immunochemical studies reveal that the Tangier α-lipoprotein, in both its lipidrich and its delipidated form, is not antigenically identical to normal α lipoprotein.[150] Thus, it has been given the separate designation, Tangier α lipoprotein; it is present in the plasma of patients with Tangier disease in about one twelfth of the concentration of α lipoprotein in normal subjects (about 30 mg. vs. 360 mg. per 100 ml.) and is the only form of α lipoprotein that can be identified by immunochemical technics. The heterozygous relatives of the patients have both Tangier α lipoprotein α_1 and α lipoprotein.

The β-lipoproteins in Tangier disease appear to be normal on immunophoresis. Their phospholipid content is high, however, and some float at the abnormally low density of 1.006.

The lipoprotein pattern in postabsorptive plasma from patients with Tangier disease (Fig. 6) is unique. The paper electrophoretogram alone immediately permits a presumptive diagnosis that needs only to be confirmed by immunochemical analyses.

In contrast to abeta-lipoproteinemia the patients with Tangier disease absorb fat normally from the intestine and make chylomicrons that behave physically like the normal ones. Their ability to release endogenous glyceride into the circulation in response to a dietary carbohydrate load is also unimpaired.[78] This endogenous hyperlipemia is associated, however, with peculiar triglyceride-laden lipoproteins of density less than 1.006 that appear as a broadened β band on electrophoresis (Fig. 6). This phenomenon provides a convincing demonstration that the normal pre-β mobility of the very-low-density lipoproteins depends upon the presence of α lipoproteins in the complex.[78]

The ability of patients with severe α-lipoprotein deficiency to move both endogenous and exogenous glyceride into the plasma implies that α lipoproteins are not essential in this phase of glyceride transport. That they may have another role in facilitating the passage of glycerides and other lipids from plasma to tissues is suggested by 2 consistent observations in Tangier disease. Plasma glyceride levels in the fasting state usually are abnormally high on regular diets. Whenever either endogenous or exogenous hyperglyceridemia is induced by appropriate diets the maximum glyceride concentrations and the duration of the hyperlipemia are greater than normal. How α lipoproteins assist in the exodus of glyceride from plasma is still open to speculation.

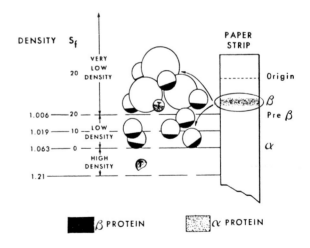

FIGURE 6. *Lipoprotein Pattern in Tangier Disease (α-Lipoprotein Deficiency).*

The small quantity of α lipoprotein is marked with a "T" to indicate that the molecule is abnormal. Clinical features are low cholesterol, normal or elevated triglycerides, enlarged tonsils and hepatosplenomegaly due to cholesterol-ester storage and autosomal recessive inheritance.

As best as can be determined from immunochemical studies the reticuloendothelial tissues in patients with Tangier disease do not seem to contain α lipoproteins in unusual quantities, and there is no evidence that the cholesterol-ester infiltration arises because cells have engorged α lipoproteins. A single study has revealed no increase in cholesterol synthesis in the Tangier tonsil. It seems more likely that α lipoprotein enhances the stability of the circulating particles containing glyceride and other lipids. When the lipoprotein is missing, the unstable particles may be more susceptible to removal by phagocytic cells. The cholesterol esters may represent the steadily increasing residue of such an uptake.

Recapitulation

Information derived from the observation of patients with lipoprotein deficiency combined with other information permits several hypotheses concerning the participation of 2 particular proteins in fat transport. These are briefly summarized as follows. The liver and intestine, and perhaps other tissues, have the capacity to synthesize proteins with a special affinity for lipids. In extracellular fluid these proteins appear in association with characteristic and different amounts of phospholipids and sterols to form 2 independent kinds of lipoproteins. These α and β lipoproteins not only provide a means for keeping their constituent lipids in solution but also assist in the stabilization of more lipids when they must be transported in plasma. The glycerides, one of the major forms in which fats destined for ultimate caloric use are carried, seem to depend upon lipoproteins for their movement out of cells and delivery to sites of removal. The B protein, backbone of β lipoprotein, appears to have a special function in making it possible for intestinal and liver cells to deliver glyceride into the extracellular fluids. How and at which cellular sites or surfaces it acts in this capacity is not known. In man, at least, the A protein, which forms the α lipoproteins, cannot perform this function. Its absence is reflected in somewhat poorer removal of glyceride from plasma and tremendous and progressive cholesterol accumulation in tissues.

Many control mechanisms must operate to maintain plasma lipoprotein concentrations. Ultimately, these affect the rates of synthesis and catabolism of the lipoprotein proteins, but they probably are more directly responsive to changing requirements for lipid transport. The constantly shifting demand for glyceride transport requires a quick response. Other requirements, such as the need for stepped up movement of cholesterol when this lipid is ingested or synthesized in increased amounts, perhaps allow more time for adaptation. The states of metabolism of carbohydrate and protein also influence lipoprotein concentrations, and the total number of genetic and environmental factors at play is obviously large.

If even the least subtle of all the possible controls on lipoprotein metabolism were completely clarified it would be much easier to discuss the clinical problem of hyperlipoproteinemia. As it is we must take up that topic in the next section, employing terms more descriptive and less mechanistic than one would desire.

(To be continued)

REFERENCES

102. Kuo, P. T., and Carson, J. C. Dietary fats and diurnal serum triglyceride levels in man. *J. Clin. Investigation* **38**:1384-1392, 1959.
103. Bierman, E. L., Hayes, T. L., Hawkins, J. N., Ewing, A. M., and Lindgren, F. T. Particle-size distribution of very low density plasma lipoproteins during fat absorption in man. *J. Lipid Research* **7**:65-72, 1966.
104. Smith, E. B. Lipoprotein patterns in myocardial infarction: relationship between components identified by paper electrophoresis and in ultracentrifuge. *Lancet* **223**:910-914, 1957.
105. Gordis, E. Demonstration of two kinds of fat particles in alimentary lipemia with polyvinylpyrrolidone gradient columns. *Proc. Soc. Exper. Biol. & Med.* **110**:657-661, 1962.
106. Frazer, A. C. Blood plasma lipo-proteins, with special reference to fat transport and metabolism. *Discussions of Faraday Soc.* **6**:81-97, 1949.
107. Kunkel, H. G., and Slater, R. J. Lipoprotein patterns of serum obtained by zone electrophoresis. *J. Clin. Investigation* **31**:677-684, 1952.
108. Bierman, E. L., Gordis, E., and Hamlin, J. T., III. Heterogeneity of fat particles in plasma during alimentary lipemia. *J. Clin. Investigation* **41**:2254-2260, 1962.
109. Salt, H. B., and Wolff, O. H. Applications of serum lipoprotein electrophoresis in paediatric practice. *Arch. Dis. Childhood* **32**:404-412, 1957.
110. Straus, R., and Sunderman, F. W. Method for fractionation of lipoproteins in serum by paper electrophoresis. In *Lipids and the Steroid Hormones in Clinical Medicine*. Edited by F. W. Sunderman and F. W. Sunderman, Jr. 207 pp. Philadelphia: Lippincott, 1960. P. 66.
111. Lees, R. S., and Hatch, F. T. Sharper separation of lipoprotein species by paper electrophoresis in albumin-containing buffer. *J. Lab. & Clin. Med.* **61**:518-528, 1963.
112. Hatch, F. T. Serum lipoproteins. In *Serum Proteins and the Dysproteinemias*. Edited by F. W. Sunderman and F. W. Sunderman, Jr. 461 pp. Philadelphia: Lippincott, 1964. P. 223.
113. Gustafson, A., Alaupovic, P., and Furman, R. H. Studies on composition and structure of serum lipoproteins: separation and characterization of phospholipid protein residues obtained by partial delipidization of very low density lipoproteins of human serum. *Biochemistry* **3**:632-640, 1966.
114. Walton, K. W., and Darke, S. J. Immunochemical characteristics of human low-density lipoproteins. *Immunochemistry* **1**:267-277, 1964.
115. Havel, R. J., and Goldfien, A. Role of liver and of extrahepatic tissues in transport and metabolism of fatty acids and triglycerides in dog. *J. Lipid Research* **2**:389-395, 1961.
116. Havel, R. J., Felts, J. M., and Van Duyne, M. Formation and fate of endogenous triglycerides in blood plasma of rabbits. *J. Lipid Research* **3**:297-308, 1962.
117. Havel, R. J. Metabolism of lipids in chylomicrons and very low density lipoproteins. In *Handbook of Physiology. Section 5: Adipose tissue.* Edited by A. E. Renold and G. F. Cahill, Jr. 824 pp. Baltimore: Waverly Press, Inc., 1965. P. 499.
118. Steinberg, D., and Vaughan, M. Release of free fatty acids from adipose tissue in vitro relation to rates of triglyceride syntheses and degradation. In *Handbook of Physiology. Section 5: Adipose tissue.* Edited by A. E. Renold and G. E. Cahill, Jr. 824 pp. Baltimore: Waverly Press, Inc., 1965. Chapter 34. Pp. 335-347.
119. Watkin, D. M., Froeb, H. F., Hatch, F. T., and Gutman, A. B. Effects of diet in essential hypertension. II. Results with unmodified Kempner rice diet in fifty hospitalized patients. *Am. J. Med.* **9**:441-493, 1950.
120. Hatch, F. T., Abell, L. L., and Kendall, F. E. Effects of restriction of dietary fat and cholesterol upon serum lipids and lipoproteins in patients with hypertension. *Am. J. Med.* **19**:48-60, 1955.
121. Nichols, A. V., Dobbin, V., and Gofman, J. W. Influence of

dietary factors upon human serum lipoprotein concentrations. *Geriatrics* **12**:7-17, 1957.

122. Antonis, A., and Bersohn, I. Influence of diet on serum-triglycerides in South African white and Bantu prisoners. *Lancet* **1**:3-9, 1961.

123. Ahrens, E. H., Jr., Hirsch, J., Oette, K., Farquhar, J. W., and Stein, Y. Carbohydrate-induced and fat-induced lipemia. *Tr. A. Am. Physicians* **74**:134-146, 1961.

124. Lees, R. S., and Fredrickson, D. S. Carbohydrate induction of hyperlipemia in normal man. *Clin. Research* **13**:327, 1965.

125. Friedberg, S. J., and Estes, E. H., Jr. Tissue distribution and uptake of endogenous lipoprotein triglycerides in rat. *J. Clin. Investigation* **43**:129-137, 1964.

126. Gage, S. H., and Fish, P. A. Fat digestion and assimilation in man and animals as determined by dark-field microscope, and fat-soluble dye. *Am. J. Anat.* **34**:1-85, 1924.

127. Rodbell, M. N-terminal amino acid and lipid composition of lipoproteins from chyle and plasma. *Science* **127**:701, 1958.

128. Rodbell, M., and Fredrickson, D. S. Nature of proteins associated with dog and human chylomicrons. *J. Biol. Chem.* **234**:562-566, 1959.

129. Wathen, J. D., and Levy, R. S. Composition of protein from dog lymph chylomicrons and dog serum high density lipoprotein. *Biochemistry* **5**:1099-1103, 1966.

130. Senior, J. R. Intestinal absorption of fats. *J. Lipid Research* **5**:495-521, 1964.

131. Nestel, P. J. Relationship between plasma triglycerides and removal of chylomicrons. *J. Clin. Investigation* **43**:943-949, 1964.

132. Fehs, J. M., and Mayes, P. A. Lack of uptake and oxidation of chylomicron triglyceride to carbon dioxide and ketone bodies by perfused rat liver. *Nature* (London) **206**:195, 1965.

133. Ontko, J. A., and Zilversmit, D. B. Utilization of chylomicrons by liver. *Federation Proc.* **25**:209, 1966.

134. Robinson, D. S. Clearing factor lipase and its action in transport of fatty acids between blood and tissues. *Advances in Lipid Research* **1**:133-182, 1963.

135. Fredrickson, D. S., McCollester, D. L., and Ono, K. Role of unesterified fatty acid transport in chylomicron metabolism. *J. Clin. Investigation* **37**:1333-1341, 1958.

136. Vogel, W. C., and Zieve, L. Post-heparin phospholipase. *J. Lipid Research* **5**:177-183, 1964.

137. Rodbell, M. Localization of lipoprotein lipase in fat cells of rat adipose tissue. *J. Biol. Chem.* **239**:753-755, 1964.

138. LeQuire, V. S., Hamilton, R. L., Adams, R., and Merrill, J. M. Lipase activity in blood from hepatic and peripheral vascular beds following heparin. *Proc. Soc. Exper. Biol. & Med.* **114**:104-107, 1963.

139. Condon, R. E., Tobias, H., and Datta, D. V. Liver and postheparin plasma lipolytic activity in dog and man. *J. Clin. Investigation* **44**:860-869, 1965.

140. Kessler, J. I. Effect of diabetes and insulin on activity of myocardial and adipose tissue lipoprotein lipase of rats. *J. Clin. Investigation* **42**:362-367, 1963.

141. Isselbacher, K. J., Scheig, R., Plotkin, G. R., and Caulfield, J. B. Congenital β-lipoprotein deficiency: hereditary disorder involving defect in absorption and transport of lipids. *Medicine* **43**:347-361, 1964.

142. Wolff, O. H. A-beta-lipoproteinemia. *Ergebn. d. inn. Med. u. Kinderh.* **23**:191-201, 1965.

143. Farquhar, J. W., and Ways, P. Abetalipoproteinemia. In *The Metabolic Basis of Inherited Disease.* Second edition. Edited by J. B. Stanbury, J. B. Wyngaarden and D. S. Fredrickson. 1434 pp. New York: McGraw-Hill, 1966. P. 509.

144. Bassen, F. A., and Kornzweig, A. L. Malformation of erythrocytes in case of atypical retinitis pigmentosa. *Blood* **5**:381-387, 1950.

145. Salt, H. B., et al. On having no beta-lipoprotein: syndrome comprising a-beta-lipoproteinaemia, acanthocytosis, and steatorrhoea. *Lancet* **2**:325-329, 1960.

146. Kuo, P. T., and Basset, D. R. Blood and tissue lipids in family with hypo-beta-lipoproteinemia. *Circulation* **26**:660, 1962.

147. van Buchem, F. S. P., Pol, G., de Gier, J., Böttcher, C. J. F., and Pries, C. Congenital β-lipoprotein deficiency. *Am. J. Med.* **40**:794-804, 1966.

148. Lewis, L. A., Robertson, A., Mars, H., and Williams, G., Jr. Lipid and cytological abnormalities in familial hypobetalipoproteinemia. *Circulation* **34** (Supp. III):19, 1966.

149. Fredrickson, D. S. Inheritance of high density lipoprotein deficiency (Tangier disease). *J. Clin. Investigation* **43**:228-236, 1964.

150. Levy, R. I., and Fredrickson, D. S. Nature of alpha lipoproteins in Tangier disease. *Circulation* **34** (Supp. III):156, 1966.

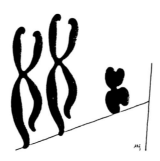

148 THE NEW ENGLAND JOURNAL OF MEDICINE Jan. 19, 1967

MEDICAL PROGRESS

FAT TRANSPORT IN LIPOPROTEINS — AN INTEGRATED APPROACH TO MECHANISMS AND DISORDERS (Continued)*

DONALD S. FREDRICKSON, M.D.,† ROBERT I. LEVY, M.D.,‡ AND
ROBERT S. LEES, M.D.§

BETHESDA, MARYLAND

HYPERLIPOPROTEINEMIA

Definitions

Up to this point we have concentrated on laying the support for 2 generalizations. The first is that, with the exception of free fatty acid concentrations, which have no lipoprotein equivalents, all abnormalities in plasma lipid concentrations or *dyslipidemia* can be translated into *dyslipoproteinemia*. The second is that the shift of emphasis to lipoproteins offers distinct advantages in the recognition and management of such disorders. We have already discussed the relatively few cases in which *hypolipoproteinemia* is a clinical problem, and the remainder of the review will be devoted to *hyperlipoproteinemia*.

Hyperlipoproteinemia (hyperlipidemia) falls into 2 major subdivisions from the standpoint of differential diagnosis on the basis of etiology. The *secondary* kind is an expression of altered metabolism due to some other recognizable disease, such as the nephrotic syndrome or hypothyroidism. One deals with the disease and ignores the symptom; hyperlipoproteinemia will go away if the underlying disease is successfully managed. *Primary* hyperlipoproteinemia includes all that is left. It is either *familial* or *sporadic*. The term *heritable* is less commonly used than familial, but it is more accurate if there is good evidence of genotypic variation. Familial hyperlipoproteinemia obviously need not be inheritable if it is due, for example, to patterns of excess in diet or alcohol intake that have been acquired by close relatives.

In a desire to use more specific terminology certain durable nouns from the "lipid era" should not be discarded. *Hypercholesterolemia* and *hyperglyceridemia* convey exact meaning, as does *hyperlipemia* (hyperglyceridemia severe enough to cause lactescence in plasma). *Exogenous hyperlipemia* is synonymous with *fat-induced hyperlipemia*. *Endogenous hyperlipemia* is sometimes *carbohydrate induced*, but these terms are not necessarily synonymous. Two venerable modifiers, *essential* and *idiopathic*, must be laid to rest. Their use no longer defines specific diseases and merely conceals heterogeneity. A diagnosis of "essential hyperlipemia," for example, should no longer be acceptable to either physician or patient.

Sorting out the Abnormals

There is no single test or maneuver that infallibly separates all those who have hyperlipoproteinemia from those who do not. The majority of laboratories still employ a combination of chemical measurements of plasma lipid concentrations for this purpose.

Lipid Determinations

The simplest screening method is a measurement of the total lipid content of plasma. Useful methods are available.[151] Some are relative, such as those depending on turbidity[152]; others, like the measurement of total fatty acids,[153,154] are more specific but also more complicated. All need careful standardization. Sometimes, laboratories report "total lipid" concentrations that are less than the sum of the concentrations of several lipid classes reported concomitantly. Measurement of total lipids alone never provides a specific diagnosis, and occasionally abnormal but reciprocal changes in cholesterol and glyceride concentrations can occur without throwing total lipid concentrations into a clearly abnormal range.

Combination of lipid analyses. Methods for determining cholesterol concentrations are widely available[155] and have even been successfully automated.[156] One should be included in any simple scheme for screening for hyperlipoproteinemia. It should be used in combination with 1 of 3 other tests or maneuvers: inspection of the serum for turbidity (a gross test for hyperglyceridemia); or the determination of either total lipids or glycerides. The best combination is measurement of cholesterol and of glyceride concentrations.[157,158] If both are *clearly* within normal limits, hyperlipoproteinemia is ruled out with a degree of precision that is quite adequate for current use.

Phospholipids. The addition of a determination of the total phospholipid concentration to plasma lipid analyses is not difficult. When the ratio of plasma cholesterol to phospholipids is high it indicates a

*From the Laboratory of Molecular Diseases, National Heart Institute.
†Director and chief, Laboratory of Molecular Diseases, National Heart Institute.
‡Head, Section on Lipoproteins, Laboratory of Molecular Diseases, National Heart Institute.
§Assistant professor and associate physician, Rockefeller University.

relative preponderance of β lipoproteins. It is relatively low in the great excesses of α lipoprotein that may accompany obstructive liver disease. Phospholipid determinations do not offer unique information about most other types of hyperlipoproteinemia, however, and they do not supplement cholesterol and glyceride determinations in such a way as to eliminate the added value of lipoprotein determinations. Plasma phospholipid concentrations[159] have therefore not been included in this review.

Lipoprotein Patterns

The 4 major groups of lipoproteins offer more variables than lipid determinations do. The patterns that these form can be used to diagnose several specific lipoprotein deficiency states already discussed and to segregate at least 5 different syndromes or groups of diseases associated with hyperlipoproteinemia (Table 2). Of all the methods for obtaining lipoprotein patterns only 2 kinds have the necessary range to achieve this segregation. The first are those based on flotation and use either the preparative ultracentrifuge alone or in combination with the analytical model. The latter comes closest to the ideal of defining hyperlipoproteinemia by a single operation or, more accurately, a series of such operations.[64] As now adapted the analytical ultracentrifuge has the ability to draw a continuous plot of the concentrations of lipoproteins in flotation (S_f)

classes differing by very-small-density increments.[39] Such instrumentation is not generally available.

The preparative ultracentrifuge can also be used to obtain quantitative lipoprotein patterns.[34,160,161] To do so in a single plasma sample requires 3 or 4 serial runs and subsequent lipid determinations. The premium for adaptation of either the analytical or the preparative ultracentrifuge to the study of many patients is thus high in terms of both instrument cost and operational time.

Electrophoresis is less quantitative but much more convenient and economical. It is adaptable to the screening of large numbers of subjects at relatively low cost. Visual inspection of properly stained strips permits the immediate recognition of most normal patterns and certain abnormal ones of specific types. The definition of borderline abnormalities and the resolution of different types is achieved by ancillary determinations. Four additional steps have been adopted by us for sequential employment as they may be required to interpret the paper electrophoretogram. These include a determination of plasma cholesterol and glycerides, the precipitation of all lower-density lipoproteins and, occasionally, a single run in the preparative ultracentrifuge. The last is required to determine the quantity of β lipoproteins and whether the lipoproteins of β mobility have normal density.

The features of the electrophoretogram along with

TABLE 2. *Types of Hyperlipoproteinemia as Defined by Various Indexes to Plasma Lipoprotein Concentrations.**

Type	Appearance	Plasma Lipids		Paper Electrophoretic Bands	Analytical Ultracentrifuge	Preparative Ultracentrifuge	Particles Separated by Starch Electrophoresis or Polyvinylpyrrolidone Density Gradients	Precipitation with High-Molecular-Weight Polymers	Immuno-precipitation (Antiserum to β Lipoproteins)
		Choles-terol	Triglyc-eride						
I	Milky	↑±	↑↑↑	Chylomicrons present; all other lipoproteins ↓.	S_f 100-400 ↑	Bulk of plasma glyceride captured with centrifugation of 10^5 g/min.	Primary & secondary particles present in increased concentrations	Massive	Variable
II	Clear	↑↑↑	Normal or ↑	β ↑↑↑ Pre-β ↑±	S_f 0-12 ↑↑↑ 20-100 ↑±	Low-density lipoproteins 1.006-1.063 ↑↑↑; >1.006 ↑±.	Few, if any, particles present	Heavy	Heavy
III	Turbid	↑↑	↑	"Broad β" present; pre-β ↑± (requires ultracentrifuge to show beta lipoproteins of density <1.006).	S_f 0-12 ↓; 12-100 ↑↑ (? typical subclass pattern).	Low-density lipoproteins 1.006-1.063 ↓; <1.006 ↑ (diagnostic only if combined with electrophoresis to show beta lipoproteins of <1.006 in density).	Not known	Heavy	Heavy
IV	Turbid	↑	↑↑	Pre-β ↑↑↑	S_f 0-20 normal or ↓; 20-400 ↑↑↑	Very-low-density lipoproteins of density <1.006 ↑	Endogenous ("hyperlipemic") particles present	Heavy	Variable
V	Turbid or milky	↑	↑↑	Chylomicron band present; pre-β ↑↑.	S_f 20-400 ↑ (? typical subclass pattern)	Very-low-density lipoproteins of density <1.006 ↑	Primary, secondary, & endogenous particles present	Heavy	Variable

* ↑, increased; ↓, decreased.

the further steps to its interpretation are summarized in Figure 7. The successful definition of lipoprotein patterns by such a systematic approach depends very much upon the standardization of certain of these procedures. The current methods in use in large-scale studies of hyperlipoproteinemia at the Clinical Center have been employed in nearly 2000 plasma samples. A full description of the analytical sequence is in preparation. It will be summarized here to assure easier understanding of the interpretations that are to follow.

The plasma sample. Proper interpretation of lipoprotein patterns requires knowledge of when the patient took his last meal and whether his diet has been out of the ordinary. The following conditions have been maintained in the studies seeking definition of abnormal phenotypes by lipoprotein patterns: for 7 to 14 days before sampling the subject should take a diet sufficient to maintain stable body weight and containing foods in proportions normal for the population. For Americans this means about 40 per cent of calories as mixed fats, 50 per cent in carbohydrates and 10 to 15 per cent as proteins. No food should be taken for 12 to 14 hours before the sample is collected. Blood is mixed with ethylenediaminetetra-acetic acid (EDTA), 1 mg. per milliliter, and immediately placed in ice. The cells are removed by means of a refrigerated centrifuge whenever this is possible, and thereafter stored at 2 to 4°C. *Freezing irreversibly alters the lipoprotein pattern.* Upon storage the lipoprotein pattern slowly begins to deteriorate, the first changes being decreased sharpness of the lipoprotein bands. This deterioration is retarded by EDTA and is temperature dependent. Storage or shipment at room temperature is to be avoided. Under ideal conditions samples can be stored for several months if absolutely necessary.

Electrophoresis. Paper electrophoresis is performed at room temperature with the use of the Durrum hanging-strip method in barbital buffer of ionic strength 0.1, pH 8.6 and containing 0.001-M EDTA and 1 per cent albumin.[111] Either human or bovine albumin may be used. Electrophoresis is carried out over 16 hours at a constant voltage (120 V) with a current of 0.75 to 1.0 ma per strip. Whatman No. 1 paper yields the sharpest lipoprotein bands with the least degree of background staining. The optimal lipoprotein separations require equilibration of the strips for 3 to 4 hours in the closed cell before sample application, maintenance of the same level of buffer in both parts of the cell and periodic check of the pH of the buffer. Aging of the buffer is associated with a fall in pH below 8.2, and with daily use, the buffer must be changed every 1 or 2 months. We have the impression that the vertical (hanging-strip) method yields better lipoprotein separations than horizontal electrophoresis.

After electrophoresis the strips are dried in an oven at 95°C. for 20 minutes and stained by immersion in a supersaturated alcoholic solution of Oil-red-O (Allied Chemical Corporation) for 4 to 6 hours at 40°C. The samples are then rinsed with water and dried. The dye is made up by addition of 1.5 liters of ethyl alcohol, 1.0 liter of water, and 1 gm. of Oil-red-O, to a round-bottom flask fitted with a reflex condenser. The flask is heated with a heating mantle until the mixture comes to a boil and is then allowed to cool until the solution can be conveniently placed *without* filtering in a staining vessel kept in an oven at 37 to 40°C. The intensity of the staining of the strips is a function of the age and degree of saturation of the dye, and control strips must be run regularly for comparisons.

A series of related determinations are required for clarification of certain lipoprotein patterns (Fig. 7). It includes the quantification of α, β and pre-β lipoproteins in terms of their cholesterol content and establishment of whether all the lipoproteins of β mobility on paper are of the normal density (more than 1.006).

Ultracentrifugation. The lipoproteins and particles of density over 1.006 are isolated from 5-ml. aliquots of plasma by a standard technic employing ultracentrifugation of plasma at its own density for 16 hours at 100.000 × g.[5] The infranatant of density greater than 1.006, which contains the normal α and β lipoproteins, is returned to a volume of 5 ml. by the addition of 0.15-M saline solution.

Precipitation. The particles and all the lipoproteins containing β lipoprotein are separated from a 3-ml. aliquot of plasma by the addition of 0.15 ml. of 1.0-M manganese chloride and 6 mg. of sodium heparin.[42] A precipitate is allowed to develop over 15 minutes at 4°C. and is removed by ordinary centrifugation for 15 minutes at 4°C. The supernatant contains only α lipoproteins; its cholesterol content is equivalent to that in the fraction of density over 1.063 isolated by the ultracentrifuge (HDL).[78]

Quantification. The cholesterol content of the original plasma sample, the fraction of greater than 1.006 density and the supernatant of the heparin-manganese precipitation are determined. The concentrations of the several groups of lipoproteins as obtained directly or by difference are expressed in terms of cholesterol (in milligrams per 100 ml.). The plasma cholesterol less the fraction greater than 1.006 in density gives the concentration of pre-β lipoproteins and chylomicrons; the fraction of density greater than 1.006 less the α lipoproteins gives the concentration of β lipoproteins; the α lipoproteins represent the supernatant of the precipitation step. The entire set of procedures can be performed on all but very lipemic serums, in which the heparin and manganese may not precipitate the largest particles.

Electrophoresis. The fractions of density greater and less than 1.006 separated in the ultracentrifuge are also subjected to paper electrophoresis, and the mobility of their lipoprotein bands compared with each other and that of the lipoproteins in the whole plasma.

The cholesterol concentrations shown in Table 3 were measured by both the Abell modification[155] and the Autoanalyzer technic.[156] There was no significant difference between results obtained with the 2 methods. Triglycerides were determined by 3 technics.[157,158,162] There were no significant differences among results obtained by these 3 methods.

Quantification from paper strips. Many workers have shown that the α-lipoprotein and β-lipoprotein bands can be quantified from paper electrophoretic strips, either directly or after elution.[30,32] This has not been demonstrated for the pre-β and chylomicron bands. We have preferred to use the strips only for qualitative patterns. With experience one can estimate from the appearance of the strips the plasma cholesterol and glyceride concentrations to within 10 to 15 per cent of the chemical determinations. For purposes of comparison each day's electrophoresis run always includes a sample from a control subject whose lipoprotein concentrations are well known.

Setting Normal Limits

The interpretation of the lipoprotein pattern depends upon standards for normal concentrations of the lipoproteins. The setting of "limits of normal" for biologic quantities is often arbitrary. What is "usual" for one population may not be for another and is not necessarily healthy for either. Multiple modes of distribution for the concentration of plasma lipids or lipoproteins have rarely been demonstrated, and one is usually forced to rely on fiducial limits that assume a normal distribution.[163] The standards differ with age and sometimes with sex.

A set of cut-off points that help to define the usual limits of plasma concentration of the variables needed to interpret lipoprotein patterns is presented in Table 3. These are approximations, and for practical purposes, some of the limits have been com-

TABLE 3. *Plasma Lipid and Lipoprotein Concentrations in Normal Subjects.*

AGE	SEX	TOTAL CHOLESTEROL[†]	TRIGLYCERIDE[†]	PRE-BETA CHOLESTEROL[†‡]	BETA CHOLESTEROL[†‡]	ALPHA CHOLESTEROL[†]		NO. OF SUBJECTS
yr.		mg./100 ml.	mg./100 ml.	mg./100 ml.	mg./100 ml.	mg./100 ml.		
0-19	M	172 ± 34	61 ± 34	9 ± 7	108 ± 33	49 ± 11		43
	F	179 ± 33	73 ± 34	11 ± 8	108 ± 10	53 ± 12		38
20-29	M	183 ± 37	73 ± 32	11 ± 8	111 ± 30	53 ± 11		41
	F	179 ± 35	62 ± 29	12 ± 10	115 ± 31	52 ± 9		37
30-39	M	210 ± 33	78 ± 39	21 ± 13	143 ± 27	48 ± 11		50
	F	204 ± 37	67 ± 48	14 ± 10	119 ± 31	58 ± 13		32
40-49	M	230 ± 55	90 ± 41	21 ± 9	128 ± 28	49 ± 10		67
	F	217 ± 35	80 ± 42	14 ± 9	130 ± 24	62 ± 14		44
50-59	M	240 ± 48	104 ± 45	29 ± 8	152 ± 22	47 ± 15		28
	F	251 ± 49	83 ± 46	23 ± 8	147 ± 36	59 ± 15		41
Suggested "normal limits"§:						MALES	FEMALES	
0-19		120-230	10-140	5-25	50-170	30-65	30-70	
20-29		120-240	10-140	5-25	60-170	35-70	35-75	
30-39		140-270	10-150	5-35	70-190	30-65	35-80	
40-49		150-310	10-160	5-35	80-190	30-65	40-85	
50-59		160-330	10-190	10-40	80-210	30-65	35-85	

*Population sample is derived from subjects with no evidence of metabolic disease or family history of hyperlipoproteinemia whose triglycerides <200 mg./100 ml.; all samples obtained 12-14 hr. after evening meal.

†Mean & standard deviation.

‡Obtained on smaller no. of patients varying from 13 to 27.

§Based on 95 per cent fiducial limits calculated for small samples — all values rounded to nearest 5 mg. (it will be noted that, for practical purposes, differences between sexes have been ignored except for alpha-lipoprotein concentrations).

bined for the 2 sexes even though modest but significant differences actually exist. The sex difference in α-lipoprotein concentrations has been maintained (Table 3) since the lower limits do have value in detecting heterozygotes for Tangier disease.[149] The upper (5 per cent) limits for all the quantities are relatively high because the samples from which they are calculated are rather small. This should bias interpretation of patterns in the direction of mislabeling as "normal" subjects some who have marginal hyperlipoproteinemia.

Age-related changes. Lipid and lipoprotein concentrations do not progress stepwise as suggested by Table 3 but as continuous and nonlinear function of age that is not necessarily identical for males and females.[64,164-166]

The lowest lipoprotein concentrations are those in cord blood. The mean cholesterol concentration is about 70 mg. per 100 ml.,[167,168] and the α lipoproteins are about half and the β lipoproteins about a third of the concentrations shown in Table 3 for the youngest age decrement.[67] At this time there are practically no pre-β lipoproteins. Within the first few hours after birth the infant is forced to call upon the fat reserves that he has accumulated mainly in the last trimester of pregnancy. The initially low concentrations of free fatty acids are doubled, and the respiratory quotient begins to fall.[169] The transport of endogenous glyceride, perhaps required mainly to take care of overshoot in release of free fatty acids, begins in this early period. The mechanisms for transporting exogenous glyceride are also activated with the first feedings. Therefore, the demands upon β and possibly α lipoproteins should increase very early. Indeed, the concentration of β lipoproteins doubles or trebles within the first week of life, and lesser but definite increases in α lipo-

proteins also occur.[170,171] A very slow ascent in lipoprotein and cholesterol concentrations continues until well into the third decade.[172] For practical purposes pediatricians may use the limits in Table 3 for the first two decades without any correction except for the immediate postnatal period.

In the third decade there begins a "third phase" in which concentrations of β and pre-β lipoproteins rise at a new and more perceptible rate.[164,165] These increases are probably expressions of the change in fuel economy that is taking place at this time. Physical growth is ending, and the subject becomes more sedentary; caloric excess is easier to achieve, and perhaps other environmental and humoral factors come into play.

There is no general agreement about lipoprotein concentrations after about the age of sixty. From the available data it appears that the rise is over, at least for men. One must be very careful not to overinterpret lipoprotein determinations in very old subjects, and this sometimes poses difficulties in kindreds in which a younger propositus has hyperlipoproteinemia.

Naming the Patterns

In Figure 7 the terms "Type I," "Type II" and so forth appeared without comment. These are shorthand designations that were originally used to define different phenotypes of hyperlipoproteinemia because the existing nomenclature for the familial syndromes was inadequate and frequently misleading.[159,173,174] They have proved to be of such value for ready communication both in the laboratory and in the clinic that they may be used to denote specific lipoprotein patterns whether they are associated with primary or secondary hyperlipoproteinemia. The advantage is one of convenience. The

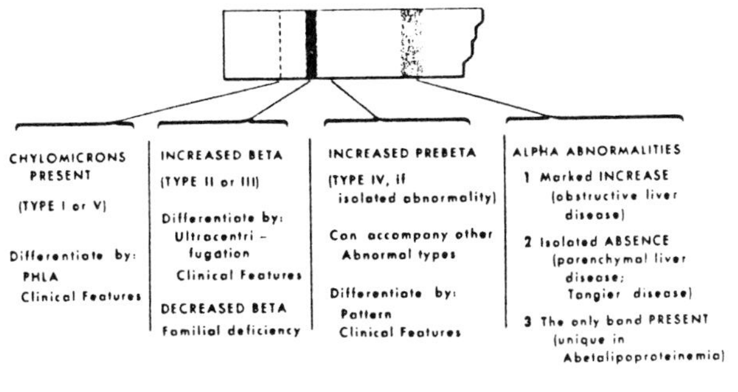

152   THE NEW ENGLAND JOURNAL OF MEDICINE   Jan. 19, 1967

FIGURE 7. *Steps in Interpreting the Paper Electrophoretogram.*

nomenclature for lipoproteins is unhandy and may be confusing when different technics are being considered. For example, the synonym "Type IV" is more convenient than either "hyperprebetalipoproteinemia" or "increased very-low-density (less than 1.006) lipoproteins." Since the clinical features associated with the different patterns tend to be specific, the type designation is frequently used here for either lipoprotein pattern or syndrome. All the nomenclature for these diseases, especially the genetically determined ones, must someday be based on a description of the responsible metabolic defect. The type system is only a temporary solution.

The numbering of the lipoprotein patterns according to type has been arranged in a mnemonically convenient way. This can be seen by comparison of Figure 5, the normal lipoprotein pattern, with similar figures that follow and show the abnormal patterns. The numbering begins at the origin of the paper electrophoretic strip, with Type I referring to the presence of chylomicrons, Type II to hyperbetalipoproteinemia and so on as the bands sequentially occur on the strip.

We may now begin to examine each of 5 abnormal types of lipoprotein patterns associated with hyperlipoproteinemia. This classification is an evolving one based on continuing studies at the Clinical Center that have emphasized genetically determined disorders.[159,173-175] It must be kept in mind that the lipoprotein patterns do not necessarily reflect genetic abnormalities, nor do they imply abnormal metabolism of the lipoproteins themselves as opposed to changing demands for fat transport. A single abnormal pattern may be the expression of one of several very different diseases. Finally, it is stressed once again that the index lipoprotein pattern for purposes of classification is that obtained on a normal diet.

TYPE I HYPERLIPOPROTEINEMIA[159]

General

Definition. The Type I lipoprotein pattern, in the system underlying this review, is characterized by the presence of chylomicrons in high concentration in plasma fourteen hours or more after the last meal of a normal diet. The chylomicrons carry dietary

glycerides and are particles so large that they scatter light and cause hyperlipemia that is properly called exogenous or fat induced. Of several theoretically possible reasons for this type of hyperlipoproteinemia there is at present good evidence concerning the existence of only one, a decrease in the activity of the enzyme lipoprotein lipase. Retarded removal of chylomicrons from plasma is associated with other disorders that may not involve decreased activity of this enzyme. Some of these will be taken up later under the mixed form of hyperlipemia, Type V.

Lipoprotein pattern. By the Type I pattern is meant hyperchylomicronemia in fairly pure form. Pre-β lipoproteins may be slightly increased. A *decrease* in α and β lipoproteins is the rule. Paper electrophoresis using the albumin-barbital buffer is at its most valuable in the quick and usually clearcut demonstration of a chylomicron band (Fig. 8). Other ways to define the Type I lipoprotein pattern are listed in Table 2.

The representation of chylomicrons in so truncated a density spectrum as available in Figure 8 is schematic in the extreme. The cut-off points used in the ultracentrifuge to separate chylomicrons are arbitrary, and a precise definition by flotation is not available. A crude and eminently practical definition is that of allowing lactescent plasma to stand overnight in the icebox. A discrete cream layer on the top usually represents chylomicrons.

Plasma lipids are helpful in detecting hyperchylomicronemia, but are not definitive. If the patient is on a regular diet the glycerides will exceed the cholesterol by a ratio (milligram per milligram) of about 8:1 or higher. The proportion of free cholesterol will be high, about 50 per cent instead of the usual 30. Under the right conditions chylomicrons

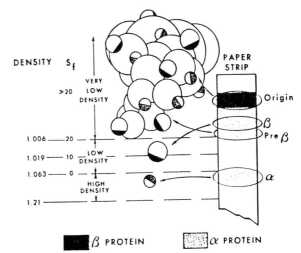

FIGURE 8. *Lipoprotein Pattern in Type I Hyperlipoproteinemia (See Also Table 3).*
The key clinical features of the familial syndrome are early expression, bouts of abdominal pain and other accompaniments of severe hyperlipemia, low postheparin lipolytic activity (PHLA) and autosomal recessive transmission.

Vol. 276 No. 3   FAT METABOLISM—FREDRICKSON ET AL.   153

are precipitable by dextran sulfate or heparin along with other low-density lipoproteins. The chylomicron precipitate often does not sediment, however, and routine precipitation technics (Table 2) yield quite variable results in severe chylomicronemia. They also cannot discriminate between exogenous and endogenous hyperlipemia.

It will be noted in Figure 8 how scanty are the amounts of α and β lipoproteins in severe hyperchylomicronemia. This is also seen with the excesses of pre-β lipoproteins or chylomicrons in Types IV and V. From evidence developed earlier it appears that these smaller lipoproteins are "bound" to or otherwise associated with the triglyceride particles so that they are no longer detectable in their usual density range or electrophoretic position.

Although concentrations of free fatty acids have not yet been proved to be helpful in diagnosis they are low in Type I and do not show the normal rise on feeding of fat. This is in accord with an assumed defect in hydrolysis of glyceride at the capillary wall.

Secondary Type I

There are cases in which abnormal chylomicronemia occurs in association with other forms of hyperlipoproteinemia. These are discussed later under Types IV and V and include difficulty in removing exogenous glyceride that appears to be secondary to such problems as uncontrolled diabetes,[176] pancreatitis[177-179] and acute alcoholism.[180] Whether hyperchylomicronemia secondary to other diseases exactly mimics the Type I pattern seen in the familial lipase deficiency is uncertain.

Primary (Familial) Type I

The most severe degree of hyperchylomicronemia is seen in patients who apparently are homozygous for a rare mutant gene regulating the activity of the clearing enzyme or enzymes. All familial Type I hyperlipoproteinemia ultimately may not turn out to represent lipoprotein lipase deficiency, but this is the only biochemical defect currently recognized.

History. The history of this syndrome has been reviewed elsewhere.[159] It is somewhat more straightforward than that of the other types of familial hyperlipoproteinemia. The manifestations are so dramatic that few if any of the earliest case reports have been ignored. The example generally accepted as the first representative of the primary familial Type I syndrome was the case of a twelve-year-old boy reported in 1932 under the title "hepatosplenomegalic lipidosis" by Bürger and Grütz.[181] The first patient with a relative who also had hyperlipemia was described in 1939 as having "idiopathic familial hyperlipemia."[182] After this description appeared many other cases were reported under the title "idiopathic" or "essential hyperlipemia," but close scrutiny of the case reports suggested that only a few of these qualify as the Type I syndrome. If fairly rigid criteria are used to define

the syndrome, about 35 acceptable case reports can be found.[159] Examples of primary Type I have been described by the following synonyms: idiopathic familial hyperlipemia; essential familial hyperlipemia; retention hyperlipemia; alimentary "hepatogenic" fat retention; familial lipemia; fat-induced hyperlipemia; and familial hyperchylomicronemia. Of these definitions only the last 2 seem acceptable. One defines the characteristic lipoprotein pattern, and the other the origin of the glycerides accumulating in plasma. All synonyms; including the shorthand term, Type I, can be replaced by a more specific one of *lipoprotein-lipase deficient familial hyperchylomicronemia* when it has been ascertained that the patient qualifies for such a diagnosis. For this one needs to have certain information beyond the lipoprotein pattern, including the patient's enzyme response to heparin.

Clinical manifestations. The important clinical manifestations summarized in the legend of Figure 8 are sufficiently reproducible to permit the synthesis of a "typical case history." It may begin at a pediatrician's office with the appearance of a mother whose one-month-old child looks healthy but has "bouts of colic" and an unusually prominent abdomen. Recently, some yellow papules with a reddish base may have broken out over the skin and oral mucosa. An enlarged liver and spleen are felt, and hospitalization for observation is recommended. Here, the intern sees nearly white retinal vessels (lipemia retinalis). As the blood sample emerges in the syringe it looks like "cream-of-tomato soup." The lipoprotein pattern is established, and the baby's formula is changed to one containing only skim milk or other fat-free sources of calories. Within three days the hyperlipemia has cleared dramatically. The xanthomas will shortly resolve, the liver and spleen will decrease in size, and the apparent attacks of abdominal discomfort will disappear.

Such a child is more fortunate than the patient with the same genotype whose abnormality is not detected until he is old enough to describe his abdominal discomfort in details that suggest one of a variety of acute surgical emergencies. He may undergo laparotomy before the nature of his syndrome has been appreciated. Although the majority of patients are discovered before the age of ten, some may be adults when the diagnosis is first made.[159]

Diabetes. Glucose intolerance is not a feature of Type I and the usual oral and intravenous tests are normal even when the patient has severe hyperlipemia. This is in contradistinction to other types of hyperlipemia, including some that are "fat-induced" (see Types IV and V).

Diagnosis. The diagnosis of this syndrome is usually not difficult and entails three steps: identification of the Type I lipoprotein pattern; ascertainment that the glyceride accumulation is immediately related to dietary fat intake; and measurement of plasma postheparin lipolytic activity (PHLA).

Within a few days of switching a patient with a Type I pattern from a regular fat intake to less than 5 gm. of fat per day, one will note a *rapid* decline in plasma glycerides or hyperlipemia. The lipoprotein pattern will evolve in a predictable fashion. Chylomicrons will disappear, the β-lipoprotein band will increase, as will the α, but the most striking change will be abnormal accumulation of pre-β lipoproteins.[7,159] The glyceride concentrations rarely become completely normal on the fat-free diet because the patient is now moderately "carbohydrate induced." Presumably, the means of removing endogenous glyceride are similarly affected by the inherited abnormality, and even the normal increase in endogenous glyceride that follows the shift to a high-carbohydrate diet causes a slightly greater hyperlipemia than normal. The paper electrophoretic technic is most helpful for observation of the fascinating and instructive changes in lipoprotein patterns in Type I with different diets.

Lipoprotein lipase activity should be assessed in all such patients.[183-185] PHLA is best assayed under in vitro conditions capable of determining maximum reaction velocity. In 12 patients from 11 kindreds we have found values from 0.04 to 0.20 (in μEq. of free fatty acids per minute per milliliter of plasma). This is below the range of values (0.24 to 0.60, mean about 0.40) found in over 100 subjects with either normal or Type II-IV lipoprotein patterns. One other patient with the familial Type I syndrome has persistently had normal PHLA, although his sibling, with an identical lipoprotein pattern, had abnormally low values.[159]

Phenocopies. Low PHLA, as defined by the assay used for the Type I patients described above, has been reported in patients with untreated diabetes[176] and hypothyroidism.[186] This activity is also low in other syndromes, and the enzyme assay is not a specific determinant of genotype. One other problem plagues the definition of the familial Type I syndrome. This is the possibility that in some of the patients the disorder has "converted" to another type of hyperlipoproteinemia because of pancreatitis, diabetes or prolonged intake of an abnormal diet. One way to be fairly certain of the diagnosis is the detection of another typical example of Type I in the patient's family.

Inheritance. In 5 kindreds with primary Type I, multiple sibs had had equally severe hyperlipemia.[159] Occasionally, very mild hyperlipemia has been present in 1 parent or 1 or more siblings. The study of kindreds has been inadequate, particularly concerning the need to demonstrate that a relative with hyperlipemia does indeed have the Type I pattern and not, for example, the much more common Type IV pattern. Both parents of an affected child may have normal lipoprotein patterns although in several kindreds at least 1 has had mild hyperlipemia. The relatively small number of involved sibs supports the assumption that a double dose of an abnormal gene accounts for the severe Type I phe-

notype and that a single dose of the gene may produce little or no detectable abnormality.

An unusually high number of parents or sibs have PHLA in or slightly below the lowest quartile of the distribution of the enzyme in normal subjects.[159] The slightly low activity may be associated with normal postabsorptive glyceride concentrations. As illustrated by the presence of the 1 homozygous abnormal patient with normal PHLA, a more specific assay for enzyme activity is needed. Attempts have been made to measure the enzyme in human adipose tissue.[187] The activities are very low. In 1 report, levels significantly lower than normal were found in a family with fat-induced hyperlipemia.[188]

Mechanism. The few well studied examples of Type I suggest that the inheritable defect in all has been a deficiency of lipoprotein lipase activity.[159,183,189] Hydrolysis of glyceride at sites of removal is decreased. This imposes severe limitation on the rate of clearing of chylomicrons and probably that of glycerides in other particles or lipoproteins. The patients with familial Type I syndrome have almost no threshold for fat removal, as though the entire normal clearing mechanism were inoperative. This presents something of a paradox, for the evidence is far from convincing that lipoprotein lipase is present in the liver. It seems either that the liver does not have an essential role in clearing chylomicrons or that lipoprotein lipase deficiency is not the basic defect in Type I. The generalized explanation of this disorder therefore hangs upon better understanding of the physiologic mechanisms of fat clearing.

There is a need to examine carefully all new examples of Type I to be certain that lipoprotein lipase deficiency is indeed present. Among other possible mechanisms, the production of abnormal chylomicrons or presence of circulating inhibitors of lipoprotein lipase has been eliminated in some patients.[159] Defects in the re-esterification or further utilization of glyceride fatty acids that theoretically could limit the rate of clearing have not been excluded, but the persistently low levels of free fatty acids in Type I argue against such possibilities.

Management. The outlook for patients with the "pure" Type I familial syndrome is not yet predictable. The well documented cases still include a relatively young group. Most have learned they must limit their daily fat intake if they are to avoid bouts of abdominal pain. The origins of the pain are still obscure, and it can occur as well in patients with other kinds of severe hyperlipemia. Sometimes, it is accompanied by the usual chemical signs of pancreatitis. It has been speculated that this organ is compromised by fat embolization or perhaps local lipolysis, giving rise to irritatingly high free fatty acid concentrations. Proof is lacking for any mechanism. On other occasions, similar pain is not associated with any rise in serum lipase or amylase content. The pain can be restricted to a single organ such as the spleen, which may be exquisitely tender. Because pregnancy may exacerbate hyperlipemia special care must be taken with these patients during this time. Several patients have delivered normal babies.

In addition to the painful attacks, the retarded removal of dietary fat has a number of side effects. Chylomicrons awaiting access to their usual sites of disposal seem to be prime targets for uptake by reticuloendothelial cells. Large foam cells appear in the bone marrow; eruptive xanthomas arise in the skin, and the liver and spleen enlarge. These changes are less dramatic but also urge limitation of fat intake in the hope of avoiding possible compromise of the functions of these and other tissues.

Atherosclerosis. In the 35 or so patients with the familial Type I syndrome there has so far been a lack of evidence of accelerated coronary-artery disease. This is not proof, of course, that a high concentration of glycerides in plasma in the form of chylomicrons represents no particular hazard for the vessel wall. The inference is tempting, however, and may be used at least in the argument against extreme limitation in fat intake. For in these patients, this will lead to accumulation of pre-β lipoproteins. The latter seem to have a less benign association with vascular disease.

Diet. The treatment of Type I, then, is *moderate* restriction of dietary fat. The best motivated of these patients will usually select about 20 to 25 gm. of fat per day. So far as the degree of saturation of the fatty acids in the dietary glycerides is concerned, the source of the fat makes no difference to the degree of hyperlipemia.

It has been popular in recent years to feed triglycerides containing medium-chain-length fatty acids (MCT) to patients with abnormal absorption or fat-induced hyperlipemia. This permits fat intake without chylomicron excess, since these fatty acids are taken into the body by a different mechanism, apparently through the portal system. This type of fat may induce higher concentrations of pre-β lipoproteins, and its long-term safety is uncertain.

Parenterally infused fluids and no oral intake are the best treatment of the acute abdominal symptoms that may accompany Type I. Intubation may be necessary to relieve distention and ileus.

Other "antihyperlipemic" medications thus far available have not been shown to have a place in treatment of this disease. All the patients have some rise in free fatty acids in response to heparin injections, and this drug will promote some intravascular lipolysis. The small amount of lipolysis is not enough to clear the plasma, however, and the use of heparin in Type I is without good rationale.

"Intermittent" Primary Forms of Type I

Examples of severe intermittent hyperlipemia resembling Type I may occur. We have examined the plasma of a twelve-year-old girl (a patient of Dr. Allen Crocker) whose severe, "fat-induced" hyper-

lipemia seemed to be intermittent even on a regular diet. She had a typical Type I pattern on one occasion and a completely normal pattern some weeks later. There was no familial hyperlipoproteinemia. Such a case is puzzling in the extreme. It can be easily calculated that if one absorbed all of a 100-gm. daily intake of fat, and the removal of this were suddenly and completely blocked, a severe hyperlipemia of the order of 3000 mg. per 100 ml. could be attained in one day. Presumably, some "toxic" factors could so interrupt the clearing process at one step or another in a transient or sporadic fashion, but there is little or no knowledge of what such factors might be. Good examples of the inheritable Type I or their equally interesting phenocopies are hard to come by. They deserve uncommon attention.

Possible lesser degrees of Type I. In our experience with paper electrophoresis even the faintest of chylomicrons is very rarely detected in apparently healthy Americans of any age after an overnight fast. In young adults the chylomicron tide has disappeared by midnight, six hours after the last meal. When the daily fat intake, spread over 3 meals, is increased to a total load that is two or three times greater than the usual American intake, chylomicrons are still briskly removed, and the lowest glyceride measurements in the daily cycle are registered just before breakfast.

Our experience that hyperchylomicronemia is extremely unusual when electrophoresis is used for screening is not necessarily at odds with other suggestions that fat tolerance may decay with age or other conditions[190] or that minor degrees of intolerance might be genetically determined.[191] The paper electrophoretic technic is relatively insensitive and may not detect very small amounts of chylomicrons. The fast for twelve to fourteen hours is also long, and some shorter sampling time after the fat feeding might provide a better discriminant. The ideal fat tolerance test has not yet been devised. At present it is not known whether there are mild degrees of inability to remove dietary fat that are genetically determined or sporadic. Only the grosser abnormalities can be reliably detected.

(To be continued)

REFERENCES

151. Sunderman, F. W., and Sunderman, F. W., Jr. *Lipids and the Steroid Hormones in Clinical Medicine.* 207 pp. Philadelphia: Lippincott, 1960.

152. Kunkel, H. G., Ahrens, E. H., Jr., and Eisenmenger, W. J. Application of turbidimetric methods for estimation of gamma globulin and total lipid to study of patients with liver disease. *Gastroenterology* 11:499-507, 1948.

153. Stern, I., and Shapiro, B. Rapid and simple method for determination of esterified fatty acids and for total fatty acids in blood. *J. Clin. Path.* 6:158-160, 1953.

154. Albrink, M. J. Microtitration of total fatty acids of serum, with notes on estimation of triglycerides. *J. Lipid Research* 1:53-59, 1959.

155. Kabara, J. J. Determination and microscopic localization of

156 THE NEW ENGLAND JOURNAL OF MEDICINE Jan. 19, 1967

cholesterol. In *Methods of Biochemical Analysis*. Vol. 10. Edited by D. Glick. 399 pp. New York: Interscience, 1962. P. 263.

156. Total cholesterol procedure N-24. In *Auto Analyzer Manual*. Chauncey, New York, Technicon Instruments Corp., 1964.

157. Van Handel, E., and Zilversmit, D. B. Micromethod for direct determination of serum triglycerides. *J. Lab. & Clin. Med.* **50**:152-157, 1957.

158. Jagannathan, S. N. Determination of plasma triglycerides. *Canad. J. Biochem.* **42**:566-570, 1964.

159. Fredrickson, D. S., and Lees, R. S. Familial hyperlipoproteinemia. In *The Metabolic Basis of Inherited Disease*. Second edition. Edited by J. B. Stanbury, J. B. Wyngaarden and D. S. Fredrickson. 1434 pp. New York: McGraw–Hill, 1966. P. 429.

160. Cornwell, D. G., Kruger, F. A., Hamwi, G. J., and Brown, J. B. Studies on characterization of human serum lipoproteins separated by ultracentrifugation in density gradient. I. Serum lipoproteins in normal, hyperthyroid and hypercholesterolemic subjects. *Am. J. Clin. Nutrition* **9**:24-40, 1961.

161. Furman, R. H., Howard, R. P., Lakshmi, K., and Norcia, L. N. Serum lipids and lipoproteins in normal and hyperlipidemic subjects as determined by preparative ultracentrifugation. *Am. J. Clin. Nutrition* **9**:73-102, 1961.

162. Jover, A. Technique for determination of serum glycerides. *J. Lipid Research* **4**:228-230, 1963.

163. Thomas, C. B., Murphy, E. A., and Bolling, D. R. Precursors of hypertension and coronary disease: statistical consideration of distributions in population of medical students. I. Total serum cholesterol. *Bull. Johns Hopkins Hosp.* **114**:290-312, 1964.

164. Keys, A., Mickelsen, O., Miller, E. v. O., Hayes, E. R., and Todd, R. L. Concentration of cholesterol in blood serum of normal man and its relation to age. *J. Clin. Investigation* **29**:1347-1353, 1950.

165. Lewis, L. A., et al. Serum lipid levels in normal persons. *Circulation* **16**:227-245, 1957.

166. Schaefer, L. E. Serum cholesterol-triglyceride distribution in "normal" New York City population. *Am. J. Med.* **36**:262-268, 1964.

167. Mortimer, J. G. Cord blood lipids of normal infants and infants of diabetic mothers. *Arch. Dis. Childhood* **39**:342-344, 1964.

168. Crowley, J., Ways, P., and Jones, J. W. Human fetal erythrocyte and plasma lipids. *J. Clin. Investigation* **44**:989-998, 1965.

169. Van Duyne, C. M., and Havel, R. J. Plasma unesterified fatty acid concentrations in fetal and neonatal life. *Proc. Soc. Exper. Biol. & Med.* **102**:599-602, 1959.

170. Lindquist, B., and Malmcrona, R. Dietary fat in relation to serum lipids in normal infant. *J. Dis. Child.* **99**:39-47, 1960.

171. Sweeney, M. J., Etteldorf, J. N., Organ, P. M., and Fisher, R. Effect of diet during first six to eight weeks of life on total concentrations of serum protein and on electrophoretic patterns of serum protein and lipoprotein. *Pediatrics* **29**:82-89, 1962.

172. Rafstedt, S. Studies on serum lipids and lipoproteins in infancy and childhood. *Acta paediat.* **44** (Supp. 102):1-109, 1955.

173. Fredrickson, D. S., and Lees, R. S. System for phenotyping hyperlipoproteinemia. *Circulation* **31**:321-327, 1965.

174. Fredrickson, D. S., Lees, R. S., and Levy, R. I. Genetically determined abnormalities in lipid transport. In *Progress in Biochemical Pharmacology*. Vol. 2. Edited by R. Paoletti, D. Kritchevsky and D. Steinberg. Basel: Karger, 1966. P. 343.

175. Fredrickson, D. S. Essential familial hyperlipidemia. In *The Metabolic Basis of Inherited Disease*. Edited by J. B. Stanbury, J. B. Wyngaarden and D. S. Fredrickson. 1477 pp. New York: McGraw–Hill, 1960. P. 489.

176. Bierman, E. L., Bagdade, J. D., and Porte, D., Jr. Concept of pathogenesis of diabetic lipemia. *Tr. A. Am. Physics* (in press).

177. Albrink, M. J., and Klatskin, G. Lactescence of serum following episodes of acute alcoholism and its probable relationship to acute pancreatitis. *Am. J. Med.* **23**:26-33, 1957.

178. Zieve, L. Jaundice, hyperlipemia and hemolytic anemia: heretofore unrecognized syndrome associated with alcoholic fatty liver and cirrhosis. *Ann. Int. Med.* **48**:471-496, 1958.

179. Kessler, J. I., Kniffen, J. C., and Janowitz, H. D. Lipoprotein lipase inhibition in hyperlipemia of acute alcoholic pancreatitis. *New Eng. J. Med.* **269**:943-948, 1963.

180. Isselbacher, K. J., and Greenberger, N. J. Metabolic effects of alcohol on liver. *New Eng. J. Med.* **270**:351-356, 1964.

181. Bürger, M., and Grütz, O. Über hepatosplenomegale Lipoidose mit xanthomatösen Veränderungen in Haut und Schleimhaut. *Arch. f. Dermat. u. Syph.* **166**:542-575, 1932.

182. Holt, L. E., Jr., Aylward, F. X., and Timbres, H. G. Idiopathic familial lipemia. *Bull. Johns Hopkins Hosp.* **64**:279-314, 1939.

183. Havel, R. J., and Gordon, R. S., Jr. Idiopathic hyperlipemia: metabolic studies in an affected family. *J. Clin. Investigation* **39**:1777-1790, 1960.

184. Fredrickson, D. S., Ono, K., and Davis, L. L. Lipolytic activity of post-heparin plasma in hyperglyceridemia. *J. Lipid Research* **4**:24-33, 1963.

185. Boberg, J., and Carlson, L. A. Determination of heparin induced lipoprotein lipase activity in human plasma. *Clin. chim. acta* **10**:420-427, 1964.

186. Porte, D., Jr., O'Hara, D. D., and Williams, R. H. Relation between postheparin lipolytic activity and plasma triglyceride in myxedema. *Metabolism* **15**:107-113, 1966.

187. Nestel, P. J., and Havel, R. J. Lipoprotein lipase in human adipose tissue. *Proc. Soc. Exper. Biol. & Med.* **109**:985-987, 1962.

188. Harlan, W. R., Winesett, P. S., Wasserman, A. J., and Hale, B. Assay of tissue lipoprotein lipase activity in familial exogenous hypertriglyceridemia. *Clin. Research* **14**:99, 1966.

189. Kuo, P., Bassett, D., DiGeorge, A., and Carpenter, G. Lipolytic activity of post-heparin plasma in hyperlipemia and hypolipemia. *Circulation Research* **16**:221-229, 1965.

190. Angervall, G. On fat tolerance test. *Acta med. Scandinav.* Supp. **424**:1-84, 1964.

191. Hirschhorn, K., Hirschhorn, R., Fraccaro, M., and Böök, J. A. Incidence of familial hyperlipemia. *Science* **129**:716-717, 1959.

MEDICAL PROGRESS

FAT TRANSPORT IN LIPOPROTEINS – AN INTEGRATED APPROACH TO MECHANISMS AND DISORDERS (Continued)*

DONALD S. FREDRICKSON, M.D.,† ROBERT I. LEVY, M.D.,‡ AND ROBERT S. LEES, M.D.§

BETHESDA, MARYLAND

TYPE II HYPERLIPOPROTEINEMIA[159,192-196]

General

Definitions. By the Type II lipoprotein pattern we mean an increase in the concentration of lipoproteins that have discrete β mobility by electrophoresis and the normal density and chemical composition of β-migrating lipoproteins. This kind of hyperbeta-lipoproteinemia must be distinguished from another in which the density of the β-migrating lipoproteins is abnormally low, giving rise to a pattern designated as Type III in this system for defining types of hyperlipoproteinemia. The bases for distinguishing the hyperbeta-lipoproteinemia of Types II and III arise from considerable clinical and genetic evidence that they are expressions of different inheritable metabolic disorders. Type II is a common pattern; it can be a resultant of diet or secondary to hypothyroidism and other diseases, and in many patients it proves to be an expression of a mutant gene or very similar genes, appearing in relatively high frequency in many populations, including the North American.

Lipoprotein pattern. The illustration of the Type II pattern in Figure 9 depicts two important features. Foremost is the discrete increase in β lipoproteins, which on the paper electrophoretic strip is visible as a sharp band taking increased amounts of lipid stain with almost malevolent intensity when one considers the clinical implications of the abnormality. This sharp band is indicative of an increase in the low-density classes of both S_f 0-12 and 12-20. Normally, the concentration of the S_f 0-12

*From the Laboratory of Molecular Diseases, National Heart Institute.

†Director and chief, Laboratory of Molecular Diseases, National Heart Institute.

‡Head, Section on Lipoproteins, Laboratory of Molecular Diseases, National Heart Institute.

§Assistant professor and associate physician, Rockefeller University.

class is about five times that of the 12-20 class, and this differential is usually maintained in the Type II pattern.[64,194,196,197]

The second feature of the Type II pattern, and one that we are anxious to clarify, is that it must not exclude a small increase in glyceride concentrations. In analyses of 100 consecutive patients with established familial Type II patterns that are in preparation for publication, the mean glyceride concentration is about 150 mg. per 100 ml., and the upper limit about 500. This is associated with a modest increase in pre-β lipoproteins or lipoproteins of S_f 20-100.[194-197]

After comparing the glyceride and β-lipoprotein concentrations associated with several hundred lipoprotein patterns, we conclude that in Type II a given increase in glycerides will be represented by about the same increase in pre-β lipoproteins. This is noteworthy, since the overwhelming concentrations of β lipoproteins in Type II might be expected to "accommodate" abnormal amounts of glyceride without the presence of a pre-β band on the electrophoretic strip. Some Type II patients have no pre-β band (or increase in S_f 20-100 lipoproteins); others may have distinct and sometimes abnormally increased amounts of pre-β lipoproteins. The current definition of Type II[174] differs from that described by us in our first publications related to phenotyping by lipoprotein patterns.[157,173] Formerly, the combination of increased β and pre-β lipoproteins was considered one kind of Type III pattern. Type III has since been more explicitly defined (as discussed below).

Determination of hyperbeta-lipoproteinemia. The age trends of plasma cholesterol concentrations in both sexes in the general population tend to parallel those of the β-lipoprotein (S_f 0-20) concentrations.[64,198] (See also Table 3.) The concentrations

216   THE NEW ENGLAND JOURNAL OF MEDICINE   Jan. 26, 1967

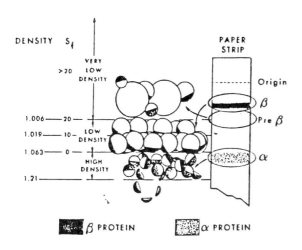

FIGURE 9. *Type II Hyperlipoproteinemia (See Also Table 3).*
The familial form is transmitted as an autosomal dominant and is usually accompanied by palpebral, tendon and tuberous xanthomas, corneal arcus and accelerated atherosclerosis. Glycerides (pre-β lipoproteins) may be modestly elevated; PHLA is normal, and glucose tolerance is usually normal.

of S_f 20-400 (pre-β) lipoproteins also rise with age.[64,198,199] Thus, an intense β-lipoprotein band on the electrophoretogram can definitely be interpreted as abnormal when the plasma cholesterol concentration is clearly beyond the upper limit of normal (Table 2) only if the triglyceride concentration is not in excess of 150 mg. per 100 ml. Instead of a triglyceride determination the plasma must therefore be observed to be perfectly clear. When there is uncertainty the quantity of β lipoproteins must be specifically determined, either as described earlier or by some comparable technic. When the native plasma or serum is perfectly clear the various chemical precipitation technics or those depending on antibodies to β lipoproteins yield their least equivocal results and provide a fairly reliable index to Type II hyperlipoproteinemia.

The establishment of any dividing line between normal and abnormal β-lipoprotein concentrations is somewhat arbitrary, as already discussed. The limits provided in Table 3 are more likely to be too high than too low, at least in the context of defining the most healthy concentrations. The suggested upper limit for any age in Table 3 is 210 mg. per 100 ml. (as lipoprotein cholesterol), and in the younger age group, it is lower. The mean β-lipoprotein concentrations for the normal levels in Table 3 are very close to those in a smaller series previously reported.[161] Sets of normal values for β lipoproteins have been obtained in larger samples by means of the analytical ultracentrifuge.[64,198] The average β-lipoprotein concentrations (S_f 0-12 plus S_f 12-20) in the latter analyses, when estimated arbitrarily in terms of cholesterol content, are slightly higher than those shown in Table 3. The mean increased with age into the sixth decade in these analyses as it does in Table 3.

Major assistance in judging what are "normal" limits has been provided by kindreds with the familial Type II syndrome. Affected adult members, on a regular diet, rarely have β-lipoprotein concentrations below 250 mg. per 100 ml. Some of the young children affected and some of the adults on strict diets may fall below 200 mg. From inspection of the data being gathered in the Clinical Center studies it appears that bimodality in the distribution of β-lipoprotein concentrations within Type II families will be demonstrable. From a few Lebanese families in which several probable homozygous abnormal members appear it seems likely that 3 modes will be demonstrable when a population sample containing a sufficient number of marriages between heterozygotes has been examined.[200] Previous attempts to show several modes of distribution of plasma cholesterol concentrations in affected American kindreds have, at the most, been only partially successful.[194,201]

Environment and the Type II pattern. The interpretation of possibly abnormal β-lipoprotein concentrations in the "gray zone" of about 175 to 225 mg. per 100 ml. (as cholesterol) is difficult. Depending on the age of the patient, the case may have to be considered primary "Type II" even though the family history is negative. Such "probable abnormal patients" are not infrequent in groups with accelerated atherosclerosis. The interpretation of their lipoprotein patterns requires special attention to their living habits. It is generally accepted from epidemiologic studies and easily demonstrable experimentally that otherwise normal subjects who eat a great deal of cholesterol[202,203] or an increased amount of saturated fats[12] generally have higher plasma cholesterol concentrations than those who eat much less of these foodstuffs. There is no consensus of whether sterol or the type of dietary glyceride is the prime determinant.[204] A β-lipoprotein concentration cannot be properly interpreted, therefore, without knowledge of the patient's diet. Although the lipoprotein level can be driven down by certain diets to much lower levels in normal subjects than in patients with the Type II pattern adequate study has not yet been made of the possibility that response to diet alone may segregate primary hyperbeta-lipoproteinemia into sporadic and inheritable forms or further subdivide patients within these main groups.

Dietary restrictions should not be imposed on a patient with a Type II pattern until the etiology has been carefully sought. The effort expended in changing a patient's food habits, and often those of his family requires that metabolic determinants other than diet be excluded and that the degree of involvement shared by the members of the family be ascertained.

Secondary Type II

Type II hyperlipoproteinemia accounts for a great deal of the "hypercholesterolemia" that the physician sees. As with other abnormal lipoprotein patterns, the most systematic approach to diagnosis and treatment first requires the elimination of certain diseases of which the hyperlipoproteinemia is a secondary manifestation.

Probably the most common of these is hypothyroidism. Next most common are some types or stages of obstructive hepatic disease and hypoproteinemias like the nephrotic syndrome; quite rarely one may encounter this pattern with myeloma, macroglobulinemia, idiopathic hypercalcemia and other unusual disorders. Obstructive jaundice usually provides a unique pattern that will be described separately. Others of these disorders will be discussed in the concluding section of this review under Type IV, the abnormal lipoprotein pattern with which they are more commonly associated.

Hypothyroidism. Myxedema may be accompanied by great increases in β-lipoprotein concentrations and a Type II pattern that mimics that due to mutation.[26,64,160,161] According to studies with ^{131}I-tagged lipoproteins there is a decreased rate of removal of β lipoproteins from circulation in hypothyroidism.[205,206] Carotene concentrations are high,[205] as they are in other forms of hypercholesterolemia.[207] In hypothyroidism this has been attributed to decreased catabolism of the β lipoprotein, the major carrier of carotene in plasma. Vitamin A levels can also be low.[205] It has not been proved that decreased conversion in the intestine of carotene to vitamin A does not occur in hypothyroidism, increasing the amount of carotene absorbed and transported. It is still not known how thyroid hormone regulates plasma levels of β lipoprotein. The assumption that such a regulatory defect may be independent of calorigenic activity of this hormone is the basis for frequent use of the dextroisomer of thyroxine in the treatment of hyperlipoproteinemia.[208] Hypothyroidism is sometimes associated with hyperlipemias as well. This will be discussed again in the differential diagnosis of Type IV.

The proof that a Type II pattern is caused by hypothyroidism rests on the demonstration of hormone deficiency and improvement in the pattern as replacement therapy is undertaken. Sometimes primary Type II is not discovered until the lipoprotein pattern fails to return to normal after a patient with myxedema has been made euthyroid.

Familial Type II[159,192-196]

One of the most common inheritable forms of hyperlipoproteinemia encountered in the world is Type II hyperbeta-lipoproteinemia. Perhaps it should be called a syndrome since it may be a group of similar diseases. For convenience it will be colloquially referred to here as "familial Type II." In addition to hundreds of affected American families there are in the literature easily identifiable examples in Caucasians and Negroes from many geographic areas. There is at least 1 report among Asiatics.[209] There are no clear-cut data on the gene frequency in any population, including the Ameri-

can, and information about its possible occurrence in some areas of the world is completely lacking. One of the major purposes of the studies that are the basis for this review has been the establishment of better criteria for ascertainment of familial Type II and the promotion of their utilization in obtaining this much needed information.

Our experience with familial Type II consists of the study, including complete lipoprotein analyses, of over 100 definitely familial examples from about 50 families and a similar number of less well studied familial cases or single patients whose lipoprotein pattern and clinical features are compatible with the syndrome. There are many other reports of single cases or whole pedigrees in the literature. A number of comprehensive studies indicate close agreement with the present description of this disorder.[192-196,200,210]

The consideration that all familial Type II may be due to a mutation at the same genetic locus is supported by the predictability of clinical expression and genetic mode in all the patients with this lipoprotein pattern. The heterozygote seems to be nearly always recognizable by lipoprotein pattern. Depending upon unknown factors that govern the degree and speed of expression, the accompanying xanthomatosis and atheromatosis frequently seen in the syndrome will develop in many heterozygotes. They usually survive the childbearing period and may have a normal life-span.

The homozygous abnormal phenotype has increases in β lipoprotein that are nearly double those seen in the usual heterozygote, quite severe xanthomatosis and often death in childhood from cardiovascular involvement. This includes endocardial deposits of lipid, sometimes causing aortic stenosis, coronary-artery disease and occlusive disease of the peripheral vessels.

History. Familial Type II seems to have entered medical history surreptitiously, possibly as long as one hundred and thirty years ago. The date will remain uncertain because xanthomas were recognized sometime before it was realized that they were due to hyperlipidemia and long before different metabolic bases for the latter were appreciated. Palpebral xanthomas (xanthelasma) are shown without comment in Rayer's[211] atlas, published in 1835. The first descriptions of tendon and tuberous xanthomas appear under the term "vitiligoidea" in *Guy's Hospital Reports* in 1851.[212] The authors, Addison and Gull, were describing lesions associated with the hyperlipoproteinemia due to obstructive biliary disease, as were the other authors of reports of xanthomas in the English and French literature for the next fifteen to twenty years. The appearance of cutaneous xanthomas in a patient free of jaundice with a relative who had the same lesions was briefly described between 1868 and 1882.[213,214] There was no mention of plasma lipids, and the descriptions of the lesions are not convincing evidence for Type II.

Synonyms for familial Type II appeared in medical writing in roughly the following order (with the omission of certain terms for similar kinds of xanthomas): hereditary xanthomatosis; familial xanthoma; hereditary xanthoma tuberosum multiplex; general xanthelasma; xanthelasma multiplex; xanthoma tendinosum; essential familial hypercholesterolemic xanthomatosis; and, most recently, essential familial hypercholesterolemia.[192] Neither "familial hypercholesterolemia," "xanthomas tendinosum" nor "familial hyperbeta-lipoproteinemia" is entirely satisfactory, however; for the quite different pattern syndromes, Types II and III, can both be included in these categorical listings. An ideal name for Type II must await elucidation of the primary abnormality.

Diagnosis. The major features of familial Type II hyperlipoproteinemia form a triad. The first component is the lipoprotein pattern in the absence of other primary disease. The second is distribution of the Type II pattern in the family according to mendelian concepts of an autosomal dominant trait. Both these components should be present for ascertainment of what, in present-day genetic studies, can be considered the familial Type II phenotype. For practical clinical purposes the first component, when coupled with florid appearance of the third feature, — xanthomatosis, — is usually adequate for diagnosis. The 3 components of this triad deserve some further, more detailed exposition.

Hyperbeta-lipoproteinemia is the first requisite. It has already been defined in detail, and stress laid on the fact that it may be accompanied by moderate hyperglyceridemia. The small pre-β-lipoprotein band appearing in many Type II patterns does not give rise to significant hyperlipemia. Therefore, *milky serum is incompatible with uncomplicated Type II.*

The observations of Type II families have not yet established whether the plasma concentration of glyceride or pre-β lipoproteins may provide an independent variable that will segregate some families as representing a different "kind" of familial Type II syndrome. In 1 large kindred glyceride concentrations in affected and nonaffected subjects were not significantly different.[196] The "sporadic" occurrence of *modest hyperprebeta-lipoproteinemia* has the earmarks of representing a "way of life" in many Americans, and one must be very cautious in considering it a discriminant for subgrouping otherwise similar diseases.

Familial appearance of the Type II pattern is the second diagnostic feature. This includes the nearly 100 per cent expectation of a similar lipoprotein abnormality in at least 1 parent and distribution of the abnormality in siblings and other blood relatives consonant with inheritance of a "highly penetrant" trait that is recognizably expressed whenever a single abnormal allele is present. One abnormal parent will theoretically affect half his progeny. With rare exceptions, the single dose of the abnormal gene is usually expressed by abnormally high β-lipoprotein concentrations in the young child. In a single case umbilical-cord-blood cholesterol has been abnormally high,[215] but from evidence in 4 other Type II children, cord-blood cholesterol levels have been normal and have increased into the abnormal range during the first year.[216] Occasionally, expression may be delayed until the second decade.[159]

Tissue lipid deposition. Xanthomas and atheromas are very common features of Type II. The most characteristic manifestation is tendinous xanthomas, located particularly in the Achilles tendons and the extensor tendons of the hands and feet. Often, there are also tuberous xanthomas, particularly over extensor surfaces, including the elbows, knees, hands and buttocks, or periorbital xanthomas (xanthelasmas). In a severely affected subject soft, tuberous xanthomas may appear at many sites over the body. A corneal arcus is common,[217] assuming greater diagnostic significance the younger the age at appearance. Accelerated arterial disease, especially involving the coronary arteries, is a life-threatening feature. Some families may be relatively free of this manifestation[196]; others are seriously affected. Occlusive peripheral or cerebrovascular disease does not seem to be as common as coronary-artery disease in Type II.[194,196]

Not typical and tending strongly to militate against the diagnosis of Type II are eruptive xanthomas, planar xanthomas in the creases of palms of the hands or tuberoeruptive xanthomas. The last term refers to raised, sometimes pedunculated and often confluent intracutaneous lesions that have the reddish, inflammatory appearance of "eruptive" xanthomas, as opposed to the saccular lesions covered by normal-looking skin that are "tuberous" xanthomas in the more accepted sense. We are unaware of any patient with a Type II pattern *and* tendon xanthomas both of whose parents have been shown clearly to have no hyperlipoproteinemia. A family history consonant with such tissue lipid deposition is therefore helpful in diagnosis if the parents cannot be sampled.

It has been shown convincingly that tissue lipid deposits increase with time and are related to the degree of abnormality in the lipoprotein pattern.[193] Homozygous abnormal subjects can have xanthomas very early in childhood and may even be born with them.

Other clinical manifestations. The legend of Figure 9 summarizes the important clinical features of Type II, most of which have already been discussed. The overall incidence of "chemical diabetes" in Type II is not obviously greater than that thought to be present in the general population. A much larger study with suitable glucose tolerance tests is needed, however, to establish the true incidence and to determine whether the *hyperprebeta-lipoproteinemia* found in some Type II subjects is related to abnormal glucose tolerance. It also is not known how the presence of other abnormal genes, such as that determining diabetes, might affect the expression of Type II.

Exaggerated carbohydrate inducibility is not a common feature of familial Type II, and most of these patients can be given diets high in carbohydrate for many weeks without marked increase in plasma glyceride concentrations. Ability to clear incoming dietary glycerides does not seem to be impaired in familial Type II, and several hundred grams of fat per day leads to no chylomicronemia in the prebreakfast sample. There has been no unusual incidence of hyperuricemia in our series; a careful study of Danish patients who very probably have Type II indicates they, too, have no unusual elevation in uric acid levels.[218] Hyperuricemia is more closely associated with hyperlipoproteinemia in which hyperglyceridemia is the prominent feature.[219,220]

Therapy. It is still an assumption, but a likely one, that the hyperbeta-lipoproteinemia in familial and other forms of Type II is a major causal factor in the accelerated atherosclerotic vascular disease that accompanies this lipoprotein pattern. If some way could be found safely to decrease the hyperlipoproteinemia on a lifetime basis it would enjoy not only universal endorsement but wide application, for the number of affected patients is not small. Many regimens have been tried; none that is simple, efficacious and entirely safe has been found. Many diets or drugs or a combination of both are in experimental trial today. Some uncertainty about the results of such trials is due to failure of the therapist to identify better the syndromes with which he is dealing. For this reason it is difficult to generalize about the response of Type II to different diets or drugs at present.

Diet. Dietary management of all forms of primary Type II is justified. The degree of dietary change from the usual depends on the age of the subject, the severity of his abnormality and the nature of the previous diet. For example, a patient with a marginal Type II pattern who has neither of the other components of the triad diagnostic for the familial syndrome and who has a high intake of foods rich in cholesterol and saturated fats warrants dietary advice, for the expectation is good that he will respond. A young patient with familial Type II likewise is at such high hazard for vascular complications that dietary restrictions that do not neglect normal growth requirements are in order. In very young patients with Type II, appropriate diets can significantly lower the plasma cholesterol. For a patient over fifty years of age with a Type II pattern, there is less justification for difficult diet changes that may radically alter his way of life.

The 2 components in dietary treatment of the Type II abnormality are limited intake of cholesterol and the substitution of polyunsaturated for saturated fats. Cholesterol and saturated (usually animal) fats occur together in foods, and many therapists today are more concerned with their elimination than with the achievement of any particular ratio of polyunsaturated to saturated fats in the diet. Substitution of skim-milk for whole-milk products, severe restriction or even elimination of egg yolks and reduction in meat intake for a daily intake of about 100 mg. of cholesterol and 20 to 30 gm. of fat is one of the most effective dietary regimens.[202] Most Type II patients (provided they have normal glucose tolerance) can tolerate carbohydrate intakes of approximately 4 or 5 gm. per kilogram of body weight per day without significant rise in their glyceride concentrations. To avoid any possible carbohydrate induction, however, as well as to increase the palatability of the diets, polyunsaturated fats are often added, to make a total fat intake of 30 to 45 per cent of calories. The sources of most polyunsaturated fats also contain plant sterols, which have an independent cholesterol-lowering action.[12,221]

Body weight and expression of familial hyperbeta-lipoproteinemia have not been shown to bear a relation. Perhaps partly in anticipation of coronary insufficiency and other cardiac manifestations, it is reasonable to urge such patients to keep thin. A diet low in cholesterol and high in vegetable fats and maintenance of ideal weight, then, are the basic regimen for Type II.

Whatever the diet, there is always a margin of excess β lipoproteins in familial Type II patients that is persistently maintained. For example, 1 of our patients is a sixteen-year-old girl with familial Type II who, on a regular diet containing 800 mg. of cholesterol per day, has a plasma cholesterol concentration of 400 mg. per 100 ml.; 80 per cent of this is in β lipoproteins. On a restricted diet her plasma cholesterol can be dropped to about 220 mg. per 100 ml. A normal subject of the same age and on the same diet, however, will have a cholesterol concentration of about 100 mg.

Drugs.[222] Many drugs have been used in treatment of hypercholesterolemia. The 5 agents that are most commonly being tried in Type II patients are as follows, listed in descending order according to their probable effectiveness in lowering β-lipoprotein concentrations:

Cholestyramine[223] is administered by mouth in doses of 12 to 30 gm. daily. This drug binds bile acids and prevents their reabsorption. This increases the catabolism of cholesterol and may also interfere with its absorption. The dosage must be adjusted to avoid serious malabsorption of fat, and some patients find its bulk and taste quite unpleasant.

β-sitosterol,[224] in doses of 12 to 18 gm. daily by mouth, interferes with cholesterol absorption; one of the older medications still in use, it has effects that are rarely dramatic, but it has few if any important side effects.

D-thyroxine,[208] in a usual dose of 4 to 8 mg. daily by mouth, sometimes lowers cholesterol, possibly by increasing its catabolism; it is still debatable whether this action is independent of an increase in metabolic rate, which can be a serious side effect if coronary-artery disease is present.

Nicotinic acid,[225-227] in adult doses of 3 to 6 gm., daily by mouth, is capable of lowering cholesterol and glycerides by modes of action that are still to be determined but include inhibition of free fatty acid release from adipose tissue; side effects include flushing, pruritus, abdominal discomfort, increased uric acid and blood sugar and usually reversible abnormalities in liver-function tests. Its effect is greater in hyperlipemia.

Chlorophenoxyisobutyric acid,[228] usually given by mouth in doses of 2 gm. daily, is dramatically effective in some kinds of hyperglyceridemia; its mode of action is still unknown. It has thus far proved to have little toxicity and is now being used in several large-scale field trials; the available literature suggests that this drug has little effect on Type II, but experience is still meager.

Hormones. Estrogens have been shown to increase the concentration of α lipoproteins and decrease the concentration of β lipoproteins in man and lower animals.[222,228] Androgens have the reverse effect. Side effects, including gynecomastia, loss of libido and impotence, have frequently made continued therapy with high doses of estrogen impractical.[229]

In familial Type II all these agents are not likely to produce normal lipoprotein concentrations, and rebound may occur. In some patients, most tragically in severely affected children, they may have no effect. Drug therapy in Type II is therefore still experimental, even with older drugs already licensed. After appropriate attempts to classify the etiology of the Type II pattern — excluding any of the treatable causes of secondary hyperlipoproteinemia — the physician properly may elect to try one of the agents listed above, provided he closely follows the plasma lipids. There is no justification for maintaining the administration of any drug unless it clearly decreases the plasma cholesterol within a few weeks. It should also be discontinued if the cholesterol level returns to its abnormal pretreatment state or if signs of significant toxicity appear.

There is no adequate information about the response of familial Type II disease to radical procedures for upsetting cholesterol metabolism such as ileal bypass.[196,230] Since such a procedure presumably should be performed in early childhood to be maximally effective in familial Type II, it seems almost forbiddingly heroic.

The Future of Type II

Phenotyping. Just as specific therapy is urgently needed for Type II, so is wider application of means to ascertain the trait and to search for knowledge of the aberrant mechanisms. There are important questions of gene frequency and distribution, some of which could very probably be answered now if existing technics were widely used. They have direct and immediate importance in genetic counseling. The rare marriage of 2 homozygous persons portends disastrous consequences for their offspring. Counseling in such cases can be fairly definite. Marriages between heterozygotes or between a normal subject and a heterozygote make predictions more difficult, partly because phenotyping the partners is subject to more error. Physicians advising such couples about the genetic hazard to their progeny have to keep in mind the limitations of available tests for ascertainment and the fact that heterozygous offspring often have a normal life-span. Despite these uncertainties, the possibilities for identification and rational follow-up study and management of Type II families is greater than is often recognized today.

Biochemical defect. The variability of the course in different families affected with familial Type II invites some skepticism concerning the genetic homogeneity of this syndrome. The explanation may be no more than capricious variation in location of an atheroma, but both the severity and the timing of xanthomas, as well as the concentrations of β lipoproteins, vary considerably among patients. The question will be settled ultimately when the biochemical lesions that gain expression in the Type II pattern have been specifically determined. For years the search for these has been narrowly confined to consideration of the pathways for making and disposing of cholesterol. Experimental studies of cholesterol metabolism in Type II have been summarized elsewhere[159,175,196]; they have not revealed the defect. Actually, there is no more reason for suspecting that in familial Type II the mutation affects cholesterol metabolism than that of the phospholipids or β apoprotein found in the β lipoproteins. Since the latter is unique for the lipoprotein, and the lipids not so, the metabolism of the protein remains a prime suspect. Just as the sterol and phosphatides in plasma in Type II have not been shown to be chemically different from those in normal subjects, the β protein has not been shown to be abnormal, but published data are far from complete.

The differences between the β-lipoprotein concentrations in normal subjects and in those assumed to have single and double doses of the abnormal gene for Type II suggest that the mutation or mutations responsible for the disease have affected genes governing the control of synthesis of the lipoprotein rather than its structure. The most effective approach to therapy for familial Type II may be a search for pharmacologic agents capable of suppressing the synthesis of B protein and thus replacing such missing genetic controls.

TYPE III HYPERLIPOPROTEINEMIA

General

Definition. In the course of the phenotyping stud

ies that form the core of this review, a lipoprotein pattern different from Type II and from Type IV, which will be discussed in the concluding section, has been found in a relatively small number of subjects. This lipoprotein anomaly has been classified as the Type III pattern. It is a feature of a clinical syndrome that was perhaps first pointed out over ten years ago[64] but is still often considered a variant of Type II. At present sufficient evidence has been gathered to indicate that the disorders associated with patterns II and III are independent. Whether the Type III pattern is the expression of a single disease or of several different metabolic disorders has not been established.

Type III hyperlipoproteinemia (Fig. 10) is an excess of lipoproteins that have β mobility but abnormally low density. It is manifested by hypercholesterolemia *and* hyperglyceridemia. A peculiar feature — and one that tips off the lipoprotein pattern if it is present — is lipid deposition in the palms of the hands. The lipoprotein anomaly may be detected in close relatives and as such is probably the expression of a double dose of an uncommon abnormal gene. We have so far examined 24 Type III patients and over 100 of their relatives, and the following discussion will be based mainly on these observations. The abnormality will be referred to as the Type III syndrome or simply as "Type III."

Lipoprotein pattern. The electrophoretic abnormality in Type III is a "broad beta band." As depicted in Figure 10, there is a broad, intensely staining lipoprotein band beginning in the normal β zone but extending continuously into the pre-β region. When the plasma is subjected without adjustment of density to ultracentrifugation for sixteen hours at 100,000 g, and the supernatant and infrana-

tant fractions again subjected to electrophoresis, most of the lipoprotein band having β mobility appears in the fraction with density less than 1.006 (Fig. 11). Normally, and in other types of hyperlipoproteinemia, all the lipoproteins of β mobility remain in the infranatant (density greater than 1.006) fraction (Fig. 11). Although adequate comparisons have not yet been made the features of the Type III pattern in the analytical ultracentrifuge can be estimated from early studies of patients who almost certainly represented the same syndrome.[64,197,231] The predominant abnormalities are lower than normal concentrations of S_f 0-12 lipoproteins, moderate increases in S_f 12-20 and marked increases in the S_f 20-100 and often the S_f 100-400 subclasses. At present a certain determination of the Type III pattern requires either the combination of electrophoresis and preparative ultracentrifugation described here or analyses in the analytical ultracentrifuge.

History. The appearance in the medical literature of the first example of Type III may never be determined. Descriptions of "mixed" hyperlipidemia have been present in many reports of heterogenous patients with severe hyperlipoproteinemia and xanthomatosis.[232-236] It is inevitable that some Type III patients, with their tendency toward tendon xanthomas, xanthelasmas and crippling atherosclerosis, should have been classified as having "essential hypercholesterolemia" (Type II). Others have been singled out by their milky plasma and yellow-red eruptions on the extremities, and these cases have been consigned to "essential hyperlipemia" — a sanctuary of the undifferentiated that one hopes will soon be abandoned. One study stands out during the period from 1950 to the present, a comparison of xanthoma type and lipoprotein patterns at the Donner Laboratory.[64,195] Two groups of patients were examined, defined as having "xanthoma tendinosum" and "xanthoma tuberosum." The first group almost certainly contained examples of familial Type II; all had marked increases in S_f 0-12 lipoproteins (hyperbeta-lipoproteinemia). The other

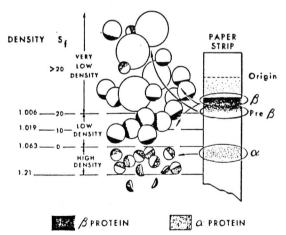

FIGURE 10. *Type III Hyperlipoproteinemia (See Also Table 3).*
Note that the key feature is β-migrating lipoproteins having abnormally low density (less than 1.006). In addition to arcus, palpebral and tendon xanthomas, there usually are palmar and "tuberoeruptive" xanthomas. Advanced atherosclerosis of peripheral and coronary arteries is common. PHLA is normal; glucose intolerance is the rule. When familial, it is inherited as a recessive.

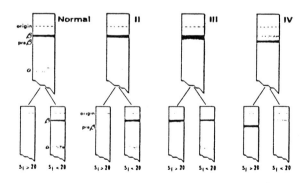

FIGURE 11. *Electrophoretic Mobility of the Lipoproteins Isolated in the Ultracentrifuge at Density 1.006.*
$S_f > 20$ represents the supernatant fraction, and $S_f < 20$ the infranate. Only in Type III do lipoproteins of β mobility appear in the 1.006-density supernate.

222 THE NEW ENGLAND JOURNAL OF MEDICINE Jan. 26, 1967

group had skin lesions on "extensor surfaces of the elbows, buttocks, extensor aspects of the knees, the hands, expecially the volar surfaces, and over the ankle malleoli, especially laterally."[197] In contrast to the patients with xanthoma "tendinosum," some of whom had lesions in childhood, all the 23 with xanthoma "tuberosum" had first noted their lesions in adulthood. Two of the latter were sibs, the only familial examples presented. In these patients the S_f 0-12 lipoproteins were lower than normal, and the S_f 12-400 classes greatly elevated.

When the classification of familial hyperlipidemia by the current system was begun at the Clinical Center, one of the objectives was the search for proof of the existence of separate phenotypes comparable to those suggested by these early studies. The present concept of Type III evolved through trial and error. In the earliest published classification by electrophoretograms[159,173] a "Type III" pattern was defined as an increase in both β and pre-β lipoproteins. It was noted that there seemed to be 2 different variations on this pattern. In 1 the 2 lipoprotein bands were intense and distinct. In the other they merged in a broad, intensely staining β band. As described above, the former pattern was eventually found to be a variant of the Type II pattern. The "broad-beta" pattern has come to define a group of patients whose familial expression and clinical features were clearly different.[174] The abnormal flotation of the β lipoproteins was noted after the quantification steps were added to the typing system. It has been observed that the β-lipoprotein anomaly is consistent and reproducible and not a technical artifact. This flotation anomaly is not a function of the absolute amounts of β lipoprotein, cholesterol or glycerides in plasma. It has never been observed in patients with Types II or IV patterns even though their plasma lipid concentrations are sometimes very similar to those seen in Type III. The important difference between the inheritance of Types II and III will be described below.

Clinical Manifestations

Plasma lipids. The plasma cholesterol concentrations in Type III vary from 200 to more than 1400 mg., and the glycerides from 175 to more than 1500 mg. per 100 ml. Extreme variability of cholesterol and glyceride concentrations is a diagnostic feature and a distinct contrast to the steady elevations in Type II. The lipoprotein levels are quite sensitive to changes in the content of the diet and the amount of total calories. If the patient is switched from a regular diet to one rich in polyunsaturated fats and containing only 100 to 200 mg. of cholesterol per day both cholesterol and glyceride concentrations may be lowered severalfold within a few weeks. The effect of negative caloric balance may be even more dramatic. Glyceride concentrations tend to rise moderately on high carbohydrate diets, but Type III is not always accompanied by carbohydrate inducibility exceeding the response of nor-

mal subjects. Carbohydrate intolerance is the rule in most patients (over 90 per cent), and the ability to handle either an oral or intravenous glucose load seems to decrease with age faster than it does in the normal state. There have been no measurements of plasma insulin levels in Type III; only 1 of 24 patients thus far has ever taken insulin or hypoglycemic agents for his mild diabetes.

The 10 patients with Type III who have been available for testing have had a small accumulation of chylomicrons after an overnight fast when they were fed more than 150 gm. of fat per day. Their hyperglyceridemia on regular diets is not exogenous, however, as witnessed by their good therapeutic response to low-cholesterol diets containing 100 gm. or more of fat. The "palmar striae" of Type III are not typical of any other type of *primary* hyperlipoproteinemia.

Xanthomas. The terms "xanthoma tendinosum" and "xanthoma tuberosum" do not accurately distinguish Types II and III. Tendon lesions occur in both, as do thickened tibial tuberosities, corneal arcus and periorbital xanthomas. The distinctive lesions in Type III are found on the palmar surfaces of the hands. The creases and sometimes the tips of the fingers or other areas, especially where rings are worn, contain yellow-white deposits that rise a little above the surface; they are often subtle changes and are sometimes overlooked by both patient and physician. So-called planar xanthomas of similar appearance but usually on the back of the hands have long been associated with obstructive liver disease; they can be seen on models constructed from jaundiced patients over a hundred years ago.[237] Such lesions are not typical of any other type of primary hyperlipoproteinemia.

On the elbows several kinds of lesions have been observed in Type III. Soft, pedunculated growths may be present, but they tend to be confluent and smaller than tuberous xanthomas usually seen in Type II and do not have the smooth normal skin cover of the latter. The Type III lesions bear the reddish, inflammatory appearance that is the trademark of skin lesions associated with hyperglyceridemia. Sometimes, they are confluent, yellow-red papules raised just above the surface. Occasionally, when they seem to be involuting they closely resemble dabs of peanut butter spread on the skin; these last two forms may commonly be amalgamated into brownish-yellow papules having a reddish base. Similar lesions in severe diabetes have been called "xanthoma diabeticorum." For all these the name "tuberoeruptive" may be helpful in suggesting their appearance of transition between tuberous and eruptive xanthomas. The lesions wax and wane, and may even disappear without obvious change in the plasma lipoprotein pattern. Similar-appearing xanthomas may appear on the buttocks or knees. In distinct contrast to Type II, thus far only 1 patient in 24 with Type III at the Clinical Center has noted any xanthomas before the age of twenty-five.

Vascular disease. Occlusive vascular disease is a serious and frequent accompaniment of Type III. In the samples observed by us occlusive peripheral vascular disease, especially of femoral and popliteal vessels with severe claudication, has been at least as frequent as coronary atherosclerosis.

Genetics

The Type III lipoprotein pattern and other clinical features occur in families, but in contrast to Type II, the distribution of affected members is not that of a trait expressed in single dosage of an abnormal gene. The 24 patients have come from 19 kindreds. In 3 of these, 2 siblings have been involved, and in 2 others, a parent and one offspring. Fourteen have been males, and 10 females. The 104 blood relatives sampled do not include complete sets of parents and siblings from all kindreds. In 3 kindreds both parents of the propositus have been sampled. One of each set was normal. One spouse had Type III, and the other 2 Type IV patterns. It is most significant that in none of the 128 relatives and patients sampled was a Type II pattern present. Conversely, complete lipoprotein analyses of 105 patients with familial Type II and 90 of their relatives (representing 50 kindreds) failed to reveal a single instance of Type III. These include three presumably homozygous abnormal examples of Type II.

From these data it is apparent that Type III and Type II are not simply different phenotypic expressions of the same genotype. They are at least 2 different diseases. A few Type IV patterns (endogenous hyperlipemia) have been noted in the Type III relatives. As will be discussed shortly, this is a frequent pattern in Americans and may be due to factors that are not genetic. Type IV patterns appear as well in some relatives of Type II patients, and any significant differences in distribution have not developed. It is conceivable, of course, that Type III and Type IV could prove to be related, including the possible expression of the "Type III heterozygote" sometimes as a Type IV pattern. The possibility that several mutant alleles determine this pattern also remains open.

Speculation on the Mechanism

Type III, with its apparent accumulation of a subclass of very-low-density lipoproteins, requires consideration of a theory of "interconversion" of plasma lipoproteins. This is inherent in the concept developed earlier in this review (Fig. 1), which in turn evolved from even more theoretical considerations.[26,23s] Briefly stated, it can be imagined that large particles containing glyceride, β and α lipoproteins are degraded in stepwise fashion. As glyceride is sequentially removed a rise and fall of lipoproteins of progressively lower S_f occurs. Metabolic block at any point in this transformation would theoretically cause accumulation of very-low-density lipoproteins of a given subclass.[26] Actually, such a

sequence has never been convincingly demonstrated during chylomicron clearance[1] and a disorder of metabolism of specific subclass of pre-β lipoproteins has likewise not been proved. The tendency today is to assume that the concentration and average density of pre-β lipoproteins is a function of the amount of circulating glyceride, which in turn is determined by the state of energy metabolism at the cellular level.

It is therefore unlikely that the peculiar Type III lipoprotein anomaly is the result of a metabolic block at a discrete point in the metabolism of otherwise normal pre-β lipoproteins. The anomaly has not been observed in other types of hyperlipoproteinemia, even when the plasma concentrations of pre-β lipoproteins are being driven up or down by extreme changes in diet. For example, the glyceride levels in Type IV patients may be changed from 100 to 5000 mg. per 100 ml., and there is never lipoprotein of discrete β mobility floating at density 1.006. The Type III anomaly therefore appears more likely to be secondary to the presence of an abnormal lipoprotein.

The Type III pattern is mimicked in the "broad beta" band seen in Tangier disease (Fig. 6); in this instance β lipoproteins and glyceride form a complex that lacks the added negative charge contributed by α lipoproteins, normally giving such complexes pre-β mobility. Although the "floating beta" of Type III is suggestive of a deficient participation of α lipoprotein in formation of the glyceride-rich complexes, dietary studies have shown that these patients make pre-β lipoproteins. Because no way has yet been found to delipidate these complexes and still obtain accurate quantification of their content of α and β lipoprotein, some obvious questions cannot be answered. The regular α and β lipoproteins (in their usual density class) react with antiserums as though normal, and the content of α (as measured after heparin precipitation) is normal. One is left at the moment with the suggestion of a peculiar affinity of Type III β lipoproteins for glyceride, for "floating beta" is present in Type III patients even when diets have brought their glycerides to within normal limits. More details of these studies will be forthcoming shortly from this laboratory; they still leave Type III as a most provocative biochemical enigma.

Management

The prognosis in Type III is uncertain. Four of our patients have reached the seventh decade. The majority have evidence of vascular disease, however, and it seems reasonable to utilize such conservative means as are available to lower plasma lipid concentrations. The latter are characteristically labile and responsive to diet alone.

Diet. Weight reduction is one key to reduction of plasma lipids in Type III and is always effective if the patient is overweight. After ideal weight is reached it may be maintained by diets containing

40 to 50 per cent of calories from fats that are as high in polyunsaturated fats and as low in cholesterol as is practicable. If the diet is carefully followed, normal or nearly normal lipid levels can be maintained for many months and the skin lesions may completely disappear. It is hoped that the vascular changes may be undergoing similar beneficial involution. The "floating" β lipoprotein will persist, however, in the lipoprotein pattern.

Drugs. It is premature to comment on drug therapy for Type III since none of the agents now being investigated have been tested adequately in this syndrome. It is our opinion that drugs tending to be more effective against hyperglyceridemia than isolated hypercholesterolemia will be more effective in Type III. Agents in this category have been discussed under Type II. Perhaps the most effective and generally useful drug will prove to be chlorophenoxyisobutyric acid. Some evidence that it may lower lipid levels in Type III has been reported.[228]

(To be concluded)

REFERENCES

192. Wilkinson, C. F., Hand, E. A., and Fliegelman, M. T. Essential familial hypercholesterolemia. *Ann. Int. Med.* **29**:671-686, 1948.

193. Piper, J., and Orrild, L. Essential familial hypercholesterolemia and xanthomatosis: follow-up study of twelve Danish families. *Am. J. Med.* **21**:34-46, 1956.

194. Guravich, J. L. Familial hypercholesteremic xanthomatosis: preliminary report. I. Clinical, electrocardiographic and laboratory considerations. *Am. J. Med.* **26**:8-29, 1959.

195. Epstein, F. H., Block, W. D., Hand, E. A., and Francis, T., Jr. Familial hypercholesterolemia, xanthomatosis and coronary heart disease. *Am. J. Med.* **26**:39-53, 1959.

196. Harlan, W. R., Jr., Graham, J. B., and Estes, H. E. Familial hypercholesterolemia: genetic and metabolic study. *Medicine* **45**:77-110, 1966.

197. Gofman, J. W., Rubin, L., McGinley, J. P., and Jones, H. B. Hyperlipoproteinemia. *Am. J. Med.* **17**:514-520, 1954.

198. Glazier, F. W., et al. Human serum lipoprotein concentrations. *J. Gerontol.* **9**:395-403, 1954.

199. Lewis, L., et al. Serum lipid levels in normal persons: findings of cooperative study of lipoproteins and atherosclerosis. *Circulation* **16**:227-245, 1957.

200. Khachadurian, A. K. Inheritance of essential familial hypercholesterolemia. *Am. J. Med.* **37**:402-407, 1964.

201. Schaefer, L. E., Drachman, S. R., Steinberg, A. G., and Adlersberg, D. Genetic studies on hypercholesteremia: frequency in hospital population and in families of hypercholesteremic index patients. *Am. Heart J.* **46**:99-116, 1953.

202. Connor, W. E., Stone, D. B., and Hodges, R. E. Interrelated effects of dietary cholesterol and fat upon human serum lipid levels. *J. Clin. Investigation* **43**:1691-1696, 1964.

203. Erickson, B. A., Coots, R. H., Mattson, F. H., and Kligman, A. M. Effect of partial hydrogenation of dietary fats, of ratio of polyunsaturated fatty acids, and of dietary cholesterol upon plasma lipids in man. *J. Clin. Investigation* **43**:2017-2025, 1964.

204. Davidson, C. S., et al. *Dietary Fat and Human Health.* 51 pp. Washington, D.C.: National Academy of Sciences, National Research Council, 1966. (Publication No. 1147.)

205. Walton, K. W., Campbell, D. A., and Tonks, E. Significance of alterations in serum lipids in thyroid dysfunction. I. Relation between serum lipoproteins, carotenoids, and vitamin A in hypothyroidism and thyrotoxicosis. *Clin. Sc.* **29**:199-215, 1965.

206. Walton, K. W., Scott, P. J., Dykes, P. W., and Davies, J. W. L. Alterations of metabolism and turnover of I¹³¹ low density lipoprotein in myxoedema and thyrotoxicosis. *Clin. Sc.* **29**:217-238, 1965.

207. Zöllner, N. Über das verhalten der carotinoide bei hypercholesterinämischen krankheiten. *Verhandl. d. deutsch. Gesellsch. f. inn. Med.* **64**:153-156, 1958.

208. Boyd, G. S., and Oliver, M. F. Effect of certain thyroxine analogues on serum lipids in human subjects. *J. Endocrinol.* **21**:33-43, 1960.

209. Aizawa, T., Goto, Y., and Nakamura, H. Study on lipid metabolism with gas-liquid chromatography — xanthoma with hyper-

210. Wheeler, E. O. Genetic aspects of atherosclerosis. *Am. J. Med.* **23**:653-660, 1957.

211. Rayer, P. P. *Traité théorique et pratique des Maladies de la Peau ondé sur de nouvelles recherches d'anatomie et de physiologie pathologiques.* 2 vol. Paris: Baillière, 1835.

212. Addison, T., and Gull, W. On certain affection of skin, vitiligoidea — a) plana, b) tuberosa with remarks. *Guy's Hosp. Rep.* **7**:265-276, 1851.

213. Fagge, C. H. Two cases of vitiligoidea associated with chronic jaundice and enlargement of liver. *Tr. Path. Soc. London* **19**:434-446, 1868.

214. Hutchinson, J., Sangster, A., and Crocker, H. R. Report on cases of xanthoma multiplex brought before Pathological Society by Mr. James Startin and Dr. Stephen Mackenzie. *Tr. Path. Soc. London* **33**:376-384, 1882.

215. Kaplan, S., Bossak, E. T., Wang, C-I., and Adlersberg, D. Pregnancy complicated by idiopathic hyperlipemia and idiopathic hypercholesteremia. *J. Mt. Sinai Hosp.* **24**:39-44, 1957.

216. Brown, H. B., Green, J. G., Lewis, L. A., and Page, I. H. Unpublished data.

217. Klatskin, G. Familial xanthomatosis and arcus senilis. *New Internat. Clin.* **3**:13-39, 1941.

218. Jensen, J., Blankenhorn, D. H., and Kornerup, V. Blood-uric-acid levels in familial hypercholesterolaemia. *Lancet* **1**:298-300, 1966.

219. Feldman, E. B., and Wallace, S. L. Hypertriglyceridemia in gout. *Circulation* **29**:508-513, 1964.

220. Berkowitz, D. Gout, hyperlipidemia, and diabetes interrelationships. *J.A.M.A.* **197**:77-80, 1966.

221. Beveridge, J. M. R., Connell, W. F., Mayer, G. A., Haust, H. L., and White, M. Plant sterols, degree of unsaturation, and hypocholesterolemic action of certain fats. *Canad. J. Biochem. & Physiol.* **36**:895-911, 1958.

222. Eder, H. A. Drugs used in prevention and treatment of atherosclerosis. In *The Pharmacological Basis of Therapeutics: A textbook of pharmacology, toxicology, and therapeutics for physicians and medical students.* Third edition. Edited by L. S. Goodman and A. Z. Gilman. 1785 pp. New York: Macmillan, 1965. P. 754.

223. Hashim, S. A., and Van Itallie, T. B. Cholestyramine resin therapy for hypercholesterolemia. *J.A.M.A.* **192**:289-293, 1965.

224. Farquhar, J. W., Smith, R. E., and Dempsey, M. E. Effect of beta sitosterol on serum lipids of young men with arteriosclerotic heart disease. *Circulation* **14**:77-82, 1956.

225. Berge, K. G., Achor, R. W. P., Christensen, N. A., Mason, H. L., and Barker, N. W. Hypercholesteremia and nicotinic acid: long-term study. *Am. J. Med.* **31**:24-36, 1961.

226. Drugs which lower blood lipids. *M. Letter* **5**:81, 1963.

227. Carlson, L. A., and Orö, L. Persistence of inhibitory effect of nicotinic acid on catecholamine-stimulated lipid mobilization during prolonged treatment with nicotinic acid. *J. Atheroscler. Research* **5**:436-439, 1965.

228. Symposium on atromid: (proceedings of conference held in Buxton, England, June 5-6, 1963). *J. Atheroscler. Research* **3**:341-755, 1963.

229. Stamler, J., et al. Effectiveness of estrogens for therapy of myocardial infarction in middle-age men. *J.A.M.A.* **183**:632-638, 1963.

230. Buchwald, H. Lowering of cholesterol absorption and blood levels by ileal exclusion. *Circulation* **29**:713-720, 1965.

231. McGinley, J., Jones, H., and Gofman, J. Lipoproteins and xanthomatous diseases. *J. Invest. Dermat.* **19**:71-82, 1952.

232. Malmros, H., Swahn, B., and Truedsson, E. Essential hyperlipaemia. *Acta med. Scandinav.* **149**:91-108, 1954.

233. Lever, W. F., Smith, P. A. J., and Hurley, N. A. Idiopathic hyperlipemic and primary hypercholesteremic xanthomatosis. I. Clinical data and analysis of plasma lipids. *J. Invest. Dermat.* **22**:33-51, 1954.

234. Adlersberg, D. Inborn errors of lipid metabolism: clinical, genetic, and chemical aspects. *Arch. Path.* **60**:481-492, 1955.

235. Borrie, P. Essential hyperlipaemia and idiopathic hypercholesterolaemic xanthomatosis. *Brit. M. J.* **2**:911-915, 1957.

236. Jobst, H., Huber, H., and Schettler, G. Essentielle familiäre hyperlipämie bei einem eineiigen Zwillingspaar. *Med. Klin.* **58**:710-716, 1963.

237. Fagge, C. H. *Catalogue of the Models of Diseases of the Skin.* 269 pp. London: Churchill, 1876. P. 170.

238. Lindgren, F. T., Freeman, N. K., Nichols, A. V., and Gofman, J. W. In Third International Conference on Biochemical Problems of Lipids. *The Blood Lipids and the Clearing Factor.* 418 pp. Brussels: Koninkl. Vlaam. Acad. Wetenschappen (Letteren on Schone Junsten Van Belgïe, Klasse der Wertenschappen), 1956. P. 224.

cholesterolemia. *Reports of General Study on Medicine* (Japan) **2**:1, 1963.

Vol. 276   No. 5   FAT TRANSPORT—FREDRICKSON ET AL.   273

MEDICAL PROGRESS

FAT TRANSPORT IN LIPOPROTEINS — AN INTEGRATED APPROACH TO MECHANISMS AND DISORDERS (Concluded)*

DONALD S. FREDRICKSON, M.D.,† ROBERT I. LEVY, M.D.,‡ AND
ROBERT S. LEES, M.D.§

BETHESDA, MARYLAND

TYPE IV HYPERLIPOPROTEINEMIA

General

Definition. The Type IV lipoprotein pattern is the hallmark of endogenous hyperlipemia. It implies that glycerides synthesized in the body, usually in the liver, have been excreted into plasma at rates exceeding the capacity for removal. The appearance of a Type IV pattern often suggests that something has gone wrong with carbohydrate metabolism or caloric balance. There is evidence that it can sometimes mean inordinate emotional stress, excessive alcoholic intake or some other conflict between the patient and his environment. The development of this type of hyperlipoproteinemia is often conditioned by genotype.

The Type IV pattern (hereafter called simply "Type IV") is a valuable indicator of metabolic imbalance; it does not describe a specific disease. It is sometimes considered synonymous with "carbohydrate-induced hyperlipemia." This is probably too narrow a concept since most patients who have this pattern on a regular diet do not lose it entirely when their diet is changed so that 10 per cent of their calories come from carbohydrate, and an occasional patient does not have an *abnormal* increase in plasma glycerides when fed 80 per cent of his calories as carbohydrate. If freed of a generic connotation, the term "carbohydrate induced"[123] has great virtue, however, for it focuses immediate attention on abnormal glucose tolerance and a family history of diabetes, both associated with Type IV with extraordinary frequency.[159,239-241] At the Clinical Center, where patient selection has recently been biased toward other lipoprotein anomalies, 15 of approximately 100 kindreds with proved familial hyperlipoproteinemia have been families in which affected members had only Type IV. The pattern has been observed in several hundred plasma samples from different individuals on a regular diet. Quantitative data from a large sample representative of the entire population are not available, but Type IV may be the most common of all types of hyperlipoproteinemia.

Lipoprotein pattern. As shown in Figure 12, endogenous hyperlipemia is manifested as hyperprebeta-lipoproteinemia. This is associated with an increase in glycerides above normal limits as defined in Table 2 and is commonly accompanied by a rise in cholesterol, on the order of about 1 mg. for each 5-mg. increase in glyceride concentration. With the use of other analytical methods Type IV is defined by increased concentrations of S_f 20-400 and sometimes S_f 400 lipoproteins in the analytical ultracentrifuge, very-low-density lipoproteins (density less than 1.006) as separated by the preparative ultracentrifuge, lipoproteins and "endogenous" particles having α_2 mobility on starch-block electrophoresis or intermediate density by polyvinylpyrrolidone fractionation, or low-density "beta" lipoproteins as measured by most precipitation technics. Concentrations of α and β lipoproteins are usually below normal in the Type IV pattern; chylomicrons are not present.

The Type IV pattern is easy to spot by the electrophoretogram when lipemia is not extreme (glycerides less than 2000 mg. per 100 ml.). In severe hyperlipemia the trail of endogenous particles from the origin is marked, and interpretation difficult. Diluting plasma onefold or twofold with saline so-

*From the Laboratory of Molecular Diseases, National Heart Institute.

†Director and chief, Laboratory of Molecular Diseases, National Heart Institute.

‡Head, Section on Lipoproteins, Laboratory of Molecular Diseases, National Heart Institute.

§Assistant professor and associate physician, Rockefeller University.

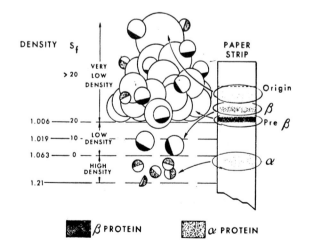

FIGURE 12. *Type IV Hyperlipoproteinemia (See Also Table 3) — Endogenous Hyperlipemia That Is Typically Carbohydrate Inducible and Accompanied by Glucose Intolerance.*

PHLA is normal, and hyperuricemia is common. There are many causes, and the pattern is often familial.

274 THE NEW ENGLAND JOURNAL OF MEDICINE Feb. 2, 1967

lution may help to distinguish any boundary between pre-β lipoproteins and chylomicrons (the two together being defined as the Type V pattern). The Type I pattern is not likely to be confused with either Type IV or Type V.

The ability of paper electrophoresis to separate endogenous from exogenous glyceride appears to depend on the comparatively greater ratio of mass to charge of the dietary particles. The distinction is not absolute, and it is likely that some fed glycerides may quickly appear in pre-β lipoproteins. Patients with even the most severe endogenous hyperlipemia, however, do not have chylomicron bands in the absence of fat in the diet. Conversely, patients with Type IV who have accumulated heavy prebeta bands on high-carbohydrate diets usually have transient hyperchylomicronemia for a few days after fat is returned to the diet. As with all other types of hyperlipoproteinemia, the pattern obtained after a week or two of a normal diet must be the index for purposes of classification.

In Type IV the concentrations of β and α lipoproteins vary with the degree of hyperlipemia. As heavy concentrations of glycerides are reduced, the 2 lipoprotein bands become progressively greater. The rise and fall in β-lipoprotein concentrations is an especially prominent feature of the transition in the Type IV pattern induced by dietary changes.

History. Observations of patients with ketosis and uncontrolled diabetes who had hyperlipemia despite malnutrition probably provided some of the earliest stimulus to a concept of endogenous hyperlipemia. Other patients with lactescent serum that did not improve markedly upon withdrawal of fat from the diet have often been observed. With the development of the concept of carbohydrate induction all doubt has been removed that excess glycerides in the plasma are frequently not of dietary origin. Interest in postabsorptive increases in plasma glycerides, or what are here called pre-β lipoproteins, has also been maintained by many studies, not always in agreement, of an uneven distribution of this phenomenon in different populations. There has been special interest in whether this abnormality is unusually common in young and middle-aged adults who have ischemic heart disease.[241-245]

What are lacking almost completely in the literature are family data in clear-cut examples of Type IV. We have summarized elsewhere a few reports of what seem likely to have been Type IV patterns occurring in siblings or in succeeding generations.[159] Exploration of the pedigrees of affected patients has been distressingly meager and must be improved if the meaning of the abnormal pattern is to become clearer.

Clinical Manifestations

It is perhaps not pertinent to discuss the clinical features of what is only a chemical indicator, but patients with Type IV tend to have certain general characteristics that can be summarized as a prelude to discussion of primary and secondary forms of this hyperlipoproteinemia.

Common features of hyperlipemia. Severe Type IV from any cause may show some abnormalities already described in exogenous hyperlipemia, such as eruptive xanthomas, lipemia retinalis and foam cells in bone marrow and other reticuloendothelial tissues. The patients are also subject to the same bouts of abdominal pain — with or without chemical signs of pancreatitis. Hyperuricemia occurs in hyperlipemia,[219,220] but its frequency in Type IV has not been established.

Obesity and glucose tolerance. Secondary Type IV can occur in thin, nondiabetic subjects. So can the primary form, but in patients with the latter, excessive body weight and abnormal glucose tolerance are extremely common. In our experience the incidence of abnormal glucose tolerance in those with familial Type IV patterns exceeds 90 per cent.

Age at detection. Plasma triglyceride concentrations rise with age (Table 2). Apparently so does the incidence of Type IV. Familial occurrence has been seen in young children, as has the secondary form, but the overall frequency in children seems much less than in adults.

Atherosclerosis. All the evidence concerning the association of coronary-artery disease and pre-β lipoproteins is retrospective; some of it is derived from plasma glyceride concentrations, and some from lipoprotein analyses. Agreement is lacking, but the consensus indicates a positive correlation at least in relatively young men.[242-246] Noteworthy is the finding of a much higher concentration of pre-β lipoproteins in males who had had a myocardial infarct than in controls.[243] The possibility that many patients with infarcts are placed on very low-fat, and hence high-carbohydrate diets may be a factor in enhancing the lipoprotein abnormalities. Our collection of about 200 kindreds with all types of familial hyperlipoproteinemia cannot yet be properly matched for age and sex for estimation of the incidence of atherosclerosis. The available experience leaves the impression that Type IV is not associated with atherosclerosis to the same extent as Types II and III. Diabetes and obesity complicate such comparisons, and only more data of the proper kind will eventually resolve this important question.

Mechanisms in Type IV

Two abnormalities may be operative in production of Type IV. A brief summary of them can be confined for simplicity to the interplay between adipose tissue and liver. The roles of both organs in normal endogenous glyceride metabolism have been discussed earlier and need not be repeated.

Excess glyceride release. The first possible abnormality is release of glycerides by the liver faster than the adipose tissue can remove them. In the steady state a new equilibrium will be established at some higher plasma level of pre-β lipoproteins. Examples in which this undoubtedly occurs include excessive flow of free fatty acids to the liver or extremely high-carbohydrate feeding. Both substrates in great excess will be turned out by the liver as glycerides that usually seek storage in the expansible reservoirs of the adipose tissue but may linger in the plasma.

To demonstrate steady or cyclical increases in flux of free fatty acids in patients is not simple; it depends in part on the determination of a plasma substance whose concentrations are notoriously labile. Increased mobilization of fatty acids has been invoked to explain clinical examples of endogenous hyperlipemia. The evidence is convincing only in diabetic ketosis but highly provocative in some examples of prolonged emotional stress.

Carbohydrate induction, on the other hand, is easy to demonstrate.[123,124,159] It may not, however, be assumed to be the defect in any patient with Type IV unless the patient's response is clearly outside the normal degree of carbohydrate inducibility – a rise in glycerides to levels as high as 300 to 400 mg. per 100 ml. after four to seven days on a diet containing 6 or 7 gm. of carbohydrate per kilogram of body weight.[124] The issue of exaggerated carbohydrate inducibility may not be solved by the use of carbohydrate loads that far exceed those the patient is usually eating when he has hyperlipemia. Isotopic technics recently refined to measure hepatic glyceride synthesis[9,247-249] are more likely to reveal the nature of the abnormalities in the presence of conventional diets. A combination of such technics with appropriate measurements of glucose turnover, plasma and tissue insulin activities, hepatic arteriovenous differences of glyceride and perhaps opportunity to measure hepatic glyceride and lipoprotein synthesis directly may be required to understand the abnormal "diversion" of substrate to glycerides that seems certain to underlie Type IV in some patients.

Decreased glyceride removal. The second possible abnormality in Type IV is a decrease in the ability of the adipose tissue to clear glyceride that is entering plasma at the normal rate. Two major stages at which abnormality might occur were discussed earlier. A deficiency of lipase activity at the capillary wall or in the cell is one, and defective glyceride resynthesis in the cell is the other. Although PHLA levels tend to go down on high-carbohydrate diets they are usually normal in patients with florid endogenous hyperlipemia on regular diets.[184] Granting the oblique nature of available assays, a deficiency in lipoprotein lipase activity is probably not the explanation for most of Type IV. Deficiencies of PHLA in diabetes[140,176] and pancreatitis[179] are perhaps more usually accompanied by mixed hyperlipemia, discussed below under Type V. Direct and correlative measurements of the capacity of adipose tissue to convert fatty acids to glyceride are not simple in man and have not been applied to the

problem of hyperlipemia. Normal glucose metabolism is essential in this process, and the abnormalities of glucose tolerance in Type IV call attention to this site. Of particular interest is the question of whether insulin activity at the level of the adipose-tissue cell may not be abnormal.

Briefly noted as a third possible abnormality in Type IV is the formation of anomalous lipoproteins, resistant to normal processes of removal. Possible examples of this in Type IV are presently limited to certain dysglobulinemias described below.

Secondary Type IV

Type IV hyperlipoproteinemia is often secondary to other known diseases. In the differential diagnosis 2 disorders outstrip all others in frequency and in confusion, for it is sometimes very difficult to determine whether the hyperlipoproteinemia or the associated disease is the underlying abnormality. These conditions are diabetes mellitus and pancreatitis.

Diabetes mellitus.[64] As a rule, diabetes that is insulin-sensitive and generally occurring in younger nonobese subjects inclined to have ketosis is considered the *cause,* and the Type IV hyperlipoproteinemia developing when control is poor the transient *resultant.* In severe uncontrolled diabetes hyperlipemia is almost universal and often accompanied by eruptive xanthomas (xanthoma diabeticorum) and the other clinical features of any hyperlipemia. Adipose-tissue stores are briskly mobilized, plasma free fatty acid concentrations are high, and hyperlipemia develops soon after ketosis. Patients with insulin-dependent diabetes may have Type IV patterns or, when exogenous hyperlipemia is superimposed on the endogenous, Type V. Hyperlipemia clears rapidly when the diabetes is brought under control.

By contrast exogenous insulin has little effect on Type IV patterns or carbohydrate intolerance in the patients with mild diabetes in whom ketosis never develops. Commonest in the obese and middle-aged, the hyperlipoproteinemia responds to caloric restriction and sometimes to orally administered hypoglycemic agents.[250,251] The abnormal mechanism is unlikely to be related to excessive transport of free fatty acids.

Pancreatitis and alcoholism.[177-180,252-254] The combination of hyperlipemia and abdominal pain has been known for nearly half a century.[255] Probably the commonest cause is pancreatitis, not infrequently in alcoholism. In a few subjects like the patients with the Type I pattern already discussed, hyperlipemia apparently antedated the pancreatitis; in the majority pancreatitis apparently preceded the hyperlipemia. In acute pancreatitis lipoprotein patterns have been described that resemble Types I, IV and V.[179,254] For the chronic hyperlipemia persisting after an attack, Type IV is perhaps most common, but the existing data are too skimpy to support a generalization. Lipoprotein patterns are therefore of little help to the physician in the immediate dilemma posed by a patient with abdominal pain and hyperlipemia that are both of uncommon severity. Several suggestions are offered for management: to stop all fat intake until the pain is gone; to check for the chemical signs of pancreatitis; regardless of the outcome of these tests, to be cautious about undertaking any exploratory surgery; and when the patient has recovered, not to neglect to seek evidence of familial hyperlipemia in his relatives. No mechanism has been proved for the hyperlipemia in pancreatitis.

Alcohol.[180,256] Oral and intravenous administration of ethanol has been shown to cause endogenous hyperglyceridemia, but the plasma glyceride concentrations are less than those frequently seen in pancreatitis. The mechanisms whereby alcohol produces hyperlipemia are still being debated.[180] In most patients with glyceride levels in excess of 1000 mg. per 100 ml. there is chemical evidence of hepatocellular damage as well as pancreatitis. Low PHLA has been reported in alcoholism.[257] Zieve[178] has described the occurrence of hemolytic anemia and hyperlipemia in alcoholism. This association could be due to 2 distinct effects of alcohol since anemia and hyperlipemia may occur singly in chronic alcoholism. There is a tendency to be empirical about intake of alcohol in patients with Type IV. Hyperlipemia observed after a "binge" usually cannot be reproduced under experimental conditions, and the association is difficult to prove.

Glycogen-storage disease. Mild to severe hyperlipemia is frequently found in several types of glycogen-storage diseases.[64,258] We have examined plasma from 4 patients with glycogenosis (Cori Type I); the Type IV pattern was present in each.

Idiopathic hypercalcemia. Hyperlipidemia[109] or hypercholesterolemia[259] has been reported to be a frequent feature of idiopathic hypercalcemia of infancy; changes in lipoproteins have been reported in only a few cases.[109] The Type IV pattern has been observed in 2 children (studied in collaboration with Dr. Sidney Levin). In 1, it was possible to demonstrate that hyperlipemia was associated with exaggerated carbohydrate induction. It is not known whether the children who have recovered from this disorder, which may be associated with premature atherosclerosis, have persistent lipoprotein abnormalities.

Hypothyroidism. Thyroid deficiency should always be considered in a patient with the Type IV pattern.[260] It can occur, but is less common than the Type II anomaly, as previously described. The relation can only be proved by therapeutic trial.

Nephrotic syndrome.[27,64,261] The nephrotic syndrome can provide a panoply of lipoprotein patterns, ranging from a discrete increase in β lipoproteins to tremendous increases in pre-β lipoproteins.[100,261,262] The severity is related to the degree of hypoalbuminemia. The mechanism by which lipoprotein concentrations are increased in nephrosis

has been much studied but not established. Suggestions have included a block in the "conversion" of pre-β lipoproteins to β lipoproteins[100] (a theoretical mechanism, also discussed under Type III) possibly associated with a decreased uptake of triglyceride by the adipose tissue.[27] Others have suggested that the hyperglyceridemia is secondary to an increased outflow of free fatty acids from adipose tissue[27] or that the proteinuria provokes increased hepatic synthesis of proteins (and lipoproteins).[261]

Dysglobulinemia.[263-270] One of the diagnoses often suggested by the sudden appearance of severe hyperlipoproteinemia is the presence of an abnormal plasma gamma globulin as in myeloma, cryoglobulinemia or macroglobulinemia. There have been an increasing number of reports of multiple myeloma associated with Type II or Type IV pattern. Xanthomas, tendinous, tuberous or eruptive in form, have sometimes been present. Xanthomatosis has been reported in multiple myeloma without definite hyperlipoproteinemia. The myeloma protein has usually been a β_{2A} globulin. Usually, there is a direct relation between the amount of abnormal protein and the degree of hyperlipoproteinemia. It has been variously considered that the abnormal protein itself serves as a lipid carrier, is complexed with β or pre-β lipoproteins in such a way as to retard their catabolism or serves as a cryoprecipitin for the lipoproteins.

Gestational hormones. Women who are taking progesterone analogues by mouth, alone or in combination with estrogens, for contraception or other purposes frequently have Type IV patterns.[271] The same thing is true of pregnancy.[272]

Other disorders. We have also observed Type IV patterns in association with gout, Niemann–Pick disease, Gaucher's disease, total lipoatrophy, Werner's syndrome and other diseases.

Primary Type IV

Doubtless, all the diseases of which Type IV may be only an accompaniment have not been distinguished. Neither have all the more subtle environmental facts that may cause sporadic appearance of the pattern in the population. Just as the incidence of primary forms of Type IV is not known, so is information meager about the number of such cases that are genetically determined. The limited experience at the Clinical Center appears to be the major source of data bearing on this last question.

In the two or three years in which phenotyping has become a more than casual activity, approximately 90 patients have been seen at the Clinical Center whose index patterns on regular diets could be classified as primary Type IV. This excludes many more in whom such a pattern has been detected in connection with collaborative studies, in analysis of pedigrees of propositi of other types or in other patients in whom obvious disorders causing secondary lipoprotein abnormalities could not be excluded. For 22 of the patients with Type IV patterns it has been possible to sample some of their parents, siblings and children. In only 5 kindreds have all parents and all sibs been available. The choice of the relatives sampled in all 22 kindreds was based solely on availability and is therefore presumably subject to only such bias as this might introduce. Familial occurrence has been detected in 15 of the kindreds. The data from this study offer some interesting insight into the familial distribution of Type IV.

Eighty-six parents, children or sibs of the 22 index patients with primary Type IV were sampled. Thirty-four (40 per cent) had Type IV patterns. If the "propositi" are added to the sample, the percentage of abnormal family members rises to 52 (56 in 108). The Type IV pattern was the only abnormal one observed in these kindreds. Both the mother and the father of 5 "propositi" were sampled. In 2 sets both were abnormal; 1 in each of 3 sets was normal, and the other had Type IV. Ten of a total of 21 parents sampled were abnormal. Of the sibs of the index patients 52 were sampled, and 21 (40 per cent) had Type IV. The remaining 13 relatives examined were some of the children of the propositi. Three of 13 had Type IV, and all the abnormal relatives were over twenty years of age. Of the 10 who were normal, 7 were still less than twenty years of age. These data are too incomplete to warrant any statistical evaluation or serious genetic interpretation. Proper controls are lacking, and doubtless more than one biochemical defect is represented. It does appear, however, that the incidence of the same lipoprotein abnormality is surprisingly high in relatives of patients with primary Type IV. "Vertical transmission" does occur, and only 1 parent may show the defect. The data expose a broad opportunity and great need for further population study.

Clinical features. The lipoprotein abnormalities in most of the familial examples of Type IV described above have been mild. A few cases have been quite severe. Examples have been described elsewhere in detail.[159] The clinical manifestations include those described above for Type IV in general. Glucose intolerance has been nearly universal, being present in 22 of 23 subjects tested so far in the overall familial sample. Some, but not all, of the familial examples have been associated with obesity. Subjects with the severest hyperlipemia have usually exceeded normal weight limits. Exaggerated carbohydrate inducibility has been present in 6 of 7 who were adequately tested.

Management. The treatment of primary Type IV presently includes weight control, avoidance of excessive dietary carbohydrate and hypolipemic agents, in that order. Obese patients with Type IV who are brought to ideal weight will have a dramatic improvement in lipoprotein patterns and, usually, in glucose tolerance. If excessive carbohydrate inducibility can actually be tested this is ideal; if not, it is reasonable to assume that most patients will have less hyperlipemia if they maintain ideal weight on a diet in which 45 to 50 per cent of calories come from fats, particularly of fairly unsaturated, low-cholesterol sources. This helps the patient keep down his craving for sugars and starches.

If the program outlined above does not lower plasma glycerides to below 400 mg. per 100 ml., drug therapy may be considered in addition. The orally administered antidiabetic agents may be of value[250,251] although they do not reduce lipoprotein patterns to normal levels in some patients. Hyperlipoproteinemia is no contraindication to their use in the management of accompanying diabetes. Certain agents promoting hypolipidemia were described in the discussion of Type II. The 2 most effective in decreasing hyperlipemia are chlorphenoxyisobutyric acid and nicotinic acid. The precautions mentioned earlier for use of these agents apply to Type IV as well. Heparin injections may temporarily reduce Type IV hyperlipoproteinemia.[222] Its chronic use in the treatment of hyperlipemia is not practical.

TYPE V HYPERLIPOPROTEINEMIA[159]

Definition

There are some patients on a regular diet who have chylomicrons *and* increased amounts of pre-β lipoproteins in the usual postabsorptive sample. The Type V pattern has been reserved to designate this combination of exogenous and endogenous hyperlipemia. The legitimacy of Type V as an indicator of a specific disease, syndrome or group of disorders may be properly questioned. It may be, for example, merely a stage of Type IV, produced by sudden imposition of a heavy load of dietary fat on clearing mechanisms intolerably burdened by endogenous glycerides. This sequence has been experimentally demonstrated in more than 1 of the patients with Type IV referred to in the last section. A Type V pattern may also appear when the severe exogenous hyperlipemia of Type I is clearing on the low-fat diets that cause modest carbohydrate induction in such patients. Type V could be a genotypic variant of Type IV, possibly in terms of homozygous expression of the same mutant (or mutants) or because of the interaction of other genes. Type IV patterns frequently occur in the few "Type V kindreds" sampled thus far. The significance of Type V, therefore, is not clear, but its recognition is important. It provides the therapist with a guide to dietary management and the experimentalist with a tool to determine the identity or separateness of clearing mechanisms for glycerides of different origin and the factors determining the rate of removal.

The incidence of patients with the Type V pattern on normal diets is not known. Twenty-one such patients have been screened at the Clinical Center. A partial sampling of the relatives of these has brought the total number of examples of Type V to 27. Our sampling of patients with acute diseases associated with hyperlipemia has been extremely limited, and the frequency of this pattern might be much greater in general hospitals.

278 THE NEW ENGLAND JOURNAL OF MEDICINE Feb. 2, 1967

There is no body of useful information about Type V in the medical literature to warrant a drawing of historical perspectives. Many examples of this abnormality have undoubtedly been reported, but it is only with the increasing use of polyvinylpyrrolidone gradients and starch-block and paper electrophoresis that the identification of mixed hyperlipemia has been sufficiently good to permit the study of patients with Type V patterns.

Lipoprotein Pattern

As shown in Figure 13, the Type V pattern is complex. Cholesterol and glyceride concentrations are elevated but in proportions too variable to be helpful in diagnosis. Simple observation of the plasma after it has sat overnight in the cold can be useful. As they do in Type I, chylomicrons appear as a cream layer at the top. However, the infranatant layer in Type V remains lactescent. In the polyvinylpyrrolidone gradient tube, top, intermediate and bottom layers of turbid particles are usually seen. On starch-block electrophoresis primary and secondary particles are accompanied by endogenous particles of α mobility.[6] On the paper electrophoretogram the pre-β lipoproteins usually leave their trail of endogenous glyceride from the origin, but the chylomicron band is identifiable as a discrete band at the point of application.[7] When the chylomicrons are few, or when both bands are very intense, the distinction can be hard and requires experience. Concentrations of α and β lipoprotein tend to be low. If precipitation technics are used, there is an increase in "low-density lipoproteins," but reliable distinction of chylomicrons from endogenous particles requires ancillary analyses.

Clinical Forms and Features

The patients with Type V patterns studied so far have many clinical features in common. Both males and females are affected. Symptoms have frequently appeared first in the late teens or the third decade. The commonest complaint is recurrent abdominal pain; this has often led to exploratory surgery, which has provided no specific diagnosis in most cases. Occasionally, the surgeons have found milky fluid in the peritoneal cavity. Sometimes, the appearance of eruptive xanthomas has been the first abnormality noted by the patient. As in Type I, these are commonly on the knees, buttocks, shoulders and back, but they may be anywhere. Lipemia retinalis, foam cells in the bone marrow and hepatosplenomegaly may be present. The patients are often obese and frequently have a family history of both diabetes and obesity. Evidence of accelerated atherosclerosis in either patients or their families has not been striking. Hyperuricemia may or may not be present. Pancreatic lipase and amylase may not be elevated even during bouts of abdominal pain. Glucose tolerance is almost invariably abnormal.

The contrast with Type I is important. Patients

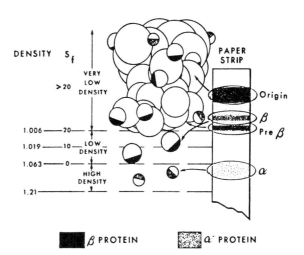

FIGURE 13. *Type V Hyperlipoproteinemia (See Also Table 3), Which Is a Mixture of Endogenous and Exogenous Hyperlipemia Uncertainly Related to Type IV.*

PHLA is normal or low; glucose tolerance is usually abnormal. Abdominal pain, eruptive xanthomas and hepatosplenomegaly are seen as in Types I and IV. The pattern is often familial, but there are "phenocopies" secondary to many disorders.

with Type I usually have symptoms beginning in infancy. There is no relation of their hyperlipemia to obesity or diabetes. The levels of PHLA in Type I are distinctly reduced. In Type V they may be somewhat low but are usually in the range of normal. The fall in hyperlipemia with a fat-free diet is usually rapid in both Types I and V, but the glyceride level is much more dependent upon the dietary fat intake in Type I. Type V hyperlipemia is much more affected by negative caloric balance. For both Types I and V one must be very cautious in refeeding fat after the patient has been on a fat-free, high-carbohydrate diet. Marked chylomicronemia and severe abdominal pain may develop in one day.

As with other types of hyperlipoproteinemia, Type V can be separated into primary and secondary forms, a distinction that for the present means simply the presence or absence of other diseases or conditions known to be associated with hyperlipemia. For example, the 21 index patients with Type V at the National Institutes of Health included 9 with what was considered to be primary and 12 with secondary. Of the latter, 3 had uncontrolled, insulin-dependent diabetes, and 5 chronic pancreatitis, and 4 were patients with history of recent heavy alcohol intake.[176] Full lipoprotein analyses have been done infrequently in cases of hyperlipemia due to alcoholic excess or pancreatitis, but many reports suggest that Type V patterns were present.

Genetic information. Of 9 "primary" examples of Type V in the Clinical Center group studied thus far (5 males and 4 females), all have proved to have at least 1 relative with hyperlipemia.

It has been possible to sample all the siblings of the propositi in 4 kindreds, and both parents of the propositi in 3. The parents of the fourth propositus are dead. All the 6 living parents had abnormal lipoprotein patterns. In 2 sets both had Type IV, and in the third, the father was Type V and the mother Type IV. The 4 propositi had 13 siblings. Four were normal; 3 had Type V, and 6 Type IV. Ten children of the propositi or their affected siblings were all normal, but none were over thirteen years of age. It is possible that the expression of the disorder is delayed, as was suggested in the discussion of Type IV, and young children should be treated separately in any population analyses until this point is clarified.

To sum up the lipoprotein patterns seen in 23 adult members of 4 kindreds of patients presenting Type V patterns, including the propositi, their siblings and parents, 8 had Type V, and 11 Type IV, and only 4 were normal. Not included in these analyses is another kindred only partially studied[159] in which at least 2 of 6 siblings have severe Type V patterns. The incidence of abnormal glucose tolerance tests in members of families with Type V and hyperlipoproteinemia (either Type IV or V patterns) is 16 of 17 subjects tested at the Clinical Center.

The sampling is so small as to make any genetic interpretations perilous. Nevertheless, it is worth comparing the data from the 4 completely sampled families with Type V just described with those obtained in relatives of propositi with Type IV described in the preceding sections.

The 4 propositi with Type V had 19 adult relatives (their sibs or parents) who were sampled. Four (20 per cent) were normal; 4 had Type V patterns, and 11 Type IV patterns. Fourteen patients who presented Type IV patterns and were then demonstrated to have primary familial hyperlipoproteinemia provided 54 adult sibs or parents for comparison. Twenty-four of these (44 per cent) were normal. All the 30 abnormal relatives were Type IV. The number of affected males and females was about equal. It is obvious that if 1 of the relatives with Type IV in the "Type V kindreds" had been seen first and had become the index patient, the distribution of patterns in the relatives of the 2 sets of propositi would have been different. This does not alter a strong impression from the available data that if the Type IV and Type V patterns represent the same genotype, such influences as determine 1 phenotype or the other seem not to be randomly distributed among all the affected families. With observation of the presence, so far, of abnormalities in both parents of the kindreds with Type V, one possibility is that Type IV and Type V are the heterozygous and homozygous genotypes, respectively, for identical mutant alleles. It is also possible that single genes for Type I and Type IV defects interact to produce Type V. The only tests of these and other possible explanations must come from the careful study of more kindreds. Very probably, the ultimate solution will require the development of better tests for genotype than these 2 lipoprotein patterns can provide.

Biochemical Mechanisms

Type V is a combination of abnormalities whose possible bases have already been discussed under Types I and IV. Speculation that the underlying lesion is comparable to that in Type IV, with the exogenous hyperlipemia a secondary feature attributable to diet, has already been mentioned. Acceptance of this theory will in part depend upon more rigorous proof than is available that chylomicrons and pre-β lipoproteins compete at identical sites for removal of their glyceride. Although this is probably so, more information will be needed to explain some of the family data just discussed.

If Type V represents the homozygous expression of Type IV one might expect that patients with V would be much more susceptible to carbohydrate induction. Adequate comparisons have not been made. If the mechanism in Type V is related to that in Type I, one would expect lipoprotein lipase deficiency to be present as detected by assay of PHLA. In 7 patients with Type V so tested the activity has varied from a low value of 0.17 in 1 patient to others clearly in the normal range during intake of regular diets. The test lacks the ability to discriminate clearly partial defects in enzyme activity as is evident in subjects assumed to be heterozygous for Type I. Tests are in progress to determine whether patients with Type V might have exaggerated de-induction of PHLA during low-fat feeding or retarded adaptation of the enzyme levels to the challenge of higher loads of dietary fat.

It has been reported that patients who have insulin-deficient diabetes, and Type V-like patterns when they are out of control, also have low PHLA activity that returns to normal when insulin is readministered and clearing of hyperlipemia occurs.[176] Patients with hyperlipemia and pancreatitis have also been reported to have decreased PHLA.[179] Diabetic animals clear ingested or infused glycerides better when treated with insulin,[273] and a similar phenomenon has been shown in man.[176,274]

Management

If one may generalize about so elusive a syndrome, Type V appears to combine the hazards of Type I and Type IV. The treatment of Type V, beyond dietary manipulation, has not been systematically developed. The secondary and primary forms may be approached similarly from the standpoint of diet. Weight reduction in the obese patient is an excellent way to decrease hyperlipemia. As in Type IV, Type V patterns that return completely to normal levels on severe caloric restriction again become abnormal when isocaloric feeding is resumed at ideal weight. The hyperlipoproteinemia is usually much improved, however. Diets that are not unusually high in fats or carbohydrates should be used in maintenance. The patients must be followed carefully, both to forestall gain in weight and to discourage intemperance in alcohol, as well as to

CLASSIC PAPERS IN HYPERLIPIDAEMIA 129

280 THE NEW ENGLAND JOURNAL OF MEDICINE 1967

observe the lipoprotein pattern for unanticipated changes. Whenever severe endogenous hyperlipemia develops, care must be taken to reduce both calories and carbohydrate until improvement results, for a sudden switch to isocaloric high-fat diets may cause an abdominal crisis. The use of drugs has not been carefully described for Type V. The same considerations as mentioned under Type IV obtain.

OTHER ABNORMAL LIPOPROTEIN PATTERNS

With the conclusion of the discussion of 5 types of lipoprotein patterns seen in patients with hyperlipoproteinemia, it will be clear to observers of other patients that some significant and perhaps diagnostic patterns have been left out of the numbering scheme. One may draw upon the experience with blood-clotting factors for encouragement to limit the entries in any numbered system. New patterns will inevitably be discovered as representative of other syndromes, and better technics will fragment the existing Types I through V. The nomenclature will evolve as it must. Nothing has been said of chemical abnormalities in the constituent lipids of the lipoproteins, such as the quantities of phytanic acid that appear in Refsum's syndrome[275] or small increases in cerebrosides in Gaucher's disease.[276]

Some other specific lipoprotein patterns such as the absence or deficiency of α and β lipoproteins have already been discussed in this review. One other set of patterns encountered quite often remains to be described. These are the patterns in certain liver diseases.

Obstructive Liver Disease

The lipoprotein patterns and serum lipids in patients with either intrahepatic or extrahepatic biliary obstruction are unique. They are characterized by marked hypercholesterolemia and hyperphospholipidemia. The increase in serum cholesterol is mainly confined to free sterol whereas the esterified cholesterol content is normal or low. The increase of phospholipid is relatively greater than that of the cholesterol. More often than not the serum triglyceride and free fatty acid concentrations are normal, and the plasma is icteric but perfectly clear.[277,278] The content of high-density lipoproteins is severely reduced or even absent in analyses made by preparative or analytical ultracentrifugation.[26,64] There is, on the other hand, a marked increase in the lipoproteins having density between 1.019 and 1.063. Comparison of the ultracentrifugal data to early work with Cohn fractionation pointed up a seeming paradox.[278] Usually, large amounts of lipid were present in the fraction IV that contains α lipoprotein in normal serum. The increased low-density lipoproteins were also shown to be abnormal, having lower than normal ratios of protein to lipid and cholesterol to phospholipid. They also did not react to antiserums specific for β lipoproteins.[278]

We have recently found that patients with biliary cirrhosis may have tremendous increases in α lipoproteins on the electrophoretogram and by immunochemical analyses. The α lipoproteins behave as though antigenically identical to the normal lipoproteins but migrate much more slowly during paper electrophoresis. These α lipoproteins, which contain more phospholipid than normal, float in the density region 1.006 to 1.063 and swell the concentration of low-density lipoprotein. Other patients with biliary-tract obstruction may have an elevation in true β lipoprotein that also contains more phospholipid than usual. The relation of bile stasis to these abnormal lipoproteins is unclear. It has been suggested that the overall lipoprotein increase may be related to the surfactant properties of bile salts favoring disruption of lipid-protein complexes and promoting a different type of stabilization of the lipids in plasma.[277] The liver probably also releases a good deal more lipid into the plasma because the normal flow of phospholipids and cholesterol in the bile is obstructed and because interruption of the enterohepatic cycle of cholesterol has altered the synthesis of lipoproteins. The hyperlipoproteinemia does vary with the extent and degree of biliary obstruction. The drug cholestyramine has been variably successful in lowering the hyperlipoproteinemia of biliary obstruction.[279] When severe hepatocellular damage occurs in the liver there is a lowering of all lipoprotein fractions, and patients with parenchymal liver disease may have severe total deficiency of α lipoproteins.[78]

CONCLUSIONS

The plasma is often the only window from which one can see the state of intracellular metabolism. The view is limited, and all ingenuity is demanded to gain the sharpest perspectives. The plasma lipoproteins have been discussed, and the vast information about them distilled from the point of view of the clinician who seeks the most rational approach to patients with certain abnormalities in fat metabolism. The lipoproteins serve this purpose better than chemical determination of plasma lipid concentrations alone. It is hoped that the systematic way of using some of the simpler tools for lipoprotein analyses described will encourage wider application of lipoprotein patterns in clinical practice so that more specific diagnoses will replace certain of the time-worn clichés and more attention will be focused on the many basic problems of etiology that are still to be solved. Major emphasis has been placed on the use of lipoprotein patterns to seek genetic factors that produce altered plasma lipid levels. It has been one of the areas most neglected. If a pedigree chart appeared on the clinical record of every patient with hyperlipidemia, the number of unanswered questions might be reduced by half; certainly, the satisfaction that the physician gains from the study of patients with hyperlipidemia would be doubled.

REFERENCES

239. Kinsell, L. W., Walker, G., Michaels, G. D., and Olson, F. E. Dietary fats and diabetic patient. *New Eng. J. Med.* **261**:431-434, 1959.

240. Kuo, P. T., and Bassett, D. R. Primary hyperlipidemias and their management. *Ann. Int. Med.* **59**:495-507, 1963.

241. Knittle, J. L., and Ahrens, E. H., Jr. Carbohydrate metabolism in two forms of hyperglyceridemia. *J. Clin. Investigation* **43**:485-495, 1964.

242. Gofman, J. W., Glazier, F., Tamplin, A., Strisower, B., and de Lalla, O. Lipoproteins, coronary heart disease, and atherosclerosis. *Physiol. Rev.* **34**:589-607, 1954.

243. Besterman, E. M. M. Lipoproteins in coronary artery disease. *Brit. Heart J.* **19**:503-515, 1957.

244. Carlson, L. A. Serum lipids in men with myocardial infarction. *Acta med. Scandinav.* **167**:399-413, 1960.

245. Albrink, M. J., Meigs, J. W., and Man, E. B. Serum lipids, hypertension and coronary artery disease. *Am. J. Med.* **31**:4-23, 1961.

246. Brown, D. F., Kinch, S. H., and Doyle, J. T. Serum triglycerides in health and in ischemic heart disease. *New Eng. J. Med.* **273**:947-952, 1965.

247. Fine, M., et al. Incorporation of C[14] from uniformly labeled glucose into plasma triglycerides in normals and hyperglyceridemics. *Metabolism* **11**:893-911, 1962.

248. Baker, N., and Schotz, M. C. Use of multicompartmental models to measure rates of triglyceride metabolism in rats. *J. Lipid Research* **5**:188-197, 1964.

249. Farquhar, J. W., Gross, R. C., Wagner, R. M., and Reaven, G. M. Validation of incompletely coupled two-compartment nonrecycling catenary model for turnover of liver and plasma triglyceride in man. *J. Lipid Research* **6**:119-134, 1965.

250. Morris, J. H., West, D. A., and Bolinger, R. E. Effect of oral sulfonylurea on plasma triglycerides in diabetics. *Diabetes* **13**:87-89, 1964.

251. Schwartz, M. J., Mirsky, S., and Schaefer, L. E. Phenformin, serum lipids, and diabetes mellitus. *Lancet* **1**:959, 1965.

252. Poulsen, H. M. Familial lipaemia: new form of lipoidosis showing increase in neutral fats combined with attacks of acute pancreatitis. *Acta med. Scandinav.* **138**:413-420, 1950.

253. Klatskin, G., and Gordon, M. Relationship between relapsing pancreatitis and essential hyperlipemia. *Am. J. Med.* **12**:3-23, 1952.

254. Greenberger, N. J., Hatch, F. T., Drummey, G. D., and Isselbacher, K. J. Pancreatitis and hyperlipemia: study of serum lipid alterations in 25 patients with acute pancreatitis. *Medicine* **45**:161-174, 1966.

255. Feigl, J. Neue Untersuchungen zur Chemie des Blutes bei akuter Alkohol-intoxikation und bei chronischem Alkoholismus mit besonderer Berücksichtigung der Fette und Lipoide. *Biochem. Ztschr.* **92**:282-317, 1918.

256. Losowsky, M. S., Jones, D. P., Davidson, C. S., and Lieber, C. S. Studies of alcoholic hyperlipemia and its mechanism. *Am. J. Med.* **35**:794-803, 1963.

257. Jones, D. P., Losowsky, M. S., Davidson, C. S., and Lieber, C. S. Effects of ethanol on plasma lipids in man. *J. Lab. & Clin. Med.* **62**:675-682, 1963.

258. Field, R. A. Glycogen deposition diseases. In *The Metabolic Basis of Inherited Disease*. Second edition. Edited by J. B. Stanbury,

J. B. Wyngaarden and D. S. Fredrickson. 1434 pp. New York: McGraw-Hill, 1966. P. 141.

259. Joseph, M. C., and Parrott, D. Severe infantile hyperglicemia with special reference to facies. *Arch. Dis. Childhood* **33**:385-395, 1958.

260. O'Hara, D. D., Porte, D., Jr., and Williams, R. H. Effect of diet and thyroxin on plasma lipids in myxedema. *Metabolism* **15**:123-134, 1966.

261. Baxter, J. H. Hyperlipoproteinemia in nephrosis. *Arch. Int. Med.* **109**:742-757, 1962.

262. Baxter, J. H., Goodman, H. C., and Havel, R. J. Serum lipid and lipoprotein alterations in nephrosis. *J. Clin. Investigation* **39**:455-465, 1960.

263. Lewis, L. A., and Page, I. H. Serum proteins and lipoproteins in multiple myelomatosis. *Am. J. Med.* **17**:670-673, 1954.

264. Lennard-Jones, J. E. Myelomatoses with lipaemia and xanthomata. *Brit. M. J.* **1**:781-783, 1960.

265. Marten, R. H. Xanthomatosis and myelomatosis. *Proc. Roy. Soc. Med.* **55**:318, 1962.

266. Cohen, L., Blaisdell, R. K., Ormiste, V., and Djordjevich, J. Xanthomatosis, familial hyperlipidemia, and myelomatosis. *Circulation* **30**:111-5, 1964.

267. Levin, W. C., Aboumrad, M. H., Ritzmann, S. E., and Brantly, C. γ-Type 1 myeloma and xanthomatosis. *Arch. Int. Med.* **114**:688-693, 1964.

268. Short, M. H. Multiple myeloma with xanthoma formation: report of case. *Arch. Path.* **77**:400-406, 1964.

269. Savin, R. C. Hyperglobulinemia purpura terminating in myeloma hyperlipemia and xanthomatoses. *Arch. Dermat.* **92**:679-686, 1965.

270. Lewis, L. A., Van Ommen, R. A., and Page, I. H. Association of cold-precipitability with β-lipoprotein and cryoglobulin. *Am. J. Med.* **40**:785-793, 1966.

271. Aurell, M., Cramér, K., and Rybo, G. Serum lipids and lipoproteins during long-term administration of oral contraceptive. *Lancet* **1**:291-293, 1966.

272. Pantelakis, S. N., Fosbrooke, A. S., Lloyd, J. K., and Wolff, O. H. Nature and occurrence of pre-beta-lipoprotein in diabetic children and pregnant women: electrophoretic and ultracentrifugal study of serum lipoproteins. *Diabetes* **13**:153-160, 1964.

273. Hirsch, R. L., and Perl, W. Transport of lipoprotein triglyceride in normal control and diabetic rabbit. *Circulation*

274. Krut, L. H., and Barsky, R. F. Effect of enhanced glucose utilisation on postprandial lipaemia in ischaemic heart-disease. *Lancet* **2**:1136-1138, 1964.

275. Richterich, R., Van Mechelen, P., and Rossi, E. Refsum's disease (heredopathia atactica polyneuritiformis): inborn error of lipid metabolism with storage of 3, 7, 11, 15-tetramethyl hexadecanoic acid. 1. Report of case. *Am. J. Med.* **39**:230-236, 1965.

276. Hillborg, P. O., and Svennerholm, L. Blood level of cerebrosides in Gaucher's disease. *Acta paediat.* **49**:707-710, 1960.

277. Kunkel, H. G., and Ahrens, E. H., Jr. Relationship between serum lipids and electrophoretic pattern, with particular reference to patients with primary biliary cirrhosis. *J. Clin. Investigation* **28**:1575-1579, 1948.

278. Russ, E. M., Raymunt, J., and Barr, D. P. Lipoproteins in primary biliary cirrhosis. *J. Clin. Investigation* **35**:133-144, 1956.

279. Keczkes, K., Goldberg, D. M., and Fergusson, A. G. Xanthomatous biliary cirrhosis treated with cholestyramine: report of case. *Arch. Int. Med.* **114**:321-328, 1964.

Clin. Sci. (1968) **34**, 541–548.

INCREASED HEPATIC SYNTHESIS OF CHOLESTEROL AFTER ILEAL BY-PASS IN MONKEYS

C. D. MOUTAFIS AND N. B. MYANT

Medical Research Council, Hammersmith Hospital, London

(*Received* 13 *December* 1967)

SUMMARY

1. When monkeys are submitted to an ileal by-pass operation, there is a fall in the plasma cholesterol level, followed by a return to the pre-operative value.

2. Cholesterol synthesis in the liver, as judged by the rate of incorporation of [^{14}C]acetate into digitonin-precipitable sterols in liver biopsies *in vitro*, is enhanced after the operation.

3. It is suggested that the secondary rise in the plasma cholesterol level after the operation is due to increased synthesis of cholesterol in the liver brought about by release of endogenous synthesis from end-product inhibition.

Exclusion of the ileum has been used as a method of treating essential hypercholesterolaemia (Buchwald & Varco, 1966), on the grounds that this operation leads to a fall in the plasma cholesterol level in man and in experimental animals (Buchwald, 1964). Davis *et al.* (1966), however, found that an ileal by-pass operation had only a temporary effect on the plasma cholesterol level in a girl suffering from severe essential hypercholesterolaemia. Although the cholesterol level in this patient began to fall shortly after the operation, it subsequently returned to the pre-operative value.

One of the possible causes of a secondary rise in the plasma cholesterol level after an ileal by-pass is an increased rate of synthesis of cholesterol in the liver, a major source of the endogenous cholesterol in the plasma. To test this possibility, we have measured the rate of incorporation of [^{14}C]acetate into cholesterol *in vitro* in the livers of monkeys before and after exclusion of the ileum.

METHODS

Three immature monkeys were used (see Table 1). Each animal was kept in a separate cage at a constant temperature of 23° and was given a diet *ad libitum* of mixed dog biscuits (Spillers

Correspondence: Dr N. B. Myant, Medical Research Council, Hammersmith Hospital, Ducane Road, London, W.12.

542   *C. D. Moutafis and N. B. Myant*

Ltd, London) and M.R.C. diet No. 41 (Bruce & Parkes, 1946), supplemented with fruit and vegetables. The daily intake of cholesterol was between 10 and 20 mg/monkey.

The operation

Three grams of glucose were given by intravenous injection $1\frac{1}{2}$ hr before the operation. The monkey was anaesthetized with intravenous pentothal (20 mg/kg) and the trachea was intubated with a Magill's tube. Anaesthesia was maintained throughout the operation with nitrous oxide and oxygen. As soon as the abdomen was opened, a liver biopsy was taken (see below). The small intestine was divided 22–30 cm below the duodeno-jejunal junction (see Table 1) and the distal end was closed. The proximal end was anastomosed to the appendix. After the operation, the monkey was given monthly intramuscular injections of a mixture of vitamins B (aneurin, 10 mg; nicotinamide, 40 mg; riboflavin, 4 mg; B_{12}, 100 μg).

TABLE 1. Details of monkeys with ileal by-pass operation

Monkey	Species	Sex	Weight (kg)	Site of by-pass*
1	*Macaca irus*	Male	<3.0	22
2	*M. irus*	Female	2.7	30
3	*M. mulatta*	Female	3.7	25

* Distance below duodeno-jejunal junction in centimetres.

Liver biopsy

In order to minimize variations in the glycogen content of the liver on different occasions, intravenous glucose (3 g) was given $1\frac{1}{2}$ hr before each biopsy. The animal was anaesthetized with intravenous pentothal (20 mg/kg), and the abdomen was opened under sterile conditions. Two or three samples of liver were then taken, either with a Menghini needle or by cutting out small wedges of tissue from the anterior margin of the liver. The biopsy specimens were immediately suspended in 1 ml of the bicarbonate buffer used for the incubation. Pieces of tissue were then transferred to sheets of polythene and were rapidly separated from surface moisture and from clots of blood or fibrin by teasing with a fine glass rod. If necessary, the wedges of tissue were cut into pieces of a suitable size with a razor blade. The tissue was transferred to a weighed tube containing the incubation mixture, and the weight of the tissue found from the weight of the tube, plus incubation mixture, plus tissue. The weight of tissue used for a single incubation varied from 2 to 20 mg.

Conditions of incubation

The incubation mixture was a modification of that described by Bhattathiry & Siperstein (1963). It contained Krebs–Ringer bicarbonate buffer, pH 7.4 (0.15 M), modified by equalizing the concentrations of sodium and potassium ions, potassium acetate (4.0 mM) and sodium [1-^{14}C]acetate (0.01 mM, 5 μCi/flask). The final volume was 0.5 ml. The tubes were gassed for 1 min with 95% oxygen and 5% CO_2, stoppered, and shaken in a water-bath at 37° for 3 hr. The incubations were carried out in duplicate or triplicate. The time between taking the liver biopsy and starting the incubation was not longer than 15 min.

Isolation and radioassay of cholesterol

At the end of the incubation, 0·4 ml of 40% NaOH and 2 ml of ethanol containing 2 mg of non-radioactive cholesterol were added to the incubation mixture, and the mixture was boiled under reflux for 6 hr. The cholesterol was extracted from the hydrolysate with light petroleum (b.p. 40–60°) and the extract washed with 1% acetic acid. The washed extract was taken to dryness, dissolved in acetone and the cholesterol precipitated as the digitonide. The digitonide was washed once with cold acetone and once with cold diethyl ether and was then dried at 60°. The dried digitonide was dissolved in hot methanol. One-tenth was taken for estimation of cholesterol and the remainder was transferred to a glass vial for radioassay. After evaporation of the methanol, 2 ml of ethanol were added, followed by 10 ml of toluene containing 0·4% of 2,5-diphenyl-oxazole and 0·01% of 1,4-*bis*-(2-(5-phenyl-oxazolyl))benzene. Radioactivity was assayed in a Packard TriCarb scintillation spectrometer. A known fraction of the dose of [1-^{14}C]acetate used for each incubation was assayed for radioactivity under the same conditions, so that the results could be expressed in p-moles of acetate incorporated into digitonin-precipitable sterols. The final values were corrected for the recovery of the cholesterol added to the incubation mixture. Recoveries varied from 95% to 98%. Endogenous acetate present in the biopsy sample was ignored in the calculation of the amount of [^{14}C]acetate incorporated into digitonin-precipitable sterols.

Serial blood samples (1·0–1·5 ml) were taken from the saphenous vein and 0·2 ml was transferred at once to tubes containing sodium ethylenediaminetetra-acetate for measurement of the haematocrit value. The remainder of the sample was allowed to clot and the serum taken for measurement of the serum cholesterol concentration. Duplicate 0·2-ml samples of serum were pipetted into 20 ml of chloroform–methanol (2:1) and the mixture was brought to the boil. The extract was filtered and a known fraction of the filtrate taken to dryness and assayed for total cholesterol by the fluorimetric method of Carpenter, Gotsis & Hegsted (1957).

Materials

Sodium [1-^{14}C]acetate was obtained from the Radiochemical Centre, Amersham, Bucks.

RESULTS

Before operation

Serial biopsies were taken from the livers of three monkeys over periods ranging from 20 to 225 days before the ileal by-pass was established (Figs. 1–3). In eight biopsies taken from the three monkeys before operation, the rate of incorporation of [^{14}C]acetate into cholesterol *in vitro* ranged from 3 to 208 p-moles mg fresh liver^{-1} 3 hr^{-1} incubation (Table 2). The results from monkeys 1 and 2 suggest that the taking of a liver biopsy by laparotomy, both before and after the operation, caused a temporary fall in the plasma cholesterol level (Figs. 1 and 2).

After operation

After the ileal by-pass operation there was a substantial fall in the plasma cholesterol level in monkeys 1 and 3, the values reaching a minimum within 20 days and then returning to the pre-operative level during the next 30–40 days. In monkey 2 the initial effect of the by-pass operation may have been masked by the effect of the previous biopsy, but the secondary rise was clearly seen in this monkey. The fall in the plasma cholesterol level after the operation

544   *C. D. Moutafis and N. B. Myant*

was not due to haemodilution, since the blood samples taken before and after the operation showed no significant change in haematocrit value.

In each of the three monkeys the rate of incorporation of [14C]acetate into cholesterol in

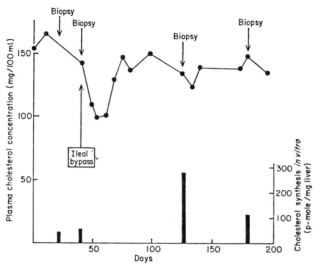

FIG. 1. Monkey 1: plasma cholesterol concentration (●) and rate of incorporation of [14C]acetate into digitonin-precipitable sterols of liver slices before and after an ileal by-pass operation.

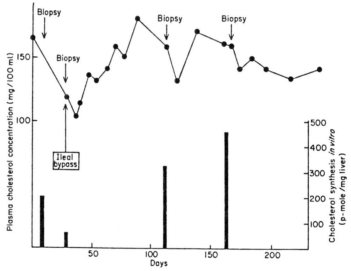

FIG. 2: Monkey 2: plasma cholesterol concentration (●) and rate of incorporation of [14C]acetate into digitonin-precipitable sterols of liver slices before and after an ileal by-pass operation.

the liver biopsies was higher after the by-pass operation than before. The most striking effect was in monkey 3, the rate of incorporation increasing by more than tenfold after the operation (Table 2).

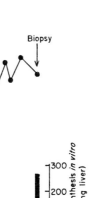

FIG. 3. Monkey 3: plasma cholesterol concentration (●) and rate of incorporation of [^{14}C]acetate into digitonin-precipitable sterols of liver slices before and after an ileal by-pass operation.

TABLE 2. Cholesterol synthesis in serial biopsies of liver before and after ileal by-pass operation

	[^{14}C]acetate incorporated into liver cholesterol (p-moles mg fresh liver^{-1} 3 hr^{-1})		
	Monkey 1	Monkey 2	Monkey 3
Before operation	41	208	10
	51	52	3
	–	–	21
	–	–	12
After operation	283	321	269
	108	458	–

DISCUSSION

The reason why exclusion of the ileum brings about a fall in the plasma cholesterol level is not completely understood. Diminished absorption of cholesterol from the intestine is probably a major factor, since removal of the ileum leads to a marked decrease in the proportion of an oral dose of [^{14}C]cholesterol absorbed (Buchwald, 1964); presumably, the reabsorption of the plasma cholesterol excreted in the bile is affected to the same extent.

In the presence of an intact intestinal tract, absorption of cholesterol is thought to take place largely from the upper small intestine (Swell *et al.*, 1958; Borgström, 1960; Simmonds, Hofmann & Theodor, 1967). It is unlikely, therefore, that the diminished absorption of cholesterol which occurs in the absence of a functioning ileum is due simply to loss of absorbing surface for cholesterol. A shortened transit time of the contents of the intestine may be a contributory factor, but a decrease in the amount of bile salt available for fat absorption in the upper small intestine is probably of greater importance. The bile salts, after participating in the absorption of fat from the jejunum, are normally reabsorbed from the ileum (Frölicher, 1936; Baker & Searle, 1960; Lack & Weiner, 1963; Borgström, Lundh & Hofmann, 1963) and are then re-excreted in the bile. When the ileum is removed, the enterohepatic circulation is interrupted and bile salts are lost from the body at a greatly accelerated rate (Playoust, Lack & Weiner, 1965; Hofmann & Grundy, 1965; Austad, Lack & Tyor, 1967). This may result in a shortage of the bile salts required for the formation of lipid micelles in the jejunum. In favour of this explanation, Hofmann & Grundy (1965) found an abnormally low concentration of micellar lipid in the jejunal juice of a patient whose ileum had been removed. It is reasonable to suppose that a similar chain of events occurs in monkeys submitted to an ileal by-pass operation.

The abnormal loss of bile salts brought about by removal or by-passing of the ileum may also help to lower the plasma cholesterol level by stimulating the formation of bile acids, since cholesterol is an obligatory intermediate in bile acid synthesis. Bergström & Danielsson (1958) have shown that bile acid synthesis is regulated by end-product inhibition, the bile salts reabsorbed from the intestine inhibiting the formation of bile acids in the liver. When the enterohepatic circulation of the bile salts is interrupted, either by making a bile fistula (Bergström & Danielsson, 1958) or by giving cholestyramine (Huff, Gilfillan & Hunt, 1963) or by removing the ileum (Hofmann & Grundy, 1965), the rate of formation of bile acids is much increased. If, as seems likely (Danielsson, Einarsson & Johansson, 1967), bile salts exert their effect on bile acid synthesis by regulating a step later than the formation of cholesterol, increased removal of bile salts from the body should stimulate the conversion of cholesterol into bile acids.

Hepatic synthesis of cholesterol in several species of animals (Gould, 1958), including monkeys (Cox *et al.*, 1954), is regulated by end-product inhibition, cholesterol inhibiting an early step in its own synthesis. Increased removal of cholesterol from the body, due either to diminished reabsorption from the intestine or to increased conversion into bile acids, might, therefore, be expected to enhance cholesterol synthesis in the liver. This may be the mechanism whereby hepatic synthesis of cholesterol is stimulated in monkeys with an ileal by-pass. An increased rate of hepatic synthesis of cholesterol may, in turn, explain the secondary rise in the plasma cholesterol level, since a substantial fraction of the endogenous cholesterol in the plasma is synthesized in the liver. If the above argument is valid, it must be supposed that in the presence of an intact enterohepatic circulation, and of a dietary intake of 10–20 mg of cholesterol per day, hepatic synthesis of cholesterol in monkeys is in a partially inhibited state and can therefore be stimulated by a decrease in end-product inhibition.

It may be noted that a situation in some ways similar to that in monkeys with an ileal by-pass has been described in bile-fistula rats (Myant & Eder, 1961) and in cholestyramine-fed rats (Huff *et al.*, 1963) and mice (Beher, Beher & Rao, 1966). In all three cases, the interruption of the enterohepatic circulation of the bile salts stimulates cholesterol synthesis from acetate in the liver.

From the clinical point of view, our finding that an ileal by-pass stimulates cholesterol synthesis in monkeys is not encouraging. It supports the suggestion of Johnston *et al.* (1967) that the secondary rise in the serum cholesterol level in their hypercholesterolaemic patient was

Cholesterol and ileal by-pass 547

due to a compensatory increase in cholesterol synthesis. In agreement with this interpretation, Moutafis & Myant (unpublished observation) found that the fractional rate of turnover of this patient's plasma cholesterol was increased after the by-pass operation, at a time when the plasma cholesterol level was rising or had returned to the pre-operative value. This is difficult to explain other than by supposing that the rate of flux of cholesterol through the plasma was higher after than before the operation. Grundy *et al.* (1966) have also observed an increased rate of synthesis of cholesterol in patients who have had ileal by-pass operations.

ACKNOWLEDGMENTS

We are much indebted to Professor I. D. A. Johnston and to Mr A. G. Cox for doing the by-pass operations, and to Mr S. Balasubramaniam and Mr R. C. Gent for technical help.

REFERENCES

AUSTAD, W.I., LACK, L. & TYOR, M.P. (1967) Importance of bile acids and of an intact distal small intestine for fat absorption. *Gastroenterology*, **52**, 638–646.

BAKER, R.D. & SEARLE, G.W. (1960) Bile salts absorption at various levels of rat small intestine. *Proc. Soc. exp. Biol. (N.Y.)*, **105**, 521–523.

BEHER, W.T., BEHER, M.E. & RAO, B. (1966) Bile acid and cholesterol metabolism in the mouse as affected by cholestyramine. *Proc. Soc. exp. Biol. (N.Y.)*, **122**, 881–884.

BERGSTRÖM, S. & DANIELSSON, H. (1958) On the regulation of bile acid formation in the rat liver. *Acta physiol. scand.* **43**, 1–7.

BHATTATHIRY, E.P.M. & SIPERSTEIN, M.D. (1963) Feedback control of cholesterol synthesis in man. *J. clin. Invest.* **42**, 1613–1618.

BORGSTRÖM, B. (1960) Studies on intestinal cholesterol absorption in the human. *J. clin. Invest.* **39**, 809–815.

BORGSTRÖM, B., LUNDH, G. & HOFMANN, A. (1963) The site of absorption of conjugated bile salts in man. *Gastroenterology*, **45**, 229–238.

BRUCE, H.M. & PARKES, A.S. (1946) Feeding and breeding of laboratory animals. II. Growth and maintenance of rabbits without fresh green food. *J. Hyg. (Lond.)*, **44**, 501–507.

BUCHWALD, H. (1964) Lowering of cholesterol absorption and blood levels by ileal exclusion. Experimental basis and preliminary clinical report. *Circulation*, **29**, 713–720.

BUCHWALD, H. & VARCO, R.L. (1966) Ileal bypass in patients with hypercholesterolemia and atherosclerosis. *J. Amer. med. Ass.* **196**, 627–630.

CARPENTER, K.J., GOTSIS, A. & HEGSTED, D.M. (1957) Estimation of total cholesterol in serum by a micro method. *Clin. Chem.* **3**, 233–238.

COX, G.E., NELSON, L.G., WOOD, W.B. & TAYLOR, C.B. (1954) Effect of dietary cholesterol on cholesterol synthesis in monkeys' tissue in vitro. *Fed. Proc.* **13**, 31.

DANIELSSON, H., EINARSSON, K. & JOHANSSON, G. (1967) Effect of biliary drainage on individual reactions in the conversion of cholesterol to taurocholic acid. *Europ. J. Biochem.* **2**, 44–49.

DAVIS, J.A., JOHNSTON, I.D.A., MOUTAFIS, C.D. & MYANT, N.B. (1966) Ileal bypass in hypercholesterolaemia. *Lancet*, **ii**, 971–972.

FRÖLICHER, E. (1936) Die Resorption von Gallensäuren aus verschiedenen Dünndarmabschnitten. *Biochem. Z.* **283**, 273–279.

GOULD, R.G. (1958) Biosynthesis of cholesterol. *Cholesterol: Chemistry, Biochemistry and Pathology* (Ed. by R. P. Cook), pp. 209–235. Academic Press, New York.

GRUNDY, S.M., HOFMANN, A.F., DAVIGNON, J. & AHRENS, E.H., JR (1966) Human cholesterol synthesis is regulated by bile acids. *J. clin. Invest.* **45**, 1018–1019.

HOFMANN, A.F. & GRUNDY, S.M. (1965) Abnormal bile salt metabolism in a patient with extensive lower intestinal resection. *Clin. Res.* **13**, 254.

548   *C. D. Moutafis and N. B. Myant*

HUFF, J.W., GILFILLAN, J.L. & HUNT, V.M. (1963) Effect of cholestyramine, a bile acid binding polymer on plasma cholesterol and fecal bile acid excretion in the rat. *Proc. Soc. exp. Biol. (N.Y.)*, **114**, 352–355.

JOHNSTON, I.D.A., DAVIS, J.A., MOUTAFIS, C.D. & MYANT, N.B. (1967) Ileal by-pass in the management of familial hypercholesterolaemia. *Proc. roy. Soc. Med.* **60**, 746–748.

LACK, L. & WEINER, I.M. (1963) Intestinal absorption of bile salts and some biological implications. *Fed. Proc.* **22**, 1334–1338.

MYANT, N.B. & EDER, H.A. (1961) The effect of biliary drainage upon the synthesis of cholesterol in the liver. *J. Lipid Res.* **2**, 363–368.

PLAYOUST, M.R., LACK, L. & WEINER, I.M. (1965) Effect of intestinal resection on bile salt absorption in dogs. *Amer. J. Physiol.* **208**, 363–369.

SIMMONDS, W.J., HOFMANN, A.F. & THEODOR, E. (1967) Absorption of cholesterol from a micellar solution: intestinal perfusion studies in man. *J. clin. Invest.* **46**, 874–890.

SWELL, L., TROUT, E.C., HOPPER, J.R., FIELD, H., JR & TREADWELL, C.R. (1958) Mechanism of cholesterol absorption. II. Changes in free and esterified cholesterol pools of mucosa after feeding cholesterol-4-C^{14}. *J. biol. Chem.* **233**, 49–53.

Circulation

APRIL   1970
VOL. XLI   NO. 4
SUPPLEMENT NO. I

AN OFFICIAL JOURNAL of the AMERICAN HEART ASSOCIATION

Summary

IN AN international cooperative study on the epidemiology of coronary heart disease (CHD), international teams examined 12,770 men aged 40 through 59 years in Finland, Greece, Italy, Japan, the Netherlands, the United States, and Yugoslavia. Strictly standardized methods and criteria were used, and all items that could be measured and analyzed centrally were handled at the University of Minnesota—all tabulations and statistical work, classification of electrocardiograms, diagnoses and causes of death, chemical analyses of a serum cholesterol, dietary items, and menu composites.

The 12,770 men included 11 cohorts of 500 to 1,000 men each in rural Yugoslavia (three), Finland (two), Italy (two), Greece (two), and Japan (two), the men examined comprising an average of more than 95% of all men aged 40–59 living in geographically defined areas. In Yugoslavia there were two additional cohorts of men aged 40–59, one comprising men in a small agricultural center with some food-processing industry (Zrenjanin), the other comprising members of the faculty of the University of Belgrade. In the Netherlands the cohort was a statistically drawn sample of four out of nine men aged 40–59 in Zutphen, a small commercial town with light industry in central Holland. In the United States the cohort of 2,571 men was made up of employees of railroad companies in the northwestern sector of the country, the eligible men being drawn by sampling the companies, locations, and occupations. For comparison, a sample of 768 railroad men aged 40–59 was enrolled in Italy.

The examination procedure included standardized questionnaires on family status, work, personal habits and medical history, anthropometry, including subcutaneous fat measurements, physical examination by internists using a standardized protocol and record forms, 12-lead ECG, three-minute exercise test with ECG repeated immediately thereafter, blood sample, and qualitative urinalysis. Frequent exchange of professional personnel between national teams and diagnostic guidelines were provided to assure maximum comparability of examinations and diagnoses.

Average diets of all cohorts except the railroad men were estimated from surveys on random samples of the cohorts. The dietary surveys involved weighing all items consumed during seven days of the survey and were repeated in different seasons. Nutrients were estimated from chemical analyses of composites of replicate meals and menus as well as from tables of food composition developed to cover local foodstuffs. The diets of the U.S. railroad men were estimated by calculation from dietary interview and recall records, supplemented by visits to the homes of a small subsample.

After entry examination the men were followed, with checks by an internist on mortality and major morbidity several times a year, and then were re-examined, as at entry, after five years. Complete five-year re-examinations covered 94.2% of all survivors, and at least some information about health status was obtained for almost all of the other men; fewer than 0.5 of 1% were lost to follow-up.

Prevalence of Coronary Heart Disease

Great differences between cohorts in age-standardized prevalence rate of CHD were observed at entry, ECG evidence of old myocardial infarction being many times higher in the U.S. and in Finland than in Yugoslavia, Greece, Italy, and Japan, with Zutphen being intermediate. Angina pectoris and CHD diagnosed on "softer" clinical and ECG criteria tended to show similar population differences. The prevalence rates of CHD of the cohorts tended to be directly related to characteristics of the cohorts in regard to blood pressure and serum cholesterol but not in regard to relative body weight or body fatness or smoking habits of the cohorts.

Supplement 1 to Circulation, Vols. XLI and XLII, April 1970

Editorial Note: Extracts only of 'Coronary Heart Disease in Seven Countries' are reproduced.

CORONARY HEART DISEASE IN SEVEN COUNTRIES

Prevalence at Entry—Prognosis

Among 129 men with a diagnosis of definite old myocardial infarction at entry, at the end of five years 27 were dead from CHD, or 13.6 times the CHD death rate of men judged CHD-free at entry of the same age in the same cohorts. Prevalence cases of angina pectoris and of CHD diagnosed on softer clinical and ECG criteria experienced, respectively, 4.7 and 6.8 times the CHD death rate of the men without evidence of CHD at entry. CHD accounted for 72% of all deaths among men with any diagnosis of CHD at entry. Among 87 men with a diagnosis of definite old myocardial infarction at entry and who were alive five years later, 29 did not meet criteria for evidence of CHD at the five-year re-examination. Of 100 five-year survivors among men who at entry had less definite clinical and ECG signs of CHD or who had classic angina pectoris, 41 met no criteria for CHD five years later. The five-year prognosis of men with CHD at entry showed no clear relationship to relative body weight, blood pressure, or serum cholesterol.

Deaths

During five years there were 588 deaths in the entire study population, 158 from CHD. Figure S1 summarizes the age-standardized death rates, cohorts being combined by countries. Among the U.S. railroad men 62 of 125 deaths were due to CHD; in Finland 38 of 111 deaths were due to CHD; in the Netherlands 16 out of 50 deaths were thus accounted for. For all other cohorts combined, only one out of eight deaths was due to CHD. That low proportion did not reflect a high death rate ascribed to other, non-CHD causes.

In most of the cohorts, low CHD death rates were associated with low all-causes deaths, the standard basis of comparison for CHD and all-causes deaths being the deaths expected to match the five-year experience of equal numbers of white men in the United States with the same age distribution, the expected numbers being calculated from life tables and death rates in U.S. vital statistics for 1962 (approximately in the middle of the five-year follow-up).

The least favorable all-causes death rates, expressed as ratios of observed deaths to deaths expected to match U.S. experience, were east Finland (O/E = 1.34); Slavonia, Yugoslavia (O/E = 1.22); west Finland (O/E = 0.96); Crevalcore, Italy (O/E = 1.00); Zutphen, Netherlands (O/E = 0.95); and U.S. railroad men (O/E = 0.82). The unfavorable mortality in Slavonia was accounted for by death causes scarcely seen in the other cohorts—tuberculosis, suicide, cirrhosis of the liver, and acute alcoholism. The U.S. railroad men, being fully employed at entry were expected to have a lower death rate than U.S. white men in general. The other ten cohorts were expected to provide 344.7 deaths; the observed number was only 188 deaths, O/E = 0.545.

Great differences in CHD death rate accounted for most but not all of the differences in all-causes deaths. In the same ten cohorts for which all-causes death rate gave O/E = 0.545, the ratio of observed to expected CHD deaths was 24/139.2, or O/E = 0.172. In these ten cohorts there were 157 fewer all-causes deaths than expected; the relative rarity of CHD in those cohorts accounted for 115 of the 157 expected total deaths that did not occur. In contrast, in the other six cohorts combined, all-causes deaths were 98.4% of those expected to match the general population of U.S. white men.

Among U.S. railroad men age-standardized death rates from all causes were higher among switchmen (physically active) than men in sedentary occupations while the reverse was true of CHD deaths, but in neither case was the difference statistically significant. The same was true when comparison was made of men free of CHD at entry.

Incidence of Coronary Heart Disease

Among 12,529 men judged to be free from CHD at the entry examination, the five-year CHD experience, in a hierarchy of mutually exclusive diagnostic categories, was as follows: 116 deaths from CHD, 113 nonfatal

Figure S2

Age-standardized average yearly CHD incidence rates per 10.000 of 12.529 men aged 40-59, judged to be free of CHD at the outset, followed for five years. Non-fatal CHD incidence in Japan is not precisely indicated because the relevant 5-year clinical and ECG records were not independently reviewed at the University of Minnesota center.

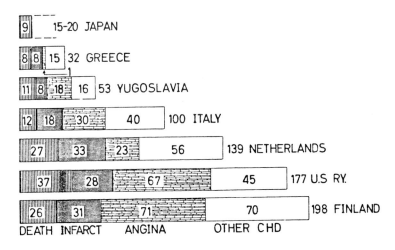

MEN 40-59, CHD-FREE AT ENTRY
CHD INCIDENCE / 10,000 / YEAR

CORONARY HEART DISEASE IN SEVEN COUNTRIES   I-189

definite myocardial infarctions, 219 cases of classic angina pectoris, and 113 men given the diagnosis of CHD on the basis of less rigid and specific clinical and ECG criteria. The crude average annual rate for all CHD incidence in these men initially CHD-free was 102.3 per 10,000. For CHD incidence meeting the hardest criteria—deaths and definite infarcts—the corresponding rate was 36.5 per 10,000 men.

The age-standardized CHD incidence rate for men CHD-free at entry differed greatly in the several cohorts, the extremes being in Finland and the U.S. on the high side with the cohorts in Japan, Greece, and Yugoslavia on the low side. Figure S2 summarizes the data for the cohorts combined by countries. Within countries there were no significant differences between cohorts in CHD rates except for rural Finland where the total CHD incidence rate in the east (272 ± 59) was definitely higher than in the west (130 ± 39). The difference in rate, east minus west Finland, was 142 cases

per 10,000 with 95% confidence limits of +6 and +278.

In general, the several categories of CHD diagnosis tended to show much the same picture for differences in rates between cohorts, but the rates for angina pectoris were not in close conformity with the rates for the objective and standardized diagnoses of CHD death and nonfatal infarction. In the Netherlands angina pectoris apparently contributed a lower proportion of total CHD incidence than in the other areas; there is no way of deciding whether this apparent peculiarity reflects a difference in the manifestation of the disease or diagnostic conservatism of the responsible cardiologist.

Differences Between Cohorts—Risk Factors

Examination of the representation in the several cohorts of the so-called risk factors shows that most of those factors, whatever may be their influence within cohorts, cannot explain the observed differences in the incidence of CHD. Figure S3 shows that cigarette

Figure S3

Percentage of men regularly smoking at least 10 cigarettes every day. The lengths of the narrow solid bars are proportional to the age-standardized CHD incidence rates among men CHD-free at entry as given in Figure S2.

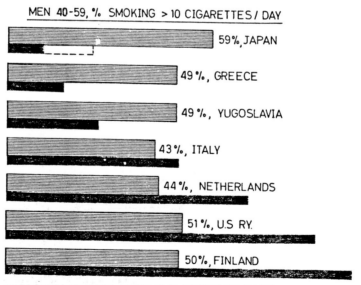

MEN 40-59, % SMOKING > 10 CIGARETTES / DAY

59%, JAPAN

49%, GREECE

49%, YUGOSLAVIA

43%, ITALY

44%, NETHERLANDS

51%, U.S RY.

50%, FINLAND

NARROW, SOLID BARS SHOW CHD INCIDENCE RATE

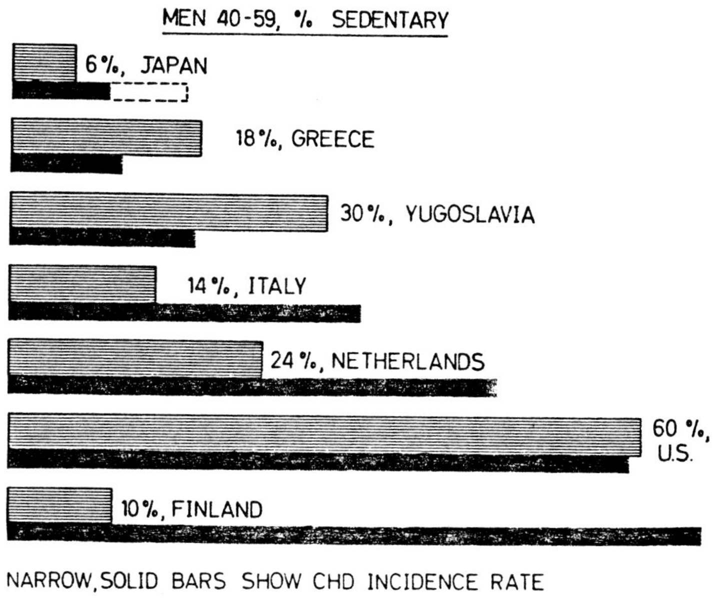

MEN 40-59, % SEDENTARY

6%, JAPAN

18%, GREECE

30%, YUGOSLAVIA

14%, ITALY

24%, NETHERLANDS

60%, U.S.

10%, FINLAND

NARROW, SOLID BARS SHOW CHD INCIDENCE RATE

Figure S4

Percentage of men sedentary or engaged only in very light physical activity.

Figure S5

Percentage of men with relative body weight of 110 or more.

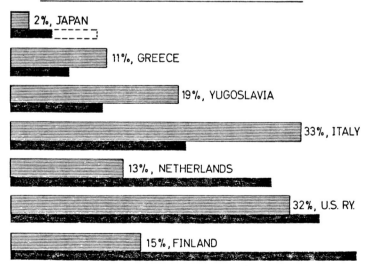

MEN 40-59, % WITH RELATIVE WEIGHT >110%

2%, JAPAN

11%, GREECE

19%, YUGOSLAVIA

33%, ITALY

13%, NETHERLANDS

32%, U.S. RY.

15%, FINLAND

NARROW, SOLID BARS SHOW CHD INCIDENCE RATE

Supplement I to Circulation, Vols. XLI and XLII, April 1970

CORONARY HEART DISEASE IN SEVEN COUNTRIES   I-191

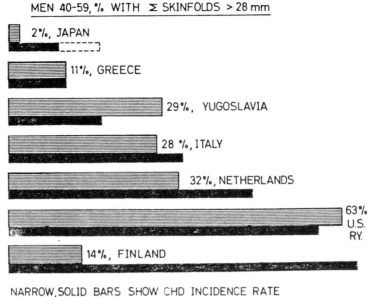

Figure S6

Percentage of men with values of 28 or more mm for the sum of the skinfolds over the triceps muscle and over the tip of the scapula.

smoking cannot be involved as an explanation; cigarette smoking habits do not differ much between the various cohorts or cohorts combined by country as in figure S3.

Differences between the cohorts in the proportion of the men who are sedentary or physically inactive do not explain the differences between the cohorts in the incidence of CHD. The data are summarized by countries in figure S4.

There were large differences between cohorts in body fatness and relative body weight, but as illustrated by figures S5 and S6, consideration of neither obesity nor relative weight helps to explain the population differences in CHD incidence. The U.S. railroad men tend to be relatively much heavier and fatter than the men in any of the other groups, but the thin and relatively lightweight Finns match the Americans in CHD incidence. The Italians were the most often overweight and, although less fat than the Americans, were certainly far more obese than the Finns, yet

they were much less prone to CHD than either the Finns or the Americans. The conclusion is that the group trends in these variables have nothing to do with the group trends in CHD incidence.

Blood pressure and the prevalence of hypertension are more interesting, as shown by figures S7 and S8. There is some tendency for the incidence of CHD to be related to the prevalence of hypertension in the cohorts; at least hypertension was less common in the cohorts with the lowest incidence of CHD. It is not possible, of course, to insist that the blood pressures recorded for the several cohorts are strictly comparable, especially for diastolic pressure. Common instructions were issued about recording blood pressure, but uncertainties remain in the absence of identity of the environment and of a measuring device without human intervention. The role of blood pressure in CHD incidence is more reliably examined within cohorts.

Figure S9 indicates that the incidence rate

Supplement I to Circulation, Vols. XLI and XLII, April 1970

Figure S7

Age-standardized percentage of men with resting systolic blood pressure of 160 mm or more.

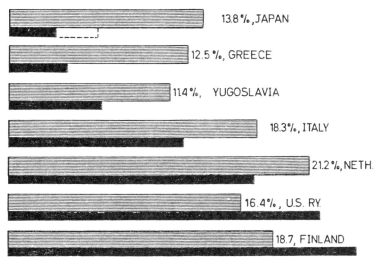

MEN 40-59, % MEN WITH SYSTOLIC B.P. ≥160

13.8 %, JAPAN

12.5 %, GREECE

11.4 %, YUGOSLAVIA

18.3 %, ITALY

21.2 %, NETH.

16.4 %, U.S. RY.

18.7, FINLAND

NARROW, SOLID BARS SHOW CHD INCIDENCE RATE

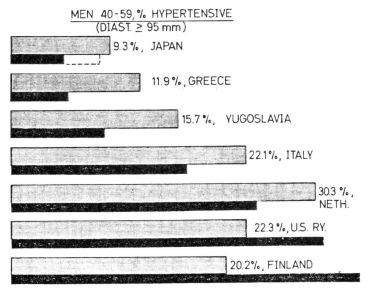

MEN 40-59, % HYPERTENSIVE
(DIAST. ≥ 95 mm)

9.3 %, JAPAN

11.9 %, GREECE

15.7 %, YUGOSLAVIA

22.1 %, ITALY

30.3 %, NETH.

22.3 %, U.S. RY.

20.2 %, FINLAND

NARROW, SOLID BARS SHOW CHD INCIDENCE RATE

Figure S8

Age-standardized percentage of men with resting diastolic blood pressure of 95 mm or more.

Supplement I to Circulation, Vols. XLI and XLII, April 1970

CORONARY HEART DISEASE IN SEVEN COUNTRIES   I-193

Figure S9

Percentage of men with serum cholesterol values over 250 mg per deciliter.

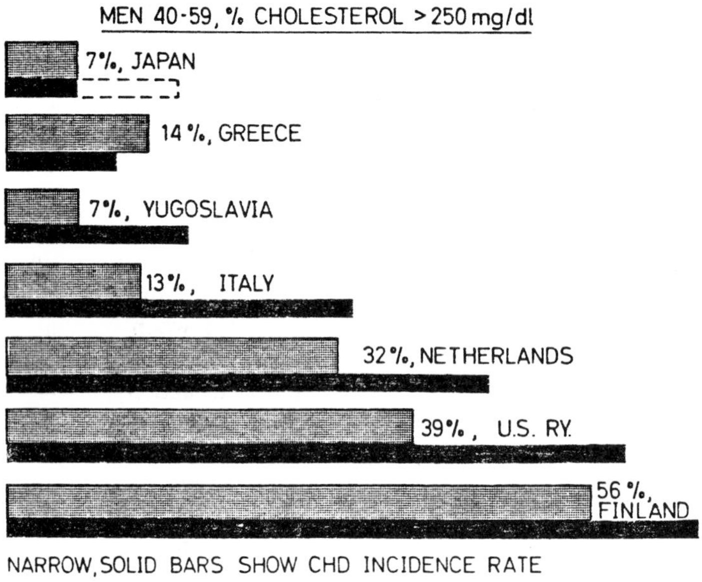

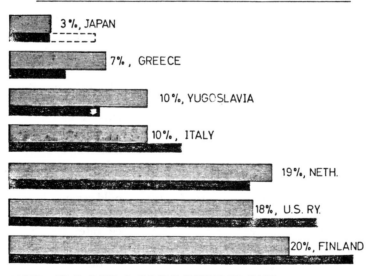

Figure S10

Average percentage of total dietary calories provided by saturated fatty acids.

Supplement I to Circulation, Vols. XLI and XLII, April 1970

of CHD tends to be directly related to the distributions of serum cholesterol values. Since the average serum cholesterol values of the cohorts tended to be directly related to the average proportion of calories provided by saturated fats in the diet, it is not surprising to find the picture shown in figure S10. The CHD incidence rates of the cohorts are just as closely related to the dietary saturated fatty acids as to the serum cholesterol level. Serum cholesterol averages and CHD incidence rates were not found to be related to the percentage of calories provided by protein or polyunsaturated fatty acids in the diet and were only slightly related to total fat calories.

Average relative body weight, as well as average body fatness, tended to be inversely related to the average dietary calories per unit of body mass. It was indicated that, on the average, relative obesity and overweight is more a reflection of underexpenditure of calories rather than of overconsumption.

Risk Factors Within Cohorts

The analysis of the relationships within cohorts consistently indicated the importance of blood pressure and serum cholesterol. When "hard" criteria of CHD death and infarction were used for diagnosis, CHD incidence was not significantly related to either relative body weight or to body fatness. When all CHD diagnoses were used in computing incidence rate, there was a weak tendency for the rate to be related to relative body weight as well as to body fatness. That tendency was not statistically significant when the confounding influence of blood pressure was removed.

CHD incidence was significantly related to smoking habits in the U.S. railroad men but not in the European cohorts. All-causes death rate was also related to smoking habits in the U.S. railroad men but not in the other cohorts.

In the U.S. railroad cohort the CHD incidence rate of the men in sedentary occupations was about 16% higher than the rate of the physically more active switchmen, but the difference was not statistically significant. In the other cohorts no statistically

significant relationships between habitual physical activity and any measure of CHD incidence rate were found. If there were a true excess of 15 to 20% CHD among sedentary men, the present material would be too small to prove it.

Analysis was made of the relationship, in men judged to be CHD-free at entry, between CHD incidence and certain ECG abnormalities at entry. Ischemic type of ST depression after exercise was associated with a CHD incidence rate more than double the rate in men without that abnormality. The bad outlook for men with that ECG abnormality persisted when matching was done on blood pressure, relative weight, serum cholesterol, physical activity, smoking habits, and age. Other post-exercise ECG abnormalities investigated included junctional ST depression, negative T waves, and various arrhythmias, none of which proved to be associated with significantly more CHD incidence than could easily occur by chance. On the other hand, among men not judged as CHD-free, later CHD deaths were significantly increased when the entry ECG showed large Q waves, negative T waves, or atrial fibrillation.

Multivariate Differences Between Cohorts

The coefficients for the multiple logistic equation for CHD risk, obtained by Truett et al. (1967) from Framingham data, were tested with the present material. Comparison of absolute numbers of CHD cases with those "predicted" is improper because of lack of identity in the diagnostic methods and the question of comparing five-year observed rates with predictions based on 12 years of follow-up. However, analysis in terms of ratios of rates would seem to be reasonable to consider. When both observed and predicted CHD incidence rates for the various cohorts are expressed as ratios of the observed and predicted rates of the U.S. railroad men, the correspondence between observed and predicted ratios was unexpectedly good; the coefficient of correlation was $r = 0.83$. A detailed multivariate analysis with new solutions to the multiple logistic is in progress. Besides the approach of Truett et al. (1967), which assumes multivariate normality and equality of variances and covariances, that of Walker and Duncan (1967) without those assumptions is being used.

Total Mortality and Coronary Heart Disease

There was no indication that the incidence of CHD was inversely related to the incidence of any other disease or that, in effect, rarity of CHD in a cohort was compensated by an excess of other affliction. In general, the total all-causes death rate reflected the death rate from CHD with the result that the all-causes death rate was remarkably low in several of the cohorts with the lowest incidence of CHD. In Slavonia, an apparent exception, unusual causes of death were involved.

In spite of the bad experience in Slavonia, for all five Yugoslav cohorts combined, all-causes deaths totaled 123 compared with 175.5 expected for age-matched white men in the United States, $O/E = 0.70$. The all-causes mortality of the three Italian cohorts was also favorable with $O/E = 0.80$ (114 deaths observed, 142.3 expected to match U.S. white men), as was that of the Japanese men with $O/E = 0.78$ (47 deaths, 60.3 expected). The Greeks had by far the best experience with only 21 deaths instead of 70.5 expected, $O/E = 0.30$. CHD was relatively much less common in all of these cohorts than in the Finns, the men of Zutphen, and the U.S. railroad men.

Supplement 1 to Circulation, Vols. XLI and XLII, April 1970

References

ADELSON S, KEYS A: Diet and some health characteristics of 123 business and professional men. U. S. Department of Agriculture Publ ARS 6211, 1962

ANDERSON JT, GRANDE F, MATSUMOTO Y, ET AL: Glucose, sucrose and lactose in the diet and blood lipids in man. J of Nutrition 79: 349, 1963

ANTONIS A, BERSOHN P: Influence of diet on serum lipids in South African white and Bantu prisoners. Amer J Clin Nutr 10: 484, 1962

ARAVANIS C, DONTAS AS, LEKOS D, ET AL: Rural populations in Crete and Corfu, Greece. Acta Med Scand (suppl) 460: 209, 1967

Association Medico-actuarial Mortality Investigations, vol. 1. New York, Assoc Life Insurance Med Dir and Actuarial Soc Amer, 1912

BLACKBURN H, KEYS A, SIMONSON E, ET AL: The electrocardiogram in population studies: A classification system. Circulation 21: 1160, 1960.

BLACKBURN H, PARLIN RW, AND KEYS A: The interrelations of electrocardiographic findings and physical characteristics of middle-aged men. Acta Med Scand Suppl 460: 316, 1967

BLOOM WL, EIDEX MF: Inactivity as a major factor in adult obesity. Metabolism 16: 679, 1967

BRONTE-STEWART B, KEYS A, BROCK JF: Serum-cholesterol, diet and coronary heart disease. Lancet 2: 1103, 1955

BRONTE-STEWART B, ANTONIS A, GALES L, ET AL: Effect of feeding different fats on serum-cholesterol level. Lancet 1: 521, 1956

BROZEK J, AND ALEXANDER H: A note on estimation of the components of variation in a two-way table. Amer J Psych 60: 629, 1947

BROZEK J, BUZINA R, MIKIC F: Population studies on serum cholesterol and dietary fat in Yugoslavia. Amer J Clin Nutr 5: 279, 1957

VANBUCHEM FSP, DALDERUP L: Town of Zutphen, the Netherlands. Acta Med Scand (suppl) 460: 191, 1967

BULLEN BA, REED RB, MAYER J: Physical activity of obese and non-obese adolescent girls appraised by motion picture sampling. Amer J Clin Nutr 14: 211, 1964

BUZINA R, FERBER E, KEYS A, ET AL: Diets of rural families and heads of families in two regions of Yugoslavia. Voeding 25: 629, 1964

BUZINA R, KEYS A, BRODAREC A, ET AL: Dietary surveys in rural Yugoslavia: II. Chemical analyses of diets of Dalmatia and Slavonia. Voeding 27: 31, 1966

BUZINA R, KEYS A, BRODAREC A, ET AL: Dietary survey in rural Yogoslavia: III. Comparison of three methods. Voeding 27: 99, 1966

BUZINA R, KEYS A, MOHACEK I, ET AL: Rural men in Dalmatia and Slavonia. Acta Med Scand (suppl) 460: 147, 1967

CHAPMAN JM, GOERKE LS, DIXON W, ET AL: Clinical status of a population group in Los Angeles under observation for two to three years. Amer J Public Health 47 (pt 2): 33, 1957

CHIANG BN, PERLMAN LV, OSTRANDER LD JR, ET AL: Relationship of premature systoles to coronary heart disease and sudden death in Tecumseh epidemiologic study. Ann Intern Med 70: 1159, 1969

Committee on the Coronary Circulation: Statistical review of cases with clinically diagnosed myocardial infarction and with anginal pains in several districts in Japan. Jap Circ J 21: 1, 1957

DAVENPORT CB: Body build and its inheritance. Carnegie Institute, Washington, D. C., publ no 329, 1923

DAWBER TR, MOORE FE, MANN GV: Coronary heart disease in the Framingham Study. Amer J Public Health 47 (pt 2): 4, 1957

DJORDJEVIC B, JOSIPOVIC V, NEDELJKOVIC SI, ET AL: Men in Velika Krsna, a Serbian village. Acta Med Scand (suppl) 460: 267, 1967

DJORDJEVIC B, SIMIC B, SIMIC A, ET AL, WITH THE HELP OF THE STATISTICIAN TODOROVIC, P: Dietary studies in connection with epidemiology of heart diseases: Results in Serbia. Voeding 26: 117, 1965

DOYLE JT, HESLINS S, HILLEBOE HE, ET AL: Prospective study of degenerative cardiovascular disease in Albany. Report of three years' experience. 1. Ischemic heart disease. Amer J Public Health 47 (pt 2): 25, 1957

DREYFUSS F: Incidence of myocardial infarction in various communities in Israel. Amer Heart J 45: 749, 1953

DREYFUSS F, TOOR M, AGMON J, ET AL: Observations on myocardial infarction in Israel. Cardiologia 30: 387, 1957

FIDANZA F, FIDANZA ALBERTI A, FERRO-LUZZI, G, ET AL: Dietary surveys in connection with the epidemiology of heart disease: Results in Italy. Voeding 25: 502, 1964

FIDANZA F, AND FIDANZA ALBERTI A: Dietary surveys in connection with the epidemiology of heart disease: Reliability, sources of variation and other data from nine surveys in Italy. Voeding 28: 244, 1967

FIDANZA F, PUDDU V, DEL VECCHIO A, AND KEYS A: Men in rural Italy. Acta Med Scand Suppl 460: 116, 1967

GRIZZLE JE: Continuity correction in the X^2-test for 2 x 2 tables. American Statistician 21: 28, 1967

Supplement I to Circulation, Vols. XLI and XLII, April 1970

denHartog C, Van Schaik Th FSM, Dalderup LM, et al: Diet of volunteers participating in a long term epidemiological field survey on coronary heart disease at Zutphen, Netherlands. Voeding 26: 184, 1965

denHartog C, Buzina R, Fidanza F, et al Eds: Dietary Studies and Epidemiology of Heart Disease. The Hague, Sticht. Wetensch. Voorlichting Voedingsgebied, 1968

Huenemann RL, Hampton MC, Shapiro LR, et al: Adolescent food practices associated with obesity. Fed Proc 25 (pt I): 4, 1966

Kannel WB, Dawber TR, Kagan A, et al: Factors of risk in the development of coronary heart disease—six year follow-up experience, the Framingham Study. Ann Intern Med 55: 33, 1961

Karvonen MJ, Blomqvist G, Kallio V, et al: Men in rural east and west Finland. Acta Med Scand (suppl) 460: 169, 1967

Keys A, Brozek J: Body fat in adult man. Physiol Reviews 33: 245, 1953

Keys A: Cholesterol problem. Voeding 13: 539, 1952 (a)

Keys A, et al: Epidemiological studies related to coronary heart disease: characteristics of men aged 40-59 in seven countries. Acta Med Scand Suppl 460, 392 pp, 1967

Keys A: Human atherosclerosis and the diet. Circulation 5: 115, 1952 (b)

Keys A, Kimura N: Diets of middle-aged farmers in Japan. Amer J Clin Nutr, 1970. In press

Keys A: Atherosclerosis: A problem in newer public health. J Mount Sinai Hosp NY 20: 118, 1953 (a)

Keys A: Prediction and possible prevention of coronary disease. Amer J Public Health 43: 1399, 1953 (b)

Keys A: Obesity and degenerative heart disease. Am J Public Health 44: 864, 1954

Keys A, Fidanza F, Scardi V, et al: Studies on serum cholesterol and other characteristics on clinically healthy men in Naples. Arch Intern Med (Chicago) 93: 328, 1954

Keys A: Weight changes and the health of men. Chapter 8, pp 108-118, in Weight Control (ES Eppright, P Swanson, and CA Iverson, eds.) Iowa State College Press, Ames, Iowa, 1955

Keys A: Diet and the epidemiology of coronary heart disease. JAMA 164: 1912, 1957

Keys A, Kimura N, Kusukawa A, et al: Serum cholesterol in Japanese coal miners: A dietary experiment. Amer J Clin Nutr. 5: 245, 1957

Keys A, Kimura N, Kusukawa A, et al: Lessons from serum cholesterol studies in Japan, Hawaii and Los Angeles. Ann Intern Med 48: 83, 1958

Keys A, Karvonen MJ, Fidanza F: Serum-cholesterol studies in Finland. Lancet 2: 175, 1958

Keys A, Taylor HL, Blackburn HW, et al: Coronary heart disease among Minnesota business and professional men followed fifteen years. Circulation 28: 381, 1963

Keys A, and Grande F: Body weight, body composition and calorie status. Pp 13-43 in Modern Nutrition in Health and Disease (MG Wohl, and RS Goodhart, eds.) Lea and Febiger, Philadelphia, 1964

Keys A: Dietary survey methods in studies on cardiovascular epidemiology. Voeding 26: 464, 1965

Keys A, Anderson JT, Grande F: Serum cholesterol response to changes in the diet. Metabolism 14: 747, 1965

Keys A, Aravanis C, Sdrin H: Diets of middle-aged men in two rural areas of Greece. Voeding 27: 575, 1966

Keys A, Parlin RW: Serum cholesterol response to changes in dietary lipids. Amer J Clin Nutr. 19: 175, 1966

Keys A: Blood lipids in man—a brief review. J Amer Diet Ass 51: 508, 1967

Keys A: Current status of research on the epidemiology of coronary heart disease. Jap Circ J 32 (No. 12): 1669, 1968

Keys A: Serum cholesterol and the question of "normal." Pp 147-170 in Multiple Laboratory Screening (PS Strandjord and E Benson, eds.) Academic Press, New York, 1969

Keys A, Vivanco F, Rodriguez-Minon JL, et al: Studies on the diet, body fatness and serum cholesterol in Madrid, Spain. Metabolism 3: 195, 1954

Kimura N: A farming and a fishing village in Japan—Tanushimaru and Ushibuka. Acta Med Scand (suppl) 460: 231, 1967

Kimura N: Analysis of 10,000 post-mortem examinations in Japan. In World Trends in Cardiology: I. Cardiovascular Epidemiology, edited by A Kevs and PD White, Hoeber-Harper, New York, 1956, p 22-33

Lindberg HA, Berkson DM, Stamler J, et al: Totally asymptomatic myocardial infarction: Estimate of it in the living population. Arch Intern Med (Chicago) 106: 628, 1960

Lyle AM: Coronary disease as an underwriting problem. Trans Soc Actuaries 15: 324, 1963

Malmros H: Relation of nutrition to health—a statistical study of the effect of war-time on arteriosclerosis, cardiosclerosis, tuberculosis and diabetes. Acta Med Scand (suppl) 246: 137, 1950

Mantel N, Haenszel W: Statistical aspects of the analysis of data from retrospective studies of disease. J Nat Cancer Inst 22: 719, 1959

Mantel N: Chi-square tests with one degree of freedom: Extensions of the Mantel-Haenszel procedure. J Am Stat Assoc 58: 690, 1963

Mantel N, Greenhouse SW: What is the continuity correction? American Statistician 22: 27, 1968

Master AM, Rosenfeld I: Exercise as an estimation

of cardiac function. J Amer Coll Chest Physicians 51: 347, 1967

MATHEWSON FAL, BRERETON DC: A-V block: U. of Manitoba follow-up study reports—series 1963. Trans Ass Life Insur Med Dir Amer 48: 210, 1964

MAYER J: Overweight—causes, cost and control. Prentice-Hall, Englewood Cliffs, New Jersey, 213 pp, 1968

METROPOLITAN: Metropolitan Life Insurance Co Statist Bull. No 23, 1942

MORRIS JN, KAGAN A, PATTISON DC, ET AL: Incidence and prediction of ischaemic heart disease in London busmen. Lancet 2: 553, 1966

MORRIS JN, MARR JW, HEADY JA, ET AL: Diet and plasma cholesterol in 99 bank men. British Med J 1: 571, 1963

NATIONAL HEALTH SURVEY: Weight by height and age of adults, United States, 1960-62. U.S. Dept. H.E.W., Nat Center Health Stat Ser 11, No 14, 1966

NEW YORK HEART ASSOCIATION: Diseases of the heart and blood vessels. Nomenclature and criteria for diagnosis. Sixth edition. Little, Brown and Co., Boston, 463 pp, 1964

OŠANCOVA K, AND HEJDA S: Dietary studies in connection with epidemiology of heart diseases: Results of surveys in Czechoslovakia. Voeding 26: 71, 1965

PAUL O, LEPPER MH, PHELAN WH, ET AL: A longitudinal study of coronary heart disease. Circulation 28: 20, 1963

PEARSON ES: Choice of statistical test illustrated on the interpretation of data classed in a 2 x 2 table. Biometrika 34: 139, 1947

PEKKARINEN M: Chemical analysis in connection with dietary surveys in Finland. Voeding 28: 609, 1967

PEKKARINEN M, KIVIOJA S, JORTIKKA L: Comparison of the food intake of rural families estimated by one-day recall and precise weighing methods. Voeding 28: 470, 1967

PLACKETT RL: Continuity corrections in 2 x 2 tables. Biometrika 51: 427, 1964

REMINGTON RD, SCHORK MA: Determination of number of subjects needed for experimental epidemiologic studies of the effect of increased physical activity on incidence of coronary heart disease—preliminary considerations. In Physical Activity and the Heart, edited by MJ Karvonen, AJ Barry. Springfield, Ill, Charles C Thomas, 1967, p 311-319

RION JW: The development of height weight tables from life insurance data. Manuscript in the Division of Chronic Disease, U.S. Public Health Service, Washington, D. C., 1952

ROINE P, PEKKARINEN M, KARVONEN MJ, ET AL: Diet and cardiovascular disease in Finland. Lancet 2: 173, 1958

ROINE P, PEKKARINEN M, KARVONEN MJ: Dietary studies in connection with epidemiology of heart diseases: Results in Finland. Voeding 25: 384, 1964

ROSE GA, BLACKBURN H: Cardiovascular survey methods. WHO Monograph Series no. 56, 1968

SCHORNAGEL HE: Connection between nutrition and mortality from coronary sclerosis during and after World War II. Documenta de Medicina Geographica et Tropica (Amsterdam) 5: 173, 1953

SELTZER CC: Some re-evaluations of the Build and Blood Pressure Study, 1959, as related to ponderal index, somatotype and mortality. New England J Med 284: 254, 1966

SOCIETY OF ACTUARIES: Build and Blood Pressure Study. Society of Actuaries, Chicago, Illinois, 1959

STAMLER J, LINDBERG HA, BERKSON DM, ET AL: Prevalence and incidence of coronary heart disease in strata of the labor force of a Chicago industrial corporation. J Chronic Dis 11: 405, 1960

STAMLER J: Cardiovascular diseases in the United States. Amer J Cardiol 10: 319, 1962

STEFANIK PA, HEALD FP JR, MAYER J: Caloric intake in relation to energy output of obese and non-obese adolescent boys. Amer J Clin Nutr 7: 55, 1959

STRØM A, JENSEN AR: Mortality from circulatory diseases in Norway. Lancet 1: 126, 1951

TAYLOR HL, KLEPETAR E, KEYS A, ET AL: Death rates among physically active and sedentary employees of the railroad industry. Amer J Public Health 52: 1697, 1962

TAYLOR HL, PARLIN RW, BLACKBURN H, ET AL: Problems in the analysis of the relationship of coronary heart disease to physical activity or its lack, with special reference to sample size and occupational withdrawal. In Physical Activity in Health and Disease, edited by K Evang, K Lange Andersen. Oslo, Universitetsforlaget, 1966, p. 242-261

TAYLOR HL, MONTI M, PUDDU V, ET AL: Railroad employees in Rome. Acta Med Scand (suppl) 460: 250, 1967

TAYLOR HL, BLACKBURN H, BROZEK J, ET AL: Railroad employees in the United States. Acta Med Scand (suppl) 460: 55, 1967

TOOR M, KATCHALSKY A, AGMON J, ET AL: Serum lipids and atherosclerosis among Yemenite immigrants in Israel. Lancet 1: 1270, 1957

TRUETT J, CORNFIELD J, KANNEL W: Multivariate analysis of the risk of coronary heart disease. J Chronic Dis 20: 511, 1967

VARTIAINEN I, KANERVA K: Arteriosclerosis and wartime. Ann Med Intern Fenn 36: 748, 1947

WALKER SH, DUNCAN DB: Estimation of the probability of an event as a function of several independent variables. Biometrika 54: 167, 1967

YANO L, UEDA S: Coronary heart disease in Hiroshima, Japan. Yale J Biol Med 35: 504, 1963

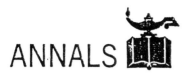

ANNALS

of Internal Medicine

JANUARY 1971 · VOLUME 74 · NUMBER 1

Published Monthly by the American College of Physicians

Serum Cholesterol, Lipoproteins, and the Risk of Coronary Heart Disease

The Framingham Study

WILLIAM B. KANNEL, M.D., WILLIAM P. CASTELLI, M.D., TAVIA GORDON, and

PATRICIA M. MCNAMARA, Framingham, Massachusetts; and Bethesda, Maryland

Risk of coronary heart disease over 14 years was examined prospectively in 2,282 men and 2,845 women according to their antecedent cholesterol and lipoprotein status. An increased risk proportional to antecedent serum cholesterol was found whether or not it was associated with elevated S_f 20-400 prebeta lipoprotein. When adjustment was made for the concomitant prebeta lipoprotein concentration and other factors related both to coronary heart disease risk and to blood lipids, a residual gradient of coronary heart disease risk proportional to the serum cholesterol was still evident. On the other hand, when risk of coronary heart disease was examined according to prebeta lipoprotein concentration, adjusting for cholesterol, no residual risk gradient remained in men. In women over 50, however, prebeta lipoprotein was superior to cholesterol in discriminating potential coronary heart disease cases. Risk of coronary heart disease in men can be estimated using any of the lipids evaluated; however, none proved more useful than an accurate total serum cholesterol.

► From the Heart Disease Epidemiology Study, Framingham, Mass.; and the National Heart and Lung Institute, National Insitutes of Health, Bethesda, Md.

V IRTUALLY EVERY lipid and lipid-bearing substance encountered in the blood has been incriminated in atherogenesis, but none has been more substantially implicated than cholesterol. As a result of a considerable research into the details of lipid metabolism in relation to atherosclerosis, the pathogenetic mechanisms involved are being clarified. A series of presumably genetic lipoprotein disorders that are associated with precocious atherosclerosis have lately been identified (1).

There is evidence that the common type of modest "hypercholesterolemia" encountered in the general population may not be a homogeneous entity (1-5).

Neither cholesterol nor any other lipid occurs in the blood in a free state but is linked with protein for transport. Each major lipoprotein fraction carries cholesterol. This report examines prospectively the risk of coronary heart disease in a general population over 14 years, according to antecedent serum cholesterol and lipoprotein status.

Methods

At the time of the initial examination in Framingham 2,282 men and 2,845 women aged 30 to 62, examined and found free of coronary heart disease, were classified into subgroups according to the level of a variety of serum lipids at the time of the first 2 biennial examinations. The rate of development of initial clinical manifestation of coronary heart disease over 14 years of follow-up in the population so classified was determined. This allowed an estimate of the risk in relation to antecedent serum lipid content.

The Framingham Study has been in continuous operation since 1949, following a reasonably representative sample of the adult population of the town for the development of coronary heart disease. The derivation and composition of the population sample under study has been described in detail previously (6-9). After exclusion of those persons with any evidence of coronary heart disease on the initial examination, a study was undertaken to identify factors related to the onset of first events of clinical coronary heart disease. At the time of the initial examinations a variety of lipid determinations were made in the Framingham Study laboratory, including serum cholesterol (by the method of Kendall-Abell) and phospholipids (by the method of Youngberg), and the various lipoprotein fractions were determined by ultracentrifugal analysis at the Donner Laboratory, courtesy of Dr. John Gofman (2, 6, 10). Cholesterol values were determined at each biennial examination. Beta (S_f0-20) and prebeta (S_f20-400) lipoprotein fractions were determined only on the first two biennial examinations owing to the technical complexity of the analyses. All specimens were casual and obtained on subjects initially free of coronary heart disease. The cholesterol and S_f0-20 *beta* lipoprotein concentrations are not materially affected by recent meals.

The average S_f20-400 prebeta lipoprotein level is higher postprandially than fasting, and this should be taken into account when considering casual S_f20-400 values. For men in this population, however, it has been determined that the casual S_f20-400 lipoproteins and a fasting triglyceride done 18 to 20 years later were positively correlated. Men and women generally came in for examination as spouse pairs at the same time of day, so there is little likelihood of systematic sampling differences to explain differences between men and women with respect to S_f20-400 lipoprotein determinations.

A casual blood sugar was determined by the method of Somogyi-Nelson. Blood pressure determination, vital capacity, weight relative to the median for specified heights, uric acid, and history of cigarette smoking were also obtained.

DIAGNOSTIC CRITERIA

Criteria used for the diagnosis of coronary heart disease have been described in some detail elsewhere (8, 9). In brief, these included the clinical manifestations of angina pectoris, myocardial infarction, the coronary insufficiency syndrome, and sudden unexpected death. A diagnosis of *angina pectoris* required the concurrence of two observers that the minimum criteria of substernal discomfort of brief duration definitely precipitated by exercise or excitement and promptly relieved by rest were present. The diagnosis of *myocardial infarction* was made only in the presence of serial electrocardiographic evidence of infarction or of abnormal serum enzyme levels consistent with myocardial necrosis in a suitable clinical setting. All hospital records and electrocardiograms were reviewed by the study investigators. Where available (in approximately 40% of those who died), autopsy information was used to confirm a clinical diagnosis of acute myocardial infarction. A diagnosis of *coronary insufficiency* was made in subjects presenting with a history compatible with a myocardial infarction and associated with transient ischemic ECG changes but with no evidence of myocardial necrosis either by ECG or serum enzymes. *Sudden death* was attributed to coronary heart disease when the history indicated that it had very likely occurred in a matter of minutes (documented within 1 hr) and could be attributed to no other cause in subjects not suffering from a potentially fatal illness.

FOLLOW-UP

Of the original study group free of coronary heart disease on the initial examination it was possible to re-examine 80% at the clinic on the eighth biennial examination, representing 14 years of follow-up. Another 8% were known to have died before this examination, and in each instance cause of death was determined. From observation of the population sample at subsequent clinic examination, routine daily surveillance of admission to the only local general hospital, and inquiry made of physicians and relatives it was possible to reach a conclusion about the state of health with respect to coronary heart disease for another 10%. It is considered unlikely that a significant number of new coronary heart disease events have been missed in the 14 years of follow-up. Less than 2% of the population sample were completely lost to follow-up.

Results

In the 14 years of follow-up 323 men and 169 women between the ages of 30 and 62 years at initial examination developed for the first time some clinical manifestation of coronary heart disease. The incidence increased with age in both sexes with a striking male predominance in younger victims but a closing gap in incidence with advancing age. The mean level of each of the major serum lipids and lipoproteins was higher at the initial examination in those who went on to develop coronary heart disease than in their cohorts, who remained free of clinical manifestations of the disease over the 14-year period of observation. The levels of cholesterol observed in this population were generally high compared with those reported from other areas in the world, where low coronary heart disease rates have been reported (11, 12). The distributions of all the lipids examined, comparing subjects who did and did not develop the disease, overlapped to such an extent that no concentration of any lipid was characteristic of either group (6).

Reexamination of the relation of the level of each of the major blood lipids and lipoproteins under consideration after 14 years of biennial follow-up continues to show a distinct and striking increment in risk proportional to the antecedent lipid concentration. The relationship was generally stronger in younger than in older persons. It might be expected that the biochemical substance closest to the responsible metabolic defect would show a more striking association with the disease than that secondarily, or less fundamentally, related. Although differences in measurement precision may obscure the comparisons, risk of subsequent coronary heart disease over 14 years was thus studied in the 5,127 men and women participating in the Framingham Study in relation to their antecedent lipoprotein and lipid status, as determined at the time of their first 2 biennial examinations.

Graphing the incidence of coronary heart disease developing in portions of the population grouped by quartiles of the distribution of cholesterol and the lipoprotein fractions measured provides a valid visual comparison of the differences in risk between the first and fourth quartile of the antecedent level of each lipid. Risk was proportional to the concentration of each lipid (Figure 1). The gradients of risk so demonstrated were not identical, but the differences

observed were not great enough to suggest one particular lipid as most basic to the development of this atherothrombotic disease.

Designating values in the fourth quartile of each lipid and lipoprotein under consideration as "abnormal," each lipid appears to be contributing to risk of coronary heart disease, with the incidence proportional to the number of lipid "abnormalities" so defined (Figure 2). Whether this is a fact or a statistical artifact cannot, however, be discerned from these data. Since these lipids are positively correlated, the mean level of each particular lipid also rises with the number of lipid abnormalities present (Table 1).

Hence, a more detailed examination of the relation of serum cholesterol to risk of coronary heart disease, using a more sophisticated type of analysis, is required. First, the relationships of serum lipids to coronary heart disease do not vary with the type of coronary heart disease so far as can be judged from the available data. The net contribution of cholesterol and $S_f 20$-400 prebeta lipoprotein is about the same for uncomplicated angina as it is for other coronary heart disease. Cholesterol, as indicated by the size of the coefficient in Table 2, carries most of the weight as a contributor to coronary heart disease in men, whether manifested as angina or some more serious form of the disease. For women, numbers allow an examination of the net effect of the lipids only for angina.

Risk of each particular clinical manifestation of coronary heart disease (including angina, myocardial infarction, and sudden death) proved proportional to the antecedent serum cholesterol level in men of all ages studied. The net effect appears to decline with age in both sexes, and in women beyond 50 little relationship can be shown. In men and younger women

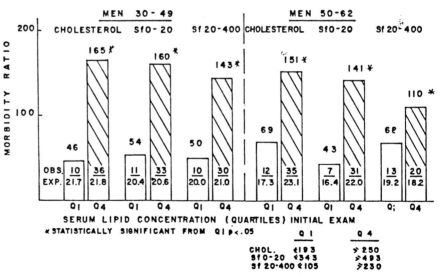

Figure 1. Risk of myocardial Infarction (14 years) according to serum lipid content: men, age 30 to 62 at entry. Framingham Heart Study.

Kannel et al. • Risk of Coronary Heart Disease   3

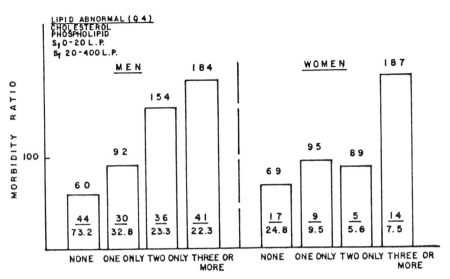

Figure 2. Risk of coronary heart disease (14 years) according to number of abnormal lipids: men and women, age 30 to 49 at entry. Framingham Study.

the risk simply rose in proportion to the antecedent serum cholesterol concentration from the lowest to highest values recorded in this population sample (Figure 3). There was nothing to suggest that some particular level was "critical." Hence, it does not appear logical to examine the relation of cholesterol to risk of coronary heart disease in terms of "hypercholesterolemia" but rather in terms of the actual concentration of cholesterol in the plasma.

Examination of the risk of developing coronary heart disease according to the actual serum cholesterol concentration of each subject grouped into quartiles showed an increase in risk proportional to the antecedent cholesterol concentration, not only in the general population but in persons free of factors believed associated both with hypercholesterolemia and with coronary heart disease (Figure 4). Even after excluding persons with hypertension, diabetes,

ECG abnormalities, and the cigarette habit, a distinct gradient of risk proportional to the cholesterol concentration can be demonstrated. This tends to brand the lipid, not associated variables, as the culprit. This is also shown in discriminant analysis accounting for the presence and the values of some of these associated variables in the entire population. As shown in an earlier analysis, a net effect of cholesterol is clearly apparent in men of all ages (13).

A discriminant analysis was also made of the relation of various lipids measured in the study to incidence of coronary heart disease after 8 years. The net effect of each of the lipids, including cholesterol, phospholipid, and the lipoprotein fractions (S_f0-12, 12-20, 20-100, and 100-400), was assessed. According to this analysis the dominant effect was assigned to serum cholesterol, with an insignificant contribution of the other lipids (6). In multivariate discrimi-

Table 1. Mean Lipid and Lipoprotein Content According to Number of Lipid "Abnormalities": Men and Women 30 to 49 Years Old at Entry

Number of Lipid Abnormalities	Number of Subjects	Mean Serum Lipid Content			
		S_f20-400 Lipoprotein	S_f0-20 Lipoprotein	Serum Cholesterol	Serum Phospholipid
		mg/100 ml			
In men 30 to 49					
0	746	126.7	363.6	197.2	143.8
1	309	189.8	434.9	222.5	178.7
2	211	259.5	479.1	248.0	200.0
3	136	339.7	501.2	285.4	236.5
4	65	345.9	567.2	293.0	249.9
In women 30 to 49					
0	1,112	75.3	338.6	194.0	144.2
1	325	136.6	412.1	224.0	185.1
2	170	162.4	485.8	254.7	203.9
3	121	171.4	539.6	282.9	221.9
4	62	255.5	594.0	307.7	252.7

Table 2. Risk of Specified Manifestations of Coronary Heart Disease According to Serum Cholesterol and S₂20-400 Prebeta Lipoprotein: Men 30 to 62 Years Old at Entry

Lipid Variable	Coronary Heart Disease Other Than Angina Pectoris			Uncomplicated Angina Pectoris		
	Number of Subjects	Coefficient	SE	Coefficient	SE	Number of Subjects
Age 30 to 39	42					7
Cholesterol		0.01377	0.0039	0.01364	0.0089	
S₂20-400 lipoprotein		0.00086	0.0012	−0.00451	0.0044	
Age 40 to 49	83					50
Cholesterol		0.00920*	0.0027	0.00835*	0.0038	
S₂20-400 lipoprotein		0.00029	0.0008	0.00081	0.0013	
Age 50+	108					32
Cholesterol		0.00864*	0.0028	0.00853	0.0035	
S₂20-400 lipoprotein		0.00026*	0.0010	0.00075	0.0011	

* Statistically significant at 5% level.

nation involving a number of highly correlated variables, however, a slight statistical advantage in one of these variables will lead to a marked depression of the discriminant weights assigned to the other variables. It would be incorrect to dismiss this effect as a mere statistical artifact; rather it indicates that the analytical question cannot be satisfactorily explored with the data in hand and that either the question should be reformulated or other kinds of data should be collected.

Since it was not feasible to retrospectively collect other data, a reduced question was put to the data—namely, does the S₂20-400 lipoprotein fraction tell us something about the risk of coronary heart disease over and above what is already shown by the serum cholesterol level? These two determinations are not highly correlated since the bulk of serum cholesterol is ordinarily carried in other lipoprotein fractions, whereas the S₂20-400 fraction carries a sizable amount of triglyceride as well as cholesterol.

For the purposes of this analysis persons free of disease at examinations 2, 4, or 6 were assigned to coronary heart disease or noncoronary heart disease categories as they did or did not develop disease in the ensuing 4 years. Although a person may appear in a specified age group only once, he may appear as a noncase in three different age groups, provided he came in for the second, fourth, or sixth biennial examination and was free of disease at the beginning of these three examination periods. Although levels of characterization according to serum lipids and other related variables differed somewhat from one examination to another, both subsequent cases and noncases were measured in the same way and are therefore always directly comparable. For the computation of mean differences all cases and all noncases were pooled without any weighting, it being assumed that age-specific incidence after each of the examinations was the same. Variances and covariances, however, were computed separately for each

of the cohorts; and then the within-cohort variances and covariances were combined, thus achieving a slight gain in sensitivity. It is apparent that in men cholesterol accounts for more of the total distance between those who developed and those who remained free of the disease than does S₂20-400 *prebeta* lipoprotein in all but the oldest subjects. The use of both was little better than cholesterol alone in discriminating potential coronary heart disease cases (Table 3). The standardized mean deviations were in general substantially larger for cholesterol than S₂20-400 *prebeta* lipoprotein, and all were positive in the men.

Among younger women the same appeared to hold. In older women, however, S₂20-400 *prebeta* lipoprotein appears to discriminate distinctly better than cholesterol. Beyond age 55 the standardized mean deviations were larger, and the S₂20-400 *prebeta* lipoprotein also accounted for most of the generalized distance between those with and those free of coronary heart disease (Table 3). Again, both do little better than the appropriate lipid alone in discriminating future coronary heart disease.

The meaning of this analysis may be a little clearer

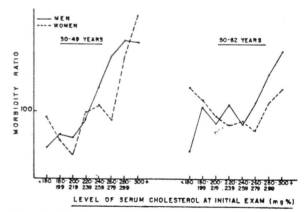

Figure 3. Risk of coronary heart disease (14 years) according to cholesterol level: men and women age 30 to 62 at entry. Framingham Study.

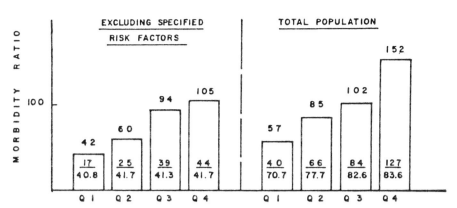

Figure 4. Risk of coronary heart disease (14 years) according to serum cholesterol concentration excluding persons with other risk factors: men, age 30 to 62 at entry. Framingham Study.

SERUM CHOLESTEROL CONCENTRATION – QUARTILES, INITIAL EXAMINATION

*OTHER RISK FACTORS EXCLUDED:– E C G ABNORMALITY, DIABETES, HIGH BLOOD PRESSURE, CIGARETTES > I PKG.
55 PERSONS WITH UNKNOWN ATTRIBUTES NOT INCLUDED

from an examination of Figures 5 and 6. These show the relative risk of coronary heart disease according to the concentration of each of these lipid values after adjustment for the level of the other lipid and the values of the other associated variables. An expected number of coronary heart disease events was obtained from a computed "risk function" derived from the values of each of the other variables for each subgroup of the lipid under consideration. This was compared with the number of cases actually observed in each lipid subgroup. The ratio of the observed to the expected number of cases times 100 (morbidity ratio) gives an expression of the relative

risk with the standard risk set at 100. For cholesterol in men a strong residual effect remains after accounting for the level of $S_f 20$-400 lipoprotein and the other factors (Figure 5). This independent effect, however, is much more modest than noted without such adjustment. In younger, but not older, women distinctly higher cholesterol values may also contribute independently to risk (Figure 6).

On the other hand, when risk of coronary heart disease is examined according to $S_f 20$-400 prebeta lipoprotein level, adjusting for cholesterol and the other factors, it is difficult to discern any residual risk gradient in men (Figure 5). In older women there

Table 3. Discriminant Analysis Relation of Serum Cholesterol and $S_f 20$-400 Lipoprotein to Subsequent Coronary Heart Disease: Men and Women 38 to 69 Years Old

Age	Standardized Mean Deviation		Generalized Distance			Number of Cases
	Cholesterol	$S_f 20$-400	Cholesterol	$S_f 20$-400	Both	
yr						
Men						
38-41	1.17	0.74	16.26*	6.39†	16.48*	12
42-45	0.54	0.20	7.59*	1.08	7.71*	27
46-49	0.87	0.72	18.26*	12.48*	21.78*	25
50-53	0.65	0.21	17.68*	1.80	17.80*	44
54-57	0.25	0.05	3.28	0.14	3.46	56
58-61	0.27	0.32	3.29	4.84†	5.82†	50
62-65	0.22	0.08	1.19	0.16	1.19	26
66-69	0.06	0.33	0.04	1.30	1.39	13
Average	0.45	0.27				253
Women						
38-41	—	—	—	—	—	1
42-45	0.73	−0.30	4.21†	0.71	7.13*	8
46-49	1.10	0.06	8.49*	0.02	9.57*	7
50-53	0.84	0.10	7.65*	0.12	8.23*	11
54-57	0.06	0.23	0.07	1.10	1.12	21
58-61	0.17	0.29	1.03	2.90	3.11	37
62-65	−0.04	0.43	0.03	4.30†	5.08†	24
66-69	0.53	0.77	5.60†	11.97*	13.88*	22
Average	0.32	0.32				130

* Statistically significant at 1% level (14-year follow-up).
† Statistically significant at 5% level (14-year follow-up).

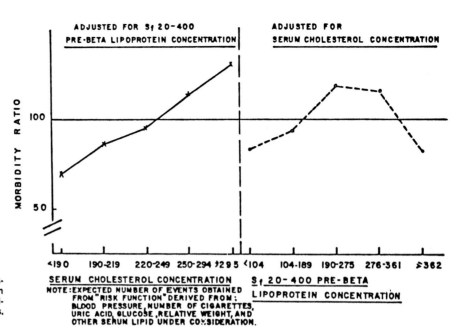

Figure 5. Risk of coronary heart disease (14 years) according to serum lipid adjusted for associated variables: men, age 38 to 69 years. Framingham Study.

may be an independent residual effect of S_f20-400 prebeta lipoprotein, although an inverse relationship, if anything, appeared to exist in younger women (Figure 6). If one puts a further question to the data and asks if by adjusting the S_f20-400 by S_f0-20 lipoproteins the risk gradient is also made to disappear, the answer is yes, suggesting that in the general population the people with high S_f20-400 often tend to have high S_f0-20 or cholesterol levels that may well explain their subsequent higher risk of coronary heart disease.

Traditionally, it has been held that a high concentration of cholesterol is more serious when not accompanied by a commensurate elevation of phospho-

lipid. The cholesterol to phospholipid ratio has long been advocated as an index of atherogenesis. Prospective examination of this hypothesis among persons with modest "hypercholesterolemia" as it occurs in the general population showed no clear trend of increased risk proportional to the cholesterol to phospholipid ratio (Figure 7).

As regards risk of coronary heart disease in relation to serum cholesterol concentration, the concomitant blood pressure had a more pronounced effect than either the lipoprotein pattern or the phospholipid content of the serum. Elevated serum lipid content, whether it be the cholesterol or the S_f20-400 pre-beta lipoprotein value, is considerably more

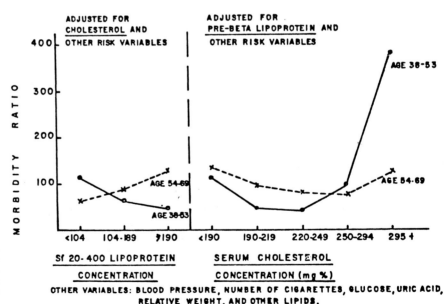

Figure 6. Risk of coronary heart disease (14 years) according to serum cholesterol and S_f20-400 lipoprotein adjusted for associated variables: women, age 38 to 69. Framingham Study.

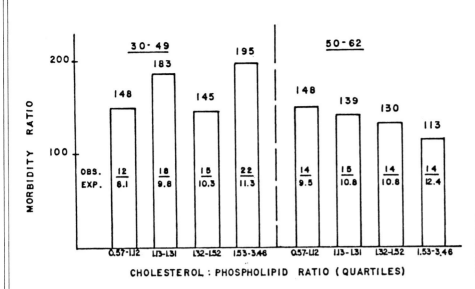

Figure 7. Risk of coronary heart disease (14 years) in hypercholesterolemic subjects according to cholesterol to phospholipid ratio: men, age 30 to 62 at entry. Framingham Study.

ominous in hypertensive than in normotensive individuals. The risk at any lipid level varies over a wide range, depending on the associated blood pressure. The converse was also true, and at any level of blood pressure risk was markedly influenced by the associated lipid value (Figure 8).

Discussion

Multiple interrelated factors, both host and environmental, have been shown to play a role in the evolution of this disease in various general population samples (14-19). Of all the identified host factors associated with increased susceptibility to coronary heart disease, the blood lipids are among the strongest. The accumulated evidence from epidemiologic studies, clinical observations, laboratory research, and animal experiments permits the logical conclusion

that lipids must play at least a contributory role in atherogenesis. If there is in fact a single common denominator through which the multiple interrelated predisposing factors in coronary heart disease operate, an abnormal accumulation or handling of blood lipids would appear the most likely candidate.

Since the discovery over a century ago that cholesterol was a prominent constituent of the atherosclerotic plaque (20) and that this same substance was also present in the blood, a huge volume of research has been directed toward obtaining a better understanding of the precise nature of the relationship of cholesterol to atherogenesis. Subsequent research has shown that cholesterol from the blood does actually enter into intimal atheromas (21-24) and that inducing a high blood cholesterol content in a variety of ways has resulted in an accelerated development of

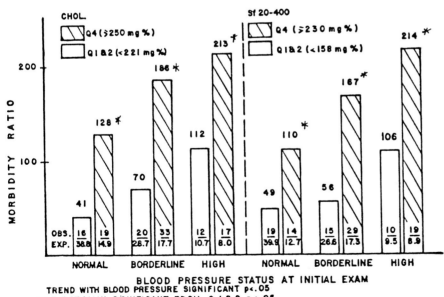

Figure 8. Risk of coronary heart disease (14 years) according to serum lipid and blood pressure status: men, age 30 to 49 at entry. Framingham Study.

atherosclerotic lesions in a number of animal species (25-28). Reduction of the concentration of cholesterol in the blood in some animal experiments appears to reverse the process (29, 30). In addition, populations with a high average level of serum cholesterol tend to have a high reported mortality from coronary heart disease. Conversely, lower death rates and less extensive atherosclerosis at postmortem have been reported from areas where substantially lower indigenous cholesterol levels are found (12). That this is not simply a racial difference has been demonstrated in migrants of the same race from a low to a high cholesterol area who appear to correspondingly change their cholesterol levels and propensity to coronary heart disease mortality (11). More direct epidemiologic evidence has been provided by prospective studies that have repeatedly demonstrated, in a variety of population samples, that risk of subsequent disease is directly related to the antecedent serum cholesterol values of individuals within the population (31, 14-18).

Depending on the age group studied, clinicians have often (32-34), but not always (35-37), found a higher concentration of cholesterol in the blood of coronary patients than in suitable controls. Based on a comparison of serum lipids in persons already afflicted with coronary heart disease with some group labeled a "control," it has been claimed that one or another lipid or lipoprotein vehicle is more specific for the disease than is cholesterol. These investigators have found significant differences in the blood content of a variety of lipids and have implicated the total fasting triglyceride, beta and prebeta lipoprotein, alpha to beta cholesterol ratio, cholesterol to phospholipid ratio, and fatty acids (1, 2, 32, 37-42). These findings have generated a vast amount of research into the details of lipid metabolism in general and its relation to atherosclerosis in particular. It has been pointed out that lipids other than cholesterol are also present in the atherosclerotic plaque (43, 44) and that none of the major blood lipids, including cholesterol, phospholipid, triglyceride, or nonesterified fatty acid, circulate in the blood in a simple state. They are transported as part of various lipoprotein complexes or in association with albumin. It has been suggested that faulty lipid transport may be more fundamental in atherogenesis and that the lipoproteins more accurately mirror the underlying metabolic defect.

Each major lipoprotein fraction carries cholesterol. The S_f0-20 *beta* lipoprotein fraction is the principal carrier in most normal persons. The S_f20-400 *"prebeta"* lipoprotein fraction also carries a modest amount of cholesterol. On occasion a high serum cholesterol content may result primarily from a pronounced increase in this lipoprotein fraction. The common variety of "hypercholesterolemia" seen in the general population is, however, often associated with a modest elevation of both beta and prebeta lipoprotein fractions. "Elevation" of the *prebeta* lipoprotein without a concomitant "elevation" (in the fourth quartile of each) of *beta* lipoprotein is relatively uncommon, occurring in less than 10% of the "hypercholesterolemia" in the Framingham population.

A general population such as encountered in the Framingham Study includes few persons with serum cholesterol levels greater than 400 mg/100 ml and few xanthomatous individuals. There were 6 xanthomatous individuals in the Framingham population sample of 5,127 men and women. All had serum cholesterol values exceeding 400 mg/100 ml and a strong family history of coronary heart disease, and within the follow-up period all six died of coronary heart disease before their fiftieth birthdays.

The distribution of serum cholesterol values that has been reported in such persons clearly belongs to a different universe than that which has been observed in general population samples such as Framingham (Figure 9). Moderate serum cholesterol elevations between 250 and 350 mg/100 ml constitute the bulk of "hypercholesterolemias" that appear to be predisposing to the abundance of coronary heart disease as it occurs in the general population. Such levels constitute the upper quartile of the distribution of cholesterol in this general population sample. Moderate elevations in this range, depending on age and sex, are associated with a risk of coronary heart disease two to five times higher than is noted with values below the average of about 220 mg/100 ml (Table 4). This modest level of "hypercholesterolemia" therefore represents both a potent and a common factor contributing to risk of coronary heart disease.

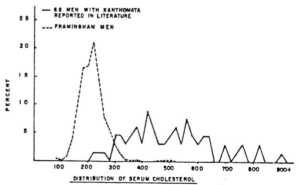

Figure 9. Frequency distribution of serum cholesterol level: men age 30 to 62 years. Subjects from the Framingham Study versus xanthomatous patients.

Kannel et al. • Risk of Coronary Heart Disease   **9**

Table 4. Factor of Increased Risk of Coronary Heart Disease Over 14 Years According to Antecedent Serum Cholesterol Concentration*: Men and Women 35 to 64 Years Old

Age	Relative Risk	
	Men	Women
yr		
35 to 44	5.5	5.0
45 to 54	2.4	1.5
55 to 64	1.7	1.3
All ages	2.5	1.5

* Cholesterol level of 265 mg/100 ml or higher versus cholesterol level of under 220 mg/100 ml.

Current investigations raise the possibility that it may be useful to determine the lipoprotein pattern in order to select more specific corrective therapy in those with marked hypercholesterolemia (1, 45). This information may also be useful in treating the common moderate degrees of hypercholesterolemia encountered in the general population. On the other hand, the observation of the lack of a relation of the cholesterol to phospholipid ratio to risk of coronary heart disease among "hypercholesterolemic" persons suggests that the phospholipids as a group play little role in atherogenesis, either protective or otherwise. This does not preclude a powerful effect of some particular component of the phospholipid group such as the cephalins (40).

One can properly view triglyceride and S_f20-400 prebeta lipid determinations obtained in the nonfasted state with skepticism, although this skepticism may be exaggerated in view of the correlation in population samples between fasting and nonfasting specimens. Unfortunately, it is seldom feasible to obtain fasting specimens in large voluntary general population studies where subjects have to be seen in the evening in order to obtain cooperation. The data presented in this study do not necessarily reflect on the issue of a possible association of fasting endogenous triglyceride or fasting prebeta lipoprotein on incidence of coronary heart disease. In medicine these days, however, dynamic tests of function are replacing static ones that are often much less sensitive. Metabolic tests may be normal in the fasted state but distinctly abnormal after a load. Such tests in the fasted state do not necessarily reflect the usual metabolic state of persons in the course of daily living. Despite or because of the fact that these specimens were casual, risk of coronary heart disease was strikingly related to antecedent S_f20-400 prebeta values.

It remains to be clarified whether the moderate hypercholesterolemia so prevalent in the general population and so potent a contributor to coronary heart disease morbidity and mortality is principally a het-

erozygous state for one or more inborn errors of lipid metabolism or simply an acquired state caused by overnutrition. It is possible that both play a role. Although it seems likely that the blood lipid content, enhanced by increased blood pressure, is related in a fundamental way to the rate of general deposition of lipid in the intima, local factors appear to determine the site of deposition. These local factors include damage to the intima (46), the caliber of the vessel (47), dynamics of flow (48), factors promoting fibrin deposition (49), and possibly metabolic factors in the vessel wall (24, 44). Factors promoting thrombus formation, so important in determining whether an occlusion occurs, must also play a prominent role in determining whether these atheromatous lesions prove lethal. They may also participate in initiating the lipid-laden atheromatous lesion (49, 50). Also, transient tides in the blood lipid content may enhance blood clotting and sludging (51).

Many questions remain concerning the details of atherogenesis. Promising new analytical techniques developed by Fredrickson, Levy, and Lees (1) are under active investigation. Such investigations may throw a new light on the entire subject. These uncertainties should not be allowed to obscure the firmly established striking association between high blood lipid content in general, and cholesterol in particular, and coronary atherosclerotic disease. Evidence is beginning to accumulate to suggest that effective lowering of the serum cholesterol level may be followed by a corresponding reduction in coronary morbidity and mortality (52-57).

Prospective data concerning the risk of coronary heart disease in relation to antecedent lipoprotein status are quite scarce. Those relating to lipoprotein types (as proposed by Fredrickson and colleagues) are nonexistent since this concept has been too recently introduced. Prospective data relating lipoprotein status to coronary heart disease in women are nonexistent. The data herein reported provide some indication of the contribution of lipids and lipoproteins to risk of coronary heart disease within the scope of contemporary concepts.

In men, knowledge of both the serum lipoprotein levels and the cholesterol concentration appears to provide no better discrimination of potential coronary victims than can be deduced from an accurate serum cholesterol value alone. Any one of the lipids or lipoproteins examined, and, by inference, a triglyceride as well, can be used effectively for assessing vulnerability to coronary heart disease. None, however, would appear superior to the more convenient serum cholesterol determination for this purpose. Specific tables describing the relation of serum cholesterol to coronary heart disease incidence in absolute rather than relative terms appear in other Framingham reports (58).

In women, however, the picture appears to be somewhat different. In women under the age of 50, as in men, high cholesterol values and not S_f20-400 prebeta lipoprotein appear to be associated with an increased risk. In older women, on the other hand, cholesterol appears to have no predictive value, and S_f20-400 prebeta lipoprotein actually appears to be superior to cholesterol for estimating risk.

The data presented suggest that in men the moderately elevated cholesterol values commonly encountered in the general population, regardless of the metabolic aberration responsible or how it is transported or partitioned among the lipoproteins, are associated with increased risk of coronary heart disease. Elevated endogenous triglyceride values appear significant in coronary atherogenesis only when accompanied by high cholesterol values. Knowledge of the associated lipoprotein pattern in "hypercholesterolemic" men may be important for determining the nature of the responsible metabolic defect and for selecting the most efficacious therapy, but its contribution to assessing risk of coronary heart disease remains to be determined. In older women, on the other hand, S_f20-400 prebeta lipoprotein, or by inference a fasting triglyceride, may be the only lipid capable of prognosticating coronary heart disease.

ACKNOWLEDGMENTS: Received 12 June 1970; revision accepted 30 September 1970.

► Requests for reprints should be addressed to William B. Kannel, M.D., National Heart Institute, 25 Evergreen St., Framingham, Mass. 01701

References

1. FREDRICKSON DS, LEVY RI, LEES RS: Fat transport in lipoproteins—an integrated approach to mechanisms and disorders. *New Eng J Med* 276:34-44, 94-103, 148-156, 215-224, 273-281, 1967
2. GOFMAN JW, YOUNG W, TANDY R: Ischemic heart disease, atherosclerosis, and longevity. *Circulation* 34:679-697, 1966
3. AHRENS EH JR, HIRSCH J, OETTE K, et al: Carbohydrate-induced and fat-induced lipemias. *Trans Ass Amer Physicians* 74:134-146, 1961
4. KUO PT: Current metabolic-genetic interrelationship in human atherosclerosis. With therapeutic considerations. *Ann Intern Med* 68:449-466, 1968
5. KRITCHEVSKY D, TEPPER SA, ALAUPOVIC P, et al: Cholesterol content of human serum lipoproteins obtained by dextran sulfate precipitation and by preparative ultracentrifugation. *Proc Soc Exp Biol Med* 112:259-262, 1963
6. KANNEL WB, DAWBER TR, FRIEDMAN GD, et al: Risk factors in coronary heart disease. *Ann Intern Med* 61:888-899, 1964
7. GORDON T, MOORE FE, SHURTLEFF D, et al: Some methodologic problems in the long-term study of cardiovascular disease: observations on the Framingham Study. *J Chronic Dis* 10:186-206, 1959
8. FRIEDMAN GD, KANNEL WB, DAWBER TR, et al: An evaluation of follow-up methods in the Framingham Heart Study. *Amer J Public Health* 57:1015-1024, 1967

9. DAWBER TR, KANNEL WB, LYELL LP: An approach to longitudinal studies in a community: the Framingham Study. *Ann N Y Acad Sci* 107:539-556, 1963
10. DeLALLA OF, GOFMAN JW: Ultracentrifugal analysis of serum lipoprotein, in *Methods of Biochemical Analysis*, vol. 1, edited by GLICK D. New York, Interscience, 1954, pp. 459-478
11. KEYS A, KIMURA N, KUSUKAWA A, et al: Lessons from serum cholesterol studies in Japan, Hawaii and Los Angeles. *Ann Intern Med* 48:83-94, 1958
12. BRONTE-STEWART B, KEYS A, BROCK JF: Serum-cholesterol, diet, and coronary heart disease; an inter-racial survey in the Capo peninsula. *Lancet* 2:1103-1108, 1955
13. TRUETT J, CORNFIELD J, KANNEL WB: A multivariate analysis of the risk of coronary heart disease in Framingham. *J Chronic Dis* 20:511-524, 1967
14. DOYLE JT, HESLIN AS, HILLEBOE HE, et al: Measuring the risk of coronary heart disease in adult population groups: a prospective study of degenerative cardiovascular disease in Albany: report of three years' experience. I. Ischemic heart disease. *Amer J Public Health* 47(suppl April):25-32, 1957
15. CHAPMAN JM, GOERKE LS, DIXON W, et al: Measuring the risk of coronary heart disease in adult population groups: clinical status of a population group in Los Angeles under observation for two to three years. *Ibid.*, pp. 33-42
16. STAMLER J, LINDBERG HA, BERKSON DM, et al: Prevalence and incidence of coronary heart disease in strata of the labor force of a Chicago industrial corporation. *J Chronic Dis* 11:405-420, 1960
17. KEYS A, TAYLOR HL, BLACKBURN H, et al: Coronary heart disease among Minnesota business and professional men followed 15 years. *Circulation* 28:381-395, 1963
18. PAUL O, LEPPER MH, PHELAN WH, et al: A longitudinal study of coronary heart disease. *Ibid.*, pp. 20-31
19. SHAPIRO S, WEINBLATT E, FRANK CW, et al: The H. I. P. study of incidence and prognosis of coronary heart disease: preliminary findings on incidence of myocardial infarction and angina. *J Chronic Dis* 18:527-558, 1965
20. VOGEL J: *The Pathological Anatomy of the Human Body*, 1st ed. Philadelphia, Lea and Blanchard, 1847, p. 531
21. CHOBANIAN AV, HOLLANDER W: Body cholesterol metabolism in man. 1. The equilibration of serum and tissue cholesterol. *J Clin Invest* 41:1732-1737, 1962
22. SIMONTON JH, GOFMAN JW: Macrophage migration in experimental atherosclerosis. *Circulation* 4:557-562, 1951
23. BIGGS MW, KRITCHEVSKY D: Observations with radioactive hydrogen in experimental atherosclerosis. *Ibid.*, pp. 34-42
24. SIPERSTEIN MD, CHAIKOFF IL, CHERNICK SS: Significance of endogenous cholesterol in arteriosclerosis: synthesis in arterial tissue. *Science* 113:747-749, 1951
25. ANITSCHKOW N, CHALATOW S: Ueber experimentelle cholesterinsteatose und ihre Bedeutung fuer die Entstehung einiger pathologischer Prozesse. *Centralbl Allg Path Anat* 24:1-9, 1913
26. IGNATOWSKI A: Ueber die Wirkung des tierischen Eiweisses auf die Aorta und die parenchymatosen Oregane der Kaninchen. *Virchow Arch Path Anat* 198:248-270, 1903
27. KATZ LN, STAMLER J: *Experimental Atherosclerosis*. Springfield, Ill., Charles C Thomas, Publisher, 1953
28. ROBERTS JC, STRAUS R (editors): *Comparative Atherosclerosis*. New York, Hoeber Medical Division, Harper & Row, Publishers, Inc., 1965
29. HORLICK L, KATZ LN: Retrogression of atherosclerotic lesions on cessation of cholesterol feeding in the chick. *J Lab Clin Med* 34:1427-1442, 1949
30. ARMSTRONG ML, WARNER ED, CONNOR WE: Regression of coronary atheromatosis in rhesus monkeys (abstract). *Circ Res* 27:59, 1970
31. KANNEL WB, CASTELLI WP, McNAMARA PM: The coronary profile: 12 year follow-up in the Framingham Study. *J Occup Med* 9:611-619, 1967
32. GERTLER MM, GARN SM: Lipid interrelationship in health and in coronary artery disease. *Science* 112:14-16, 1950
33. STEINER A, DOMANSKI B: Serum cholesterol level in coronary arteriosclerosis. *Arch Intern Med (Chicago)* 71:397-402, 1943
34. LERMAN J, WHITE PD: Metabolic changes in young people with coronary heart disease. *J Clin Invest* 25:914, 1946
35. GROEN JJ, TIJONG KB, KOSTER M, et al: The influence of nutrition and ways of life on blood cholesterol and the prev-

alence of hypertension and coronary heart disease among Trappist and Benedictine Monks. *Amer J Clin Nutr* 10:456-470, 1962

36. EPSTEIN FH, SIMPSON R, BOAS EP: The epidemiology of atherosclerosis among a random sample of clothing workers of different ethnic origins in New York City. II. Associations between manifest atherosclerosis, serum lipid levels, blood pressure, overweight, and some other variables. *J Chronic Dis* 5:329-341, 1957

37. ALBRINK MJ, MEIGS JW, MAN EB: Serum lipids, hypertension and coronary artery disease. *Amer J Med* 31:4-23, 1961

38. ANTONIS A, BERSOHN L: Serum-triglyceride levels in South African Europeans and Bantu and in ischaemic heart disease. *Lancet* 1:998-1002, 1960

39. HATCH FT, REISSEL PK, POON-KING TMW, et al: A study of coronary heart disease in young men. Characteristics and metabolic studies in the patients and comparison with age-matched healthy men. *Circulation* 33:679-703, 1966

40. NOTHMAN MM, PROGER S: Cephalins in the blood. Patients with coronary heart disease and patients with hyperlipemia. *JAMA* 179:40-43, 1962

41. SANDLER M, BOURNE GH: Some new observations on human aortic atheroma. The possible role of essential fatty acids in its development. *Ibid.*, pp. 43-46

42. CASTELLI WP, NICKERSON RJ, NEWELL JM, et al: Serum NEFA following fat, carbohydrate and protein ingestion, and during fasting as related to intracellular lipid deposition. *J Atheroscler Res* 6:328-341, 1966

43. BUCK RC, ROSSITER RJ: Lipids of normal and atherosclerotic aortas chemical study. *Arch Path (Chicago)* 41:224-237, 1951

44. ZILVERSMIT DB, McCANDLESS EL, JORDAN PH JR, et al: The synthesis of phospholipids in human atheromatous lesions. *Circulation* 23:370-375, 1961

45. AHRENS EH JR: Differential diagnosis and treatment of hyperglyceridemia. *JAMA* 207:763-764, 1969

46. COX GE, TRUEHART RE, KAPLAN J, et al: Atherosclerosis in rhesus monkeys. IV. Repair of arterial injury—an important secondary atherogenic factor. *Arch Path (Chicago)* 76:166-176, 1963

47. YOUNG W, GOFMAN JW, TANDY R, et al: The quantitation of atherosclerosis. I. Relationship to artery size. *Amer J Cardiol* 6:288-293, 1960

48. TEXON M: The hemodynamic concept of atherosclerosis. *Amer J Cardiol* 5:291-294, 1960

49. DUGUID JB: Thrombosis as a factor in the pathogenesis of coronary atherosclerosis. *J Path Bact* 58:207-212, 1946

50. PATERSON JC, MOFFATT T, MILLS J: Hemosiderin deposition in early atherosclerotic plaques. *Arch Path (Chicago)* 61:496-502, 1956

51. O'BRIEN JR: Fat ingestion, blood coagulation, and atherosclerosis. *Amer J Med Sci* 234:373-390, 1957

52. TURPEINEN O: Diet and coronary events. *J Amer Diet Ass* 52:209-213, 1968

53. LEREN P: Effect of plasma cholesterol lowering diet in male survivors of myocardial infarction. *Acta Med Scand* (suppl) 466:1-92, 1966

54. DAYTON S, PEARCE ML, HASHIMOTO S, et al: A controlled clinical trial of a diet high in unsaturated fat in preventing complications of atherosclerosis. *Circulation* 40 (suppl II): 1-63, 1969

55. Controlled trial of soya-bean oil in myocardial infarction: report of a research committee to the Medical Research Council. *Lancet* 2:693-699, 1968

56. BIERENBAUM ML, GREEN DP, FLORIN A, et al: Modified-fat dietary management of the young male with coronary disease. A five-year report. *JAMA* 202:1119-1123, 1967

57. CHRISTAKIS G, RINZLER SH, ARCHER M, et al: The anti-coronary club: a dietary approach to the prevention of coronary heart disease—a seven-year report. *Amer J Public Health* 56:299-314, 1966

58. *The Framingham Study. An Epidemiological Investigation of Cardiovascular Disease.* Sections 10 and 23. Washington, D.C., U. S. Government Printing Office, 1969

Proc. Nat. Acad. Sci. USA
Vol. 70, No. 10, pp. 2804–2808, October 1973

Familial Hypercholesterolemia: Identification of a Defect in the Regulation of 3-Hydroxy-3-Methylglutaryl Coenzyme A Reductase Activity Associated with Overproduction of Cholesterol

(cholesterol synthesis/hyperlipidemia/low-density lipoproteins/enzyme regulation/ coronary heart disease)

JOSEPH L. GOLDSTEIN AND MICHAEL S. BROWN

Divisions of Medical Genetics and Gastroenterology-Liver, Department of Internal Medicine, University of Texas Southwestern Medical School, Dallas, Tex. 75235

Communicated by E. R. Stadtman, June 20, 1973

ABSTRACT The homozygous form of the autosomal dominant disorder, familial hypercholesterolemia, is characterized by the presence in children of profound hypercholesterolemia, cutaneous planar xanthomas, and rapidly progressive coronary vascular disease that usually results in death before age 30 years. Cultured skin fibroblasts from three unrelated subjects with this disorder showed 40- to 60-fold higher activity of 3-hydroxy-3-methylglutaryl coenzyme A reductase (EC 1.1.1.34), the rate-controlling enzyme in cholesterol biosynthesis, when compared with fibroblasts of seven control subjects. Enhanced enzyme activity resulted from a complete absence of normal feedback suppression by low-density lipoproteins, which led to a marked overproduction of cholesterol by the mutant cells. The demonstration of apparently identical kinetic properties of the reductase activity of control and mutant cells, coupled with the evidence that this enzyme is normally regulated not by allosteric effectors but by alterations in enzyme synthesis and degradation, suggests that the primary genetic abnormality does not involve the structural gene for the enzyme itself, but a hitherto unidentified gene whose product is necessary for mediation of feedback control by lipoproteins. The fibroblasts of two obligate heterozygotes, the parents of one of the homozygotes, showed a pattern of enzyme regulation intermediate between that of controls and homozygotes.

Familial hypercholesterolemia is transmitted in humans as an autosomal dominant trait (1–4). Although heterozygotes are born with an elevated level of plasma cholesterol, they usually remain clinically asymptomatic until the third–sixth decade of life, at which time they may manifest tendinous xanthomas and coronary heart disease of varying severity (1–5). Subjects who are homozygous for the familial hypercholesterolemia gene uniformly develop: (*a*) a profound elevation in plasma cholesterol often exceeding 800 mg/dl; (*b*) cutaneous planar xanthomas appearing in the first several years of life; (*c*) rapidly progressive coronary, cerebral, and peripheral vascular occlusive disease occurring in childhood and associated with widespread accumulation of cholesterol in atheromatous plaques; and (*d*) death from myocardial infarction, often before the age of 30 (1, 2, 5).

Despite the unique phenotype of the homozygous form of familial hypercholesterolemia and the relatively high population frequency of individuals with the heterozygous form of

the disease (6), very little is known about the fundamental physiological or biochemical defect in this disorder. For example, there is no agreement as to whether cholesterol accumulates in familial hypercholesterolemia because of increased synthesis (7–9) or because of defective degradation either of cholesterol itself (10) or of the plasma low-density lipoprotein (LDL) to which it is bound (11).

Studies of Siperstein and other workers have demonstrated that the rate of cholesterol synthesis in mammalian liver is controlled by the activity of 3-hydroxy-3-methylglutaryl coenzyme A reductase (HMG CoA reductase; EC 1.1.1.34), the enzyme catalyzing the first step unique to the cholesterol biosynthetic pathway (reviewed in ref. 12). We have recently developed a method for studying regulation of the activity of this enzyme in cultured human-skin fibroblasts and have found that the enzyme activity in normal cells is under a sensitive form of feedback control mediated specifically by LDL and very low-density lipoproteins (13).

In the present studies, we used this model system to characterize regulation of HMG CoA reductase activity in fibroblasts from subjects with the homozygous and heterozygous forms of familial hypercholesterolemia. Our studies indicate that cells of these patients have a genetic defect in regulation of HMG CoA reductase activity by lipoproteins and that this abnormality results in a marked increase in their rate of cholesterol synthesis.

MATERIALS AND METHODS

Human Subjects. J.P. is a 12-year-old Caucasian girl with the classic phenotypic and genetic features of the homozygous form of familial hypercholesterolemia (1, 2, 5). She has diffuse cutaneous planar xanthomas present since age 2 years, tendinous xanthomas, bilateral arcus corneae, and generalized atherosclerosis manifest by angina pectoris, aortic stenosis, and a myocardial infarction at age 11 years. Her total plasma cholestrol has ranged between 700 and 1000 mg/dl, and her fasting plasma triglyceride has been repeatedly below 100 mg/dl. Both her father (M.P., age 40 years) and her mother (P.C., age 38 years) have the phenotypic features of the heterozygous form of familial hypercholesterolemia (1–5). Her father's total plasma cholesterol has averaged 350 mg/dl, and his fasting plasma triglyceride has been consistently below 140 mg/dl. Her mother, who had a documented myocardial infarction at age 31 years, has a total plasma cholesterol ranging between

Abbreviations: HMG CoA reductase, 3-hydroxy-3-methylglutaryl coenzyme A reductase; LDL, low-density lipoproteins.

Proc. Nat. Acad. Sci. USA 70 (1973) HMG CoA Reductase in Familial Hypercholesterolemia 2805

400 and 490 mg/dl and a fasting plasma triglyceride that has always been below 140 mg/dl except for one value of 190 mg/dl.

Fibroblasts derived from two other homozygotes were also studied. L.L., a 10-year-old boy, and A.C., a 23-year-old woman, each had a clinical phenotype identical to that of J.P., and both had pedigree evidence consistent with homozygosity for the familial hypercholesterolemia gene.

The control subjects consisted of six healthy individuals of various ages (D.S., newborn boy; D.C., 6-year-old boy; T.L., 9-year-old girl; G.W., 24-year-old woman; G.C., 25-year-old woman; L.G., 28-year-old woman) and one patient with a nonfamilial form of hyperlipidemia (E.S., 44-year-old woman) whose disorder was manifest clinically by a type-V lipoprotein pattern (1), total plasma cholesterol of 463 mg/dl, and fasting plasma triglyceride of 2173 mg/dl.

Cells. Skin biopsies were obtained with informed consent, and fibroblast cultures were established in our laboratory for all subjects except for T.L., a control subject whose cells were obtained from the American Type Culture Collection, Rockville, Md. Cell lines were maintained in a humidified CO_2 incubator at 37° in 75-cm² flasks (Falcon) containing 10 ml of Eagle's minimum essential medium (Gibco, Cat. no. F-11), supplemented with penicillin (100 units/ml), streptomycin sulfate (100 μg/ml), 50 mM Tricine (pH 7.4) (Sigma), 0.05 g/100 ml of $NaHCO_3$, 1% (v/v) nonessential amino acids (Gibco), and 10% (v/v) fetal-calf serum (Flow Laboratories). For all experiments, cells from the stock flasks were dissociated with trypsin-EDTA solution (13) and were seeded (day 1) at about 2.5×10^5 cells per dish into 60×15-mm dishes (Falcon) containing 3 ml of the above growth medium with 10% fetal-calf serum. On day 3 the medium was replaced with fresh growth medium containing 10% fetal-calf serum. On day 6 when the cells were confluent, the medium was removed and the cellular monolayer was washed with 1.5 ml of Puck's saline A (Gibco), after which 3 ml of fresh medium containing either 10% fetal-calf serum or 5% lipoprotein-deficient human plasma was added as indicated.

Extracts. Cells were harvested by scraping, collected by centrifugation, washed, and frozen at −196° as described (13). Cell extracts were prepared by dissolving the thawed pellet in 0.1 ml of buffer containing 50 mM potassium phosphate (pH 7.4)–5 mM dithiothreitol–5 mM EDTA–0.2 M KCL–0.25% Kyro EOB (13). After incubation for 10 min at 37°, the suspension was centrifuged for 1 min at 12,000 rpm in a Beckman Microfuge, and aliquots of the supernatant were assayed for HMG CoA reductase activity and protein content.

HMG CoA Reductase Activity was measured by a described method (13). Aliquots of the cell extract (20–100 μg of protein) were incubated for 120 min at 37° in a final volume of 0.2 ml containing 0.1 M potassium phosphate (pH 7.5), 20 mM glucose-6-phosphate, 2.5 mM TPN, 0.7 unit of glucose-6-phosphate dehydrogenase, 5 mM dithiothreitol, and 30 μM DL-[3-¹⁴C]HMG CoA (5.26 Ci/mol) (14). The [¹⁴C]-mevalonate formed was isolated by thin-layer chromatography and counted, with an internal standard of [³H]mevalonate to correct for incomplete recovery (13, 14). The amount of extract was adjusted so that mevalonate formation was always linear with time and protein concentration (13). The

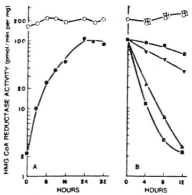

FIG. 1. HMG CoA reductase activity in fibroblasts of a control subject (*closed symbols*) and a patient with homozygous familial hypercholesterolemia, J.P. (*open symbols*). (*A*) Cells were grown in dishes containing 10% fetal-calf serum. On day 6 (0 time), the medium was replaced with 3 ml of fresh medium containing 5% human lipoprotein-deficient plasma. At the indicated time, extracts were prepared and HMG CoA reductase activity was measured. (*B*) 24 hr after addition of 5% human lipoprotein-deficient plasma, 0.1 ml of buffer A containing human LDL was added to give the indicated concentration: (○,●) None; (▽,▼) 2 μg/ml; (△,▲) 10 μg/ml; (□,■) 20 μg/ml. HMG CoA reductase activity was measured at the indicated time.

mean variation in HMG CoA reductase activity between duplicate dishes was ±5.1%.

Measurement of Cholesterol Synthesis. Fibroblasts were grown to confluence, and the growth medium was replaced with 2 ml of Krebs-Ringer phosphate buffer (pH 7.0) containing either 0.6 mM [2-¹⁴C]sodium acetate (New England Nuclear Corp., 53.4 Ci/mol) or 0.1 mM [2-¹⁴C]potassium mevalonate (Amersham Searle, 10 Ci/mol). Each dish was incubated 2 hr at 37° in a humidified atmosphere of 95% air–5% CO_2. The medium was then removed, and the cells were scraped with a rubber policeman into 1 ml of water. Each dish was further washed with 2 ml of water; the medium, the cells, and both washes were pooled in a final volume of 5 ml, to which was added 0.5 ml of 90% KOH and 1 mg of nonradioactive cholesterol. [¹⁴C]Cholesterol was isolated and quantitated by digitonin precipitation followed by thin-layer chromatography (15, 16).

Lipoproteins from normolipidemic subjects and from J.P. were isolated from plasma collected in EDTA (1 mg/ml) after a 15-hr fast. They were fractionated by sequential flotation and dialyzed into buffer A containing 0.15 M NaCl–0.3 mM EDTA (pH 7.4) (13). The fraction of density 1.019–1.063 g/ml is referred to as LDL. The fraction of density >1.215 g/ml is referred to as lipoprotein-deficient plasma.

Protein concentrations were determined by a modification of the method of Lowry *et al.* (17), with bovine-serum albumin as a standard.

RESULTS

In control fibroblasts grown to confluence in medium containing 10% fetal-calf serum, HMG CoA reductase activity was relatively low (Fig. 1*A*, 0 time). We previously showed that this low enzyme activity is due to suppression of the enzyme by lipoproteins present in fetal-calf serum (13). When fetal-calf serum was replaced with human lipoprotein-

2806   Genetics: Goldstein and Brown   *Proc. Nat. Acad. Sci. USA 70 (1973)*

TABLE 1. *Synthesis of [14C]cholesterol from [14C]acetate and [14C]mevalonate by fibroblasts from a control subject and a patient with homozygous familial hypercholesterolemia (J.P.)*

Growth conditions	[14C]Acetate → [14C]Cholesterol (pmol/2 hr per mg of protein)		[14C]Mevalonate → [14C]Cholesterol (pmol/2 hr per mg of protein)		HMG CoA reductase activity (pmol/min per mg of protein)	
	Control	Homozygote	Control	Homozygote	Control	Homozygote
A. 10% Fetal-calf serum	12.2	960	149 (446)	266 (798)	4.2	123
B. 5% Lipoprotein-deficient human plasma	251	878	188 (564)	208 (624)	74.0	158
C. 5% Lipoprotein-deficient human plasma + LDL	96	1828	187 (562)	195 (584)	—	—

Cells were grown in dishes containing 10% fetal-calf serum. On day 6 (0 time), the medium was removed, the cells were washed, and 3 ml of fresh medium containing either 10% fetal-calf serum (A) or 5% lipoprotein-deficient human plasma (B and C) was added. 24 hr later cells in group C received LDL at a final protein concentration of 12 μg/ml (20 μg/ml of cholesterol). Incorporation of [14C]acetate and [14C]mevalonate into [14C]cholesterol and measurement of HMG CoA reductase activity were determined at either 24 hr (A and B) or 30 hr (C). Each value represents the mean of duplicate determinations on duplicate dishes. The protein content of the dishes ranged between 0.16 and 0.24 mg per dish. Since each molecule of mevalonate originates from three molecules of acetate, the values in parentheses indicate the number of pmol of acetate represented by the [14C]mevalonate incorporated into [14C]cholesterol.

deficient plasma, the specific activity of HMG CoA reductase progressively increased by about 40-fold, reaching a plateau at 24 hr (Fig. 1A). At this point addition of human LDL resulted in a time- and concentration-dependent decrease in HMG CoA reductase activity (Fig. 1B). Fibroblasts from a patient with the homozygous form of familial hypercholesterolemia (J.P.) showed no such regulation (Fig. 1). In the presence of 10% fetal-calf serum, HMG CoA reductase activity in the mutant cells was about 60-fold higher than in normal cells grown under identical conditions (Fig. 1A, 0 time). Moreover, this activity did not change either when fetal-calf serum was replaced with lipoprotein-deficient plasma (Fig. 1A) or when LDL was added (Fig. 1B). When extracts from normal and mutant cells, both grown in the presence of fetal-calf serum, were mixed, the activity of HMG CoA reductase was additive, indicating that the mutant cells did not lack an intracellular inhibitor of this enzyme.

If HMG CoA reductase activity is the rate-controlling step in cholesterol synthesis in human fibroblasts as it is in other mammalian tissues (12), then the failure of regulation of this enzyme should result in defective regulation of cholesterol synthesis from acetate but not mevalonate. That this was indeed the case is shown by the data in Table 1. Cholesterol synthesis from acetate in control fibroblasts increased by about 20-fold when fetal-calf serum was replaced with lipoprotein-deficient plasma and it decreased by 62% when LDL was added. In contrast, in the presence of fetal-calf serum, mutant fibroblasts synthesized cholesterol from acetate at a rate that was nearly 80-times greater than that of control cells; in addition, the mutant cells showed no response to alterations in the lipoprotein content of the medium. Mevalonic acid, the product of the HMG CoA reductase reaction, was incorporated into cholesterol at a similar rate in control and mutant cells and this rate was unaffected by alterations in lipoprotein content of the medium (Table 1). Although the experiments in Table 1 represent a valid comparison of the relative rates of cholesterol synthesis at one arbitrary concentration of either acetate or mevalonate, these substrate concentrations were such that maximal rates were not necessarily obtained. Consequently, stoichiometric comparisons between the rates of cholesterol synthesis from acetate and mevalonate in intact cells or a comparison of either of these rates with HMG CoA reductase activity in cell free extracts was not possible.

After we demonstrated that normal plasma LDL had no effect on cells of the homozygote, it was of interest to ascertain whether plasma LDL of the homozygote was capable of depressing HMG CoA reductase activity in normal cells. When equal concentrations of LDL isolated from a normolipidemic subject and from the homozygote J.P. were added to normal fibroblasts that had been previously grown in lipoprotein-deficient plasma, both LDL preparations reduced HMG CoA reductase activity in an identical manner (Fig. 2). In other experiments not shown, both types of LDL were identical in their inability to depress the HMG CoA reductase activity of the cells of J.P.

HMG CoA reductase activity from mutant and control cells showed identical Michaelis constants for the two substrates, HMG CoA and TPNH (Fig. 3). These kinetic data suggest that the increased HMG CoA reductase activity in the cells of the homozygote is not due to an enhanced affinity of the enzyme for one of its substrates.

To determine whether regulation of HMG CoA reductase activity in fibroblasts from heterozygotes with familial hypercholesterolemia was abnormal, the enzyme activity was studied in cultured cells of the parents of J.P., who are obligate heterozygotes for this disorder. In the presence of fetal-calf serum, the enzyme activity of the two heterozygotes resembled that of seven control lines (Fig. 4). However, when lipoproteins were removed, enzyme activity of the two heterozygotes became abnormally elevated and approached the levels seen in three unrelated homozygotes. A more clear-cut abnormality in these heterozygotes was demonstrated by the experiments in Fig. 5, in which the inhibitory response to LDL was compared in cell lines from two controls, two heterozygotes, and a homozygote. The heterozygotes showed a partial and intermediate defect in regulation of HMG CoA reductase activity by LDL.

DISCUSSION

In the experiments reported in this paper, cultured skin fibroblasts from three subjects with the homozygous form of familial hypercholesterolemia were shown to have a marked increase in the activity of the rate-controlling enzyme in cholesterol biosynthesis, HMG CoA reductase, when compared with cells from seven control subjects. The enhanced activity of the enzyme, which resulted from a complete absence of its normal regulation by lipoproteins, led to overproduction of cholesterol by the mutant cells. In fibroblasts

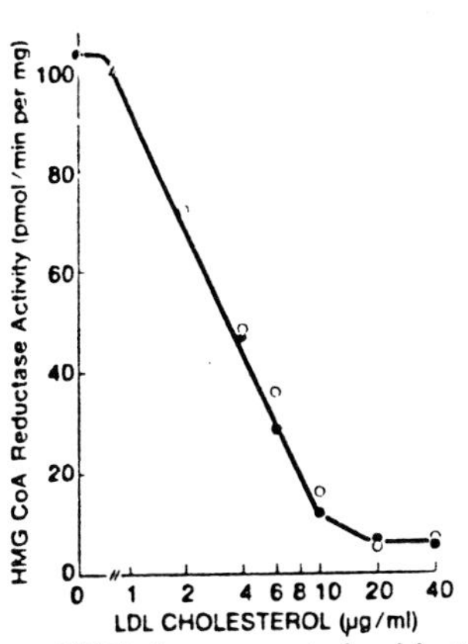

Proc. Nat. Acad. Sci. USA 70 (1973) HMG CoA Reductase in Familial Hypercholesterolemia 2807

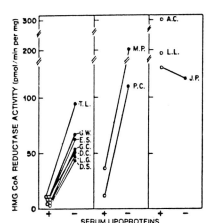

FIG. 2. Effect of LDL from a control subject and LDL from a patient with homozygous familial hypercholesterolemia (J.P.) on HMG CoA reductase activity of control fibroblasts. Cells were grown in dishes containing 10% fetal-calf serum; on day 6 the medium was replaced with 3 ml of fresh medium containing 5% human lipoprotein-deficient plasma. After 24 hr 0.1 ml of buffer A containing LDL from a control subject (●) or LDL from the homozygote J.P. (○) was added to give the indicated concentration. 6 hr later extracts were prepared and assayed for HMG CoA reductase activity.

FIG. 4. Regulation of HMG CoA reductase activity in fibroblasts from control subjects (*left*) and patients with the heterozygous (*middle*) and homozygous (*right*) forms of familial hypercholesterolemia. Cells were grown in dishes containing 10% fetal-calf serum; on day 6 the medium was replaced with 3 ml of fresh medium containing either 10% fetal-calf serum (0) or 5% human lipoprotein-deficient plasma (●). 18 hr later, extracts were prepared and assayed for HMG CoA reductase activity. Each value represents the mean enzyme activity of duplicate dishes. The initials of each subject correspond to those given in *Methods*.

from two obligate heterozygotes, HMG CoA reductase activity was higher than in controls and these cells showed a partial defect in enzyme regulation by LDL.

The failure of regulation of HMG CoA reductase activity in the mutant cells could be due either to a mutation in a structural gene for the enzyme itself or to a mutation in a gene that specifies an hitherto unidentified protein critical for normal regulation of the enzyme activity by lipoproteins. Two lines of evidence suggest that a mutation in a structural gene for the enzyme is not responsible for the observed defect. First, the normal process of regulation of this enzyme does not appear to

depend upon a property of the enzyme itself since no direct allosteric effects on the isolated enzyme can be demonstrated (13, 14); rather, its regulation appears to be mediated by alterations in enzyme synthesis and degradation (13). This observation implies that a genetically determined abnormality in the structure of HMG CoA reductase would produce a result different from that reported here in that it would lead to altered activity of the enzyme without affecting the process of its regulation (18). Second, the demonstration of apparently identical kinetic properties of the enzyme from normal and mutant cells also suggests that the enzyme itself may not be

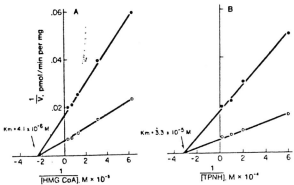

FIG. 3. Kinetic properties of HMG CoA reductase activity from fibroblasts of a control subject and a patient with homozygous familial hypercholesterolemia (J.P.). Cells were grown in dishes containing 10% fetal-calf serum; on day 6 the medium was removed and 3 ml of fresh medium containing 10% fetal-calf serum was added to the cells of the homozygote (○) and medium containing 5% human lipoprotein-deficient plasma was added to the cells of the control subject (●). 24 hr later, extracts were prepared and aliquots containing 22 μg of protein (homozygote) or 45 μg of protein (control) were assayed for HMG CoA reductase activity as described in *Methods* except that the concentrations of HMG CoA (*A*) and TPNH (*B*) were varied as indicated.

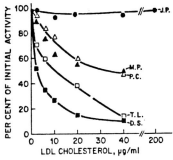

FIG. 5. Effect of LDL on HMG CoA reductase activity in fibroblasts from control subjects (*squares*), heterozygotes (*triangles*), and a homozygote (*circles*). Cells were grown in dishes containing 10% fetal-calf serum; on day 6 the medium was replaced with 3 ml of fresh medium containing 5% human lipoprotein-deficient plasma. After 24 hr, 0.1 ml of buffer A containing LDL from a control subject was added to give the indicated concentration. 6 hr later extracts were prepared and assayed for HMG CoA reductase. Results are plotted as the percentage of HMG CoA reductase activity of cells receiving only buffer A without LDL (initial activity). These values, expressed in pmol/min per mg were: J.P., 227; M.P., 211; P.C., 162; D.S., 65.4; T.L., 93.3.

2808 Genetics: Goldstein and Brown

Proc. Nat. Acad. Sci. USA 70 (1973)

altered. If further studies support the hypothesis that the mutation in these patients' cells involves a protein other than HMG CoA reductase, then identification of this putative gene product should provide new insight into the normal mechanism of regulation of cholesterol biosynthesis.

Our studies of cultured fibroblasts indicate that subjects with familial hypercholesterolemia of the type reported in this paper carry in all cells of the body an abnormal gene that has the potential to induce excessive cholesterol production. The tissues in which this abnormal gene is expressed *in vivo* and the conditions governing its expression cannot be determined from these cell-culture studies, since human cells of a given type in culture may express genes *in vitro* that they do not express *in vivo* (19). However, our data would seem to warrant the suggestion that accumulation of cholesterol in subjects with this disorder is due to a genetically determined defect in regulation of cholesterol synthesis at the level of HMG CoA reductase.

Dr. H. Peter Chase of the John F. Kennedy Child Development Center, the B. F. Stolinsky Research Laboratories, University of Colorado Medical Center, Denver, Colo., is the physician of J.P.; we thank him for calling our attention to this patient and for allowing us to obtain a skin biopsy from her and her parents. Dr. Jean D'Avignon of the Institut de Recherches Cliniques, Montreal, Canada, is the physician of L.L. and A.C.; we thank him for allowing us to obtain skin biopsies from them. Dr. Jean D. Wilson was of invaluable aid in the experiments in which cholesterol synthesis was measured. Suzanna E. Dana, Gwendolyn Fidler, Mary Jo Harrod, and Jean Helgerson provided excellent assistance. This research was supported by grants from the American Heart Association (72629) and the National Institutes of Health (GM 19258, CA 08501, and 5 TO1 AM05490). J.L.G. is the recipient of a USPHS Research Career Development Award 1K4-GM-70, 227-01.

1. Fredrickson, D. S. & Levy, R. I. (1972) in *The Metabolic Basis of Inherited Disease*, eds. Stanbury, J. B., Wyngaarden, J. B. & Fredrickson, D. S. (McGraw-Hill Book Co., New York), pp. 545–614.
2. Khachadurian, A. K. (1964) *Amer. J. Med.* 37, 402–407.
3. Nevin, N. C. & Slack, J. (1968) *J. Med. Genet.* 5, 9–28.
4. Schrott, H. G., Goldstein, J. L., Hazzard, W. R., McGoodwin, M. M. & Motulsky, A. G. (1972) *Ann. Intern. Med.* 76, 711–720.
5. Goldstein, J. L. (1972) *Birth Defects, Orig. Artic. Ser.* 8, 202–208.
6. Goldstein, J. L., Schrott, H. G., Hazzard, W. R., Bierman, E. L. & Motulsky, A. G. (1973) *J. Clin. Invest.* 52, 1544–1568.
7. Khachadurian, A. K. (1969) *Lancet*, ii, 778–780.
8. Myant, N. B. (1970) *Sci. Basis Med.* 10, 230–259.
9. Chida, N. & Okamura, T. (1971) *Tohoku J. Exp. Med.* 105, 147–155.
10. Miettinen, T. A., Pelkonen, R., Nikkila, E. A. & Heinonen, O. (1967) *Acta Med. Scand.* 182, 645–650.
11. Langer, T., Strober, W. & Levy, R. I. (1972) *J. Clin. Invest.* 51, 1528–1536.
12. Siperstein, M. D. (1970) in *Current Topics in Cellular Regulation*, eds. Stadtman, E. & Horecker, B. (Academic Press, New York), Vol. 2, p. 65.
13. Brown, M. S., Dana, S. E. & Goldstein, J. L. (1973) *Proc. Nat. Acad. Sci. USA* 70, 2162–2166.
14. Brown, M. S., Dana, S., Dietschy, J. M. & Siperstein, M. D. (1973) *J. Biol. Chem.*, 248, 4731–4738.
15. Wilson, J. D. (1972) *J. Clin. Invest.* 51, 1450–1458.
16. Dietschy, J. M. & Siperstein, M. D. (1967) *J. Lipid Res.* 8, 97–104.
17. Lowry, O. H., Roseborough, N. J., Farr, A. L. & Randall, R. J. (1951) *J. Biol. Chem.* 193, 265–275.
18. Yoshida, A. (1970) *J. Mol. Biol.* 52, 483–490.
19. Uhlendorf, B. M. & Mudd, S. H. (1968) *Science* 160, 1007–1008.

Hyperlipidemia in Coronary Heart Disease

I. LIPID LEVELS IN 500 SURVIVORS OF MYOCARDIAL INFARCTION

Joseph L. Goldstein, William R. Hazzard, Helmut G. Schrott,
Edwin L. Bierman, and Arno G. Motulsky with the assistance of
Mary Jo Levinski and Ellen D. Campbell

*From the Departments of Medicine (Division of Medical Genetics, University
Hospital, and Division of Metabolism and Gerontology, Veterans Administration
Hospital) and Genetics, University of Washington, Seattle, Washington 98195*

A B S T R A C T Plasma cholesterol and triglyceride levels were measured after an overnight fast in 500 consecutively studied 3-mo survivors of myocardial infarction. Virtually all patients under 60 yr of age (95% ascertainment) and a randomly chosen group of older survivors admitted to 13 Seattle hospitals during an 11 mo period were included. A comparison of their lipid values with those of 950 controls demonstrated that 31% had hyperlipidemia. These lipid abnormalities were most commonly found in males under 40 yr of age (60% frequency) and in females under 50 yr of age (60% frequency). Elevation in triglyceride levels with (7.8%) or without (15.6%) an associated elevation in cholesterol levels was three times more common in survivors than a high cholesterol level alone (7.6%). These results raise the possibility that hypertriglyceridemia may be as an important a risk factor for coronary atherosclerosis as hypercholesterolemia. The identification of hyper-

This work was presented in part at the 85th Session of the Association of American Physicians, Atlantic City, N. J., 2–3 May 1972, and published in the Transactions (1).

Dr. Goldstein was supported by Special National Institutes of Health Fellowship GM 4784-01 and is now a Research Career Development Awardee (1-K4-GM 70, 277-01) from the National Institute of General Medical Sciences. His present address is the Division of Medical Genetics, Department of Internal Medicine, University of Texas Southwestern Medical School, Dallas, Tex. 75235. Dr. Hazzard was the recipient of a Clinical Investigatorship of the Veterans Administration and is now an Investigator of the Howard Hughes Medical Institute. Dr. Schrott was supported by Special National Institutes of Health Fellowship HE-48 695. His present address is the Mayo Clinic and Mayo Foundation, Rochester, Minn. 55901.

Received for publication 20 September 1972 and in revised form 19 February 1973.

lipidemic survivors of myocardial infarction provided a unique source of probands for family studies designed to disclose the genetic origin of hyperlipidemia in coronary heart disease.

INTRODUCTION

It is generally recognized that coronary heart disease shows a tendency to aggregate in certain families (2–4). In his monograph on angina pectoris published in 1897, Osler emphasized the importance of genetic factors in the pathogenesis of this disorder (5). Yet despite early recognition of the influence of heredity on atherosclerosis, the nature of the underlying genetic mechanisms has remained obscure. The observed familial aggregation may reflect genetically determined risk factors such as hyperlipidemia, diabetes mellitus, and hypertension (6, 7). Hypercholesterolemia and hypertriglyceridemia, as predisposing factors to atherosclerosis, have received the most recent attention (7, 8). Hence, genetic analysis of families with elevations in these plasma lipids should contribute to an understanding of the inheritance of coronary atherosclerosis and ultimately provide clues for determining the underlying biochemical lesions. Certain forms of hypercholesterolemia and hypertriglyceridemia are known to be inherited (9–11). However, it is not known whether hereditary hyperlipidemia is usually determined by simply inherited (monogenic) factors or by more complex (polygenic) mechanisms, and whether classification of hyperlipidemia by lipoprotein phenotyping provides genetically useful information.

The present study was undertaken to answer these questions by carrying out a detailed genetic analysis of the fasting plasma cholesterol and triglyceride levels in the families of probands selected for hyperlipidemia from 500 consecutively studied survivors of myocardial infarction. The results are reported in three parts. This first paper discusses the criteria for diagnosis of hyperlipidemia, compares its frequency in survivors of myocardial infarction with that in controls, examines the effect of age and sex on its occurrence, and relates the presence of hypercholesterolemia and hypertriglyceridemia to other risk factors. The second paper (12) reports the analysis of family members, presents evidence for a newly recognized inherited disorder (combined hyperlipidemia), and suggests an approach to classifying hyperlipidemia on the basis of plasma lipid levels in relatives. The third paper (13) examines the genetic significance of lipoprotein phenotyping by determining the lipoprotein characteristics of survivors with different genetically defined lipid disorders.

METHODS

Ascertainment of hospital admissions for myocardial infarction. Two of us (J. L. G. and H. G. S.) examined the records of virtually all patients admitted to the coronary care units of 13 metropolitan Seattle hospitals from 1 November 1970, to 1 October 1971. The 13 hospitals involved are known to admit about 95% of all local patients with acute myocardial infarction (14, 15). The diagnosis of myocardial infarction was accepted when two of these three criteria were met: (*a*) compatible clinical history; (*b*) serial electrocardiograms showing development of a diagnostic Q wave or S–T segment elevation followed by T wave inversion (16); and (*c*) characteristic changes in activity of glutamic-oxalacetic transaminase, lactic dehydrogenase, and/or creatine phosphokinase (17) in serially drawn blood samples. Of the 2793 patients admitted to the 13 coronary care units during the period of the study, 1166 (41.8%) satisfied two of the above criteria. (Of these 1166 survivors, 1049 [90%] fulfilled all three criteria.) For each case, information about coronary heart disease, diabetes mellitus, thyroid disease, peripheral and cerebrovascular disease, hyperlipidemia, hypertension, smoking and drinking habits, weight change, dietary restrictions, and drug therapy was recorded on a

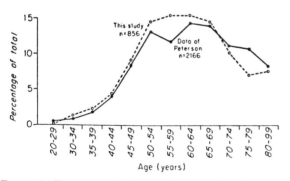

FIGURE 1   Frequency distribution of the number of hospital admissions for acute myocardial infarction in men of different ages, comparing the results of two different methods of ascertainment. The data of Peterson were collected from the same hospitals as our 11 mo study, but over a more extended period of time (31 December 1967 to 31 December 1969).

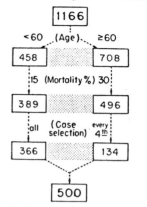

Admissions for Myocardial Infarction

Survivors Studied at 3 Months

FIGURE 2   Method of selection of 500 survivors of acute myocardial infarction for lipid studies. Details are described in the Methods.

standardized medical history form. The age distribution of all male cases identified during the 11 mo of our study was compared with that of a 24 mo epidemiologic study in this area, covering all hospital admissions for myocardial infarction (14, 15).[1] The close agreement between the two sets of data (Fig. 1) indicated that our ascertainment was valid.

Selection of survivors for lipid study. Of the 1166 patients with acute myocardial infarction, 885 were still alive at 3 mo after hospital admission,[2] and 500 were selected for study, as shown in Fig. 2. An attempt was made to study all survivors under 60 yr of age. Of the 389 survivors under 60 yr of age, 366 (95%) were included. The remaining 23 survivors in this age group were not studied either because they could not be located (9 patients), were psychiatrically unstable (3 patients), or were unwilling to cooperate (11 patients). No attempt was made to study all 496 3-mo survivors 60 yr of age and older. Random selection of 134 of this latter group was made by choosing every fourth consecutively admitted survivor. Whenever a survivor in this older age group either refused to participate (15 patients) or could not be located (5 patients), an alternate was selected on the basis of a similar time of hospital admission.

Survivors. Informed constant was obtained from each patient and his private physician. Survivors were seen 3–4 mo after the acute episode of myocardial infarction by one of two public health nurses (M. J. L. and E. D. C.). They determined the patient's weight and height, recorded a medical history on a standardized form, and collected 30 ml of blood after 12–14 h overnight fast. Before the interview, each survivor had been contacted four times: first by letter, explaining the general nature of the study; second by telephone, fixing the date and place of the interview; third by letter, confirming the date of the interview; and fourth by

---

[1] These data were made available by Donald R. Peterson, M.D., Professor of Epidemiology, School of Public Health and Community Medicine, University of Washington, Seattle, Wash.

[2] The mortality rate for 3-mo survivors of acute myocardial infarction was strikingly dependent on age. The highest mortality (30%) occurred in survivors age 60 and above, while only 15% of the survivors below age 60 expired within 3 mo. Below age 45 the mortality rate was 8%.

telephone, on the day before the interview. Participants were instructed to remain on their usual diet, and the importance of obtaining a *fasting* blood specimen (no food after 6 p.m.) was repeatedly emphasized. Interviews were conducted between 8 and 10 a.m. either in the patient's home (70%) or in the clinics of the University Hospital or the Veterans Administration Hospital (30%).

None of the 500 survivors selected was excluded from the study. However, at the time of sampling, 11 were taking clofibrate because hyperlipidemia had been previously diagnosed; of these 11, 5 had normal lipid levels when tested by us. No survivors were taking cholestyramine, nicotinic acid, d-thyroxine, or other hypolipidemic agents. Medications taken by the 99 female survivors included estrogens (14%), thyroid (11%), oral contraceptives (2%), and estrogens and thyroid (1%). 8 of the 500 survivors had disorders known to cause secondary elevations in blood lipids: 5 with uncontrolled diabetes mellitus (fasting plasma glucose level greater than 200 mg/100 ml) and 1 each with idiopathic nephrotic syndrome, chronic glomerulonephritis and uremia, and parenteral hyperalimentation after a small bowel resection. Three additional survivors had a previous diagnosis of primary hypothyroidism; all were receiving thyroid replacement therapy at the time of the study and were euthyroid on the basis of thyroid function tests. 44% of the 500 survivors said they were conscientiously following a diet low in content of cholesterol and fat, but there was no apparent correlation between dietary intake and levels of plasma lipids. The mean ±SD for adjusted cholesterol and triglyceride levels, respectively, was 233±56 and 143±114 mg/100 ml in those on a low fat diet, as compared with 239±51 and 129±74 mg/100 ml in those on an unrestricted diet. To determine weight stability, 129 hyperlipidemic and 27 normolipidemic survivors were weighed on two occasions averaging 3 mo apart. The mean change in weight was less than 0.4 kg for both groups (13).

Controls. The controls consisted of 550 adult women and 400 adult men selected from the nonblood relatives of the survivors. 125 were the spouses of the survivors and 825 were spouses of their relatives. All but 1% were white. None of these subjects was excluded as a control, but 4% had a history of previous myocardial infarction or were being treated with nitroglycerin for angina pectoris. 7.8% of controls indicated on a standardized medical history form that they had been diagnosed previously as having hyperlipidemia; only one of these individuals was on hypolipidemic drug therapy. 2.4% of controls claimed that they were conscientiously following a diet low in content of cholesterol and fat. One male control without known hyperlipidemia was taking clofibrate as part of another study. Drug therapy among the 550 female controls included estrogens (18.4%), thyroid (7.8%), oral contraceptives (9.2%), and both estrogens and thyroid (5.3%).

Collection of blood specimens. Fasting blood specimens from controls were obtained in one of two ways: (a) If the individual lived in the greater Seattle area, he was contacted and interviewed as described for survivors (see above) with the exception that each person filled out his own standardized medical history form. (b) Subjects living outside the Seattle area were initially contacted by telephone by J. L. G. or H. G. S., who explained the study, after which they were sent by mail the following items: (a) two tubes each containing 10 mg of ethylenediaminetetraacetic acid (EDTA) and one tube without EDTA; (b) a set of instructions addressed to a physician or technician collecting the blood sample; and (c) a standardized medical history form to be filled out by the individual. The instructions stated that 10 ml of blood was to be collected into each of the two tubes after a 12–14 h overnight fast and that the two EDTA tubes were to be centrifuged and the plasma placed in the empty tube for return to Seattle at ambient temperature by air mail, special delivery, in the stamped mailing container provided. The physician or technician was asked not to return specimens obtained on nonfasting subjects. Out-of-town specimens usually arrived at the Seattle laboratory within 24–36 h of collection and immediately refrigerated at 4°C until further processed.

The validity of this method of collection for out-of-town samples was established in a pilot study in which the distribution of fasting plasma cholesterol and triglyceride levels of 100 consecutively studied out-of-town controls was compared with that of 100 consecutively studied Seattle controls. Mean ±SD for age and sex-adjusted cholesterol values was 223±41 and 225±46 mg/100 ml for out-of-town and Seattle controls, respectively. Mean ±SD for age and sex-adjusted triglyceride values was 94±64 and 94±59 mg/100 ml for out-of-town and Seattle controls, respectively.

Analyses of plasma lipids, glucose, and uric acid. All analyses were performed on fasting venous blood samples collected in tubes containing EDTA (10 mg/10 ml blood). Samples obtained in Seattle were centrifuged at 3000 rpm for 15 min within 2 h of collection. Out-of-town plasma samples were recentrifuged in a similar fashion. All plasma samples were kept frozen at −20°C until analysis.

All lipid analyses were performed in the laboratory of the Division of Metabolism and Gerontology under the supervision of W. R. H. and E. L. B. Plasma cholesterol and triglyceride concentrations were measured from separate portions of a single chloroform: methanol (2:1 vol:vol) extract. Cholesterol was measured by AutoAnalyzer method N-24a (18) and triglyceride by a semiautomated method modified from the procedure of Carlson (19, 20). This laboratory had previously passed phase I of the triglyceride standardization program of the U. S. Center for Disease Control (Atlanta, Ga.) with a coefficient of variation of 5% and accuracy within 10% of the true value. Reproducibility of these methods was determined periodically throughout the 15 mo of analyses by repeated checking (n = 128) of portions from a frozen standard plasma pool. Results (mean ±SD) for this standard were: cholesterol, 244±9.5 mg/100 ml and triglyceride, 90±3.7 mg/100 ml. Coefficients of variation were 3.9 and 4.3%, respectively. Similar results were also obtained by using a lower standard cholesterol plasma (level of 164 mg/100 ml) and a higher standard triglyceride plasma (level of 234 mg/100 ml). Samples from controls and survivors were analyzed simultaneously throughout the study.

The glucose and uric acid levels, measured on the fasting plasma samples of survivors, were determined by AutoAnalyzer methods N-2b and N-13b respectively (21) at the Pathology Central Laboratory, Seattle, Wash. Reproducibility of these methods was checked periodically throughout the 2 wk of analyses by examining a frozen plasma standard. Results (mean ±SD) for these standards were 109±0.84 mg/100 ml for glucose (n = 50) and 5.4±0.1 mg/100 ml for uric acid (n = 50). Coefficients of variation were 0.8 and 1.8%, respectively.

Processing, transformation, and analysis of data. Data processing was performed on the CDC 6400 computer at the University of Washington Computer Center. Initial input was by key punched cards with permanent storage of the raw and transformed data on magnetic tape.

Hyperlipidemia in Coronary Heart Disease 1535

To allow comparison of cholesterol and triglyceride levels of controls and survivors of different age and sex, lipid levels were transformed by using control means derived by linear regression analysis. This transformation was based on the following principle (22): For each individual the deviation of his lipid level from that of the control mean for his or her age and sex was given a positive or negative sign according to whether it was above or below the mean value. This deviation was then adjusted to a reference age at which the mean and standard deviation was the same for the two sexes; in this way the lipid values were adjusted also for sex. The formula used was as follows: adjusted lipid value = (observed lipid value − control mean lipid value of appropriate age and sex) + mean lipid value at age 45 yr of appropriate sex. Control mean lipids values for men and women at different ages were derived from the regression equations for the appropriate sex: $y = ax + b$, where y = mean cholesterol concentration or mean $\log_{10}$ triglyceride concentration; x = age in years; a = average annual change of cholesterol or $\log_{10}$ triglyceride concentration; and b = cholesterol or $\log_{10}$ triglyceride concentration when $x = 0$. The constants for a (coefficient of linear regression) and b (y intercept) used in the calculation of the adjusted lipid values are summarized in Table I.[3] Under these conditions of the regression equations, mean lipid values for both men and women were nearly equivalent at age 45 yr. Since the logarithms of triglyceride levels in controls were found to be distributed more normally than the corresponding skewed, untransformed values, the log scale was used for age and sex adjustments of triglyceride with subsequent reconversion to the arithmetic scale.

Data were analyzed by the following procedures: (a) Estimates of various population parameters, such as means, standard deviations, and correlation coefficients, were made with standard statistical package programs such as XTAB (Computer Programs for Biomedical Data Processing)[4] and BMD (Biomedical Computer Programs).[5] (b) Frequency distributions of plasma cholesterol and triglyceride concentrations were plotted on relative frequency histograms with interval widths of 10 mg/100 ml. Smooth distribution curves for both the adjusted cholesterol and adjusted triglyceride values of the control group were drawn with a CalComp Plotter.[6] The plotted values were calculated by a method developed by Tarter and Kronmal, which uses the or-

thogonal polynomial to derive nonparametric density estimates for the distributions (23). (c) Upper percentile lipid values (i.e., 90th, 95th, and 99th percentile cut-off points) in the controls were computed from the adjusted mean and standard deviation values of their respective normal distributions (Fig. 4) in conjunction with a table of cumulative standardized normal values (24). The actual mean and standard deviation values used were 219 and 40 for cholesterol and 1.922 and 0.202 for $\log_{10}$ triglyceride. Since the logarithms of the triglyceride of controls were more normally distributed than the corresponding untransformed, skewed values, percentile values for triglyceride were derived from the sex and age-adjusted $\log_{10}$ values. For clarity of presentation, all log percentile values were reconverted to the arithmetic scale. Therefore, our computed upper percentile cut-off values for triglyceride (Table II) are not directly applicable to untransformed triglyceride data. However, they can be used as approximate guidelines for "upper limits of normal" if the untransformed values are increased by 10–15 mg/100 ml.[7] In other words, the 95th percentile cut-off point for the untransformed triglyceride level of a 45-yr old man or women would be about 175 mg/100 ml (165 + 10) and the corresponding 99th percentile value would be about 215 mg/100 ml (200 + 15) (Table II).

RESULTS

Plasma lipid levels in controls. The age and sex composition of the 950 controls and their unadjusted and untransformed lipid values grouped by decade are shown in Table III. These figures were remarkably similar to those reported in other studies (25, 26).

A plot of unadjusted control cholesterol levels against age (Fig. 3 A) showed that in both sexes cholesterol concentration increased with age up to about 60 yr, that the rate of increase with age (coefficient of linear regression) was higher in women than in men (Table I), and that the standard deviations of cholesterol at different ages were nearly identical. Above age 60 the cholesterol level in men fell sharply, suggesting the possibility that hypercholesterolemic men die prematurely. A comparable fall in female levels was not seen until after age 70. At age 45 the mean cholesterol values for men and women, as determined from the regression equations, were equal (220 mg/100 ml).

Triglyceride levels in controls also increased with age (Fig. 3 B and Table I), especially in women (Table I). Unlike the constant variation pattern seen for cholesterol, the standard deviations of triglyceride differed markedly at different ages, especially above age 40. However, when the triglyceride data were converted to the logarithmic scale (Fig. 3 C), this age variation was much less apparent. At age 45, the mean $\log_{10}$ value for triglyceride levels in both sexes was nearly equal (1.921 and 1.937, respectively). In contrast to the cholesterol data, no

---

[3] Although the relationship between age and cholesterol for men fit a quadratic function better than a linear function (Fig. 3), age and sex-adjustments were carried out on the linear scale for the following reasons: (a) assuming that the fall that is observed in cholesterol levels in men above age 60 (and to some extent in triglyceride levels in men above 60) occurs because older hyperlipidemic men die prematurely, the adjustment on a fitted curvilinear regression line would result in a false elevation of the values of the surviving older individuals; and (b) as compared with adjustment on a fitted curvilinear line, adjustment by linear regression had the overall effect of underestimating, rather than overestimating the absolute levels of cholesterol or triglyceride in older men and hence the data were not biased in favor of high values. Patterson and Slack also found linear regression to be a satisfactory method for age and sex adjustment of lipid levels (26).

[4] University of Washington Computer Center Manual, Seattle, Wash. 1968.

[5] University of California Press, Berkeley, Calif. 1968.

[6] California Computer Products, Inc., Anaheim, Calif.

[7] For a skewed distribution in which the sample mean is greater than the median, the antilog of the geometric mean (i.e., the mean of the log values comprising the sample) is always lower than the arithmetic mean of the corresponding antilog values.

TABLE I

Summary of Data in 950 Controls as Derived from Regression Analyses

Plasma lipid	Correlation with age	Coefficient of linear regression	Y intercept‡	Mean lipid level at age 45	Standard deviation about regression line
		mg/100 ml per yr	mg/100 ml	mg/100 ml	
Cholesterol					
Women, n = 550	+0.41*	1.450	155	220	44.6
Men, n = 400	+0.21*	0.610	193	220	43.6
Triglyceride					
Women	+0.32*	1.294	35	94	52.0
Men	+0.23*	0.759	63	97	50.5
Log₁₀ triglyceride					
Women	+0.33*	0.0057	1.66	1.921	0.205
Men	+0.27*	0.0037	1.77	1.937	0.207

* Denotes statistical level of significance at <0.001 using t test.
‡ See Fig. 3.

significant decrease in triglyceride levels was noted in older individuals. Carlson and Lindstedt have reported that the mean triglyceride levels in "healthy" individuals (i.e., those without obesity, coronary heart disease, and hypertension) decrease markedly after age 60 (27). The difference in our data may be related to the fact that all of our spouse controls would not be considered "healthy," since no spouses were excluded because of obesity, hypertension, coronary artery disease, diabetes mellitus, or because they were taking medications known to raise triglyceride levels (e.g., estrogens [28]).

A summary of the data derived from the regression analyses of plasma lipids with age in the 950 controls is presented in Table I. As noted in the previous section, both the cholesterol and triglyceride regression lines of male and female controls crossed each other at age 45 yr, so that adjustment of all values to this age avoided the need for correction for sex. Furthermore, since the standard deviations about the cholesterol and log₁₀ tri-

glyceride regression lines were the same in both sexes at different ages, no additional corrections were necessary.

The frequency distribution of the adjusted lipid values in the 950 controls is shown in Fig. 4. The adjusted cholesterol levels appeared normally and unimodally distributed (Fig. 4 A), so that transformation of the data was not necessary for calculation of percentile values. The 90th, 95th, and 99th percentile values were 270, 285,

TABLE II

Estimated Upper Percentile Values for Sex and Age-Adjusted Plasma Lipids in Controls

Plasma lipid	Upper percentiles		
	90th	95th	99th
	mg/100 ml		
Cholesterol	270	285	314
Triglyceride	147	165	200

Percentile values were computed from the mean and standard deviation estimates of the respective normal distributions of adjusted cholesterol and adjusted log₁₀ triglyceride as described in the Methods.

TABLE III

Unadjusted Plasma Lipid Levels in Controls

Age range	No.	950 Spouse controls	
		Cholesterol Mean ±SD	Triglyceride Mean ±SD
yr		mg/100 ml	mg/100 ml
Men			
15–19	13	168±27	53±22
20–29	13	192±33	76±37
30–39	62	212±34	92±56
40–49	116	226±43	101±47
50–59	85	239±42	109±58
60–69	51	226±39	103±58
70–79	24	200±39	98±43
80–89	6	169±21	98±19
Total	400		
Women			
15–19	11	183±17	71±27
20–29	47	199±36	79±40
30–39	88	196±39	73±38
40–49	168	215±42	87±46
50–59	162	238±43	107±55
60–69	55	250±49	98±47
70–79	19	230±32	146±78
Total	550		

Hyperlipidemia in Coronary Heart Disease   1537

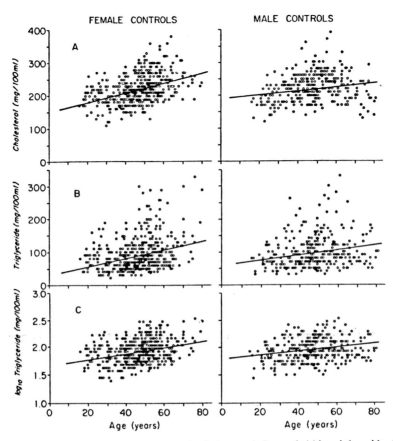

FIGURE 3   Relation between age and the levels of plasma cholesterol (A), triglyceride (B), and log₁₀ triglyceride (C) in controls. The female data consist of the lipid values determined for the first 400 consecutively studied individuals of a total female control group of 550. The male data consists of the lipid values determined for the first 300 consecutively studied individuals of a total male control group of 400. The triglyceride values of four controls (301, 450, 680, 850 mg/100 ml), although included in the calculation of the regression equations, are not shown in panels B and C.

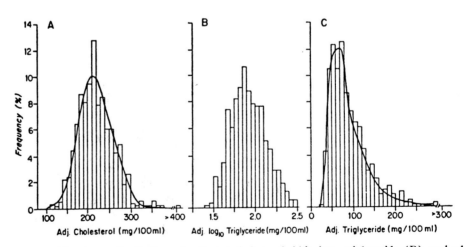

FIGURE 4   Frequency distributions of adjusted cholesterol (A), log₁₀ triglyceride (B), and adjusted triglyceride (C) levels in 950 controls. The smooth curve represents a nonparametric density estimate of the distribution and was plotted as described in the Methods.

TABLE IV

Age and Sex Composition of 500 Survivors of Myocardial Infarction

Age range	500 Survivors	
	No. of men	No. of women
yr		
30–39*	23	2
40–49*	88	19
50–59*	199	35
60–69‡	57	18
70–79‡	24	19
80–89‡	10	6
Total	401	99

* Represents virtually complete ascertainment of 3-mo survivors of myocardial infarction.

‡ Represents a randomly chosen group of 3-mo survivors of myocardial infarction (one out of four selected).

and 314 mg/100 ml, respectively (Table II). Since the adjusted log₁₀ triglyceride levels appeared normally and unimodally distributed (Fig. 4 B), estimations of percentile values for this lipid class were carried out in logarithms, and the values were reconverted to their antilogs and expressed as adjusted triglyceride values. The 90th, 95th and 99th percentile values were 147, 165, and 200 mg/100 ml, respectively (Table II). The distribution of the adjusted triglyceride levels was skewed to the higher values (Fig. 4 C).

Plasma lipid levels in survivors. The age and sex composition of the 500 survivors of acute myocardial infarction is shown in Table IV. 92.2% were non-Jewish white, and 5% were Jewish; 1.4% were black; and the remaining 1.4% were either Indian, Filipino, Puerto Rican, Japanese, or Arab.

Figs. 5 and 6 show that distribution of adjusted lipid levels in the survivors of myocardial infarction. In the males the distributions of cholesterol (Fig. 5 A) and triglyceride (Fig. 6 A) appeared unimodal, although both curves showed a deficiency of low values and an excess of high values as compared with those of controls. In the females the lipid distributions appeared more abnormal and were suggestive of bimodality, especially with regard to triglyceride (Figs. 5 B and 6 B).

Since bimodality could not be unequivocally demonstrated in these lipid distributions, arbitrary cut-off values had to be established for classifying survivors as hyperlipidemic or normal. The proportion of survivors exceeding several upper limits of normal for plasma lipids are shown in Table V. From these comparisons of the distribution of lipids in survivors and controls, a number of points are evident: (*a*) hypertriglyceridemia was more

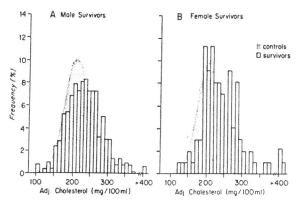

FIGURE 5 Frequency distributions of adjusted cholesterol levels in male (A) and female (B) survivors of myocardial infarction. The distribution is divided into increments of 10 mg/100 ml. The smooth stippled curve represents a nonparametric density estimate of the control distribution.

common among survivors than hypercholesterolemia no matter which upper limits of normal were used to define hyperlipidemia; (*b*) the separation between controls and survivors was greatest at the 99.9th percentile for both cholesterol and triglyceride, there being a 36-fold difference for cholesterol and an 80-fold difference for triglyceride in the observed/expected ratio of the two groups; and (*c*) although the 99.9th percentile value was associated with the highest ratio of survivors/controls for both plasma lipids, a clear-cut excess of survivors/controls was also apparent when the 99th, 95th, and 90th percentile values were used as cut-off levels for hyperlipidemia.

Frequency of hyperlipidemia in survivors. When the 95th percentile was used to separate normals and affected, 157 (31.0%) of the 500 survivors were consid-

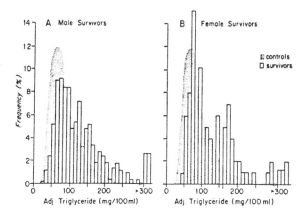

FIGURE 6 Frequency distribution of adjusted triglyceride levels in male (A) and female (B) survivors of myocardial infarction. The distribution is divided into increments of 10 mg/100 ml. The smooth stippled curve represents a nonparametric density estimate of the control distribution.

TABLE V

Comparison of Hyperlipidemia in 500 Survivors and 950 Controls

Percentile of controls	Adjusted cholesterol*			Adjusted triglyceride*		
	Expected‡	Observed§	Observed/Expected	Expected‡	Observed§	Observed/Expected
	%	%		%	%	
80th	20	33.8	1.7	20	42.2	2.1
90th	10	22.2	2.2	10	32.2	3.2
95th	5	15.4	3.1	5	23.5	4.7
99th	1	6.8	6.8	1	14.3	14.3
99.9th‖	0.1	3.8	38.0	0.1	8.0	80.0

* Independent of level of other plasma lipid.

‡ Expected = percent of controls with plasma lipid level equal to or exceeding indicated percentile.

§ Observed = percent of survivors with plasma lipid level equal to or exceeding indicated percentile.

‖ 99.9th percentile for adjusted cholesterol = 342 mg/100 ml and for adjusted tryglyceride = 245 mg/100 ml.

ered hyperlipidemic (Table VI). 78 (15.6%) showed hypertriglyceridemia without associated hypercholesterolemia; 41 (7.8%) showed both hypercholesterolemia and hypertriglyceridemia; and 38 (7.6%) showed hypercholesterolemia without associated hypertriglyceridemia.

The relation between the frequency of hyperlipidemia and the age and sex of survivors is shown in Fig. 7. The highest frequency (60%) was found in male survivors below age 40 and female survivors below age 50. With increasing age, the proportion of males with hyperlipidemia decreased markedly and by age 70 was almost zero. However, in the women hyperlipidemia remained at relatively high frequencies in the older ages, and about 30% of women between ages 70 and 79 had elevated levels.

TABLE VI

Overall Frequency of Hyperlipidemia in 500 Survivors

Lipid elevation	Frequency	
	Number	Percentage
		%
Hypercholesterolemia alone		
Adjusted cholesterol ≥ 285 mg/100 ml	38	7.6
Adjusted triglyceride < 165 mg/100 ml		
Hypertriglyceridemia alone		
Adjusted cholesterol < 285 mg/100 ml	78	15.6
Adjusted triglyceride ≥ 165 mg/100 ml		
Both		
Adjusted cholesterol ≥ 285 mg/100 ml	41	7.8
Adjusted triglyceride ≥ 165 mg/100 ml		
Total	157*	31.0

* This total becomes 162 (32%) if five normolipidemic survivors who were taking clofibrate for previously diagnosed hyperlipidemia had been included.

Risk factors in hyperlipidemic and normolipidemic survivors. To determine the relation between hyperlipidemia and other risk factors for coronary heart disease, the frequency of diabetes mellitus, hypertension, obesity, hyperuricemia, and excessive smoking among normolipidemic and hyperlipidemic survivors was compared (Table VII). Obesity was significantly more frequent among hyperlipidemic survivors than among those with normal lipids. This increase in obesity in the hypercholesterolemic group was apparently independent of any associated hypertriglyceridemia, since hypercholesterolemic survivors with triglyceride values below 165 mg/100 ml (n = 38) had a similar proportion of obesity (23.8%). Both diabetes mellitus and hypertension occurred more commonly in the hypertriglyceridemic survivors than in either the hypercholesterolemic or normolipidemic survivors. Hyperuricemia and excessive smoking appeared equally common among hypercholesterolemic, hypertriglyceridemic, and normolipidemic survivors.

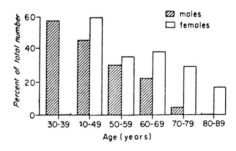

FIGURE 7 Relation between frequency of hyperlipidemia and age and sex of survivors. The number of survivors in each age and sex category is indicated in Table IV.

TABLE VII

Frequency of Risk Factors in Normolipidemic and Hyperlipidemic Survivors‡

	Frequency			
Risk factor	All survivors (n = 500)	Normolipidemic survivors (n = 343)	Hypercholesterolemic survivors§ (n = 78)	Hypertriglyceridemic survivors§ (n = 118)
			%	
Diabetes mellitus‖	12.6	11.1	11.5	18.6
Hypertension¶	15.4	13.4	16.6	21.2*
Obesity**	17.2	14.0	25.5*	*24.5*
Hyperuricemia‡‡	13.8	13.1	14.1	19.5
Excessive smoking§§	39.5	38.5	44.0	40.8

* Denotes statistical level of significance at 0.05 (italicized number denotes 0.01) using Chi-square test to compare proportion with risk factor in hyperlipidemic with that in normolipidemic group.

‡ 95th percentile values used to define hyperlipidemia.

§ Independent of level of other plasma liquid.

‖ Diagnosed if one of two criteria fulfilled: (*a*) survivor taking either insulin or an oral antihyperglycemic medication; or (*b*) fasting plasma glucose >120 mg/100 ml.

¶ Considered present if past history of specific treatment with antihypertensive drug therapy. Frequency of hypertension by same criterion in controls was 6.2%.

** Weight in excess of 125% of ideal body weight by criteria of Metropolitan Life Insurance Company tables (51). Frequency of obesity by same criteria in controls was 16.8%.

‡‡ Plasma uric acid ≥ 7.0 mg/100 ml in women and ≥ 8.0 mg/100 ml in men (52).

§§ More than 20 cigarettes per day. Frequency of excessive smoking by same criterion in controls was 10.0%.

DISCUSSION

The extensive epidemiological investigations in the last decade have established an association between coronary heart disease and elevated levels of plasma cholesterol and triglyceride (6–8, 29–32). Less certain, however, is the frequency of lipid abnormalities and the nature of the different types of hyperlipidemia in carefully defined patients with coronary heart disease, such as survivors of myocardial infarction or patients with angiographically proven coronary heart disease. Although in a number of recent investigations the plasma lipids in such patients have been measured (33–47), most of these studies were performed either on small numbers of patients, often without adequate control data, or on biased, nonrandom groups of patients. However, Patterson and Slack's recent investigation was carefully designed and had few biases in patient ascertainment (26). They found that about one-fourth of survivors of myocardial infarction were hyperlipidemic as defined by a cholesterol or triglyceride level exceeding 2 SD of control values. Their study included a total of 193 patients, representing about 50% of all their consecutively ascertained hospital survivors of myocardial infarction (26).

The design of our study differs from all previous investigations. A large control group consisting of 950 spouses was obtained for direct comparisons of plasma lipid levels with survivors and their relatives (12). We studied virtually all 3-mo survivors under age 60 in a large metropolitan area (population estimated at 700,000) during an 11 mo period. One-fourth of the other survivors who were aged 60 and older were selected at random and also included in the study. This approach permitted a more rigorous and less biased measurement of the frequency and characterization of hyperlipidemia in patients with myocardial infarction.

The results of the present study show that when the 95th percentile of controls was used as a cut-off level, hyperlipidemia was found in 31% of the 500 consecutively studied survivors of myocardial infarction. Moreover, the presence of hyperlipidemia in survivors was critically dependent on both age and sex. The highest frequency of hyperlipidemia (60%) was found in male survivors below age 40 and in female survivors below age 50.

The finding that hypertriglyceridemia with or without associated hypercholesterolemia occurred in survivors at nearly three times the frequency of hypercholesterolemia alone raises the possibility that the level of plasma triglyceride may be as important a risk factor for coronary atherosclerosis as is the level of plasma cholesterol.

In this respect, these data are in close agreement with the studies of Albrink, Meigs, and Man (31) and Carlson (33, 34, 37, 48), who have stressed the importance of triglyceride as a predictor of coronary artery disease. An alternative explanation for the high frequency of triglyceride elevations observed among our survivors may be related to the dietary alterations applied to subjects surviving a myocardial infarction. Since a diet low in content of cholesterol and fat can reduce cholesterol and often elevate triglyceride levels (49), the effect of such a diet may have minimized the prevalence of hypercholesterolemia and maximized the prevalance of hypertriglyceridemia in the survivors as a group. However, this possibility seems unlikely in view of the family data reported in the next paper in this series (12), which demonstrate that as a whole elevations in triglyceride were more common than elevations in cholesterol among the presumably "healthy" relatives of these hyperlipidemic survivors of myocardial infarction.

Another interesting finding emerged from comparing the frequencies of nonlipid risk factors (viz., hypertension, diabetes mellitus, smoking, obesity, and hyperuricemia) among the normolipidemic, hypercholesterolemia, and hypertriglyceridemic survivors. Among hypertriglyceridemic survivors, there was significantly more obesity, hypertension, and diabetes mellitus than in either the hypercholesterolemic or normolipidemic survivors. This unique aggregation of metabolic abnormalities in certain patients with coronary heart disease has been noted previously (50).

The single most important result of this study was the identification of a large number ($n = 157$) of hyperlipidemic survivors of myocardial infarction who represented unselected patients with coronary heart disease and provided probands for investigating the genetics of hyperlipidemia. As demonstrated in the next paper in this series (12), the genetic approach to hyperlipidemia in coronary heart disease offers a powerful tool for classifying lipid disorders and for clarifying basic mechanisms.

ACKNOWLEDGMENTS

We are indebted to the following colleagues for their able assistance in carrying out these studies: Stanley Albert for computer programming; Martha Salsburg, Susan Mar, and Kathryn Bakeman for clerical help; Martha Kimura, Y.-L. Lee Lum, and Marilyn Vogel for lipid analyses; Dr. Pat Wahl of the Department of Biostatistics for statistical analyses; Dr. Donald R. Peterson of the Department of Epidemiology and International Health for epidemiological consultation; Dr. Joseph Felsenstein of the Department of Genetics, University of Washington, Seattle, and Dr. Newton Morton, Population Genetics Laboratory, University of Hawaii, Honolulu, for statistical consultation; and Dr. Eloise R. Giblett for critical review of the manuscript.

This work was supported by U. S. Public Health Service Grants GM 15253, AM 06670, and HD 04872; by a grant from the Washington State Heart Association; by National Institutes of Health contract NHLI 71-2157; and by the Veterans Administration.

REFERENCES

1. Goldstein, J. L., W. R. Hazzard, H. G. Schrott, E. L. Bierman, and A. G. Motulsky. 1972. Genetics of hyperlipidemia in coronary heart disease. *Trans. Assoc. Am. Physicians Phila.* 85: 120.

2. Gertler, M. M., and P. D. White. 1954. Coronary Heart Disease in Young Adults: A Multidisciplinary Study. Harvard University Press, Cambridge, Mass.

3. Thomas, C. B., and B. H. Cohen. 1955. The familial occurrence of hypertension and coronary heart disease, with observations concerning obesity and diabetes. *Ann. Intern. Med.* 42: 90.

4. Slack, J., and K. A. Evans. 1966. The increased risk of death from ischemic heart disease in first degree relatives of 121 men and 96 women with ischemic heart disease. *J. Med. Genet.* 3: 239.

5. Osler, W. 1897. Lectures on Angina Pectoris and Allied States. Appleton-Century-Crofts, New York. 24.

6. Epstein, F. H., and L. D. Ostrander, Jr. 1971. Detection of individual susceptibility toward coronary disease. *Prog. Cardiovasc. Dis.* 13: 324.

7. Adlersberg, D. 1951. Hypercholesteremia with predisposition to atherosclerosis: an inborn error of lipid metabolism. *Am. J. Med.* 11: 600.

8. Kannel, W. B., W. P. Castelli, T. Gordon, and P. M. McNamara. 1971. Serum cholesterol, lipoproteins, and the risk of coronary heart disease. *Ann. Intern. Med.* 74: 1.

9. Fredrickson, D. S., and R. I. Levy. 1972. Familial hyperlipoproteinemias. *In* The Metabolic Basis of Inherited Disease. J. B. Stanbury, J. B. Wyngaarden, and D. S. Fredrickson, editors. McGraw-Hill Book Company, New York. 3rd edition. 545.

10. Slack, J., and N. C. Nevin. 1971. Hereditary aspects of hyperlipidemic states. *In* Treatment of the Hyperlipidemic States. H. R. Casdorph, editor. Charles C. Thomas, Publisher, Springfield, Ill. 121.

11. Epstein, F. H. 1967. Risk Factors in coronary heart disease: environmental and hereditary influences. *Isr. J. Med. Sci.* 3: 594.

12. Goldstein, J. L., H. G. Schrott, W. R. Hazzard, E. L. Bierman, and A. G. Motulsky. 1973. Hyperlipidemia in coronary heart disease. II. Genetic analysis of lipid levels in 176 families and delineation of a new inherited disorder, combined hyperlipidemia. *J. Clin. Invest.* 52: 1544.

13. Hazzard, W. R., J. L. Goldstein, H. G. Schrott, A. G. Motulsky, and E. L. Bierman. 1973. Hyperlipidemia in coronary heart disease. III. Evaluation of lipoprotein phenotypes of 156 genetically defined survivors of myocardial infarction. *J. Clin. Invest.* 52: 1569.

14. Most, A. S., and D. R. Peterson. 1969. Myocardial infarction surveillance in a metropolitan community. *J. Am. Med. Assoc.* 208: 2433.

15. Peterson, D. R., D. J. Thompson, and N. Chinn. 1972. Ischaemic heart disease prognosis: a community-wide assessment (1966–1969). *J. Am. Med. Assoc.* 219: 1423.

16. Rose, G. A., and H. Blackburn. 1968. Cardiovascular survey methods. *W. H. O. Monogr. Ser.* 56: 1.

17. Friedberg, C. K. 1966. Diseases of the Heart. W. B. Saunders Company, Philadelphia. 810.

18. Technicon Instrument Corporation. 1965. Total cholesterol procedure N-24a. Autoanalyzer Manual. Tarrytown, N. Y.
19. Carlson, L. A. 1959. Determination of serum glycerides. *Acta Soc. Med. Ups.* **64**: 208.
20. Bierman, E. L., and J. T. Hamlin, III. 1961. The hyperlipiemic effect of a low-fat, high-carbohydrate diet in diabetic subjects. *Diabetes.* **10**: 432.
21. Technicon Instrument Corporation. 1965. Glucose procedure N-2b. Uric acid procedure N-13b. Autoanalyzer Manual. Tarrytown. N. Y.
22. Hamilton, M., G. W. Pickering, J. A. F. Roberts, and G. S. C. Sowry. 1954. The aetiology of essential hypertension. 4. The role of inheritance. *Clin. Sci. (Oxf.).* **13**: 273.
23. Tarter, M. E., and R. A. Kronmal. 1970. On multivariate density estimates based on orthogonal expansions. *Ann. Math. Stat.* **41**: 718.
24. Snedecor, G. W., and W. G. Cochran. 1967. Statistical Methods. Iowa State University Press, Ames, Iowa. 6th edition. 548.
25. Johnson, B. C., F. H. Epstein, and M. O. Kjelsber. 1965. Distributions and familial studies of blood pressure and serum cholesterol levels in a total community—Tecumseh, Michigan. *J. Chronic Dis.* **18**: 147.
26. Patterson, D., and J. Slack. 1972. Lipid abnormalities in male and female survivors of myocardial infarction and their first degree relatives. *Lancet.* **1**: 393.
27. Carlson, L. A., and S. Lindstedt. 1968. The Stockholm prospective study. 1. The initial values for plasma lipids. *Acta Med. Scand. Suppl.* **493**: 1.
28. Hazzard, W. R., M. J. Spiger, J. D. Bagdade, and E. L. Bierman. 1969. Studies on the mechanism of increased plasma triglyceride levels induced by oral contraceptives. *N. Engl. J. Med.* **280**: 471.
29. Stamler, J., H. A. Lindberg, D. M. Berkson, A. Shaffer, W. Miller, and A. Poindexter. 1960. Prevalence and incidence of coronary heart disease in strata of the labor force of a Chicago industrial corporation. *J. Chronic Dis.* **11**: 405.
30. Ostrander, L. D., Jr., B. J. Neff, W. D. Block, T. Francis, Jr., and F. H. Epstein. 1967. Hyperglycemia and hypertriglyceridemia among persons with coronary heart disease. *Ann. Intern. Med.* **67**: 34.
31. Albrink, M. J., J. W. Meigs, and E. B. Man. 1961. Serum lipids, hypertension, and coronary artery disease. *Am. J. Med.* **31**: 4.
32. Brown, D. F., S. H. Kinch, and J. T. Doyle. 1965. Serum triglycerides in health and in ischaemic heart disease. *N. Engl. J. Med.* **273**: 947.
33. Carlson, L. A. 1960. Serum lipids in men with myocardial infarction. *Acta Med. Scand.* **167**: 399.
34. Havel, R. J., and L. A. Carlson. 1962. Serum lipoproteins, cholesterol and triglycerides in coronary heart disease. *Metab. (Clin. Exp.).* **11**: 195.
35. Kroman, H., J. Nodine, S. Bender, and A. Brest. 1964. Lipids in normals and patients with coronary artery disease. *Am. J. Med. Sci.* **248**: 571.
36. Hatch, F. T., P. K. Reissell, T. M. W. Poon-King, G. P. Canellos, R. S. Lees, and L. M. Hagopian. 1966.

A study of coronary heart disease in young men. *Circulation.* **33**: 679.
37. Carlson, L. A., and F. Wahlberg. 1966. Serum lipids, intravenous glucose tolerance, and their interrelation studied in ischemic cardiovascular disease. *Acta Med. Scand.* **180**: 307.
38. Cramer, K., S. Paulin, and L. Werko. 1966. Coronary angiographic findings in correlation with age, body weight, blood pressure, serum lipids, and smoking habits. *Circulation.* **33**: 888.
39. Rifkind, B. M., D. Lawson, and M. Gale. 1968. Diagnostic value of serum lipids and frequency of lipoprotein patterns in myocardial infarction. *J. Atheroscler. Res.* **8**: 167.
40. Fredrickson, D. S. 1969. The role of lipids in acute myocardial infarction. *Circ. Suppl.* **39**: IV-99.
41. Heinle, R. A., R. I. Levy, D. S. Fredrickson, and R. Gorlin. 1969. Lipid and carbohydrate abnormalities in patients with angiographically documented coronary artery disease. *Am. J. Cardiol.* **24**: 178.
42. Blankenhorn, D. H., H. P. Chin, and F. Y. K. Lau. 1968. Ischemic heart disease in young adults. *Ann. Intern. Med.* **69**: 21.
43. Shanoff, H. M., J. A. Little, and A. Csima. 1970. Studies of male survivors of myocardial infarction. XII. Relation of serum lipids and lipoproteins to survival over a 10-year period. *Can. Med. Assoc. J.* **103**: 927.
44. Enger, S. C., and S. Ritland. 1970. Serum lipoprotein pattern in myocardial infarction. *Acta Med. Scand.* **187**: 365.
45. Dyerberg, J., H. O. Bang, and J. A. Nielsen. 1970. Plasma lipids and lipoproteins in patients with myocardial infarction and in control material. *Acta Med. Scand.* **187**: 353.
46. Falsetti, H. L., J. D. Schnatz, D. G. Greene, and I. L. Bunnell. 1970. Serum lipids and glucose tolerance in angiographically proved coronary artery disease. *Chest.* **58**: 111.
47. Masarei, J. R., M. Summers, D. H. Curnow, K. J. Cullen, M. G. McCall, N. S. Stenhouse, and T. A. Welborn. 1971. Lipoprotein electrophoretic patterns, serum lipids, and coronary heart disease. *Br. Med. J.* **1**: 78.
48. Carlson, L. A., and L. E. Böttiger. 1972. Ischaemic heart disease in relation to fasting value of plasma triglycerides and cholesterol. *Lancet.* **1**: 865.
49. Wilson, W. S., S. B. Hulley, M. I. Burrows, and M. Z. Nichaman. 1971. Serial lipid and lipoprotein responses to The American Heart Association Fat-Controlled Diet. *Am. J. Med.* **51**: 491.
50. Kuo, P. T. 1968. Current metabolic-genetic interrelationship in human atherosclerosis. *Ann. Intern. Med.* **68**: 449.
51. Metropolitan Life Insurance Company. 1959. Rise in mortality last year. *Stat. Bull. Metrop. Life Insur. Co.* **40**: 1.
52. Wyngaarden, J. B., and W. N. Kelley. 1972. Gout. *In* The Metabolic Basis of Inherited Disease. J. B. Stanbury, J. B. Wyngaarden, and D. S. Fredrickson, editors. McGraw-Hill Book Company, New York, 3rd edition. 889.

Hyperlipidemia in Coronary Heart Disease

II. GENETIC ANALYSIS OF LIPID LEVELS IN 176 FAMILIES AND DELINEATION OF A NEW INHERITED DISORDER, COMBINED HYPERLIPIDEMIA

JOSEPH L. GOLDSTEIN, HELMUT G. SCHROTT, WILLIAM R. HAZZARD, EDWIN L. BIERMAN, and ARNO G. MOTULSKY with the technical assistance of ELLEN D. CAMPBELL and MARY JO LEVINSKI

From the Departments of Medicine (Division of Medical Genetics, University Hospital, and Division of Metabolism and Gerontology, Veterans Administration Hospital) and Genetics, University of Washington, Seattle, Washington 98195

ABSTRACT To assess the genetics of hyperlipidemia in coronary heart disease, family studies were carried out in 2520 relatives and spouses of 176 survivors of myocardial infarction, including 149 hyperlipidemic and 27 normolipidemic individuals. The distribution of fasting plasma cholesterol and triglyceride values in relatives, together with segregation analyses, suggested the presence of five distinct lipid disorders. Three of these—familial hypercholesterolemia, familial hypertriglyceridemia, and familial combined hyperlipidemia—appeared to represent dominant expression of three different autosomal genes, occurring in about 20% of survivors below 60 yr of age and 7% of all older survivors. Two other disorders—polygenic hypercholesterolemia and sporadic hypertriglyceridemia—each affected about 6% of survivors in both age groups.

This work was presented in part at the 85th Session of the Association of American Physicians, Atlantic City, N. J., 2–3 May 1972, and published in the Transactions (1).

Dr. Goldstein was supported by Special National Institutes of Health Fellowship GM 4784-01 and is now a Research Career Development Awardee 1-K4-GM 70, 277-01 from the National Institute of General Medical Sciences. His present address is the Division of Medical Genetics, Department of Internal Medicine, University of Texas Southwestern Medical School, Dallas, Tex. 75235. Dr. Hazzard is the recipient of a Clinical Investigatorship of the Veterans Administration and is now an Investigator of the Howard Hughes Medical Institute. Dr. Schrott was supported by Special Institutes of Health Fellowship HE 48 695. His present address is The Mayo Clinic and Mayo Foundation, Rochester, Minn. 55901.

Received for publication 20 September 1972 and in revised form 19 February 1973.

The most common genetic form of hyperlipidemia identified in this study has hitherto been poorly defined and has been designated as familial combined hyperlipidemia. Affected family members characteristically had elevated levels of both cholesterol and triglyceride. However, increased cholesterol or increased triglyceride levels alone were also frequently observed. The combined disorder was shown to be genetically distinct from familial hypercholesterolemia and familial hypertriglyceridemia for the following reasons: (a) the distribution pattern of cholesterol and triglyceride levels in relatives of probands was unique; (b) children of individuals with combined hyperlipidemia did not express hypercholesterolemia in contrast to the finding of hypercholesterolemic children from families with familial hypercholesterolemia; and (c) analysis of informative matings suggested that the different lipid phenotypes owed their origin to variable expression of a single autosomal dominant gene and not to segregation of two separate genes, such as one elevating the level of cholesterol and the other elevating the level of triglyceride.

Heterozygosity for one of the three lipid-elevating genes identified in this study may have a frequency in the general population of about 1%, constituting a major problem in early diagnosis and preventive therapy.

INTRODUCTION

The hyperlipidemias comprise a heterogeneous group of disorders whose characteristic expression is an elevation in the plasma concentration of cholesterol and/or triglyceride (2–4). These lipid disorders may occur in familial or nonfamilial form (3). Presumably, each variety of familial hyperlipidemia could arise from the action of a single gene (monogenic or Mendelian inheritance) or could reflect the interaction of several genes at many different loci (polygenic inheritance) (5, 6). Nonfamilial hyperlipidemias are often secondary to such factors as diet, alcohol intake, estrogen therapy, or to diseases such as diabetes mellitus, hypothyroidism, or nephrosis (3). In some cases, neither hereditary nor identifiable environmental factors can be implicated, and such cases are referred to in this paper as sporadic hyperlipidemia.[1]

Current laboratory tests used to define hyperlipidemia and to distinguish among the monogenic, polygenic, sporadic, and secondary disorders include measuring the plasma levels of total cholesterol, low density lipoprotein (LDL)—cholesterol, and total triglyceride (2). However, none of these measurements directly reflects the primary action of genes as do the measurements of proteins and enzymes in such disorders as the hemoglobinopathies. Instead, they are the result of combined genetic and environmental influences.

Monogenic and polygenic causes of hyperlipidemia most likely differ in the underlying biochemical lesion and in the response to diet and drug therapy. Assessing the importance of genetic factors requires a detailed study of cholesterol and triglyceride levels in relatives of hyperlipidemic probands. In hyperlipidemia transmitted as an autosomal dominant trait, lipid levels in first-degree relatives would be composed of two distinct distributions—one reflecting the presence of normal relatives and the other that of affected relatives. This distribution of lipid values would result in a bimodal curve. Bimodality is most easily detected if the mean of the quantitative parameter under study differs significantly between normals and affected, if the spread or variance of the values is not too dissimilar in the two groups, and if the proportion of relatives in each group is nearly equal (7). With dominant inheritance, a characteristic vertical pedigree pattern would be found in both near and distant relatives. In polygenic inheritance the quantitative parameter being studied is continuously distributed, and no distinct separation

---

[1] The term "polygenic" has been used in the broad sense to imply a multifactorial mechanism, in which observed familial variations could be determined either by multiple genetic factors, by a single genetic locus with one or many alleles interacting with environmental variation, or exclusively by environmental variation. In the strict genetic sense, a sporadic case of hyperlipidemia could be the result of a new autosomal dominant mutation, autosomal recessive inheritance, incomplete penetrance in autosomal dominant inheritance, or a nongenetic entity.

between normals and affected is evident (8, 9). Thus, the lipid levels in relatives of individuals with polygenic hyperlipidemia would form a single distribution with a mean higher than that of controls. Affected family members are most frequently found among first-degree relatives such as sibs, parents, and children, and would be considerably less frequent in more distant relatives (8, 9). In sporadic hyperlipidemia, lipid levels in relatives of all degrees should be identical with those of controls.

Utilizing as probands for detailed family studies the hyperlipidemic survivors of myocardial infarction identified in the accompanying paper (10), the present investigation was undertaken with the following aims: to delineate the different forms of familial and nonfamilial hyperlipidemia in patients with myocardial infarction, to characterize the mechanisms of inheritance of any familial disorders, and to determine their frequency.

METHODS

Selection of survivors as probands for family studies. Of the 500 survivors of myocardial infarction investigated in the accompanying paper (10), 176 were selected as probands for family studies as follows: (a) An attempt was made to investigate the families of all hyperlipidemic survivors whose level of adjusted plasma cholesterol and/or triglyceride equaled or exceeded the 95th percentile value of controls. Of 157 such survivors, family studies were carried out in 131. The remaining 26 hyperlipidemic survivors had either no living first-degree relatives (13 survivors) or fewer than three available first-degree relatives (13 survivors). (b) Because 95th percentile cut-off values represented an arbitrary way of distinguishing between normolipidemic and hyperlipidemic individuals, 13 survivors whose plasma cholesterol and/or triglyceride values lay above the 92.5th percentile were included for family study. (c) All 11 survivors who were taking clofibrate at the time of examination were considered hyperlipidemic regardless of their lipid values and were included for family study. Of these 11, 5 had lipid values at the time of study below the 95th percentile (10). (d) 27 normolipidemic survivors whose plasma cholesterol and triglyceride were both below the 90th percentile were also included as probands and the lipid values of their relatives were used as control family data.

Family studies. Family histories were taken and pedigrees were constructed to include every first-degree relative for each of the 500 survivors of myocardial infarction studied in the accompanying paper (10). Permission to verify causes of death in first-degree relatives was obtained from each of the 500 survivors. From the 176 survivors selected as probands, permission to contact all living first-degree relatives as well as more distant relatives when indicated was requested. A total of 2520 family members were tested, including 1695 blood relatives and 825 spouses. A fasting blood sample and a medical history were obtained from 913 of the 960 living first-degree relatives (age 6 and above) of the 176 probands (95% ascertainment). Similarly tested were 643 second-degree, 135 third-degree, and 4 fourth-degree relatives, as well as 825 spouses of these relatives. Blood specimens from local and out-of-town relatives were collected as described in the accompanying paper (10). The decision to contact the more

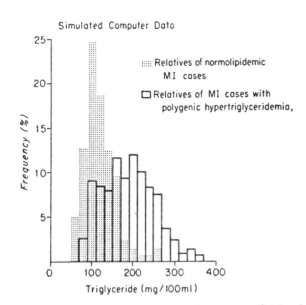

FIGURE 1 Frequency distribution of computer-simulated triglyceride levels in relatives of 60 normolipidemic and 60 hypertriglyceridemic probands. These data were derived from a polygenic model and were generated by a special computer program described in the Methods. The total number of relatives comprising each curve was 300.

distant relatives in a given family was made if one or more first-degree relatives had lipid values equal to or exceeding the 95th percentile cut-off values or if one or more first-degree relatives were said to have died of myocardial infarction. Except for their availability and willingness to cooperate, no other special selection was used in obtaining blood samples from the distant relatives.

Analyses of plasma lipids. Fasting plasma levels of cholesterol and triglyceride were measured as described in the accompanying paper (10). Lipoprotein quantification and phenotyping were performed on repeat plasma samples using methods described in the accompanying paper (11).

Control data. The levels of cholesterol and triglyceride were obtained from 950 spouse controls and adjusted for differences in age and sex as described in the accompanying paper (10).

Classification of hyperlipidemia in families. Classification of the lipid disorders was based on an analysis of the cholesterol and triglyceride levels among relatives of probands. In the absence of knowledge regarding the basic defects in the different hyperlipidemias, no method of sorting data for heterogeneity based on quantitative variation alone can be considered completely unbiased. However, in an attempt to minimize bias, the following approach was developed: Each of the hyperlipidemic families was initially separated into one of two groups depending on whether (group A) or not (group B) the family contained at least one relative besides the proband who would be considered unequivocally hyperlipidemic (i.e., whose lipid level was ≥99th percentile for adults of 20 yr of age and older or ≥95th percentile for younger individuals).[2] Families in group A were further subdivided depending on whether the predominant lipid elevation

[2] Four families in which the index case was shown to have type III hyperlipidemia were placed in a special group (see accompanying paper [11]).

in the family occurred in cholesterol alone (group A-1 or familial hypercholesterolemia); in triglyceride alone (group A-2 or familial hypertriglyceridemia); or in both lipids (group A-3 or familial combined hyperlipidemia). For the individual family this assignment to a specific group was determined by inspecting the pedigree and assessing the distribution of percentile values of the adjusted cholesterol and triglyceride levels. Analysis of one 11 member family is given for illustration:

Percentile Distribution of Lipid Levels of Each Family Member (Number)

	10th	20th	30th	40th	50th	60th	70th	80th	90th	95th	99th
Cholesterol		1	2	1	1	1	2			②	①
Triglyceride	1	2		1	1	2		1 -	①		③

Since this family showed values in the 90th–99th percentile range for both cholesterol and triglyceride, it was assigned to the category of familial combined hyperlipidemia (group A-3). This system was generally useful for classification except for occasional instances of familial hypercholesterolemia and xanthomatosis, where several affected family members had elevations in both plasma lipids (e.g., cholesterol = 410 mg/100 ml and triglyceride = 200 mg/100 ml). However, such affected individuals almost always had a cholesterol/triglyceride ratio greater than 2 (2), so it was easy to make a correct assignment to the category of familial hypercholesterolemia (group A-1). An objective method to confirm our qualitative assessment was sought by calculating a weighted variance[3] for both adjusted cholesterol and triglyceride values of adult relatives in each family. A high variance for cholesterol but not for triglyceride would be expected in familial hypercholesterolemia (group A-1); conversely, a high variance for triglyceride but not for cholesterol would be expected in familial hypertriglyceridemia (group A-2).

Our classification into family groups A-1, A-2, and A-3 on the basis of at least one affected relative could theoretically create artificial bimodality in the lipid distribution of relatives and lead to spurious conclusions regarding monogenic inheritance. To rule out this possibility, we set up a series of simulation experiments using a special computer program developed in collaboration with Dr. Joseph Felsenstein. In these experiments, the inheritance of hyperlipidemia was assumed to be polygenic (heritability = 1), and a lipid value was assigned to each member of a hypothetical family including a mother, a father, and each of their four children, the first child being designated as the proband. Lipid values for father, G_1, and mother, G_2, were chosen from a set of random variates with a distribution having a mean and variance, σ^2, identical with those of our control data. Lipid values for the four offspring were assigned by drawing at random each value from a distribution whose mean was = $(G_1 + G_2)/2$ and variance = $\sigma^2/2$. In this way the values in the offspring

$$[3]\ \sigma^2 = \frac{\Sigma (x_1 - \mu)^2 + 0.5\,\Sigma (x_2 - \mu)^2 + 0.25\,\Sigma (x_3 - \mu)^2}{n_1 + 0.5\,n_2 + 0.25\,n_3 - 1}$$

where σ^2 = family variance weighted as to class of relative being considered, in which the weighting factor was proportional to the number of genes in common among relatives, (i.e., first-degree relatives of proband = 1, second-degree relatives = 0.5, and third-degree relatives = 0.25); x_1, x_2, x_3 = adjusted lipid level (cholesterol or triglyceride) in first-, second-, and third-degree relatives, respectively. μ = adjusted mean lipid level of controls; n_1, n_2, n_3 = number of first-, second-, and third-degree relatives, respectively. The proband of each family was excluded from analysis.

reflected polygenic inheritance (9). Thousands of such simulated families were computer generated. The first 60 families fulfilling the criteria of having a hyperlipidemic index case (≥95th percentile) and at least 1 unequivocally hyperlipidemic relative (≥99th percentile) were selected for genetic analysis. When the frequency distributions of lipid values in relatives of these artificially generated data were plotted, the curves for both cholesterol and triglyceride appeared unimodal and significantly shifted to the right of the control curve. An example of such simulated computer data for triglyceride is shown in Fig. 1. Since these simulated family data did not give results resembling monogenic inheritance (i.e., no bimodality), it seemed reasonable to conclude that the approach used in these studies to sort families for heterogeneity did not create artifical bimodality.

Analysis of data. In addition to the methods described in the accompanying paper (10), the following procedures were used in the genetic analysis. It was necessary for testing the single gene hypothesis to decompose each of the frequency distributions of lipid values of affected and normal relatives from the various family groups into two components with the most likely overlapping Gaussian distributions. Initial estimates of the parameters of the respective components were obtained by dissecting the plots of the cumulative frequency distribution on probability paper (probit analysis) by the graphical method of Harding (12). Using these initial values, maximum likelihood estimates of μ_1, μ_2, σ_1, and σ_2 (where μ_1 and σ_1 were the mean and standard deviation of the ith component [$i = 1,2$]) were obtained with the aid of a computer program using a standard iterative method (13, 14). Murphy and Bolling have discussed the applications of this technique to the testing of single locus hypotheses where there is incomplete separation of the phenotypes (15).[4]

Documentation of coronary heart disease in relatives. Copies of 90% of all requested death certificates were obtained for first-degree relatives over 35 yr of age. Death was attributed to myocardial infarction whenever one of the following conditions was listed as a direct cause of death: myocardial infarction, coronary occlusion, coronary atherosclerosis, coronary thrombosis, arteriosclerotic cardiovascular disease, or sudden death. Less specific terms such as organic heart failure, degenerative heart disease, congestive heart failure, and chronic myocarditis were not considered sufficiently indicative of coronary heart disease. Myocardial infarction was accepted in living relatives when their medical history form indicated hospitalization for "myocardial infarction," "coronary thrombosis," or "heart attack."

---

[4] Although Murphy and Bolling indicated that sometimes convergence of the estimates is not possible when the variances in the two components are not equal (15), this problem did not occur in our data, possibly as the result of the nearly precise initial estimates which greatly reduced the number of iterations (and hence the chance of encountering a point of singularity in the likelihood function) and also because we used less stringent convergence criteria. Occasionally, a small number of outliers with triglyceride values greater than 600 mg/100 ml (<2% of the total sample) severely affected the mean and standard deviation estimates in the second component. For these particular family groups three components were estimated, with the outliers contained in the last component. This proved to be a more effective way of handling the outlying values than winsoring (i.e., making all values greater than 600 mg/100 ml equal to 600), since the winsored values also affected the parameters of the second component.

RESULTS

Lipid levels in relatives of normolipidemic survivors. The mean and SD of age and sex-adjusted cholesterol and triglyceride levels in 113 adult relatives of 27 normolipidemic survivors were 215±39 and 94±54 mg/100 ml, respectively; as compared with the control values of 218±41 and 93±48. Furthermore, the frequency distributions for both cholesterol and triglyceride in these 113 normal relatives appeared unimodal and were identical with those of the controls. This excellent agreement confirmed the validity of the control values and indicated that any differences in the lipid distributions between controls and relatives of hyperlipidemic survivors could not be attributed to obtaining fasting blood samples from many relatives located in diverse geographic areas.

Lipid levels in spouse pairs. To determine whether any familial similarities in lipid levels could result from environmental similarities between family members, plasma lipids in the first 440 consecutively studied husband-wife pairs (including hyperlipidemic and normolipidemic spouses) were compared. Since no significant correlations were found for either cholesterol ($r = -0.023$) or triglyceride ($r = +0.098$), it was concluded that dietary and other environmental factors common to spouse pairs could not account for familial elevations in plasma lipids. Therefore, no corrections were necessary for nongenetic familial effects.

Lipid levels in relatives of hyperlipidemic survivors. Lipid levels in 645 adult first-degree relatives of all 149 hyperlipidemic survivors were compared with those of controls. The age and sex-adjusted values for both cholesterol and triglyceride (mean±SD) were significantly higher ($P < 0.001$) in relatives (235±53 and 126±174, respectively) than in controls (218±41 and 93±48). These differences became more striking when the hyperlipidemic survivors were separated into groups: those with hypercholesterolemia with or without an associated elevation in triglyceride (n = 81) and those with hypertriglyceridemia with or without an associated elevation in cholesterol (n = 107). (36 of these survivors showed an elevation in both lipids and therefore were included in both groups.) The mean±SD value for cholesterol in the adult first-degree relatives (n = 379) of the hypercholesterolemic survivors was 247±56 mg/100 ml (control, 218±41) whereas the mean±SD value for triglyceride in the adult first-degree relatives (n = 434) of the hypertriglyceridemic survivors was 140±200 mg/100 ml (control, 93±48). These data indicated that familial factors play an important role in the etiology of hyperlipidemia in patients with coronary heart disease. The absence of correlations in lipid levels between husband-

TABLE I
Classification of Families

Group	Number of families	Relatives per family* (mean ±SEM)	Adjusted cholesterol		Adjusted triglyceride	
			Weighted variance‡	Observed/ Expected§	Weighted variance‡	Observed/ Expected§
A-1						
Familial hypercholesterolemia	16	8.4±1.0	11,332	5.40	3,240	0.68
A-2						
Familial hypertriglyceridemia	23	10.1±1.2	1,569	0.78	31,803	6.63
A-3						
Familial combined hyperlipidemia	47	11.2±1.2	4,972	2.36	45,166	9.42
B						
Sporadic and polygenic hyperlipidemia	59	8.4±1.1	1,971	0.94	2,595	0.54
C						
Relatives of normolipidemic survivors	27	8.1±1.2	2,103	1.00	4,794	1.00

* Does not include spouses.
‡ Represents a group mean determined by averaging the individual weighted variances of each family comprising a group. The weighted variance of each family was estimated as described in the Methods.
§ Observed/expected = weighted variance of indicated group/weighted variance of group C.

wife pairs suggested that these familial factors were primarily genetic in origin.

Classification of hyperlipidemic families and development of a genetic hypothesis. In order to search for the presence of major genes contributing to hyperlipidemia, families were sorted for heterogeneity as described in the Methods. The resultant classification is shown in Table I. Group A-1 or familial hypercholesterolemia consisted of 16 families. An abnormally high mean variance was calculated for cholesterol levels in these families as compared with the mean variance for

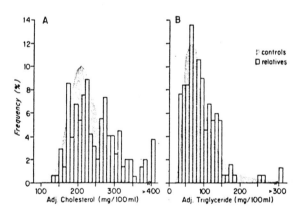

FIGURE 2 Frequency distribution of adjusted lipid levels in 132 near and distant relatives of 16 survivors with familial hypercholesterolemia. Included in this analysis were 68 first-degree, 44 second-degree, 18 third-degree, and 2 fourth-degree relatives. 49 of the 132 relatives were between the ages of 6 and 20. Age and sex-adjustments were carried out as described in the accompanying paper (10). The distribution is divided into increments of 10 mg/100 ml. The smooth strippled curve represents a nonparametric density estimate of the control distribution.

cholesterol of the normolipidemic control families (group C). Group A-2 or familial hypertriglyceridemia consisted of 23 families, with the predominant lipid elevation again reflected in an abnormally high mean variance. Group A-3 or familial combined hyperlipidemia consisted of 47 families in which elevation of both plasma lipids was reflected in high mean variances. Group B consisted of 59 families in which the mean variances in plasma lipids were not significantly higher than those in the control families (group C).

Since the variation in plasma cholesterol and/or triglyceride among relatives in Groups A-1, A-2, and A-3 was 5 to 9 times greater than that of the control families, we tested the genetic hypothesis that the hyperlipidemia in each of these three groups was determined by a different major gene.

Group A-1: familial hypercholesterolemia. The frequency distribution of adjusted lipid levels in 132 relatives of 16 hypercholesterolemic survivors (13 men, 3 women) is shown in Fig. 2. As compared with that of controls, the distribution of cholesterol was suggestive of bimodality—the first mode corresponding to controls and containing the normal relatives and the second mode containing the affected relatives (Fig. 2A). More quantitative evidence for bimodality was obtained by plotting the cumulative frequency distribution on normal probability paper (Fig. 3A). The plot of control values yielded one straight line, indicating a single Gaussian curve (12). The plot of the relatives' values contained two straight line segments, suggesting two Gaussian curves—one for normal relatives and the other for affected relatives (12). The break in the plot (i.e., the nonstraight line segment) reflected the apparent antimode of the two overlapping distributions;

its upper limit corresponded approximately to the 90–95th percentile range of controls. Since these data suggested a mixture of two normal distributions, the best fitting two-distribution mixture was obtained by the maximum likelihood computer procedure described in the Methods. The mean±SD of 214.2±28.5 mg/100 ml for the first component was very close to that of controls (218); the mean of the second component was 299.2±58.3.[5]

The mean±SD for triglyceride of relatives (89.7 ±53.1 mg/100 ml) was not significantly different from that of controls (93±48), and the distributions shown in Figs. 2B and 3B were unimodal.

The pedigrees of each of the 16 families in this group are presented in Fig. 4. Vertical transmission of hypercholesterolemia is evident from the frequent expression in offspring of affected individuals. Although hypertriglyceridemia was observed in some of these hypercholesterolemic individuals, their whole plasma ratio of cholesterol/triglyceride was almost always greater than 2, a finding not observed in individuals with other forms of familial hyperlipidemia (2,3). Finally, at least seven of these families had one or more affected members known to have tendinous xanthomas (viz., families 45, 120, 289, 292, 314, and 497).

In order to determine the pattern of inheritance of the hypercholesterolemia in these 16 families, segregation analyses were carried out. In the absence of a complete separation between the cholesterol distributions of normal and affected phenotypes, relatives were classified as affected or normal depending on whether or not the adjusted cholesterol level equaled or exceeded the 95th percentile of controls (285 mg/100 ml). This value closely reflected the physiologic separation between affected and unaffected relatives as determined both in this study (Figs. 2A and 3A) and in an independent study of familial monogenic hypercholesterolemia (5).[6]

Sib analysis is probably the method of choice for analyzing family lipid data of the type collected in this study. Sibs are usually of a similar age range as probands and will express a given lipid disorder which may not be apparent in children (see below). Furthermore, other methods of segregation analysis, which

[5] The Chi-square goodness of fit was significantly better for a mixture of two overlapping distributions ($P > 0.5$) than for a single distribution ($P < 0.025$).

[6] The cut-off value for separating normal and affected individuals can be derived by at least four methods (reviewed by Murphy [16]), but each of these methods gives approximately the same dividing point when the two component populations are nearly equal size, as is the case in our data. We placed the cut-off point for cholesterol at the 95th percentile of controls, so that the number of normal individuals who are misclassified as affected are minimized and the total number of affected family members is underestimated.

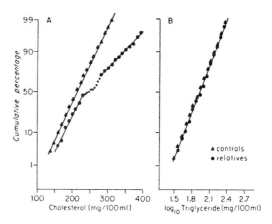

FIGURE 3 Cumulative frequency distribution of adjusted lipid levels in 132 near and distant relatives of 16 survivors with familial hypercholesterolemia. The composition of the relatives group is identical with that described for Fig. 2. The cholesterol and $\log_{10}$ triglyceride values were age and sex-adjusted as described in the accompanying paper (10).

consider phenotypes of living parents, are more likely to show a deficiency in the number of affected living relatives since many affected hyperlipidemic parents may have already died of myocardial infarction (17).

The finding of an apparently bimodal distribution in the levels of cholesterol and not triglyceride in relatives, together with the results of the sib analysis showing that about one-half of living sibs were hypercholesterolemic (Table II), are consistent with autosomal dominant inheritance. On the assumption that affected individuals die prematurely (17), one might expect a deficiency in affected sibs. The lack of such a deficiency in our data presumably reflects the relatively young age (mean = 46 yr) of the probands and their sibs. The analysis of the proportion of affected first- and second-degree relatives (Table III) further confirmed autosomal dominant inheritance and demonstrated nearly complete expression of the hypercholesterolemia gene in affected children. The finding of a higher than expected number of affected second-degree adult relatives is probably a reflection of an ascertainment bias due to the small total number of relatives tested (n = 24) in this category.

Group A-2: familial hypertriglyceridemia. The frequency distribution of adjusted lipid levels in 132 adult relatives of 23 hypertriglyceridemic survivors (18 men, 5 women) is shown in Fig. 5. As compared with that of controls, the distribution of triglyceride was suggestive of bimodality (Fig. 5B). When the cumulative frequencies of these data were examined on log probability paper, the plot of the relatives contained two straight line segments, indicating two Gaussian curves (Fig. 6B). The upper limit of the break in the plot (i.e., the antimode for separation of normal and

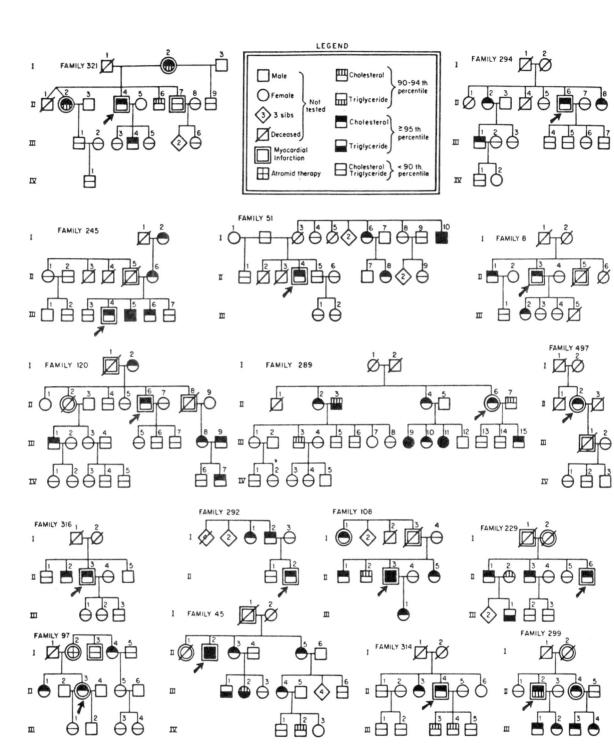

FIGURE 4 Composite showing the pedigrees of 16 families with familial hypercholesterolemia. The legend is shown in the middle of the first row of pedigrees. The proband for each family is indicated by an arrow. Spouses belonging to matings for which there were no data available for the offspring have been omitted from the pedigrees. Although family 497 does not meet the criterion of having at least one relative of the proband with a 99th percentile cholesterol value, it has been included in this group because the proband's son (III, 1) died at age 48 yr of myocardial infarction and was known to have hypercholesterolemic xanthomatosis. Identification and lipid data for each family member are available upon request. These data have been deposited with the National Auxiliary Publications Service (ID no. 02057).

TABLE II

Analysis of Sibships of 16 Survivors with Familial Hypercholesterolemia

| | Sibs (no.) | | | | | Number affected | |
| | Total | Dead | | Living | Tested | Observed‡ | Expected§ |
		By all causes	By MI*				
Brothers	24	8	2	16	15	5	7.5
Sisters	27	4	2	23	19	14	9.5
Total	51	12‖	4	39	34	19	17.0

* Deaths by myocardial infarction (MI) were documented by death certificates.
‡ Relatives were considered affected if the age and sex-adjusted plasma cholesterol level was equal to or exceeded the 95th percentile of controls.
§ Expected number of affected relatives by the hypothesis of autosomal dominant inheritance, assuming no effect of the gene on mortality at the ages tested.
‖ 5 of these 12 deaths occurred before age 35 yr.

TABLE III

Proportion of Affected Relatives of 16 Survivors with Familial Hypercholesterolemia

| Age of relatives and degree of relation | No. tested | Affected relatives | | |
| | | Observed | | Expected‡ |
		90th percentile	95th percentile	
		%	%	%
A. ≥ Age 25				
1st degree	44	54.6	50.0	50.0
2nd degree	24	41.7	37.5	25.0
B. < Age 25				
1st degree	22	45.5	38.1	50.0
2nd degree	23	26.1	21.7	25.0

* Relatives were considered affected if the age and sex-adjusted plasma cholesterol level was equal to or exceeded the indicated percentile of controls.
‡ Expected proportion of affected relatives on the hypothesis of autosomal dominant inheritance, assuming no effect of the gene on mortality of the ages tested and assuming no introduction of the gene by those marrying into the family.

TABLE IV

Analysis of Sibships of 23 Survivors with Familial Hypertriglyceridemia

| | Sibs (no.) | | | | | Number affected | |
| | Total | Dead | | Living | Tested | Observed‡ | Expected§ |
		By all causes	By MI*				
Brothers	47	19	6	28	25	12	12.5
Sisters	38	8	0	30	26	12	13.0
Total	85	27‖	6	58	51	24	25.5

* Deaths by myocardial infarction (MI) were documented by death certificates.
‡ Relatives were considered affected if the age and sex-adjusted plasma triglyceride level was equal to or exceeded the 95th percentile of controls.
§ Expected number of affected relatives by the hypothesis of autosomal dominant inheritance, assuming no effect of the gene on mortality at the ages tested.
‖ 17 of these 27 deaths occurred before age 35 yr.

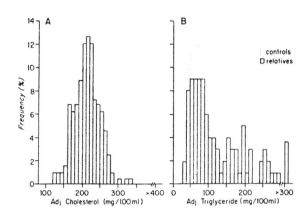

FIGURE 5 Frequency distribution of adjusted lipid levels in 132 adult (≥20 yr of age) relatives of 23 survivors with familial hypertriglyceridemia. Included in this analysis were 90 first-degree relatives, 30 second-degree relatives, and 12 third-degree relatives. Age and sex-adjustments were carried out as described in the accompanying paper (10). The distribution is divided into increments of 10 mg/100 ml. The smooth strippled curve represents a nonparametric density estimate of the control distribution.

affected relatives) corresponded to the 90th to 95th percentile range of controls. The best fitting two-distribution mixture, obtained by the maximum likelihood method, indicated that the mean±SD of normal relatives was 76.2±21.2, while the mean for affected relatives was 180.1±65.3.[7]

Cholesterol levels in these same relatives were distributed as one mode that corresponded to controls (Figs. 5A and 6A). The mean±SD for cholesterol in relatives (217±36 mg/100 ml) was almost identical with that of controls (218±41).

The pedigrees of each of the 23 families in this group are presented in Fig. 7. The inspection of these pedigrees indicates vertical transmission, but with only occasional expression of hypertriglyceridemia in children (about 12% of those at risk), and a high frequency of death by myocardial infarction in presumed carriers of the hypertriglyceridemia gene, such as parents of probands.

All these findings, as well as the results of the sib analysis (Table IV), are consistent with an autosomal dominant mechanism of inheritance. As in familial hypercholesterolemia, no deficiency in affected sibs was noted, suggesting that any effect of the gene on mortality might be delayed until the latter part of the 5th decade of life. Table V analyzes the proportion of affected first-degree relatives (including parents and

[7] The Chi-square goodness of fit was significantly better for a mixture of two overlapping distributions ($P > 0.5$) than for a single distribution ($P < 0.005$).

children as well as sibs) and second-degree relatives. The slight deficiency in the expected number of affected adult first-degree relatives (40% observed; 50% expected) was due to a deficiency in the number of affected living parents.

Group A-3: familial combined hyperlipidemia. A large number of families had affected members who expressed different combinations of elevated cholesterol and elevated triglyceride levels. Thus, affected members of the same family showed either an elevated cholesterol level with a type IIa lipoprotein pattern, an elevated triglyceride level with a type IV or type V pattern, or they showed both elevated cholesterol and triglyceride levels with a type IIb pattern (11). The pedigree of a large family with combined hyperlipidemia (family 41) is shown in Fig. 8, and the lipid data for each family member in Table VI. In this family the hyperlipidemia appeared to be transmitted as a simple Mendelian autosomal dominant trait. All offspring of normals were unaffected, and on the average one-half the offspring of affected were hyperlipidemic.

Among 157 hyperlipidemic survivors identified in the accompanying paper (10), 47 (36 men, 11 women) had pedigrees in which the combined disorder appeared to be present. Fig. 9 shows the frequency distribution of adjusted lipid levels in their 234 adult first-degree relatives. As compared with that of controls, the distribution of triglyceride was suggestive of bimodality (Fig. 9B). The cumulative frequency when plotted on log probability paper confirmed the presence of two distributions (Fig. 10B). The best fitting two-distribution mixture, obtained by the maximum likelihood method, indicated that the mean±SD of the normal distribution was 74.0±20.5 mg/100 ml, whereas the

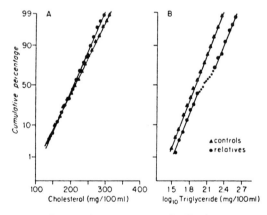

FIGURE 6 Cumulative frequency distribution of adjusted lipid levels in 132 adult (≥20 yr of age) relatives of 23 survivors with familial hypertriglyceridemia. The composition of the relatives group is identical with that described for Fig. 5. The cholesterol and log₁₀ triglyceride values were age and sex-adjusted as described in the accompanying paper (10).

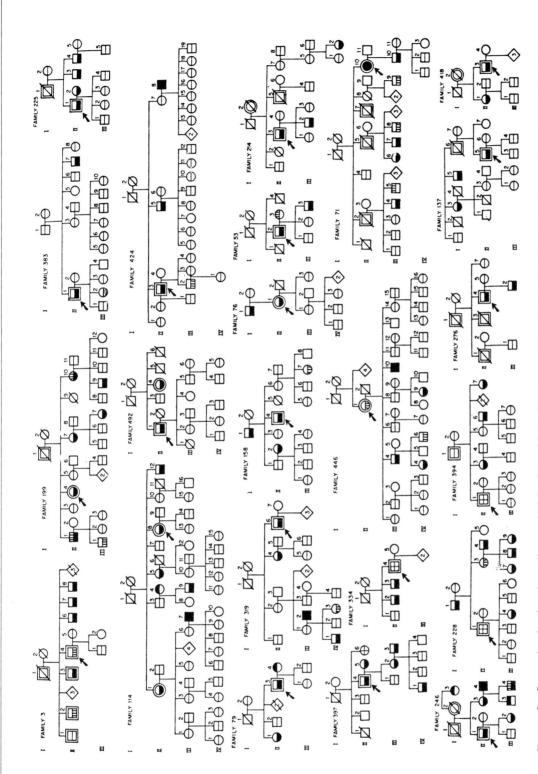

FIGURE 7 Composite showing the pedigrees of 23 families with familial hypertriglyceridemia. The legend for these pedigrees is identical with that shown for Fig. 4. The proband for each family is indicated by ⭧. Two individuals (II, 10 in family 71 and III, 10 in family 446) who showed elevations in cholesterol as well as triglyceride had hyperchylomicronemia. Spouses belonging to matings for which there were no data available for the offspring have been omitted from the pedigrees. Identification and lipid data for each family member are available upon request (deposited with the National Auxiliary Publications Service [ID no. 02057]).

TABLE V

Proportion of Affected Relatives of 23 Survivors with Familial Hypertriglyceridemia

Age of relatives and degree of relation	No. tested	Affected relatives		
		Observed*		Expected‡
		90th percentile	95th percentile	
		%	%	%
A. ≥ Age 25				
1st degree	83	42.2	36.2	50.0
2nd degree	31	29.0	20.0	25.0
B. < Age 25				
1st degree	30	16.7	13.3	50.0
2nd degree	68	10.3	10.3	25.0

* Relatives were considered affected if the age and sex-adjusted plasma cholesterol level was equal to or exceeded the indicated percentile of controls.

‡ Expected proportion of affected relatives on the hypothesis of autosomal dominant inheritance, assuming no effect of the gene on mortality at the ages tested and assuming no introduction of the gene by those marrying into the family.

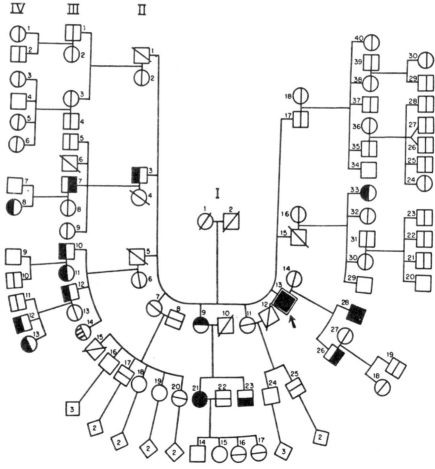

FIGURE 8 Pedigree of a family with familial combined hyperlipidemia. The legend for this pedigree is identical with that shown for Fig. 4. The proband is indicated by an arrow. The kindred is referred to elsewhere as family 41. A summary of the plasma lipid values in relatives and spouses is shown in Table VI.

TABLE VI
Summary of Plasma Lipid Values in Members and Spouses of Family 41

Pedigree position	Sex	Age	Unadjusted lipid levels		Lipoprotein type‡	Pedigree position	Sex	Age	Unadjusted lipid levels		Lipoprotein type‡
			Cholesterol	Triglyceride					Cholesterol	Triglyceride	
			mg/100 ml						*mg/100 ml*		
I 1	F	87	Cause of death unknown			23	M	55	229	200	
2	M	86	Cause of death unknown			25	M	47	252	152	
						26	M	48	248	225	IV
II 1	M	50	Cancer*			27	F	51	212	104	
2	F	79	226	186		28	M	42	328	165	IIb
3	M	84	258	453	IV	30	F	37	239	40	
5	M	47	Cancer*	—		31	M	40	209	59	
6	F	75	252	145		32	F	31	229	72	
7	F	79	251	111		33	F	26	268	95	
8	M	78	151	84		35	M	37	146	104	
9	F	75	364	196		36	F	37	163	58	
11	F	67	288	115		37	M	29	211	79	
13	M	65	341	268	IIb	38	F	34	168	46	
14	F	67	268	128		39	M	37	232	66	
15	M	47	Trauma*	—		40	F	15	111	28	
16	F	59	210	105		IV 1	F	28	186	72	
17	M	60	238	81		2	M	26	195	85	
18	F	55	197	64		3	F	33	202	57	
						5	F	28	235	60	
III 1	M	58	228	135		6	F	19	162	45	
2	F	56	201	116		8	F	23	222	124	
3	F	56	280	162		10	M	15	177	72	
4	M	59	220	36		11	M	29	179	83	
5	M	54	231	93		12	M	24	187	190	
6	M	40	Smoke inhalation*	—		13	F	22	178	166	
7	M	52	293	85	IIa	16	F	27	180	95	
8	F	50	234	153		17	F	25	194	80	
9	F	45	219	56		18	F	19	206	104	
10	M	51	239	215	IV	19	M	14	151	40	
11	F	45	274	171		21	M	17	144	30	
12	M	52	259	198		22	M	15	123	25	
13	F	51	224	86		23	M	13	189	28	
14	F	46	230	152		24	F	14	143	44	
15	M	36	Trauma*	—		25	M	13	146	38	
17	M	34	251	86		26	M	12	145	175	
20	F	27	240	90		27	M	12	137	47	
21	F	58	366	300	IIb	28	M	8	164	60	
22	M	45	219	56		29	M	9	147	30	
						30	F	8	146	39	

* Cause of death.
‡ Lipoprotein quantification and typing were determined by methods described in the accompanying paper (11).

mean of the abnormal distribution was 172.3±76.6 mg/100 ml.[8]

In these same relatives the distribution of cholesterol was not bimodal but appeared unimodal and shifted to the right of controls (Figs. 9A and 10A). Its mean±SD (250±56 mg/100 ml) was significantly higher than that of the controls (218±41) ($P < 0.001$). Fig. 11 indicates that this apparently unimodal curve was actually composed of two overlapping distributions —a normal cholesterol distribution in relatives whose triglyceride levels were normal (<90th percentile) and a shifted cholesterol distribution in relatives whose triglyceride levels were elevated (≥90th percentile).

[8] The Chi-square goodness of fit was significantly better for a mixture of two overlapping distributions ($P > 0.5$) than for a single distribution ($P < 0.005$).

The difference in mean±SD of these two distributions (238±50 and 277±60 mg/100 ml, respectively), although highly significant ($P < 0.001$), was not great enough to be resolved as a bimodal curve unless the triglyceride level was used as a discriminant (Fig. 9A). It should be noted that while the distribution and median of the cholesterol levels in the normotriglyceridemic relatives resembled those of controls (Fig. 11), the actual mean±SD of the cholesterol levels of the normotriglyceridemic relatives (238±50) was significantly higher than that of the controls (218±41) ($P < 0.01$). This higher mean value in the normotriglyceridemic relatives was due to the cholesterol values of about 6% of relatives who showed hypercholesterolemia without hypertriglyceridemia. These data suggested that familial combined hyperlipidemia

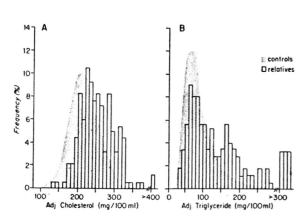

FIGURE 9 Frequency distribution of adjusted lipid levels in 234 first-degree adult (≥20 yr of age) relatives of 47 survivors with familial combined hyperlipidemia. Age and sex-adjustments were carried out as described in the accompanying paper (10). The distribution is divided into increments of 10 mg/100 ml. The smooth strippled curve represents a nonparametric density estimate of the control distribution.

is determined by a single gene whose primary action is on triglyceride metabolism with secondary effects on cholesterol metabolism. This interpretation comes from the generalization that when several phenotypic effects of a gene are considered, discrimination into distinct genetic classes becomes increasingly evident as one gets closer to the primary effect of the gene (18). As a control, similar analyses of the cholesterol curve of the adult relatives of the familial hypertriglyceridemic disorder were done. These data indicated that although the mean cholesterol of the hypertriglyceridemic relatives (228 mg/100 ml) was slightly higher than that of the unaffected relatives (211 mg/100 ml) ($P < 0.1$, but > 0.05), neither the hypertriglyceridemic nor the unaffected relatives had cho-

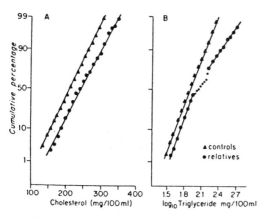

FIGURE 10 Cumulative frequency distribution of adjusted lipid levels in 234 first-degree adult (≥20 yr of age) relatives of 47 survivors with familial combined hyperlipidemia. The cholesterol and log₁₀ triglyceride values were age and sex-adjusted as described in the accompanying paper (10).

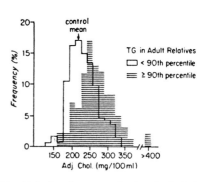

FIGURE 11 Relation between the level of cholesterol and triglyceride in 234 first-degree adult (≥20 yr of age) relatives of 47 survivors with familial combined hyperlipidemia. The 234 relatives were divided into two groups depending on whether their triglyceride level fell above (n = 98) or below (n = 136) the 90th percentile of controls. The mean value for adjusted cholesterol levels in controls (218 mg/100 ml) is indicated by the arrow at the top of the figure.

lesterol levels that were significantly different from those of controls ($P > 0.05$).

The pedigrees of 46 of the 47 families in this group are presented in Figs. 12A and 12B. (The data for the 47th family are shown in Fig. 8 and Table VI). Inspection of these pedigrees demonstrates the following: vertical transmission of hyperlipidemia; the rare occurrence of hypercholesterolemia in children; occurrence of hypertriglyceridemia in about 9% of children at risk; a striking degree of variability in the lipid phenotypes among affected relatives in the same family; and the almost complete absence of hyperlipidemic segregants among the offspring of two normolipidemic parents.

Table VII presents the results of a sib analysis of the 47 survivors with familial combined hyperlipidemia. The proportion affected with hyperlipidemia (nearly 50%) is consistent with an autosomal dominant mechanism of inheritance and excludes the segregation of two genes (one elevating cholesterol and one elevating triglyceride). With segregation of two genes, 75% of sibs would have been expected to manifest hyperlipidemia (i.e., 25% normal, 25% hypercholesterolemic, 25% hypertriglyceridemic, and 25% both). In Table VII, the expected proportion of affected sibs (50% of those tested) assumes that there is no effect of this gene on mortality at the ages tested. However, this assumption is not completely valid, since 10 out of the 24 sib deaths above the age of 35 yr were caused by myocardial infarction (Table VII). Assuming that each of these 10 dead sibs carried the gene for combined hyperlipidemia and that the other 14 sibs were noncarriers, then the ratio of affected to normal would be 61 + 10 = 71 affected as compared with 65 + 14 = 79 normal. It is, of course, possible that some family

TABLE VII

Analysis of Sibships of 47 Survivors with Familial Combined Hyperlipidemia

| | | Sibs (no.) | | | | Number affected | |
| | | Dead | | | | | |
	Total	By all causes	By MI*	Living	Tested	Observed‡	Expected§
Brothers	95	24	9	71	60	30 (9, 7, 14)¶	30
Sisters	89	14	1	75	66	31 (7, 11, 13)¶	33
Total	184	38‖	10	146	126	61	63

* Deaths by myocardial infarction (MI) were documented by death certificates.

‡ A relative was considered affected if either his cholesterol or his triglyceride level or both equaled or exceeded the 95th percentile values for cholesterol and triglyceride.

§ Expected number of affected relatives by the hypothesis of autosomal dominant inheritance, assuming no effect of the gene on mortality at the ages tested.

‖ 14 of these 38 deaths occurred before age 35 yr.

¶ Distribution (no.) of phenotypes of affected relatives are indicated in parenthesis in the following order: hypercholesterolemia alone, hypertriglyceridemia alone, and both hypercholesterolemia and hypertriglyceridemia.

members who died of causes other than myocardial infarction also carried this gene. However, this would have no significant effect on the segregation ratio. This distribution of lipid phenotypes among affected adult relatives (Tables VII and VIII) showed about one-third with the characteristic elevation in both cholesterol and triglyceride, one-third with elevated cholesterol alone, and one-third with elevated tri-glyceride alone. Affected children with hyperlipidemia had hypertriglyceridemia either with or without hypercholesterolemia, but they almost nerver had hypercholesterolemia alone (Table VIII). The sex ratio (male/female) of all affected relatives was 1.06. Similar to the data in familial hypertriglyceridemia, the observed deficiency in first-degree relatives above age 25 reflected a dearth of affected older relatives,

TABLE VIII

Proportion of Affected Relatives of 47 Survivors with Familial Combined Hyperlipidemia

| | | Affected relatives | | |
| Age of relatives and degree of relation | No. tested | Observed* | | Expected‡ |
		90th percentile	95th percentile	
		%	%	%
A. ≥ Age 25				
1st degree	212	50.0§ (13.5, 16.2, 20.3)	41.7 (10.9, 13.5, 17.3)	50.0
2nd degree	77	37.7 (11.7, 18.2, 7.8)	31.1 (10.4, 16.8, 3.9)	25.0
B. < Age 25				
1st degree	76	15.8 (2.6, 9.2, 4.0)	9.2 (0.0, 7.9, 1.3)	50.0
2nd degree	143	16.1 (3.5, 7.0, 5.6)	13.3 (1.4, 8.4, 3.5)	25.0

* A relative was considered affected if either his cholesterol or his triglyceride level or both equaled or exceeded the indicated percentile value.

‡ Expected proportion of affected relatives on the hypothesis of autosomal dominant inheritance, assuming no effect of the gene on mortality at the ages tested and assuming no introduction of the gene by those marrying into the family.

§ Distribution (percent) of phenotypes of affected relatives are indicated in parenthesis in the following order: hypercholesterolemia alone, hypertriglyceridemia alone, and both hypercholesterolemia and hypertriglyceridemia.

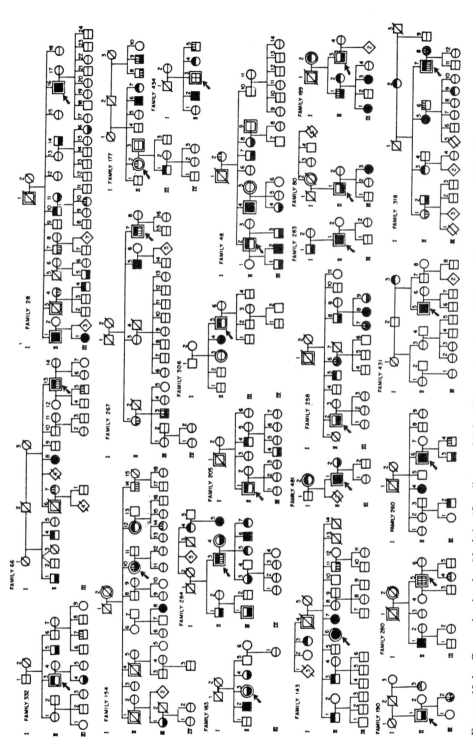

FIGURE 12 A Composite showing 23 of the 47 pedigrees with familial combined hyperlipidemia. The remaining 24 families are shown in Figs. 8 and 12 B. The legend for these pedigrees is identical with that shown for Fig. 4. The proband for each family is indicated by an arrow. Spouses belonging to matings for which there were no data available for the offspring have been omitted from these pedigrees. Identification and lipid data for each family member are available upon request (deposited with the National Auxiliary Publications Service [ID no. 02057]).

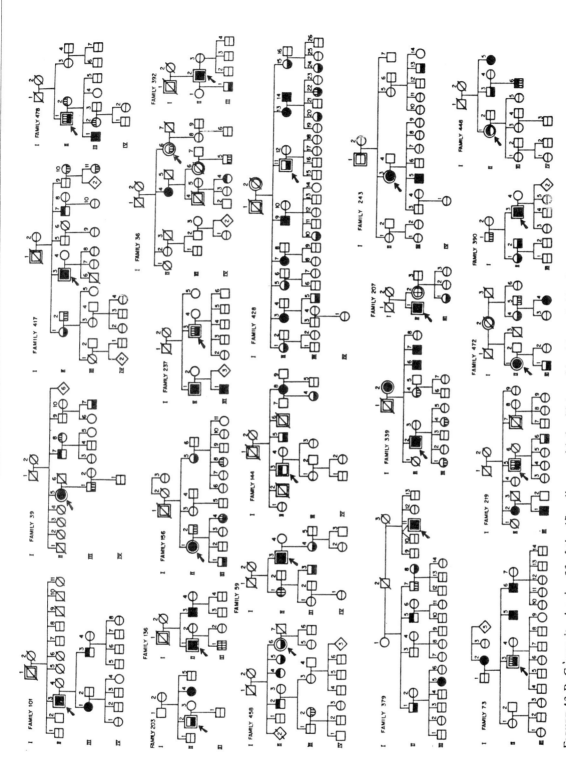

FIGURE 12 B Composite showing 23 of the 47 pedigrees with familial combined hyperlipidemia. The remaining 24 families are shown in Figs. 8 and 12 A. The legend for these pedigrees is identical to that shown for Fig. 4. The proband for each family is indicated by an arrow. Spouses belonging to matings for which there were no data available for the offspring have been omitted from these pedigrees. Identification and lipid data for each family member are available upon request (deposited with the National Auxiliary Publications Service [ID no. 02057]).

TABLE IX

Analysis of 22 Informative Matings from 20 Families with Familial Combined Hyperlipidemia*

Mating type (no.)	Distribution of phenotypes in offspring (no.)			
	Normal	↑Cholesterol	↑Triglyceride	↑Both
↑Cholesterol × normal (6)	4	1	3	2
↑Triglyceride × normal (9)	10	1	6	5
↑Both × normal (7)	10	0	8	3

* Parents and offspring were considered affected if the indicated lipid level equaled or exceeded the 95th percentile of controls. This analysis includes all matings from families with combined hyperlipidemia which met both of these criteria: (a) the parental mating type was affected × normal and (b) at least one offspring was affected.

such as parents, whose deaths by myocardial infarction might be ascribed to the effect of the gene.

Further evidence suggesting that familial combined hyperlipidemia is determined by a single gene with variable expression is indicated in Table IX, an analysis of 22 informative matings from 20 of the 47 families. Note the hypertriglyceridemic offspring (elevation in triglyceride alone or in both lipids) from hypercholesterolemic × normal matings and also the hypercholesterolemic offspring (elevation in cholesterol alone or in both lipids) from hypertriglyceridemia × normal matings. In 14 other matings between a hypercholesterolemic and a normal parent, there was a complete absence of hypercholesterolemia among 32 children, a finding quite different from that observed in families with familial hypercholesterolemia (5, 19, 20). In 20 additional matings between two normal individuals, only 2 out of 49 offspring (over half of which were above 20 yr of age) were hyperlipidemic.

Comparison of lipids in relatives, ages 6–20, in familial hypercholesterolemia, familial hypertriglyceridemia, and familial combined hyperlipidemia. Fig. 13 compared the distribution of *unadjusted* plasma lipids in first-, second-, and third-degree relatives, ages 6–20, from families with familial hypercholesterolemia (Fig. 13A), familial hypertriglyceridemia (Fig. 13B), and familial combined hyperlipidemia (Fig. 13C). Unadjusted values were used in this analysis since plasma lipid levels in 110 control individuals (ages 6–20) showed no significant correlation with age (see legend to Fig. 13 and reference 21). The cholesterol distribution was bimodal in the young relatives of probands with familial hypercholesterolemia (Fig. 13A, left). The cholesterol curve in relatives of probands with combined hyperlipidemia was predominantly unimodal, although there was a slight suggestion of a second mode involving about 2% of the total sample (Fig. 13C, left). The triglyceride distribution in familial hypercholesterolemia was unimodal (Fig. 13A, right), but appeared bimodal in familial hypertriglyceridemia (Fig. 13B, right) and in familial combined hyperlipidemia (Fig. 13C, right). These data provide further evidence that familial combined hyperlipidemia is genetically distinct from familial hypercholesterolemia and demonstrate

TABLE X

Analysis of Sibships of 31 Survivors with Sporadic Hypertriglyceridemia

	Sibs (no.)					Number affected	
		Dead					
	Total	By all causes	By MI*	Living	Tested	Observed‡	Expected‡
Brothers	57	28	4	29	23	1	11.5
Sisters	52	15	1	37	34	0	17.0
Total	109	43‖	5	66	57	1	28.5

* Deaths by myocardial infarction (MI) were documented by death certificates.
‡ Relatives were considered affected if the age and sex-adjusted plasma triglyceride level was equal to or exceeded the 95th percentile of controls.
§ Expected number of affected relatives by the hypothesis of autosomal dominant inheritance.
‖ 16 of these 43 deaths occurred before age 35 yr.

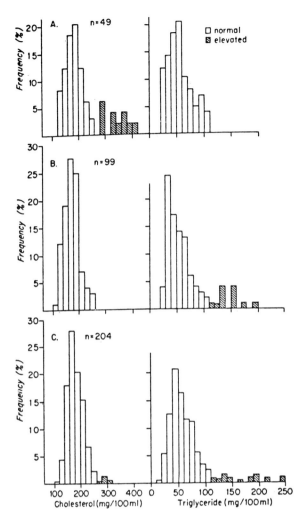

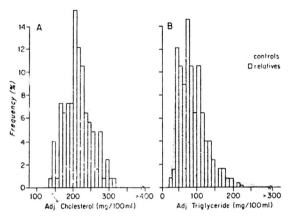

FIGURE 14 Frequency distribution of 158 near and distant adult (≥20 yr of age) relatives of 31 survivors with sporadic hypertriglyceridemia. Included in this analysis were 105 first-degree, 44 second-degree, and 9 third-degree relatives. Age and sex-adjustments were carried out as described in the accompanying paper (10). The distribution is divided into increments of 10 mg/100 ml. The smooth strippled curve represents a nonparametric density estimate of the control distribution.

FIGURE 13 Frequency distribution of unadjusted lipid levels in near and distant relatives, age 6–20, of 16 probands with familial hypercholesterolemia (A), 23 probands with familial hypertriglyceridemia (B), and 47 probands with familial combined hyperlipidemia (C). The number of relatives tested for each disorder is indicated in the appropriate panel. No age and sex-adjustments were applied to these data since no significant correlation with age was observed in values from 110 controls, ages 6–20 (see below). Moreover, when these data were reanalyzed using the age and sex-adjustments described in the accompanying paper (10), identical profiles in the lipid distributions were observed for each disorder. The only difference produced by the adjustment to age 45 was that the absolute lipid levels of each individual was higher. The arbitrary designation of normal and elevated was made from a consideration of the lipid levels in the 110 controls, ages 6–20, whose values were collected as part of the family studies of the 27 normolipidemic survivors. Since the highest unadjusted cholesterol and triglyceride values observed in these controls were 250 and 115 mg/100 ml, respectively, these values were arbitrarily considered as maximum upper limits of normal for the age range.

that the earliest manifestation in affected individuals with combined hyperlipidemia is hypertriglyceridemia alone.

Group B: sporadic hypertriglyceridemia and polygenic hypercholesterolemia. In addition to the 86 survivors of myocardial infarction with monogenic forms of hyperlipidemia (groups A-1, A-2, and A-3,) 59 hyperlipidemic survivors (group B) were identified in whom the family lipid data did not differ significantly from that of the normolipidemic families (Table I). Since these survivors in group B consisted of a mixture of hypertriglyceridemic and hypercholesterolemic individuals, we arbitrarily divided them into two groups: those with pure hypertriglyceridemia (n = 31) and those with hypercholesterolemia with or without hypertriglyceridemia (n = 28).

The distribution of adjusted plasma lipids of 158 adult relatives of these nonfamilial pure hypertriglyceridemic survivors is shown in Fig. 14. Both the cholesterol and triglyceride curves in relatives appeared unimodal, and the mean±SD for cholesterol (211±41 mg/100 ml) and for triglyceride (93±52 mg/100 ml) were almost identical with those of controls. Analysis of the sibs of these 31 survivors (Table X) showed that less than 2% were hypertriglyceridemic. Both lines of evidence suggest that inheritance factors do not play a direct role in the pathogenesis of hyperlipidemia in these survivors. We have therefore designated them as "sporadic" cases in the nongenetic sense.

The distribution of adjusted plasma lipids of 145 adult relatives of the hypercholesterolemic survivors

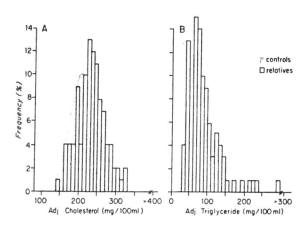

FIGURE 15 Frequency distribution of 145 near and distant adult (≥20 yr of age) relatives of 28 survivors with polygenic hypercholesterolemia. Included in this analysis were 119 first-degree, 20 second-degree, and 6 third-degree relatives. Age and sex-adjustments were carried out as described in the accompanying paper (10). The distribution is divided into increments of 10 mg/100 ml. The smooth strippled curve represents a nonparametric density estimate of the control distribution.

in group B is shown in Fig. 15. The triglyceride curve corresponds to that of controls, while the cholesterol curve is unimodal with a higher mean than that of controls and was shifted to higher values (Fig. 15A). Such a unimodal, displaced curve in relatives of probands is compatible with the hypothesis that multiple cholesterol-elevating genes—possibly in conjunction with environmental factors—are operative in such relatives. Whereas a multifactorial or polygenic mechanism is most likely, such a curve can also be caused entirely by environmental variations, or may be generated by the action of a single genetic locus with one or many alleles. Table XI indicated that about 7% of sibs were hypercholesterolemic by the arbitrary criteria used. This interpretation of multifactorial inheritance of hypercholesterolemia is further substantiated by the finding of significant correlations in cholesterol levels of parent-child ($r = +0.200$) and sib-sib ($r = +0.354$) pairs among normolipidemic families. Such correlations, in the absence of similar husband-wife correlations ($r = -0.023$), fit the concept that one of several mechanisms produce hypercholesterolemia: polygenic, monogenic, and nongenetic.

Summary of genetic analysis of hyperlipidemic survivors of myocardial infarction. A summary of our genetic analysis is presented in Fig. 16. Of the 157 hyperlipidemic survivors of myocardial infarction identified in the accompanying paper (10), 15% could not be classified because of lack of available living relatives (see Methods). 54% had one of the three monogenic disorders, the most frequent being familial combined hyperlipidemia which was observed in about

one-third of all hyperlipidemic survivors. Except for four survivors with type III hyperlipidemia (see the accompanying paper [11]), the remaining 31% of hyperlipidemic survivors had either a polygenic or sporadic form of hyperlipidemia.

Frequency of hyperlipidemia in survivors of myocardial infarction and in the general population. Since our study involved virtually all survivors of myocardial infarction under age 60 and a randomly selected group age 60 and above who were admitted to most of the hospitals in a metropolitan area during a period of 11 mo, it was possible to estimate the overall frequencies of the various disorders identified in this study. These data are shown in Table XII. In extrapolating from our observed data in survivors under age 60 to findings in the general population, it was necessary to make several assumptions each of which tended to underestimate the heterozygote frequency of these disorders. (These assumptions are enumerated in the legend of Table XII.) Although the monogenic disorders were about three times more common in the younger (< age 60) survivors than in the older survivors, both polygenic hypercholesterolemia and sporadic hypertriglyceridemia appeared equally common (each with a frequency of about 6%) among young and old survivors. Familial hypercholesterolemia occurred in 4.1% of all consecutively studied survivors under age 60 and in 0.7% of the group of randomly studied older survivors. A rough estimate of its frequency in the general population is 0.1–0.2%. Familial hypertriglyceridemia was slightly more common, occurring in 5.2% of survivors under age 60 and 2.7% of the older group. Its population frequency is estimated at 0.2–0.3%. Familial combined hyperlipidemia occurred in 11.3% of all survivors under 60 and 4.1% of the older survivors. Its population frequency is estimated at

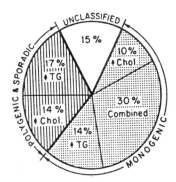

FIGURE 16 Summary of genetic analysis in 157 hyperlipidemic survivors of myocardial infarction. The unclassified category represents those hyperlipidemic survivors in whom family study was not possible because of lack of availability of at least three relatives. Type III hyperlipidemia (not included here) was identified in four, or 2.4%, of these 157 hyperlipidemic survivors (11).

TABLE XI

Analysis of Sibships of 28 Survivors with Polygenic Hypercholesterolemia

| | Sibs (no.) | | | | | Number affected | |
| | | Dead | | | | | |
	Total	By all causes	By MI*	Living	Tested	Observed‡	Expected§
Brothers	44	13	1	31	30	1	15
Sisters	58	6	0	52	44	4	22
Total	102	19‖	1	83	74	5	37

* Deaths by myocardial infarction (MI) were documented by death certificates.

‡ Relatives were considered affected if the age and sex-adjusted plasma cholesterol level was equal to or exceeded the 95th percentile of controls.

§ Expected number of affected relatives by the hypothesis of autosomal dominant inheritance.

‖ 7 of these 19 deaths occurred before age 35 yr.

0.3–0.5%. Considered together, these three monogenic disorders were present in about 20% of all survivors of myocardial infarction under age 60. It is estimated that at least 1 in 160 individuals in the general population may carry a major gene for one of these three disorders.

A summary of the major clinical, genetic, and biochemical characteristics of the five disorders identified in this study is provided in Table XIII.

DISCUSSION

The studies reported here present a genetic analysis of the lipid disorders occurring in survivors of myocardial infarction. Perhaps the simplest and least biased way to handle the data is to combine all hyperlipidemic survivors in one group and examine the lipid levels of their relatives. The results of this kind of analysis showed that relatives had significantly higher levels of both cholesterol and triglyceride as compared

TABLE XII

Frequency of Hyperlipidemia

| | Survivors of myocardial infarction | | | |
Disorder	< Age 60 (a)	≥ Age 60 (b)	Ratio a/b	General population*
	%	%		%
A. Monogenic hyperlipidemia				
Familial hypercholesterolemia	4.1	0.7	5.9	~0.1–0.2
Familial hypertriglyceridemia	5.2	2.7	1.9	~0.2–0.3
Combined hyperlipidemia	11.3	4.1	2.8	~0.3–0.5
Total	20.6	7.5		~0.6–1.0
B. Polygenic				
Hypercholesterolemia	5.5	5.5	1.0	—
C. Sporadic				
Hypertriglyceridemia	5.8	6.9	0.8	—

* These lower limit estimates of heterozygote frequency in the general population are minimal since they were made under the following assumptions: (*a*) that the prevalence rate of coronary heart disease in adults, age 30–59, is 3% (33); (*b*) that the frequency of these disorders as observed among unselected 3-mo survivors of myocardial infarction would be the same among individuals with other manifestations of coronary disease, such as angina pectoris, sudden death, and fatal myocardial infarction; and (*c*) that all heterozygotes for one of these monogenic lipid disorders manifest clinical evidence of coronary disease before age 60 yr. The upper limit estimates were made under the assumption that not all but only one-half of heterozygotes would manifest clinical evidence of coronary disease before age 60 yr.

TABLE XIII

Summary of Clinical, Genetic, and Biochemical Characteristics of Hyperlipidemic Survivors of Myocardial Infarction

Disorder	Typical age	Typical lipid level*		Lipoprotein types‡	Mode of inheritance	Penetrance below age 25§
		Cholesterol	Triglyceride			
		mg/100 ml	mg/100 ml			
Monogenic						
Familial hypercholesterolemia	M 45 F 55	353	126	IIa, IIb	Autosomal dominant	∼0.92
Familial hypertriglyceridemia	M 50 F 55	241	267	IV, V	Autosomal dominant	∼0.26
Combined hyperlipidemia	M 50 F 60	300	241	IIa, IIb, IV, V	Autosomal dominant	∼0.18
Polygenic						
Hypercholesterolemia	M 55 F 60	308	187	IIa, IIb	Polygenic	Not applicable
Sporadic						
Hypertriglyceridemia	M 55 F 60	233	243	IV, V	Nongenetic	Not applicable

* Unadjusted lipid values which represent mean levels of each group.

‡ Lipoprotein quantification and typing was determined by methods described in the accompanying paper (11).

§ Penetrance was estimated by determining the ratio of the proportion of individuals expressing with hyperlipidemia to the expected proportion on the dominant hypothesis.

with those of controls. With this clear establishment of familial factors in the etiology of hyperlipidemia in coronary heart disease, more detailed genetic analysis was undertaken.

Since previous studies had shown the hyperlipidemias to be heterogeneous disorders (2–4), we felt that any genetic analysis should be preceded by sorting the data for obvious heterogeneity. Lacking a specific and diagnostic laboratory test for each of the hyperlipidemias, our first approach was to sort the hyperlipidemias according to the pattern of variation observed in the lipid levels of relatives of affected probands. A comparison of the lipid distributions of relatives with controls should allow a distinction between genetic and nongenetic disorders. Furthermore, among the genetic disorders, autosomal dominant inheritance could be distinguished from polygenic inheritance, provided bimodality in lipid distributions (reflecting the normal and affected relatives) could be detected. Since lipid measurements are far removed from primary gene action, a perfect bimodal curve without overlap in its component distributions would not be expected.

In carrying out the analysis, it was assumed that if there is an inherited disorder in a given family, all affected relatives have the same disorder. In retrospect, such an assumption seemed justified since none of the genetic hyperlipidemic disorders detected has a population frequency of greater than 1 in 100. From the overall results, five different lipid disorders were identified

on the basis of different patterns of distribution in cholesterol and triglyceride levels of relatives.

Familial hypercholesterolemia. The disorder easiest to detect, familial hypercholesterolemia, was characterized by the finding in relatives of a normal triglyceride distribution but an apparently bimodal cholesterol distribution. Segregation analysis suggested autosomal dominant inheritance. The criterion which distinguished this disorder from the other familial hyperlipidemias was the nearly complete expression of hypercholesterolemia in affected children. In addition, almost 50% of the 16 families comprising this group were known to have one or more hypercholesterolemic members with tendinous xanthomas. Moreover, nearly all hypercholesterolemic family members manifested ratios of total plasma cholesterol/triglyceride that were greater than 2. These findings indicated that most of our 16 families with familial hypercholesterolemia closely resembled other families previously reported with this disorder (5, 19, 20). However, since all of our hypercholesterolemic families did not have affected members with xanthomatosis and with cholesterol elevations above 400 mg/100 ml, it is possible that this group of 16 families consists of several biochemically and genetically distinct subgroups that can not be further separated by current tests.

Familial hypertriglyceridemia. A second disorder identified in this study, familial hypertriglyceridemia, was characterized by the occurrence in relatives of a normal cholesterol distribution but an apparently bimodal triglyceride distribution. Segregation analysis in sibs was consistent with autosomal dominant inheritance, but was uninformative when performed on the offspring of affected subjects since hypertriglyceridemia was only expressed in about 13% of young relatives at risk. No detailed genetic analysis of familial "pure" hypertriglyceridemia has been previously published, so it is not possible to make comparisons with other studies. However, on the basis of preliminary analysis of hypertriglyceridemic probands ascertained by a different method, Fredrickson and Levy have also concluded that familial hypertriglyceridemia is determined by a Mendelian autosomal dominant mechanism and that the hypertriglyceridemia is not completely expressed in affected children (19). Moreover, we have recently investigated a large kindred (not part of this study) consisting of 74 members in whom elevated levels of triglyceride but not of cholesterol segregated as an autosomal dominant trait throughout the first-, second-, third-, and fourth-degree relatives of the proband (unpublished observations).

Familial combined hyperlipidemia. The most interesting finding in this study was the delineation of a newly recognized lipid disorder—familial combined hyperlipidemia. It was characterized by variability in expression of lipid levels among affected relatives such that any combination of elevation in LDL cholesterol and very low density lipoprotein (VLDL) triglyceride or both were observed among affected relatives. As described in the accompanying paper (11), affected individuals with this disorder manifested any one of four lipoprotein phenotypes: type IIa, type IIb, type IV, or type V patterns. In the individual family with combined hyperlipidemia, the pedigree was often puzzling and confusing because of this variability in phenotypes. But, when the family data were extensive enough and lipid levels were measured in children, the disorder was relatively easy to distinguish from both familial hypercholesterolemia and familial hypertriglyceridemia.

Several lines of genetic evidence indicate that combined hyperlipidemia is genetically distinct from both familial hypercholesterolemia and familial hypertriglyceridemia. First, the pattern of lipid distributions in relatives, showing an apparently bimodal triglyceride curve and a unimodal and shifted cholesterol curve, was unique. Second, the observation that the hypertriglyceridemic relatives with the combined disorder had abnormally elevated levels of cholesterol was not observed in the familial hypertriglyceridemic disorder in which the hypertriglyceridemic relatives had normal levels of cholesterol. Third, in contrast to the findings of familial hypercholesterolemia, elevation in cho-

lesterol alone was not observed in children of adults affected with combined hyperlipidemia. Fourth, in families with this disorder, a hypercholesterolemic × normal mating frequently gave rise to hypertriglyceridemic progeny; conversely, hypertriglyceridemic × normal matings often produced hypercholesterolemic progeny. These observations were consistent with variable expression of a single autosomal dominant gene. It remains to be seen whether all of the 47 families with combined hyperlipidemia actually have the same abnormal gene, since biochemical and genetic heterogeneity cannot be ruled out by the present studies.

Since the earliest manifestation in affected children with combined hyperlipidemia was hypertriglyceridemia alone, the primary biochemical abnormality in this disorder may involve triglyceride metabolism with secondary effects on cholesterol metabolism. Additional evidence supporting this hypothesis is the fact that triglyceride levels in relatives appeared to segregate into two distributions, whereas their cholesterol levels showed a less clear-cut bimodality. Furthermore, the recent demonstration that plasma LDL may arise physiologically from the catabolism of VLDL (22, 23) documents an interrelationship of these two lipoprotein classes and hence of plasma cholesterol and triglyceride, suggesting a possible metabolic site for the lesion in combined hyperlipidemia. In this respect, our postulation that the primary defect in combined hyperlipidemia involves triglyceride transport provides a reasonable explanation for the occurrence of either hypertriglyceridemia alone or both hypertriglyceridemia and hypercholesterolemia in affected individuals. However, the finding of hypercholesterolemia alone in a minority of affected individuals with the combined disorder cannot readily be explained by this hypothesis. Its occurrence therefore provides a challenge for additional work on the pathophysiology and biochemistry of lipoprotein metabolism.

In their recent study of lipid abnormalities in survivors of myocardial infarction, Patterson and Slack did not detect familial combined hyperlipidemia (24). However, only 39 first-degree relatives from families with all types of familial hyperlipidemia were tested, precluding the possibility of picking out this disorder. However, these authors did observe hypertriglyceridemia in relatives of probands with hypercholesterolemia and vice versa.

In keeping with our identification of combined hyperlipidemia as a genetic entity is the recent report of Rose, Kranz, Weinstock, Juliano, and Haft (25). These authors independently concluded that combined hyperlipidemia was different from either familial hypercholesterolemia or familial hypertriglyceridemia. Furthermore, one report in 1968 by Matthews of a kindred in which hypercholesterolemia and hypertriglyceridemia occurring as different phenotypic expressions of the same mutant gene (26) and another report in 1969 by Schreibman, Wilson, and Arky of a family with familial type IV hyperlipidemia (27) were both, in retrospect, probable examples of familial combined hyperlipidemia.[9] Although widely quoted as an example of familial type IV hypertriglyceridemia (and originally designated as such because of the presence in affected family members of a pre-beta band on lipoprotein electrophoresis of whole plasma), the kindred studied by Schreibman et al. (27) actually contained among the eight affected relatives two with hypercholesterolemia alone, one with hypertriglyceridemia alone, and five with both hypercholesterolemia and hypertriglyceridemia. Like the large pedigree shown in Fig. 10, both Matthews' and Schreibman's pedigrees are consistent with the present evidence for single gene inheritance of familial combined hyperlipidemia.

Problems involved in the detection of major gene effects. Although our analyses suggested that familial hypercholesterolemia, familial hypertriglyceridemia, and familial combined hyperlipidemia are each determined by a different autosomal dominant gene rather than by a polygenic mechanism, it was necessary to use arbitrary cut-off values for cholesterol and triglyceride to classify relatives as normal and affected. Consequently, there must have been misclassification of some individuals, because of the overlapping nature of the lipid distributions. However, the cut-off value chosen (95th percentile) was higher than the apparent antimode of the lipid distributions in relatives (90th percentile). This choice should have minimized the number of misclassified normal relatives, and thus any bias would be against monogenic inheritance.

In addition to the results of the segregation analyses, there are other reasons why a monogenic rather than a polygenic model is more likely for these disorders. The definite absence of unimodality and the highly suggestive presence of bimodality in the appropriate lipid distributions favored a single-gene mechanism (8). In addition, the proportion of affected relatives was higher than that predicted by a polygenic model. Assuming that the level of cholesterol or triglyceride is entirely determined by multiple genetic factors (i.e., heritability = 1) and designating those with values equal to or exceeding the 95th percentile as affected, the expected number of affected first- and second-degree relatives predicted on a polygenic

[9] Although the family reported by Matthews was originally reported as having several members affected with the type III lipoprotein pattern (26), the presence of the β-VLDL marker which characterizes this phenotype (2, 3) was not demonstrated in those individuals showing an elevation in both cholesterol and triglyceride. By current classification, these individuals would be considered to have a type IIb lipoprotein pattern.

model would be about 25 and 9%, respectively, (28, 29) rather than the observed 45–55 and 20–30%. With lower heritabilities, these estimates for the proportion of affected first- and second-degree relatives under a polygenic model would be even less (28, 29).[10] Furthermore, whereas the ratio of hyperlipidemic probands having a myocardial infarction was 4:1 (male:female), no deviation from unity in the sex ratio among hyperlipidemic relatives was noted—another argument favoring monogenic inheritance (30). Finally, in contrast to some other polygenically determined disorders where a higher proportion of relatives is affected if the proband is severely affected (28), no such phenomenon was observed in our data. For example, probands whose lipid levels fell in the 95–98th percentile range had as many relatives affected with lipid levels in the 99th percentile as did probands whose lipid levels fell in the 99th percentile (unpublished observations).

Although the above considerations seem most consistent with single gene inheritance, the evidence for major gene effects on quantitative traits such as cholesterol and triglyceride cannot be considered incontrovertible until a specific biochemical defect for each of the three disorders is identified. Alternatively, the discovery of chromosomal linkage to a known marker

[10] In studies carried out with Dr. Joseph Felsenstein, the heritability and the components of the total phenotypic variance for both the levels of cholesterol and triglyceride in these monogenic families were estimated by a maximum likelihood computer program. Covariance information between relatives was computed using all degrees of relationship, including near and distant relatives and spouses. The phenotypic variance was partitioned into the following components: additive variance, Va; dominance variance, Vd; and environmental or nongenetic variance, Ve (9). In this type of analysis, the heritability (i.e., the genetic contribution to the total variance) is defined in the broad sense as,

$$\frac{Va + Vd}{Va + Vd + Ve}.$$

Estimates of heritability in families with the monogenic disorders and in control families were as follows:

Group (Number of family members*)	Heritability	
	Cholesterol	Triglyceride
Normolipidemic families (n = 283)	0.84	0.50
Familial hypercholesterolemia (n = 189)	1.00	—
Familial hypertriglyceridemia (n = 333)	—	0.97
Familial combined hyperlipidemia (n = 734)	0.86	0.87

* Includes probands, relatives, and spouses.

gene, such as to a blood group or polymorphic enzyme, would also provide more definitive evidence for the single gene hypothesis.

In addition to the three presumably monogenic lipid disorders, two other types of hyperlipidemia were identified among survivors of myocardial infarction—polygenic hypercholesterolemia and sporadic hypertriglyceridemia. The finding of a polygenic disorder involving cholesterol but not triglyceride and of a sporadic disorder involving triglyceride but not cholesterol is in keeping with our data on familial correlations of lipid levels. These showed that among normal individuals the variation in plasma cholesterol levels is determined predominantly by genetic factors, while the variation in plasma triglyceride levels is accounted for equally by environmental and genetic factors.[10]

Frequency of hyperlipidemia. Although our calculated figures for the frequency of the three monogenic lipid disorders in the general population are indirect and represent conservative estimates, a heterozygote frequency of 0.1–0.2% for familial hypercholesterolemia agrees with the finding of the Framingham study in which about 1 in 850 individuals in the general population were observed with hypercholesterolemic xanthomatosis (31). Until detailed studies are performed on the families of hyperlipidemic individuals selected at random from the general population, the heterozygote frequencies reported here should be considered only as approximate. Assuming, however, that our estimates are correct and that no more than 1% of the general population carries a gene for one of the monogenic forms of hyperlipidemia, it is predictable that the polygenic and sporadic form of hyperlipidemia affecting 4% of the population will turn out to be the most common forms of these disorders in individuals *without* coronary heart disease. It should be pointed out, however, that the diagnosis of a polygenic disorder depends on quantitative, rather than qualitative data, requiring arbitrary cut-off values. Therefore, making a distinction between normal and affected individuals can be difficult. On the other hand, for a monogenic disorder a clear qualitative difference is ultimately obtainable and the individual diagnosis can be made more confidently.

If the data of this study can be confirmed and if familial hypercholesterolemia, familial hypertriglyceridemia, and familial combined hyperlipidemia can in fact each be proven to be determined by a separate major gene, then these genes affecting lipid metabolism and ultimately the pathogenesis of coronary heart disease are among the most common disease-producing genes in our population. Considering that at least 1 in 160 individuals may carry one of these three genes, the familial hyperlipidemic disorders are major public health problems.

It is tempting to speculate that one reason for the rising frequency of premature coronary heart disease in affluent societies may be the interaction between a genetic factor such as one of these hyperlipidemic genes whose frequency has presumably not changed over many generations and some newly introduced environmental factor(s) such as diet, stress, and/or sedentary habits. Such a mechanism would be analogous to other types of heredity-environment interaction (32) and implies that different approaches may be required in preventing the various hyperlipidemic disorders. The existence of distinct monogenic hyperlipidemias offers defined subpopulations for assessing the effects of various drugs and diets and also emphasizes the need for a vigorous search to identify the underlying metabolic defect and biochemical lesion in each disorder.

Note added in proof. E. A. Nikkila and A. Aro (1973. *Lancet.* 1: 954.) have independently reported that the most common form of familial hyperlipidemia in survivors of myocardial infarction is one in which multiple lipoprotein types are observed among about 50% of the first-degree relatives. These observations are similar to our data on the familial combined hyperlipidemia disorder.

ACKNOWLEDGMENTS

We are indebted to the following colleagues for their able assistance in carrying out these studies: Stanley Albert and Sally Zitzer for computer programming; Kathryn Bakeman, Martha Salsburg, and Susan Mar for clerical help; Martha Kimura, Y.-L. Lee Lum, and Marilyn Vogel for lipid analyses; and Dr. Pat Wahl of the Department of Biostatistics for statistical analyses and consultation. During the early phases of the study, Dr. Newton Morton, Population Genetics Laboratory, University of Hawaii, Honolulu, Hawaii, gave advice regarding approaches to genetic analyses. Throughout the study, Dr. Joseph Felsenstein of the Department of Genetics provided frequent counsel and criticism of quantitative aspects of the data. Dr. Eloise R. Giblett provided critical review of the manuscript.

This work was supported by U. S. Public Health Service Grants GM 15253, AM 06670, and HD 04872; by a grant from the Washington State Heart Association; by National Institutes of Health contract NHLI 71-2157, and by the Veterans Administration.

REFERENCES

1. Goldstein, J. L., W. R. Hazzard, H. G. Schrott, E. L. Bierman, and A. G. Motulsky. 1972. Genetics of hyperlipidemia in coronary heart disease. *Trans. Assoc. Am. Physicians Phila.* 85: 120.
2. Beaumont, J. L., L. A. Carlson, G. R. Cooper, Z. Fejfar, D. S. Fredrickson, and T. Strasser. 1970. Classification of hyperlipidemias and hyperlipoproteinemias. *Bull. W. H. O.* 43: 891.
3. Fredrickson, D. S., R. I. Levy, and R. S. Lees. 1967. Fat transport in lipoproteins: an integrated approach to mechanisms and disorders. *N. Engl. J. Med.* 276: 34, 94, 148, 215, 273.
4. Havel, R. J. 1969. Pathogenesis, differentiation, and management of hypertriglyceridemia. *Adv. Intern. Med.* 15: 117.

5. Schrott, H. G., J. L. Goldstein, W. R. Hazzard, M. M. McGoodwin, and A. G. Motulsky. 1972. Familial hypercholesterolemia in a large kindred: evidence for monogenic mechanism. *Ann. Intern. Med.* **76**: 711.
6. Jensen, J., and D. H. Blankenhorn. 1972. The inheritance of familial hypercholesterolemia. *Am. J. Med.* **52**: 499.
7. Murphy, E. A. 1964. One cause? Many causes? The argument from the bimodal distribution. *J. Chronic Dis.* **17**: 301.
8. Carter, C. O. 1969. Quantitative characters, polygenic inheritance, and environmental interactions. An ABC of Medical Genetics. Little, Brown and Company, Boston. 50.
9. Cavalli-Sforza, L. L., and W. F. Bodmer. 1971. Polygenic inheritance and common diseases. The Genetics of Human Populations. W. H. Freeman and Company, Publishers, San Francisco. 508.
10. Goldstein, J. L., W. R. Hazzard, H. G. Schrott, E. L. Bierman, and A. G. Motulsky. 1973. Hyperlipidemia in coronary heart disease. I. Lipid levels in 500 survivors of myocardial infarction. *J. Clin. Invest.* **52**: 1533.
11. Hazzard, W. R., J. L. Goldstein, H. G. Schrott, A. G. Motulsky, and E. L. Bierman. 1973. Hyperlipidemia in coronary heart disease. III. Evaluation of lipoprotein phenotypes of 156 genetically defined survivors of myocardial infarction. *J. Clin. Invest.* **52**: 1569.
12. Harding, J. P. 1949. The use of probability paper for the graphical analysis of polymodal frequency distributions. *J. Mar. Biol. Assoc. U. K.* **28**: 141.
13. Hasselblad, V. 1966. Estimation of parameters for a mixture of normal distributions. *Technometrics.* **8**: 431.
14. Hosmer, D. W., Jr. 1971. Maximum likelihood estimation of the parameters of a mixture of two normal distributions. Ph.D. Thesis. University of Washington, Seattle, Wash.
15. Murphy, E. A., and D. R. Bolling. 1967. Testing of single locus hypotheses where there is incomplete separation of the phenotypes. *Am. J. Hum. Genet.* **19**: 322.
16. Murphy, E. A. 1967. Some difficulties in the investigation of genetic factors in coronary artery disease. *Can. Med. Assoc. J.* **97**: 1181.
17. Slack, J. 1969. Risks of ischaemic heart-disease in familial hyperlipoproteinemic states. *Lancet.* **2**: 1380.
18. Penrose, L. S. 1951. Measurement of pleiotropic effects in phenylketonuria. *Ann. Eugenics.* **16**: 134.
19. Fredrickson, D. S., and R. I. Levy. 1972. Familial hyperlipoproteinemias. *In* The Metabolic Basis of Inherited Disease. J. B. Stanbury, J. B. Wyngaarden, and D. S. Fredrickson, editors. McGraw-Hill Book Company, New York. 3rd edition. 545.
20. Nevin, N. C., and J. Slack. 1968. Hyperlipidaemic xanthomatosis. II. Mode of inheritance in 55 families with essential hyperlipidaemia and xathomatosis. *J. Med. Genet.* **5**: 9.
21. Adlersberg, D., L. E. Schaefer, A. G. Steinberg, and C. I. Wang. 1954. Genetic aspects of idiopathic hypercholesterolemia: studies of parents and offspring in 200 randomly selected families. *Circulation.* **10**: 600.
22. Bilheimer, D. W., S. Eisenberg, and R. I. Levy. 1972. The metabolism of very low density lipoprotein proteins. I. Preliminary *in vitro* and *in vivo* observations. *Biochem. Biophys. Acta.* **260**: 212.
23. Gulbrandsen, C. L., R. B. Wilson, and R. S. Lees. 1971. Conversion of human plasma very-low-density to low-density lipoproteins in the squirrel monkey. *Circulation.* **44**(Suppl. II): 10. (Abstr.)
24. Patterson, D., and J. Slack. 1972. Lipid abnormalities in male and female survivors of myocardial infarction and their first-degree relatives. *Lancet.* **1**: 393.
25. Rose, H. G., P. Kranz, M. Weinstock, J. Juliano, and J. I. Haft. 1972. Inheritance of combined hyperlipoproteinemia: evidence for a new lipoprotein phenotype. *Am. J. Med.* **54**: 148.
26. Matthews, R. J. 1968. Type III and IV familial hyperlipoproteinemia: evidence that these two syndromes are different phenotypic expressions of the same mutant gene(s). *Am. J. Med.* **44**: 188.
27. Schreibman, P. H., D. E. Wilson, and R. A. Arky. 1969. Familial type IV hyperlipoproteinemia. *N. Engl. J. Med.* **281**: 981.
28. Falconer, D. S. 1965. The inheritance of liability to certain diseases, estimated from the incidence among relatives. *Ann. Hum. Genet.* **29**: 51.
29. Edwards, J. H. 1969. Familial predisposition in man. *Br. Med. Bull.* **25**: 58.
30. Carter, C. O. 1969. Genetics of common disorders. *Br. Med. Bull.* **25**: 52.
31. Kannel, W. B., W. P. Castelli, T. Gordon, and P. M. McNamara. 1971. Serum cholesterol, lipoproteins, and the risk of coronary heart disease. *Ann. Intern. Med.* **74**: 1.
32. Motulsky, A. G. 1972. Significance of genetic disease. *In* Proceeding of the Conference on Ethical Issues in Genetic Counseling and the Use of Genetic Knowledge. P. G. Condliffe, editor. Washington, D. C. In press.
33. National Center for Health Statistics. September, 1965. Coronary heart disease in adults: United States 1960–1962. Public Health Service. U. S. Government Printing Office, Washington, D. C. Series II, No. 1.

Hyperlipidemia in Coronary Heart Disease

III. EVALUATION OF LIPOPROTEIN PHENOTYPES OF 156 GENETICALLY DEFINED SURVIVORS OF MYOCARDIAL INFARCTION

WILLIAM R. HAZZARD, JOSEPH L. GOLDSTEIN, HELMUT G. SCHROTT, ARNO G. MOTULSKY, and EDWIN L. BIERMAN with the technical assistance of MARGARET R. POOLE, ELLEN D. CAMPBELL, and MARY JO LEVINSKI

From the Departments of Medicine (Division of Metabolism and Gerontology, Veterans Administration Hospital, and Division of Medical Genetics, University Hospital) and Genetics, University of Washington, Seattle, Washington 98195

A B S T R A C T Although analysis of lipoprotein phenotypes is widely used to diagnose and classify the familial hyperlipidemias, an evaluation of this system as a method for genetic classification has hitherto not been published. The present study of 156 genetically defined survivors of myocardial infarction was therefore designed to examine the relationship between lipoprotein phenotypes and genetic lipid disorders. The lipoprotein phenotype of each survivor was determined primarily by measurement of his plasma triglyceride and low density lipoprotein (LDL)-cholesterol concentrations; his genetic disorder was identified by analysis of whole plasma cholesterol and triglyceride levels in relatives.

The mean levels of LDL-cholesterol discriminated statistically among the three monogenic lipid disorders: it was highest in survivors with familial hypercholesterolemia (261±61 mg/100 ml [mean ±SD]); intermediate in those with familial combined hyperlipidemia (197± 50); and lowest in those with familial hypertriglyceridemia (155±36) (P < 0.005 among the three groups). However, on an individual basis no lipoprotein pattern proved to be specific for any particular genetic lipid disorder; conversely, no genetic disorder was specified by a single lipoprotein pattern. This lack of correlation occurred for the following reasons: (a) individual LDL-cholesterol levels frequently overlapped between disorders; (b) in many instances a small quantitative change in the level of either LDL-cholesterol or whole plasma triglyceride caused qualitative differences in lipoprotein phenotypes, especially in individuals with familial combined hyperlipidemia, who showed variable expression (types IIa, IIb, IV, or V); (c) lipoprotein phenotypes failed to distinguish among monogenic, polygenic, and sporadic forms of hyperlipidemia; (d) clofibrate treatment of some survivors with genetic forms of hyperlipidemia caused their levels of triglyceride and LDL-cholesterol to fall below the 95th percentile, thus resulting in a normal phenotype; and (e) β-migrating very low density lipoproteins (β-VLDL), previously considered a specific marker for the type III hyperlipidemic disorder, was identified in several survivors with different lipoprotein characteristics and familial lipid distributions.

These studies indicate that lipoprotein phenotypes are not qualitative markers in the genetic sense but instead are quantitative parameters which may vary among different individuals with the same genetic lipid disorder. It would therefore seem likely that a genetic classification of the individual hyperlipidemic patient with coronary

This work was presented in part at the 85th Session of the Association of American Physicians, Atlantic City, N. J., 2–3 May 1972, and published in the Transactions (1).

Dr. Goldstein was supported by Special National Institutes of Health Fellowship GM 4784-01 and is now a Research Career Development Awardee (1-K4-GM 70, 277-01) from the National Institute of General Medical Sciences. His present address is the Division of Medical Genetics, Department of Internal Medicine, University of Texas Southwestern Medical School, Dallas, Tex. 75235. Dr. Hazzard was the recipient of a Clinical Investigatorship of the Veterans Administration and is now an Investigator of the Howard Hughes Medical Institute. Dr. Schrott was supported by Special National Institutes of Health Fellowship HE-48 695. His present address is the Mayo Clinic and Mayo Foundation, Rochester, Minn. 55901.

Received for publication 20 September 1972 and in revised form 19 February 1973.

heart disease made from a quantitative analysis of lipid levels in his relatives may provide a more meaningful approach than determination of lipoprotein phenotypes.

INTRODUCTION

As knowledge of the metabolism of lipids and lipoproteins has advanced, several methods for classifying the hyperlipidemias have been proposed (2–6). The system of classification in widest current use—analysis of lipoprotein phenotypes—was originally developed by Fredrickson, Levy, and Lees (5) and has since been modified and endorsed by the World Health Organization (7). In its present form, this system is based on the level of cholesterol in low density lipoproteins (LDL),[1] the concentration of triglyceride in whole plasma, the electrophoretic mobility of very low density lipoproteins (VLDL), and the presence or absence of chylomicrons in plasma after an overnight fast (7). Six abnormal lipoprotein patterns (types I, IIa, IIb, III, IV, and V) are presently recognized. The relationship of each to different genetically defined hyperlipidemic disorders has not yet been determined except for the familial type I pattern, which results from an autosomal recessive disorder of lipoprotein lipase deficiency (8). It has been generally assumed, however, that the presence of the type IIa or IIb pattern in several members of the same family denotes the genetic disorder, familial hypercholesterolemia; that a familial type IV pattern indicates the disorder, familial hypertriglyceridemia; and that the type III and the type V patterns when occurring in familial form each indicate distinct and separate genetic disorders (5, 9).

To test the validity of these assumptions, lipoprotein phenotypes were determined in 129 hyperlipidemic and 27 normolipidemic survivors of myocardial infarction. The phenotype of each survivor was compared with his genetic diagnosis, which had been independently made on the basis of plasma lipid levels in his relatives using the approach described in the accompanying paper (10). The data from this study have also provided useful information regarding: (a) the variability of lipid levels of survivors of myocardial infarction on repeat testing, (b) diagnostic value of a simple whole plasma cholesterol measurement in reflecting its concentration in LDL, and (c) the frequency of the type III lipoprotein pattern among consecutively studied survivors of myocardial infarction.

METHODS

Selection of survivors for analysis of lipoprotein phenotypes. Lipoprotein phenotypes were determined on repeat

[1] *Abbreviations used in this paper:* LDL, low density lipoproteins; VLDL, very low density lipoproteins; HDL, high density lipoproteins; PVP, polyvinylpyrollidone.

fasting plasma specimens collected from 156 of the 176 survivors who underwent family studies (10) on the basis of an initial lipid analysis 3 mo after their myocardial infarction (11). The mean interval between initial and repeat samplings was 117 days. Of the 20 survivors who were not retested, 5 had died in the interim, 5 left the Seattle area, 1 suffered a recurrent myocardial infarction, 5 could not be located, and 4 refused to participate. The methods for collection of the repeat fasting blood sample and for the separation of plasma were identical with those used for the initial sample (11).

Laboratory procedures. To prevent changes in the lipid composition (12) and electrophoretic patterns (5) of lipoproteins which occur upon prolonged standing of plasma at ambient temperature, all plasma specimens were centrifuged in the Spinco L2-65B preparative ultracentrifuge (Beckman Instruments, Inc., Spinco Div., Palo Alto, Calif.) within 6 h after blood collection. For this procedure 6.5 ml of plasma was overlayered with an equal volume of d 1.006 saline and centrifuged overnight (> 12 h) at 48,000 rpm in the angle 50 Ti rotor at 23° so as to float all $d < 1.006$ lipoproteins (VLDL) into the upper half of the tube. The tube was then sliced in the middle, and the supernatant ($S_f > 20$, VLDL) and infranatant ($S_f < 20$, LDL plus HDL) fractions were collected quantitatively. Each fraction and a portion of whole plasma were analyzed for cholesterol and triglyceride content by methods identical to those employed for the initial plasma sample (11). The concentration of cholesterol in HDL was determined by heparin-manganese precipitation of whole plasma (13). The cholesterol content of LDL was calculated as its concentration in whole plasma less the sum of that in VLDL plus HDL (9).

Lipoprotein electrophoresis of whole plasma was performed in both agarose (14) and polyacrylamide gels (15). The supernatant ($S_f > 20$) and infranatant ($S_f < 20$) fractions were also subjected to electrophoresis in agarose gel. The presence or absence of chylomicrons in fasting plasma was assessed both by agarose gel electrophoresis and 3% polyvinylpyrrolidone (PVP) flocculation (16).

Lipoprotein phenotypes. Lipid and lipoprotein data in each survivor were analyzed by W. R. H. (with the technical assistance of Y.-L. Lee Lum) without knowledge of the survivor's genetic diagnosis. The lipoprotein phenotype of each case was assigned according to the criteria outlined in Table I. These criteria were originally developed by Fredrickson, Levy, and Lees (5) and recently modified by an advisory committee of the World Health Organization (7).

RESULTS

Variability of plasma lipid levels between initial and repeat samples. Table II contains a summary of the whole plasma and lipoprotein lipid data of the survivors of myocardial infarction in whom family studies were performed, organized according to the genetic groups delineated in the accompanying paper (10). In each of these hyperlipidemic groups, the mean level of the lipid or lipids which had been elevated in the initial plasma sample (e.g., cholesterol in familial hypercholesterolemia, triglyceride in familial hypertriglyceridemia, etc.) remained above the 99th percentile in the repeat sample (Table II). Furthermore, on an individual basis, 73% of survivors who were initially hyperlipidemic ($\geq$ 95th percentile) had lipid values in the repeat sample which

TABLE I

Criteria for Analysis of Lipoprotein Phenotypes .

Lipoprotein phenotype	Plasma lipid level		Presence of	
	Whole plasma triglyceride ≥ 95th percentile*	LDL-cholesterol >upper limit of normal‡	Fasting chylomicrons§	β-migrating VLDL‖
IIa	−	+	−	−
IIb	+	+	−	−
III¶	+ or −	+ or −	+ or −	+
IV	+	−	−	−
V	+	−	+	−

* Based on age and sex-adjusted data from 950 control subjects (11).
‡ Based on age-related 95th percentile values estimated by Fredrickson and Levy (9).
§ By PVP flocculation and agarose gel electrophoresis.
‖ By agarose gel electrophoresis (see footnote 3).
¶ Lipid composition of isolated VLDL (and of fasting chylomicrons, when present) and electrophoretic mobility of lipoproteins in whole plasma used as confirmatory diagnostic criteria for the type III pattern but by themselves were not considered sufficient for its assignment.

equalled or exceeded the 95th percentile.[2] This proportion of survivors who remained hyperlipidemic varied among the different disorders: familial hypercholesterolemia, 93%; familial hypertriglyceridemia, 78%, familial combined hyperlipidemia, 74%; polygenic hypercholesterolemia, 75%; and sporadic hypertriglyceridemia, 61%. Of the 16 survivors with monogenic hyperlipidemia whose repeat lipid levels fell below the 95th percentile (including 1 with familial hypercholesterolemia, 8 with familial hypertriglyceridemia, and 7 with familial combined hyperlipidemia), 7 were taking clofibrate at the time of retesting (Tables II and III). Although the reason for the decrease in lipid levels in the other nine survivors was not clear, their repeat values tended to fall in the range between the 75th and 94th percentiles. Of the 19 survivors with either polygenic or sporadic disorders who were normolipidemic when retested, none was taking clofibrate at the time of the repeat sample (Tables II and III). Thus, untreated subjects with monogenic disorders appeared to remain hyperlipidemic on resampling to a more consistent degree than did those with polygenic and sporadic disorders.

The mean levels for both cholesterol and triglyceride among the 27 normolipidemic survivors who were tested on two occasions remained remarkably constant (Table II). Only one of these survivors had a repeat lipid value which exceeded the 95th percentile.

Between the time of the initial and repeat samples, the mean change in weight for survivors in all genetically

---

[2] The complete data from which the mean values of Table II were based have been deposited with the National Auxiliary Publication (ID no. 02056).

defined groups was small and was not significantly different among normolipidemic survivors (− 0.49 kg), those with monogenic forms of hyperlipidemia (− 0.32 kg), and those with polygenic and sporadic disorders (− 0.46 kg).

Relationship between levels of cholesterol in whole plasma and LDL. A major rationale for the quantitative approach to the system of lipoprotein phenotypes has been the possibility that the variable contributions to the total plasma cholesterol level from VLDL and HDL may obscure a high concentration of LDL-cholesterol and thereby mask the presence of the type IIa and IIb patterns (17). To test this relationship directly, levels of whole plasma cholesterol in the repeat samples were plotted against LDL-cholesterol measured in the same samples. Statistically significant correlations ($P < 0.001$) were noted for each of the genetically defined groups: familial hypercholesterolemia, $r = + 0.921$; familial hypertriglyceridemia, $r = + 0.800$; familial combined hyperlipidemia, $r = + 0.869$; polygenic hypercholesterolemia, $r = + 0.759$; sporadic hypertriglyceridemia, $r = + 0.690$; and normolipidemic survivors, $r = + 0.905$. The correlation coefficient of the three monogenic groups considered together (Fig. 1A) ($r = + 0.918$) was significantly higher than that for the polygenic and sporadic groups (Fig. 1B) ($r = + 0.726$) ($P < 0.02$). Thus, it appeared that whole plasma cholesterol closely reflected LDL-cholesterol concentrations in most subjects, particularly those with the monogenic disorders: However, in a small number of individual cases, the LDL-cholesterol level did exceed the upper limit of normal despite a whole plasma cholesterol

TABLE II

Summary of Clinical and Biochemical Data

Disorder (No. of subjects)	Sex	Age	Height	Initial sample						
				Weight	Ideal body weight‡	Glucose§	Uric acid§	Cholesterol‖	Triglyceride‖
	M/F	yr	cm	kg	%	mg/100 ml	mg/100 ml	mg/100 ml	mg/100 ml
Familial hypercholesterolemia (16)	13/3	48±10	172±10	74.3±18.6	111±18	88±16	5.8±1.4	353±62	129±62
Familial hypertriglyceridemia (23)	18/5	52±10	172±9	77.1±14.0	118±13	103±40	6.3±1.2	241±46	266±167
Familial combined hyperlipidemia (47)	36/11	51±9	173±9	75.6±12.8	115±16	97±40	6.2±1.4	298±52	240±116
Polygenic hypercholesterolemia (28)	22/6	53±10	174±8	78.8±13.4	118±13	96±33	6.3±1.7	307±34	184±84
Sporadic hypertriglyceridemia (31)	21/10	55±12	173±10	75.4±13.0	115±13	92±28	6.4±1.2	233±31	243±102
Type III hyperlipidemia (4)	3/1	61±12	171±8	70.1±12.3	109±9	76±23	5.1±1.3	238±53	234±52
Normolipidemic survivors (27)	16/11	44±10	173±11	70.8±13.4	110±13	84±13	5.5±1.2	226±30	97±42

* The data for each disorder are expressed as mean values ±1 SD. The complete data on individual subjects from which these mean values were derived have been deposited with the National Auxiliary Publications Service (ID no. 02056).

‡ Ideal body weight was determined by criteria of the Metropolitan Life Insurance Company as described in the accompanying paper (11).

§ Glucose and uric acid levels were measured on fasting plasma samples as described in the accompanying paper (11).

‖ Unadjusted for age and sex.

¶ Δ weight = weight at time of repeat sample—weight at time of initial sample.

concentration which lay below the 95th percentile. This phenomenon occurred in only one subject with familial hypertriglyceridemia, eight with familial combined hyperlipidemia, two with polygenic hypercholesterolemia, and four with sporadic hypertriglyceridemia. It was also seen in three normolipidemic survivors (Table II).

The relationship between the content of triglyceride in whole plasma and in VLDL was also very close, with a correlation coefficient greater than + 0.959 in all genetically defined groups including the normolipidemic survivors. Thus, the simple determination of whole plasma triglyceride accurately reflected its concentration in VLDL in all survivors.

Type III lipoprotein patterns in survivors. Unequivocal evidence for the type III pattern was present in only one survivor. This individual (no. 115, Table II) manifested the typical features of this disorder (9): hypercholesterolemia; hypertriglyceridemia; β-migrating VLDL;[3] cholesterol-rich VLDL (cholesterol/triglycer-

[3] When the electrophoretic mobility of isolated VLDL from subjects with the typical type III disorder (identified in a previous study [18]) was compared on paper and agarose gel, β-VLDL migrated slightly faster in agarose to a "slow" pre-β-position. However, in the present study such mobility has been designated as 'β' to permit comparison

ide = 0.474) (18); a low level of LDL-cholesterol; and cholesterol-rich fasting chylomicrons isolated by PVP flocculation (cholesterol/triglyceride = 0.41) (19). In addition, polyacrylamide gel electrophoresis of his whole plasma revealed the characteristic trail of lipoproteins migrating in a zone intermediate between normal VLDL and normal LDL, both of which were barely detectable in this subject (Fig. 2). A type III pattern was also present in the 19 yr old son of this survivor (Fig. 2).

In addition to this case, four other hyperlipidemic survivors were judged to have β-migrating VLDL,[3] but in none was the evidence for the type III pattern completely convincing in either the survivors themselves or in their hyperlipidemic relatives. Survivors 293 and 496 had a faint band of β-migrating VLDL, but in each case the predominant VLDL on agarose gel had a normal, pre-β-mobility. Although polyacrylamide gel electrophoresis in these cases (Fig. 2) revealed lipoproteins migrating as a trail intermediate in position between normal VLDL and LDL, it also showed a more dense band in the position of LDL than has been noted in more clear-cut examples of the type III pattern. In addition,

with other reports in which paper electrophoresis had been employed (9).

on 176 Survivors of Myocardial Infarction*

Interval between samples				Repeat sample				
				VLDL			LDL cholesterol	HDL cholesterol
	Δ Weight¶	Cholesterol‖	Triglyceride‖	Cholesterol	Triglyceride	C/T		
days	kg	mg/100 ml	mg/100 ml	mg/100 ml	mg/100 ml		mg/100 ml	mg/100 ml
126±45	−0.56±2.9	349±77	167±91	38±29	99±71	0.36±0.09	261±61	43±21
115±72	−0.22±3.6	240±51	240±252	50±52	172±213	0.32±0.09	155±36	33±8
100±50	−0.31±2.7	281±45	215±174	41±33	150±95	0.31±0.23	197±50	42±16
93±37	−0.25±2.6	288±36	169±86	33±20	106±73	0.32±0.10	206±43	47±28
96±38	−0.64±2.4	249±34	214±87	45±27	144±93	0.35±0.14	164±51	37±14
86±54	−0.33±2.2	264±56	279±146	93±69	202±143	0.45±0.01	134±60	36±13
197±92	−0.49±3.6	226±35	96±38	17±8	58±29	0.32±0.12	162±32	45±12

neither of these subjects had fasting chylomicrons. Their VLDL cholesterol/triglyceride ratios lay between the ranges observed in groups of subjects with well-defined type III patterns (≥0.48) and type IV patterns (≤0.42) as determined in a previous study (18). The other two survivors (108 and 366) were of special interest because they manifested both β-migrating VLDL and high levels of LDL-cholesterol, a combination hitherto reported only in a patient with severe concurrent hypothyroidism (20) and in a single subject with a familial form of hypercholesterolemia (21). Neither of these two cases had clinical evidence of hypothyroidism; one of them (108) was the proband of a pedigree that met the diagnostic criteria for familial hypercholesterolemia (10). In both cases polyacrylamide gel electrophoresis revealed only faint bands in the position of normal LDL (Fig. 2). Of the two cases, only no. 366 (VLDL cholesterol/triglyceride ratio of 0.45) was grouped with the type III subjects in Table II. Survivor 108 was included among those with familial hypercholesterolemia on the basis of the family data and the high-normal VLDL cholesterol/triglyceride ratio of 0.40.

These data indicate that the subjects with β-VLDL in this study comprised a heterogeneous group in terms of

both genetic and lipoprotein characteristics. Moreover, if an elevated VLDL cholesterol/triglyceride ratio had been used as the sole criterion for the diagnosis of the type III pattern, the number of apparent type III subjects would have been increased by four (cases 5, 158, 316, and 339). None of these four subjects, however, showed clear-cut electrophoretic evidence of β-VLDL. Thus, neither β-VLDL nor cholesterol-rich VLDL proved to be a specific marker for a distinct genetic disorder. Because of these diagnostic uncertainties, the frequency of the type III pattern among the 500 survivors of myocardial infarction identified in the accompanying paper (11) could only be roughly estimated at between 0.2 and 1.0%.

Relationship between genetic classification and lipoprotein phenotypes. Table III shows the distribution of lipoprotein phenotypes in 133 survivors with five different genetically defined forms of hyperlipidemia (10). As indicated in the table, no lipoprotein pattern was specific for any one genetically defined lipid disorder; conversely, no genetic disorder was specified by any single lipoprotein pattern. However, there were several trends in the relationship between genetic classification and lipoprotein phenotypes. First, the most frequent lipoprotein phenotypes in survivors with the familial hyper-

TABLE III

Relationship between Genetic Classification and Lipoprotein Phenotypes in Hyperlipidemic Survivors of Myocardial Infarction

Genetic disorder	No. of subjects	Lipoprotein phenotype				
		Normal	IIa	IIb	IV	V
Monogenic						
Familial hypercholesterolemia	14	1*	7	4	2‡	0
Familial hypertriglyceridemia	22	8§	0	2‖	11	1
Familial combined hyperlipidemia	41	·7¶	13**	10	10	1
Polygenic Hypercholesterolemia	25	9	9	2	5	0
Sporadic Hypertriglyceridemia	31	10	4‡‡	2	14	1

* Taking clofibrate at the time of the repeat sample.
‡ One of these subjects was under treatment for acute hyperthyroidism with ^{131}I and prednisone at the time of the repeat sample.
§ Four were taking clofibrate.
‖ One was taking clofibrate.
¶ Two were taking clofibrate.
** Four were taking clofibrate.
‡‡ One was taking clofibrate.

cholesterolemic disorder were the type IIa and type IIb patterns. Second, the most characteristic lipoprotein phenotype in survivors with the familial hypertriglyceridemic disorder was the type IV pattern. Third, survivors with the familial combined hyperlipidemic disorder manifested the widest variety of lipoprotein patterns: types IIa, IIb, IV, and V. A similar distribution of phenotypes was observed among the affected relatives of a large kindred with familial combined hyperlipidemia (see the accompanying paper [10]).

Since the LDL-cholesterol level was an important determinant of an individual's lipoprotein phenotype, it was important to compare the distribution of the LDL-cholesterol levels of hyperlipidemic and normolipidemic survivors grouped according to their genetic diagnoses (Fig. 3). Although the individual values showed a significant variation within each genetic group and thus many instances of overlap occurred between groups, the mean LDL-cholesterol level did tend to discriminate statistically ($P < 0.005$) among the three monogenic disorders. LDL-cholesterol levels were highest in familial hypercholesterolemia (261±61 mg/100 ml [mean ±SD]), intermediate in familial combined hyperlipi-

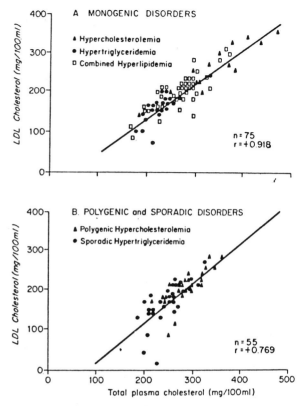

FIGURE 1 (A) Relationship between total plasma cholesterol and low density lipoprotein (LDL)-cholesterol levels in 75 survivors with monogenic lipid disorders. Included in this group of survivors were 14 with familial hypercholesterolemia, 21 with familial hypertriglyceridemia, and 40 with familial combined hyperlipidemia. Two survivors with hypertriglyceridemia associated with hyperchylomicronemia were omitted. Both the whole plasma cholesterol and the LDL-cholesterol levels were determined on the same repeat plasma sample for each survivor. (B) Relation between whole plasma cholesterol and LDL-cholesterol levels in 54 survivors with polygenic hypercholesterolemia (n = 25) and sporadic hypertriglyceridemia (n = 29). One survivor with hypertriglyceridemia associated with hyperchylomicronemia was omitted. Both the whole plasma cholesterol and the LDL-cholesterol levels were determined on the same plasma sample for each survivor.

demia (197±50), and lowest in familial hypertriglyceridemia (155±36). However, the mean LDL-cholesterol level was not significantly different between the polygenic hypercholesterolemic group (206±43) and the combined hyperlipidemic group (197±50), nor was it different between the familial (155±36) and the sporadic (164±51) hypertriglyceridemic groups. It was of note that the mean LDL-cholesterol level of the familial combined hyperlipidemic group was very close to the suggested upper limit of normal for middle-aged subjects. Thus, depending on whether one's value fell above or below this mean, an individual with familial combined hy-

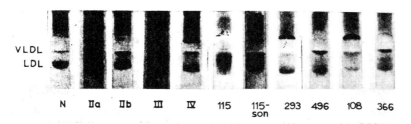

VLDL
LDL

N IIa IIb III IV 115 115-son 293 496 108 366

FIGURE 2 Whole plasma lipoprotein electrophoretic patterns in polyacrylamide gel. The positions of normal VLDL and LDL are indicated along the left margin. The first five patterns were observed in subjects not included in this study and are typical for normal (N) and IIa, IIb, III, and IV lipoprotein phenotypes, respectively. The arabic numerals designate patterns in subjects in this study according to their identification numbers (see text and Table III). 115-son is the son of case 115.

perlipidemia might show a type IIa, IIb, or IV lipoprotein pattern.

DISCUSSION

Lipoprotein phenotypes are now extensively used to diagnose and classify the familial hyperlipidemias (7). Despite this widespread acceptance and application in clinical medicine, no full evaluation of this system, based on family studies, has been published to date. Consequently, several questions have remained unanswered. For example, does lipoprotein quantification and typing provide important information beyond that obtained from the simple measurement of whole plasma lipid levels? Does each of the lipoprotein patterns reflect a different and specific genetic disorder? Do the different lipoprotein types relate to the familial distribution, pathophysiology, prognosis, and therapy of hyperlipidemia in the individual patient? Since in the present study a genetic diagnosis of a large number of hyperlipidemic survivors of myocardial infarction was determined, analysis of their lipoprotein patterns provided the opportunity to approach several of these questions.

A possible limitation in the design of this study was the determination of the lipoprotein phenotype of each survivor on a repeat rather than on the initial plasma sample. However, since 88% of the 176 survivors who underwent a family study (10) were available for repeat sample, the ascertainment bias which might have been associated with obtaining repeat samples was minimized. Furthermore, considering the variety of metabolic stresses experienced by the survivors in the interval between the two samples (e.g., alterations in diet and drug therapy, recurrence of chest pain or hospitalization), their lipid levels proved to be remarkably stable.

Perhaps the most important result of the present study was the demonstration that in the individual hyperlipidemic survivor there was no consistent relationship between lipoprotein phenotype and genetic disorder. Several factors appeared to contribute to this lack of association: First, lipoprotein phenotypes were assigned using

arbitrary 95th percentile cut-off limits for both plasma triglyceride and LDL-cholesterol. Consequently, it was not uncommon for individual survivors with genetic evidence for a familial form of hyperlipidemia to have a normal phenotype. Second, lipoprotein phenotypes failed to distinguish among the monogenic, polygenic, and sporadic forms of hyperlipidemia. Thus, determination of the lipoprotein pattern in the individual survivor did not predict whether family studies would show additional affected relatives. Third, lipoprotein phenotypes failed to separate the three monogenic disorders in the individual case because of significant overlap in LDL-cholesterol values. Fourth, since the various lipoprotein patterns differed quantitatively rather than qualitatively, a small difference in the level of either LDL-cholesterol or whole plasma triglyceride resulted in the assignment of different lipoprotein phenotypes to individuals in the

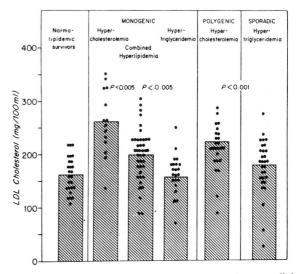

FIGURE 3 LDL-cholesterol levels in survivors of myocardial infarction grouped according to their genetic diagnosis. The LDL-cholesterol measurements were carried out on each survivor's repeat plasma sample.

same genetic group. This occurred most frequently in those with familial combined hyperlipidemia, who as a group manifested four different lipoprotein patterns: types IIa, IIb, IV, and V. Fifth, heterogeneity in both genetic and lipoprotein characteristics was also evident among survivors with the type III pattern. When the type III pattern was defined by the single criterion of the presence of β-migrating VLDL, the group of subjects so identified varied in the lipid composition of their VLDL, the level of LDL-cholesterol, the electrophoretic migration of whole plasma lipoproteins on polyacrylamide gel, the presence of cholesterol-rich fasting chylomicrons, and in their familial lipid distributions. From these data, it would appear that β-VLDL may not be a specific marker for a single and distinct lipid disorder, as has been previously suggested (9).

These studies have also served to justify the use of whole plasma lipid levels for genetic and epidemiological investigations of hyperlipidemia, since excellent correlations were observed between whole plasma and lipoprotein lipid levels in both hyperlipidemic and normolipidemic survivors. In addition, diagnosis on the basis of the family patterns derived from quantitative analysis of whole plasma lipid levels in relatives avoids the misclassification of the index case resulting from the use of arbitrary cut-off limits inherent in determining the lipoprotein phenotype. And finally, unlike the methods for analysis of lipoprotein phenotypes which require a relatively large volume of fresh or refrigerated (unfrozen) plasma, whole plasma lipid levels can be measured in small blood samples collected in diverse geographical regions and mailed at ambient temperature to a single laboratory.

Thus the present study emphasizes that lipoprotein phenotypes are not markers in the genetic sense and as such cannot be equated with specific genetic disorders. This conclusion is reinforced by three lines of previous evidence: first, variation in the lipoprotein phenotype of a given individual often occurs under varying physiological and pharmacological conditions (e.g., conversion of a type V to a type IV pattern with caloric deprivation [22]); second, different lipoprotein phenotypes often occur in several members of a single family (e.g., III and IV, I and V, IIa and IIb, II and IV, and IV and V [9]); and finally, acquired (i.e., secondary) forms of each abnormal lipoprotein pattern have been reported and cannot be distinguished by lipoprotein phenotype from genetic and sporadic forms (9).

Until the fundamental biochemical defects are identified, quantitative analysis of the variation in lipid levels in relatives of hyperlipidemic probands (10) would seem to provide a more meaningful method for genetic classification of hyperlipidemia than analysis of the lipoprotein phenotype of the individual hyperlipidemic subject. By providing patients with a genetic diagnosis, this technique offers a promising approach in the design of studies aimed at determining the underlying metabolic abnormality characteristic of each disorder.

ACKNOWLEDGMENTS

We are indebted to the following colleagues for their able assistance in these studies: Stanley Albert for computer programming; Susan Mar, Kathryn Bakeman, and Martha Salsburg for clerical help; Y.-L. Lee Lum, Karen Grams, Marilyn Vogel, and Martha Kimura for lipid analyses.

This work was supported by U. S. Public Health Service Grants GM 15253, AM 06670, and HD 04872; by a grant from the Washington State Heart Association; by National Institutes of Health contract 71-2157; and by the Veterans Administration.

REFERENCES

1. Goldstein, J. L., W. R. Hazzard, H. G. Schrott, E. L. Bierman, and A. G. Motulsky. 1972. Genetics of hyperlipidemia in coronary heart disease. *Trans. Assoc. Am. Physicians Phila.* **85**: 120.
2. Gofman, J. W., L. Rubin, J. P. McGinley, and H. B. Jones. 1954. Hyperlipoproteinemia. *Am. J. Med.* **17**: 514.
3. Thannhauser, S. J. 1958. Lipidoses: Diseases of the Intracellular Lipid Metabolism. Grune & Stratton, Inc., New York. 3rd edition. 78.
4. Ahrens, E. H., Jr., J. Hirsch, K. Oette, J. W. Farquhar, and Y. Stein. 1961. Carbohydrate-induced lipemia. *Trans. Assoc. Am. Physicians Phila.* **74**: 134.
5. Fredrickson, D. S., R. I. Levy, and R. S. Lees. 1967. Fat transport in lipoproteins—an integrated approach to mechanisms and disorders. *N. Engl. J. Med.* **276**: 32, 94, 148, 215, 273.
6. Havel, R. J. 1970. Typing of hyperlipoproteinemias. *Atherosclerosis.* **11**: 3.
7. Beaumont, J. L., L. A. Carlson, G. R. Cooper, Z. Fejfar, D. S. Fredrickson, and T. Strasser. 1970. Classification of hyperlipidemias and hyperlipoproteinemias. *Bull. W. H. O.* **43**: 891.
8. Harlan, W. R., P. S. Winesett, and A. J. Wasserman. 1967. Tissue lipoprotein lipase in normal individuals and individuals with exogenous hypertriglyceridemia and the relationship of this enzyme to assimilation of fat. *J. Clin. Invest.* **46**: 239.
9. Fredrickson, D. S., and R. I. Levy. 1972. Familial hyperlipoproteinemia. *In* The Metabolic Basis of Inherited Disease. J. B. Stanbury. J. B. Wyngaarden, and D. S. Fredrickson. McGraw-Hill Book Company, New York. 3rd edition. 545.
10. Goldstein, J. L., H. G. Schrott, W. R. Hazzard, E. L. Bierman, and A. G. Motulsky. 1973. Hyperlipidemia in coronary heart disease. II. Genetic analysis of lipid levels in 176 families and delineation of a new inherited disorder, combined hyperlipidemia. *J. Clin. Invest.* **52**: 1544.
11. Goldstein, J. L., W. R. Hazzard, H. G. Schrott, E. L. Bierman, and A. G. Motulsky. 1973. Hyperlipidemia in coronary heart disease. I. Lipid levels in 500 survivors of myocardial infarction. *J. Clin. Invest.* **52**: 1533.

12. Quarfordt, S. H., F. Boston, and H. Hilderman. 1971. Transfer of triglyceride between isolated human lipoproteins. *Biochim. Biophys. Acta.* **231**: 290.

13. Burstein, M., and J. Samaille. 1960. Sur un dosage rapide du cholesterol lié aux alpha et aux beta-lipoproteines du sérum. *Clin. Chim. Acta.* **5**: 609.

14. Noble, R. P. 1968. Electrophoretic separation of plasma lipoproteins in agarose gel. *J. Lipid Res.* **9**: 693.

15. Davis, B. J. 1959. Disc electrophoresis. II. Method and application to human serum proteins. *Ann. N. Y. Acad. Sci.* **121**: 404.

16. O'Hara. D. D., D. Porte, Jr., and R. H. Williams. 1966. Use of constant composition polyvinylpyrrolidone columns to study the interaction of fat particles with plasma. *J. Lipid Res.* **7**: 264.

17. Rifkind, B. 1970. Typing of hyperlipoproteinaemias. *Atherosclerosis.* **11**: 545.

18. Hazzard, W. R., D. Porte, Jr., and E. L. Bierman. 1972. Abnormal lipid composition of very low density lipoproteins in the diagnosis of broad-beta disease (Type III hyperlipoproteinemia). *Metab. (Clin. Exp.).* **21**: 1009.

19. Hazzard, W. R., D. Porte, Jr., and E. L. Bierman. 1970. Abnormal lipid composition of chylomicrons in broad-β disease (type III hyperlipoproteinemia). *J. Clin. Invest.* **49**: 1853.

20. Hazzard, W. R., and E. L. Bierman. 1972. Aggravation of broad-beta disease (Type III hyperlipoproteinemia) by hypothyroidism. *Arch. Intern. Med.* **130**: 822.

21. Lasser, N. L., and S. Katz. 1972. The occurrence of type II and type III hyperlipoproteinemia in a single kindred. *Clin. Res.* **20**: 549. (Abstr.)

22. Brunzell, J. D., D. Porte, Jr., and E. L. Bierman. 1971. Evidence for a common saturable removal system for dietary and endogenous triglyceride in man. *J. Clin. Invest.* **50**: 15a. (Abstr.)

Circulation

MARCH   1973
VOL. XLVII   NO. 3
SUPPLEMENT NO. 1

AN OFFICIAL JOURNAL of the AMERICAN HEART ASSOCIATION

The Coronary Drug Project

Design, Methods, and Baseline Results

By THE CORONARY DRUG PROJECT RESEARCH GROUP

SUMMARY

The Coronary Drug Project (CDP) is a nationwide collaborative clinical trial sponsored by the National Heart and Lung Institute (NHLI). The primary objective is to evaluate the efficacy of several lipid influencing drugs in the long-term therapy of coronary heart disease in men of ages 30 through 64 with ECG evidence of previous myocardial infarction. The following six treatment regimens were included for study in the CDP: Equine estrogens 2.5 mg per day and 5.0 mg per day; clofibrate 1.8 g per day; dextrothyroxine 6.0 mg per day; nicotinic acid 3.0 g per day; and lactose placebo. There are 53 clinics participating in the CDP along with a Coordinating Center, Central Laboratory, ECG Reading Center, Drug Procurement and Distribution Center, and NHLI Medical Liaison Office. A total of 8341 patients were enrolled. All patients were randomly assigned to one of the six treatment groups in a double blind fashion and are being followed for a minimum of five years. The primary response variable in the CDP is total mortality; other major response variables include cause-specific mortality and various nonfatal cardiovascular events such as recurrent myocardial infarction, acute coronary insufficiency, and others. The CDP data are reviewed periodically by a Data and Safety Monitoring Committee for evidence of adverse and beneficial treatment effects. A detailed description of the study population with respect to demographic, clinical, biochemical, electrocardiographic, and other characteristics at baseline is given. In addition, some interrelationships among these baseline characteristics are presented.

Additional Indexing Words:

Coronary heart disease   Myocardial infarction   Clinical trial   Lipid influencing drugs

Editorial Note: Extracts only of 'The Coronary Drug Project' are reproduced. A useful resume appears on page 323 i.e. paper 30.

1. Introduction

The correlation of high levels of serum cholesterol with an increased incidence and prevalence of coronary heart disease (CHD) has been demonstrated repeatedly in prospective and cross-sectional epidemiological surveys.[1-5] These findings have led to the formulation of the following questions: (1) Would long-term lowering of serum lipids in individuals free of CHD result in a reduced incidence of CHD? (2) Would long-term lowering of serum lipids in individuals with CHD have a beneficial effect on morbidity and mortality? The availability of drugs and diets which lower serum lipids makes it possible to attempt to find answers to these questions.

The Coronary Drug Project (CDP), a National Heart and Lung Institute (NHLI) collaborative clinical trial, was designed to help answer the second of these questions. The three main objectives of the CDP are (1) to evaluate the efficacy of several lipid influencing drugs in the long-term therapy of CHD in men of ages 30 through 64 with evidence of previous myocardial infarction (MI); (2) to obtain information on the natural history and clinical course of CHD; and (3) to develop more advanced methodology for the design and conduct of long-term, large, collaborative clinical trials which could be applied to other such studies.

In November, 1960 the National Advisory Heart Council invited Dr. Robert W. Wilkins of Boston to explore the desirability, feasibility, and methodology of a large-scale cooperative clinical trial of lipid lowering drugs in the treatment of atherosclerotic disease. Early in 1961, an *ad hoc* committee was formed under Dr. Wilkins' chairmanship. After a series of deliberations, the unanimous judgment was reached in March, 1961 that such a study was feasible and should be conducted. On the basis of the committee's findings and recommendations, the National Advisory Heart Council in April, 1961 expressed a definite interest in assuring the development of such a study and acted to support further development of this work.

I-8

Over the next two years a Policy Board, Steering Committee, and Coordinating Center were established, and a detailed protocol was written. In 1964 the National Advisory Heart Council recommended approval of the Coronary Drug Project and recommended implementation of the study by the National Heart Institute. In March, 1965 National Institutes of Health grants were awarded to the Coordinating Center and to the first four clinics (table 1, clinic numbers 1 to 4). Later in 1965, a Central Laboratory and a Drug Procurement and Distribution Center were established, and a fifth clinic (table 1, clinic number 5) was funded.

The first patients were enrolled in March, 1966. Twenty-nine additional clinics (table 1, clinic numbers 6 to 34) were awarded grants in 1966. In 1967 an ECG Reading Center was set up, and another 21 clinics (table 1, clinic numbers 35 to 55) were funded. Two clinics subsequently withdrew from the study, leaving a total of 53 participating clinics. Recruitment of patients was completed in October, 1969 with a total of 8341 patients enrolled.

2. Design and Methods

2.1 Major Design Features

A concise itemization of the principal features of the CDP design is given in this section. For each item the number of the section where further details can be found is given.

1. Fifty-three participating clinics plus Coordinating Center, Central Laboratory, ECG Reading Center, Drug Procurement and Distribution Center, and NHLI Medical Liaison Office (2.2).

2. Five drug groups (estrogen in two dosage levels, clofibrate, dextrothyroxine, and nicotinic acid) and a placebo group (2.3).

3. Males, 30 to 64 years old at time of entry, with ECG documented myocardial infarction (MI) at least three months prior to entry and New York Heart Association functional class I or II (2.4).

4. Patients randomly assigned to one of the six treatment groups in a double-blind fashion (2.8).

5. Follow-up visits every four months; minimum five-year follow-up on the assigned treatment (2.9).

6. Over-all mortality the primary endpoint; CHD mortality, sudden death, nonfatal MI, and nonfatal acute coronary insufficiency, other major response variables (2.11).

7. CDP data reviewed periodically by Data and Safety Monitoring Committee for evidence of adverse and beneficial treatment effects.

Table 1

Number of Patients Enrolled in the CDP, by Clinic

Clinic number and name*	No. of patients†
1. Mayo Clinic, Rochester, Minn.	105
2. USPHS Hosp., Staten Island, N.Y.	142
3. Univ. of So. Calif., Los Angeles, Calif.	284
4. Presbyterian St. Luke's Hosp., Chicago, Ill.	153
5. Albert Einstein Med. Ctr., Philadelphia, Pa.	178
6. Ann Arbor Hosp. Group, Ann Arbor, Mich.	212
7. USPHS Hosp., Baltimore, Md.	133
8. Buffalo Gen. Hosp., Buffalo, N.Y.	118
9. Palo Alto Medical Clinic, Palo Alto, Calif.	126
10. Univ. of Chicago, Chicago, Ill.	124
11. USPHS Hosp., San Francisco, Calif.	157
12. Marshfield Clinic, Marshfield, Wisc.	159
13. West Virginia Univ., Morgantown, W.Va.	173
14. St. Joseph Hosp., Chicago, Ill.	143
15. Mount Sinai Hosp., Miami Beach, Fla.	210
16. Maimonides Medical Center, Brooklyn, N.Y.	156
17. Lovelace Foundation, Albuquerque, N.M.	93
18. Mount Sinai Hosp., New York, N.Y.	155
19. V. A. Hosp., Bronx, N.Y.	142
20. Providence Hosp., Portland, Ore.	165
21. V. A. Hosp., Miami, Fla.	179
22. Case Western Reserve Univ., Cleveland, Ohio	197
23. Mount Sinai Hosp., Minneapolis, Minn.	185
24. Ochsner Clinic, New Orleans, La.	196
25. Jackson Clinic, Madison, Wisc.	191
26. Northwestern Univ., Chicago, Ill.	192
27. Grady Memorial Hosp., Atlanta, Ga.	216
29. Bryn Mawr Hosp., Bryn Mawr, Pa.	103
30. V. A. Hosp., Indianapolis, Ind.	147
31. V. A. Hosp., West Roxbury, Mass.	162
32. St. Joseph Hosp., Burbank, Calif.	249
33. Med. Univ. of South Carolina, Charlestown, S.C.	161
34. North Charles Gen. Hosp., Baltimore, Md.	161
35. V. A. Hosp., Jackson, Miss.	98
36. Univ. Dist. Hosp., Rio Piedras, P.R.	177
37. Sidney Hillman Medical Center, Philadelphia, Pa.	148
38. Univ. of Nebraska, Omaha, Neb.	147
39. Univ. of Cincinnati, Cincinnati, Ohio	119
40. Miami Heart Institute, Miami Beach, Fla.	157
41. Geisinger Medical Foundation, Danville, Pa.	148
42. Medical Associates, Chelmsford, Mass.	110
43. Greater Baltimore Medical Center, Baltimore, Md.	128
44. Montefiore Hosp., Bronx, N.Y.	143
45. Univ. of Iowa Hospitals, Iowa City, Iowa	147
46. Ogden Research Foundation, Ogden, Utah	145
47. USPHS Hosp., New Orleans, La.	103
48. Straub Medical Research Inst., Honolulu, Hawaii	150
50. Melrose-Wakefield Hosp., Melrose, Mass.	237
51. Hitchcock Clinic, Hanover, N.H.	100
52. Univ. of Utah, Salt Lake City, Utah	169
53. Santa Rosa Medical Center, San Antonio, Texas	132
54. Salt Lake Clin. Res. Found., Salt Lake City, Utah	136
55. Long Island Jewish Hosp., Jamaica, N.Y.	180
Total	8341

*Two clinics, numbers 28 and 49, withdrew early in the study.

†Includes the number of patients originally enrolled in each clinic plus or minus transfer patients from one clinic to another as of February 1, 1972.

THE CORONARY DRUG PROJECT I-9

2.2 Organizational Structure

A description of the functional units and committees of the CDP is given in this section. The members of these units and committtees are listed at the beginning of this report.

1. Fifty-three *clinics*, distributed throughout the United States and in Puerto Rico. At these clinics patients are recruited, the study drugs are administered, follow-up examinations are performed, and the information required by the study protocol is obtained. A list of these clinics and the number of patients enrolled in each is given in table 1.

2. A *Central Laboratory*, located at the Center for Disease Control in Atlanta; this center performs the routine biochemical determinations for the CDP using frozen specimens obtained from the clinics.

3. An *ECG Reading Center*, located at the University of Minnesota in Minneapolis; this center is responsible for reading and coding all of the ECG records collected in the CDP.

4. A *Coordinating Center*, located at the University of Maryland in Baltimore; this center is responsible for the collection, editing, analysis, and storage of all data from the clinics, the Central Laboratory, and the ECG Reading Center.

5. A *Drug Procurement and Distribution Center*, located at the USPHS Supply Service Center in Perry Point, Maryland; this unit is responsible for procurement and distribution of the study drugs.

6. A *Medical Liaison Office*, located at the NHLI in Bethesda, Maryland; this office provides the chief scientific link between the NHLI and the other units of the CDP.

7. A *Policy Board* which acts in a senior advisory and decision-making capacity on policy matters throughout the entire duration of the study.

8. A *Steering Committee* which provides scientific direction for the study at the operational level. Permanent members of this committee include the original principal investigators of the four initial clinics, the directors of the Coordinating Center, Central Laboratory and ECG Center, the NHLI Medical Liaison Officer, the NHLI Associate Director for Clinical Applications, the Chief of the NHLI Biometrics Research Branch, and a special statistical consultant. There are, in addition, four elected members who are investigators from the participating clinics. The term of office for these elected members is three years, with the possibility of re-election.

9. A *Technical Group* which consists of representatives from each of the 53 clinics and from the Coordinating Center, Central Laboratory, ECG Reading Center, and NHLI.

10. A *Data and Safety Monitoring Committee* which periodically reviews the study results and evaluates the treatments for beneficial and adverse effects.

11. A *Criteria Committee* which defines criteria used in recording clinical observations.

12. A *Laboratory Committee* which reviews the Central Laboratory quality control procedures and results.

13. An *Editorial Review Committee* which reviews every scientific paper using CDP data prepared for oral presentation or publication.

14. A *Statistical Committee* which reviews and makes recommendations concerning the statistical procedures used in CDP data analyses.

15. A *Natural History Committee* which plans analyses, reviews data, and writes papers on the natural history and clinical course of CHD.

16. A *Mortality Classification Committee* which reviews all death information and codes cause of death for each decedent.

17. A *Hepatology Committee* which plans analyses and reviews data relating to the effects of the study drugs on the liver.

18. A *Data Repository Committee* which reviews ancillary study proposals for acceptability of the designated data repository in order to prevent treatment unblinding.

19. An *Arrangements Committee* which is responsible for making all the arrangements for the semiannual Technical Group and Steering Committee meetings.

20. A *Resource Committee* which formulates proposals for new clinical trials utilizing the CDP resource.

21. A *Newsletter Committee* which is responsible for preparing periodic newsletters for the participating patients in the CDP.

2.3 Treatment Regimens

Six treatment regimens were included for study in the CDP: (1) mixed conjugated equine estrogens (Premarin), low dose 2.5 mg per day; (2) mixed conjugated equine estrogens (Premarin), high dose 5.0 mg per day; (3) ethyl chlorophenoxyisobutyrate (CPIB), also called clofibrate (Atromid-S), 1.8 g per day; (4) dextrothyroxine (Choloxin) 6.0 mg per day; (5) nicotinic acid 3.0 g per day; (6) lactose placebo 3.8 g per day.

All drugs, including placebo, are dispensed in identical, size no. 1, opaque gelatin capsules.

Supplement I to Circulation, Vols. XLVII and XLVIII, March 1973

The dosages given above for each of the six treatments are provided in nine capsules per day, prescribed as three capsules three times a day after meals. These dosage levels were initially reached after a stepwise increase over a period of two months. Each patient was started on one capsule three times a day, increased to two capsules three times a day after one month, and increased finally to three capsules three times a day after two months.

Apart from treatment with one of the six study drugs, no standardized regimens (such as drugs, diet, or exercise) have been imposed on the CDP patients. Neither have there been any proscriptions of any forms of therapy or prophylaxis (such as cardiac surgery or anticoagulant therapy) during a patient's follow-up period, except for the proscription of lipid-influencing drugs other than the CDP medication.

Many other drugs reported to influence serum lipids were proposed for evaluation in the study. Some of the agents considered for inclusion, but subsequently rejected for a variety of reasons, were other thyroid analogues, β-sitosterol, cholestyramine, safflower oil, linoleic acid, vitamin E, and triparanol.

A brief discussion of previous experience with each of the CDP drugs and the rationale behind their selection in 1965 follows.

Estrogens

During the late 1940's and early 1950's, extensive evidence was accumulated relating estrogens to cholesterol metabolism and suggesting a possible protective effect of these hormones against clinical atherosclerotic coronary disease.[6] It was recognized that middle-aged women with intact ovaries were remarkably resistant to atherosclerotic coronary heart disease. It was demonstrated during this period that a sex difference exists in lipoprotein patterns and that estrogens convert male patterns to female patterns. In addition, it was shown that in chickens fed with high-fat, high-cholesterol diets, estrogens prophylactically inhibited and therapeutically reversed atherosclerotic plaques in coronary arteries.

Two clinical trials carried out during the 1950's and early 1960's gave evidence suggesting that equine estrogens may be effective in reducing mortality in men with coronary heart disease if used within the proper dosage range.[7, 8] Although the evidence was not conclusive, it was sufficiently encouraging to warrant a more definitive trial.

The CDP included mixed conjugated equine estrogens at two dosage levels, 2.5 and 5.0 mg per day. These dosage levels were reached after a stepwise increase over a period of two months. The stepwise increase was predicated, in part, on data which suggested an adverse effect on survival when a 10-mg dosage of estrogen was given as the initial dosage in the early postinfarction period.[7] The 5.0 mg per day dosage was chosen in the CDP because it was feared that a lower dose might fail to influence lipids and mortality to any significant degree and thus result in a false conclusion about the efficacy of the drug. On the other hand, it was recognized that the feminizing side effects of estrogen are dose-related and that a dose of 5.0 mg per day might result in a higher dropout or nonadherence rate than that expected for the 2.5 mg dose. For this reason and because of a suggestion of possible survival benefit with the 2.5 mg per day dosage,[8] it was decided to include the 2.5 mg per day dosage of estrogen as well.*

Clofibrate

Clinical reports of the use of clofibrate were first published in the early 1960's.[10, 11] While there was a paucity of information available on this drug at the time the CDP was being planned, it was agreed that clofibrate should be included because of its significant lipid lowering effects and apparent lack of bothersome side effects and toxicity.

Dextrothyroxine

Certain thyroid analogues have been reported to be effective in lowering cholesterol without marked associated hypermetabolic effects.[12] The major concern in the use of analogues of thyroxine was the possibility that despite some dissociation of cholesterol lowering effects from calorigenic effects, hypermetabolic effects might aggravate cardiac ischemia by increasing metabolic demands on a myocardium with limited coronary perfusion. Aggravation of angina pectoris had been observed in the absence of an effect on the basal metabolism rate but had been reported only rarely in euthyroid

---

*The use of the 5.0 mg per day dose of estrogen in the CDP was discontinued in May, 1970 because of an excess incidence of recurrent nonfatal myocardial infarction, pulmonary embolism, and thrombophlebitis in this treatment group as compared with the placebo group. No such findings were evident in the group of patients taking 2.5 mg per day of estrogen, and hence, this lower dosage level continues to be used in the CDP. A detailed report of these findings is published elsewhere.[9]

THE CORONARY DRUG PROJECT   I-11

persons on less than 10 mg of dextrothyroxine daily.[13-15] There had also been reports of improvement in angina pectoris during treatment with dextrothyroxine.

A dose of 6 mg per day of dextrothyroxine was selected in the CDP. This dose was believed to have a cholesterol-lowering effect but fewer adverse effects than larger doses.*

Nicotinic Acid

Experience with the long-term use of large doses of nicotinic acid since 1955 has led to an extensive number of publications dealing with the lipid lowering effects, side effects, and other biochemical responses of this drug.[17-20] None of these studies has had sufficient numbers of patients to give any decisive evidence concerning the drug's effect on CHD. On the basis of its significant lipid lowering effects, nicotinic acid was accepted for inclusion as a study treatment.

Lactose Placebo

Placebo capsules, amounting to a daily dose of 3.8 g of lactose, are being used for the control group in the CDP. These capsules are outwardly indistinguishable from those of the other treatment groups.

2.4 Admission Criteria

In order to be enrolled in the CDP, each patient had to satisfy all of the following conditions:

1. Male between 30 and 64 years of age at time of entry into the study (i.e., at the commencement of the assigned treatment regimen).

2. ECG-documented myocardial infarction (MI) at least three months prior to entry. The patient had

---

*On the basis of early experience in the CDP, the use of dextrothyroxine was discontinued in May, 1970 in the group of 26 patients showing frequent ectopic ventricular beats on the baseline ECG. This decision was made because of an apparent excess mortality as compared with the similar subgroup of 78 placebo treated patients. A further protocol change was made in December, 1971 when the use of dextrothyroxine was discontinued in all remaining patients. This change was based principally on two factors: (1) The finding of an excess mortality in the dextrothyroxine subgroups of patients (compared with the corresponding placebo subgroups) having (a) a history at entry of two or more MI or one complicated MI, (b) a history at entry of angina pectoris, (c) a higher than average heart rate at entry, and, particularly, (d) combinations of these traits; and (2) the absence of any sustained reduction in mortality in dextrothyroxine subgroups of patients not having the foregoing traits. Detailed reports of these findings are published elsewhere.[9, 16]

Supplement 1 to Circulation, Vols. XLVII and XLVIII, March 1973

to have *either* an ECG which fulfilled one of the QRS criteria listed in item 20, CDP Form 01 (Appendix I) *or* an ECG which showed ST-T wave or T wave changes *plus* a clinical history and serum glutamic oxaloacetic transaminase (SGOT) changes indicative of an MI. Patients with myocardial infarctions probably due to coronary artery embolism, aortic dissection, and prolonged arrhythmias were excluded. Patients with "silent MI," that is, patients with ECG's satisfying the QRS criteria but without a clinical event, were included.

3. Class I (no limitation of ordinary physical activity) or class II (slight limitation) of the functional classification of the New York Heart Association.[21]

4. No previous surgery for coronary artery disease.

5. Freedom from life-limiting disease other than coronary heart disease, such as malignancy, pulmonary insufficiency, chronic hepatic disease, etc.

6. Freedom from diseases or conditions which might affect long-term follow-up, such as cerebrovascular disease with mental aberration, psychosis, alcoholism, etc.

7. Freedom from conditions which would contraindicate the use of any of the drugs under study in the CDP, such as active gastric or duodenal ulceration, hypothyroidism requiring thyroid replacement therapy, etc.

8. Not on anticoagulant therapy, lipid influencing drugs, or insulin at time of entry.

9. Willingness and ability to take the CDP medication, as determined during a two-month control period, and willing to follow the study protocol for at least a five-year period.

10. Willingness to participate in the study after attending an orientation session at which the study drugs and their characteristic side effects were discussed.

2.5 Sample Size

In deriving the required sample size for the CDP, it was first estimated that the five-year placebo death rate would be 30%. This figure was based on data from other studies giving five-year mortality rates in men surviving acute myocardial infarction and on certain assumptions about the mix of patients with respect to risk group, functional class, and other factors in the CDP population. It was also agreed that there should be a large enough sample size so that if any drug truly reduced mortality by as much as 25% (that is, from a five-year mortality rate of 30% down to 22.5%), there would be a high probability of the study detecting such a result.

Since each of the five drug groups is to be compared with the same placebo group, it is necessary that the placebo death rate be measured with greater precision than any of the drug death rates. By means of a procedure which minimizes the variance of the observed difference between the five-year death rate for a drug group and that for the placebo group,[22] it was determined that the size of the placebo group should be approximately 2.5 times as large as that of any one of the treatment groups.

Setting the Type I (α) and Type II (β) errors at 0.01 and 0.05, respectively, the total sample size was calculated to be 5865. This figure was increased by a factor of 10/7 in order to allow for as much as a 30% five-year dropout and nonadherence rate. Thus, on the basis of the given assumptions, the total required sample size was calculated to be 8379 with 2793 in the placebo group and 1117 in each of the five drug groups.* Detailed calculations are given in Appendix A.

2.6 Patient Recruitment

The types of clinics participating in the CDP include private hospitals and group practice clinics, VA and USPHS hospitals, and university hospitals. A major source of patients consisted of private patients of the investigators and other patients available within the participating institutions. Medical records in the institutions were searched in order to identify potential patients. Other sources of patients which were contacted included private physicians, other medical insitutions in the clinic's locality, and the medical departments of large business firms, industrial plants, and government agencies.

Beginning in 1968, with patient enrollment behind schedule, local publicity campaigns were mounted in some CDP clinics. With the help of the Heart Information Office of the NHLI and of local Heart Associations, press releases and 15, 30, and 60-second radio and television "spots" were prepared for use in the local press and broadcasts. This effort was highly successful. It is estimated that as many as 2000 patients were recruited in this way.

---

*The actual number of patients recruited, 8341, came remarkably close to this calculated required sample size. For administrative reasons it was necessary to set a date for ending recruitment, which is why the actual number recruited fell slightly short of the desired sample size.

It was the policy of the CDP investigators to obtain approval from the patient's private physician before admitting the patient into the study. Great care was taken to assure the private physician that it was intended that he retain responsibility for the patient's general medical care.

Table 2 shows the cumulative number and per cent of patients enrolled by month throughout the recruitment period.

Table 2

Cumulative Number of Patients Enrolled in the CDP by Month

Last day of:	No. enrolled	% enrolled
Mar. 1966	7	0.1
Apr.	10	0.1
May	25	0.3
June	44	0.5
July	74	0.9
Aug.	120	1.4
Sep.	145	1.7
Oct.	177	2.1
Nov.	277	3.3
Dec.	431	5.2
Jan. 1967	575	6.9
Feb.	682	8.2
Mar.	844	10.0
Apr.	999	12.1
May	1144	13.7
June	1289	15.5
July	1422	17.0
Aug.	1570	18.8
Sep.	1726	20.7
Oct.	1904	22.8
Nov.	2197	26.3
Dec.	2436	29.2
Jan. 1968	2735	32.8
Feb.	3055	36.6
Mar.	3452	41.4
Apr.	3869	46.4
May	4297	51.5
June	4702	56.4
July	4984	59.8
Aug.	5247	62.9
Sep.	5490	65.8
Oct.	5728	68.7
Nov.	5936	71.2
Dec.	6139	73.6
Jan. 1969	6355	76.2
Feb.	6517	78.1
Mar.	6710	80.4
Apr.	6918	82.9
May	7130	85.5
June	7401	88.7
July	7643	91.6
Aug.	8042	96.4
Sep.	8333	99.9
Oct.	8341	100.0

2.7 Informed Consent

Prior to enrollment in the study, each patient was given an orientation session in which the nature and purpose of the study were discussed and in which the known side effects of the different CDP drugs were pointed out. The patient was told that the study included a placebo treatment and that he would be randomly assigned to treatment with one of the drugs or to the placebo. After the orientation session each patient was required to sign a consent form in which he agreed to participate in the CDP and to be treated with any one of the CDP medications, including placebo. A copy of the suggested CDP Consent Form is given in Appendix I. (The clinics were given the option of using the consent form in general use at their center.) No treatment allocation was issued to a patient until the orientation session had been held and informed consent obtained.

2.8 Randomization to Treatment

Patients enrolled in the CDP were randomly assigned to one of the six treatment groups. All assignments were made by the CDP Coordinating Center, using separate randomization schedules for each clinic and for each of two risk groups within each clinic. These risk groups are defined as follows:

Risk 1—Patients with only one previous myocardial infarction and with no complications associated with that MI.

Risk 2—Patients with more than one previous MI or one MI with one or more of the following complications: sustained arrhythmia, shock, cardiac arrest, congestive heart failure, extension of infarction, pericarditis, and thromboembolism.

The treatment assignments were made in a double blind fashion, that is, with neither the patient nor the clinic personnel informed as to which drug the patient would be taking. The double blind assignment was accomplished by coding the bottles of medication with the numbers 1 through 30; four bottle numbers were randomly assigned to each of the five drug groups and ten numbers to the placebo group.

The randomization schedules were prepared and used in the following manner. First, several hundred random permutations of the numbers 1 through 30 were generated at the Coordinating Center. The randomization schedule for a given clinic and risk group consisted of from two to seven sheets of these random permutations, the number of sheets depending on the number of patients in that

clinic and risk group (an example of such a sheet is given in Appendix I). Whenever a clinic requested a treatment assignment from the Coordinating Center for a patient in a particular risk group, the patient's name and identifying number were entered after the next available bottle number on the randomization schedule for that clinic and risk group, and that allocated bottle number was sent to the clinic in a sealed envelope showing the patient's name and identifying number.

The envelope containing the allocated bottle number was not to be opened by the clinic until the patient was present for his third initial visit and a final determination had been made of the patient's eligibility for the study. The opening of the sealed bottle allocation envelope marked the patient's official and irrevocable entry into the study. That is, it meant his inclusion in all of the subsequent statistics of the study. Unopened envelopes, because of patient refusal or ineligibility for the study, were returned to the Coordinating Center, and each bottle number was assigned some time later to another patient in the same clinic and risk group.

It is evident that within a given clinic and risk group, balance among the treatment groups was achieved after every 30 allocations (i.e., ten patients assigned to placebo and four patients assigned to each of the five drug groups). Additionally, because of a special restriction applied during the generation of the random permutations, balance among the treatment groups, within a given clinic and risk group, was achieved after every 15 allocations as well (i.e., five patients assigned to placebo and two patients assigned to each of the five drug groups for every 15 treatment allocations).

The following numbers of patients were assigned to each of the six treatment groups: estrogens, 2.5 mg per day, 1101; estrogens, 5.0 mg per day, 1119; clofibrate 1103; dextrothyroxine 1110; nicotinic acid 1119; and placebo 2789.

2.9 Patient Examination Schedule and Procedures

In the original design of the CDP, each patient was to be followed for exactly five years on his assigned CDP medication. However, since patients were recruited over a 3½-year period and since all clinics recruited patients until the end of that 3½-year period, it was subsequently decided to follow all patients on their assigned medication until October, 1974. This means that all patients will be followed for a minimum of five years and some patients will be followed for as long as 8½ years.

The CDP examination schedule consists of five initial visits scheduled at one-month intervals plus three follow-up visits each year for every patient. A summary of this examination schedule is given in table 3.

Baseline Visits

The first three of the initial visits define the baseline period. During this period baseline observations were obtained, patient admissibility was assessed, and the patient was followed for two months on placebo medication (known to the physician but not the patient) to provide a baseline for drug-related complaints and to evaluate the patient's adherence to the treatment regimen. At the third initial visit a sealed envelope containing the bottle code assignment for that particular patient was opened, thus marking the patient's official entry into the study. At this visit the patient was given a prescription for one capsule three times a day of his assigned CDP medication.

Prescription Adjustment Visits

At the fourth and fifth initial visits the prescription was increased to two capsules three times a day and three capsules three times a day, respectively, unless contraindicated by side effects or other reasons. This stepwise increase of the dosage was used in order to minimize side effects and adverse reactions which might be encountered upon initiation of certain of the drug regimens.

Follow-up Visits

The follow-up visits are scheduled at four-month intervals following the patient's date of entry into the study at the third initial visit. Every third follow-up visit, performed at annual intervals following the date of entry, consists of a complete physical examination, interval medical history, resting electrocardiogram, chest x-ray, glucose tolerance test, and an extensive battery of biochemical and hematological determinations. The non-annual visits are less extensive, consisting mainly of an interval medical history, a limited physical examination, assessment of drug adherence, and determinations of serum cholesterol and certain liver function tests.

Final Visits

The final two visits for each patient, which are expected to take place in late 1974 and early 1975, will be annual-type visits, regardless of the follow-up visit numbers. During the four-month interval between these two visits, each patient will be followed without drug and observed for any change which might occur after withdrawal of the treatment regimen.

Table 3

CDP Examination Schedule

Visit name and number	Number of months before or after initial visit 3	Major features of visit
Initial Visit 1	−2	Assessment of eligibility, baseline history, physical examination, chest X-ray, laboratory determinations.
Initial Visit 2	−1	Further assessment of eligibility, laboratory determinations.
Initial Visit 3	0	Final assessment of eligibility, resting (baseline) ECG, laboratory determinations, opening of treatment allocation envelope, first prescription of study medication (three capsules/day). OFFICIAL ENTRY INTO STUDY.
Initial Visit 4	1	Increase of study medication prescription to six capsules/day.
Initial Visit 5	2	Increase of study medication prescription to nine capsules/day.
Nonannual Follow-up Visits (Follow-up Visits 1, 2, 4, 5, 7, 8, etc.)	4, 8, 16, 20 28, 32, etc.	Interval medical history, abbreviated physical examination, laboratory determinations, assessment of drug adherence.
Annual Follow-up Visits (Follow-up Visits 3, 6, 9, etc.)	12, 24, 36, etc.	Interval medical history, general physical examination, resting ECG, chest X-ray, laboratory determinations, assessment of drug adherence.

THE CORONARY DRUG PROJECT I-15

A detailed list of the information obtained at each baseline and follow-up examination is given in Appendix B. Also, copies of CDP Form 01, the Admission Form, CDP Form 02, the Initial Visit 3 Baseline Form, and CDP Form 05, the Annual Follow-up Examination Form, are included in Appendix I.

Shortly after a patient's entry into the study, an Appointment Schedule was generated at the Coordinating Center, based on the patient's date of entry into the study. This schedule gave the expected appointment dates for Initial Visits 4 and 5 and for each follow-up visit. It also gave the exact time period in which each visit was to be completed (for example, two months on either side of the expected appointment date in the case of the follow-up visits). Visits completed outside the proper time period are counted as missed visits and the resulting information is not entered into the data system for the study.

Some of the specific procedures used at these examinations are described below.

Preparation for Visits

For each of the first three initial visits and each annual follow-up visit, the patient is instructed to come to the clinic in a fasting state, that is, having eaten or drunk nothing but water since 8:00 p.m. the previous evening and having had a low fat meal and having abstained from alcohol that previous evening. For the non-annual follow-up visits the patient need not come in a fasting state, but he is instructed to avoid the intake of fats on the day of the visit. For both types of visits, the patient is not to take any of his study medication on the day of the visit until after the visit is completed. Further details are given on CDP Forms 12-A and 12-B, Dietary Instruction Sheets, found in Appendix I.

Glucose Challenge

For those visits at which a glucose challenge is given, the ECG is taken first (due to the effects of glucose on the ECG), and then a fasting blood sample is obtained from the patient. He is then given a 7-ounce drink containing 75 g of glucose. Another blood sample is obtained one hour after the glucose challenge. Special 10-ml Vacutainer tubes containing 20 mg NaF and 10 mg EDTA as a preservative for glucose are used to collect the blood for these measurements. The glucose determinations are made from the plasma obtained from these blood specimens.

Local Laboratory Determinations

The following laboratory determinations are performed at the clinic's local laboratory: hematocrit, white blood cell count, leukocyte differential (giving absolute neutrophil count), and urine glucose and protein.

Central Laboratory Determinations

Plasma, serum, and urine specimens are frozen and shipped in dry ice to the Central Laboratory where the following tests are performed (Appendix B tells which tests are done at each visit): *serum* cholesterol, triglyceride, total and direct bilirubin, glutamic oxaloacetic transaminase, alkaline phosphatase, creatine phosphokinase, uric acid, protein bound iodine, potassium, and sodium; *plasma* urea nitrogen and fasting and one-hour glucose; and *urine* pyridone of nicotinic acid and conjugate of clofibrate. Routine determinations of creatine phosphokinase, potassium, and sodium were begun in July, 1971. Each analysis is performed in duplicate. The two aliquots are analyzed in the same run but not consecutively. The duplicate determinations are used to aid in detecting reading and recording errors. The mean values of the duplicate determinations are computed and reported to the Coordinating Center for all tests. All but the lipid (cholesterol and triglyceride) and drug adherence (protein bound iodine, pyridone of nicotinic acid, and conjugate of clofibrate) results are reported to the clinic from the Central Laboratory. Any Central Laboratory results which are suggestive of possible drug toxicity are immediately reported by the Central Laboratory to the clinic by telephone. The analytical procedures used by the Central Laboratory are briefly described in Appendix C. Central Laboratory quality control procedures are discussed in section 2.10.

Electrocardiogram

Standard 12-lead resting ECG's are obtained annually and are done while the patient is in a fasting state and prior to the glucose challenge. Single channel recorders with a paper speed of 25 mm per second are used. At least a 6-inch tracing is obtained for each lead. The unmounted tracings are sent to the Coordinating Center where they are mounted in a uniform manner using a Litman Mounting Apparatus. The mounted ECG's are sent to the ECG Reading Center where they are read and coded using a modification of the 1968 revision of the Minnesota Code[23] (Appendix D) and where measurements of heart rate, QRS axis deviation, R amplitude, and T amplitude are recorded. Each ECG is read independently by two technician readers, and disagreements are adjudicated by the chief technician or a cardiologist at the Reading Center. All readings are made without knowledge of the treatment group or clinical or laboratory findings of the patient. The ECG's and the final, adjudicated readings are returned to the Coordinating Center.

Two other types of ECG's are also collected by the Coordinating Center and read by the ECG Reading Center. A qualifying ECG, that ECG which documents an MI prior to entry, is collected for all patients in the study. This ECG may either have been taken at the time of the acute MI or have been taken at the CDP clinic during a preliminary visit.

ECG's are also collected in conjunction with recurrent MI and acute coronary insufficiency (ACI) diagnosed since entry into the study. These ECG's, like the qualifying ECG's, are usually obtained from hospital records and are thus sent to the Coordinating Center already mounted. A maximum of two ECG's per event are submitted and read centrally. If the event is MI, the two ECG's are chosen which show (a) the maximum Q/QS changes and (b) the maximum ST segment elevation, respectively. If no ECG shows ST segment elevation, then the ECG showing maximum ST segment depression or maximum negativity of the T wave is chosen. If the event is ACI, the two ECG's are chosen which show (a) the maximum ST segment depression or the maximum negativity of the T wave and (b) the maximum elevation of the ST segment.

A discussion of quality control of the ECG readings is given in section 2.10.

Chest X-ray

A posteroanterior chest X-ray is taken annually and read at the clinic for evidence of possible cardiomegaly, pleural effusion, and pulmonary congestion.

Vital Signs and Physical Measurements

Height and weight measurements are made with the patient's shoes removed and with all heavy outdoor garments removed. Blood pressure is measured with the patient either lying or sitting with forearm at the level of the heart. Diastolic blood pressure is determined at the disappearance of sound.

Prescription and Adherence Records

At every follow-up visit a detailed record is filled out giving the date of any change in CDP drug prescription and the number of capsules prescribed at the change. Clinic personnel also make an assessment of the patient's adherence to his CDP drug prescription for the past four months. This is done by counting (or estimating) the number of capsules returned by the patient at that visit and by questioning the patient.

Visual Acuity

A standard distant Snellen visual acuity test is performed annually. Other procedures, such as the red reflex, are performed at the study physician's discretion.

2.10 Quality Control Procedures

There are several areas in the CDP where quality control procedures are very important: (a) bottle labeling at the Drug Procurement and Distribution Center; (b) Central Laboratory determinations; (c) ECG readings; and (d) information submitted by the clinics on the study forms. Procedures for checking the quality of information submitted by the clinics will be discussed briefly in section 2.14. The Drug Center, Central Laboratory, and ECG Reading Center all have their own internal quality control programs. In addition, external surveillance programs are being carried out by the Coordinating Center through the cooperation of some of the clinics.

External Surveillance of the Drug Center

Twice a year a new shipment of drugs is sent to each clinic. After each shipment three clinics are randomly selected by the Coordinating Center to send one bottle of each of the 30 bottle number codes (cf. section 2.8) to the Central Laboratory for analysis as a check against mislabeling.

Internal Quality Control Program of the Central Laboratory

The Central Laboratory has a quality control program which is wide in scope and utilizes all techniques commonly in use today.[24] Specimens are run in duplicate, drift standards and serum reference materials are included in every run of 36 samples (18 specimens in duplicate), and calibrations are made and rechecked several times each day. These procedures help the analyst to keep variability within prescribed limits and to detect and eliminate errors. Methods of analysis and operation of instruments are such as to yield linearity of the standard curve and minimum variability as well as accuracy.

Data from the analysis of serum reference materials are subjected to statistical analysis and review to provide surveillance in order to detect and eliminate shifts and trends. Monthly computer assisted statistical summaries of reference material analysis and patient data provide estimates of precision for each type of determination.

In addition to the above control studies, lyophilized reference materials are analyzed daily to detect temporal trends. The Central Laboratory participates in a number of reference laboratory programs including the Glucose and Urea Standardization Program and the Lipid Standardization Program of the Center for Disease Control. In the beginning all automated procedures were compared with appropriate manual methods. Frequent blind unknowns disguised as CDP patient specimens are submitted to the analyst to provide bias-free information about variability.

External Surveillance of the Central Laboratory

An external surveillance program of the Central Laboratory is carried out with the cooperation of 15 of the CDP clinics and consists of two aspects. One aspect is designed to assess the technical error or reliability of the various biochemical determinations made at the Central Laboratory. For this purpose a double volume of blood is collected from a patient, split into two sets of samples and sent to the Central Laboratory under two different identifying numbers—one the patient's own identifying number and the other the identifying number of a deceased patient (not known by the Central Laboratory to be deceased). The two sets of results, transmitted to the Coordinating Center, are evaluated there for reproducibility. The second aspect of the program is designed to detect long-term trends over time in the laboratory determinations. For this purpose a 500-ml blood specimen obtained from a blood donor is used to make several dozen vials of serum. These vials are sent to a participating clinic where they are stored at −40 C and sent at specified time points to the Central Laboratory as if they were the usual patient specimens (again using deceased patients' identifying numbers to keep the Central Laboratory blinded). This procedure is repeated several times a year for each of several clinics.

Internal Surveillance of the ECG Reading Center

A special repeat reading program is carried out every fall at the ECG Reading Center. The purpose of this special project is to check the inter-observer variation for readers recently trained during the summer months.

External Surveillance of the ECG Reading Center

Every set of 960 ECG's sent to the ECG Reading Center contains 60 records which have already been read. These repeat readings provide a basis for monitoring the ECG readings for reproducibility.

2.11 Major Response Variables

The primary response variable in the CDP is total mortality. Cause-specific mortality is also of great interest, particularly coronary and cardiovascular mortality. The classification system for cause of death is given in Appendix E. All information relating to cause of death (including death certificate, autopsy report, terminal ECG, and physician's summary) is centrally reviewed without knowledge of a patient's treatment group by the Mortality Classification Committee, and both underlying and immediate causes of death are coded by this committee. Generally, only one of the four coders on this committee does the coding for a given death, but difficult cases are reviewed by all of the coders and a uniform (or at least majority) judgment arrived at as to cause of death. Also, a certain percentage of the records are routinely resubmitted for independent review by another coder or by the same coder. In this way a continual evaluation is obtained of between reader and within reader variability in the death coding.

Other major response variables include nonfatal cardiovascular events such as recurrent MI, ACI, development of angina pectoris (AP), stroke, arrhythmias, congestive heart failure (CHF), pulmonary embolism, and others. The diagnosis of these events is established by the local CDP physician. The diagnostic criteria for these cardiovascular events are given in Appendix F.

2.12 Discontinuation or Dosage Reduction of Study Drug

During the course of a patient's participation in the CDP, it is sometimes deemed by the study physician necessary to reduce the dosage or discontinue the drug regimen temporarily for that patient. This may be due to intolerable side effects, adverse (toxic) reactions suspected to be drug-related, and intercurrent illness with or without hospitalization. In addition to dosage changes made at the discretion of the study physician, a mandatory three-month interruption of the drug regimen is required when any of the following cardiovascular events occur: definite ACI and definite or suspect MI, stroke, pulmonary embolism, pulmonary infarction, and arterial embolism. Also, if the patient is placed on a cholesterol lowering agent by his personal (non-CDP) physician, his study drug is discontinued for as long as he is taking that other drug. While patients on long-term anticoagulant therapy were excluded from the study, initiation of long-term anticoagulant therapy since entry does not require discontinuation of the study regimen.

When the patient's study drug is stopped, the patient is switched to single blind placebo capsules (that is, known to the investigator but not to the patient), whenever possible. This is done to make it easier to get the patient back on his study drug again. Continual efforts are made by the clinic investigators to get these patients to start taking their study drug again and to get them back to full dosage, except in cases of mandatory interruption of treatment as detailed above or in cases of protocol changes.

When it becomes possible to start a patient on his assigned study medication once again, if he has been off his medication for a month or longer, he is started at three capsules per day and increased to nine per day in stepwise fashion. If he has been off for less than a month, he may be started directly on nine capsules per day at the discretion of the physician.

Patients who for various reasons refuse to take any more study drug or who are advised not to do so because of a toxic reaction to the drug are urged to continue coming to the clinic for their scheduled follow-up visits.

2.13 Dropout and Transfer Patients

A dropout is defined as a patient who no longer returns to a clinic for his scheduled follow-up visits. A patient is automatically called a dropout if he misses three consecutive follow-up visits. However, a study physician can declare a patient a dropout earlier than this if he has good reason to believe the patient will no longer be returning for his scheduled follow-up visits. At yearly intervals following the date the patient was declared a dropout, the clinic is required to contact the patient or his acquaintances to obtain information on his cardiovascular history for the past year. If the clinic is unable to locate and contact the patient, the Coordinating Center assumes responsibility for the search through a professional search service. One of the benefits of keeping in contact with the dropout patient is that

he might eventually be persuaded to return to the study. A dropout patient may be reinstated in the study by completing the appropriate follow-up visit as indicated on the patient's Appointment Schedule.

Many of the dropouts are patients who moved away from the area served by their clinic, but many more patients have been saved from becoming dropouts by the provision for patient transfers from one clinic to another. If a patient moves to within commuting distance of another CDP clinic, he may continue his participation in the CDP at that clinic.

2.14 Data Collection and Monitoring of Adherence to Protocol

The completed study forms, ECG's, Central Laboratory determinations, and ECG readings are all sent to the Coordinating Center for editing, analysis, and storage. All of the data on the study forms (including written responses in catch-all categories such as "other drugs," etc.) and the ECG readings are keypunched and verified. Every two weeks, the latest batch of keypunched information is subjected to an extensive computer edit. The data are edited for completeness, internal consistency with previous data for the same patient, numerical values outside specified limits, invalid codes, illegible responses, patient identification errors, examination date errors, and CDP medication mix-ups. Errors detected in the editing process are sent to the clinics for correction. Follow-up procedures are employed to assure that all such errors get corrected and returned to the Coordinating Center.

All of the data are transferred to magnetic disk data files in card image. Included on this data file for each patient is an inventory of forms, Central Laboratory reports, ECG's, and ECG readings received by the Coordinating Center. Periodic checks are made of this inventory, and lists of delinquent records are mailed to the clinics as reminders to keep up to date in completing and mailing the records.

The CDP forms are microfilmed not less than 6 nor more than 15 months after receipt. Once a form is microfilmed and the film has been checked for accuracy and clarity, the form is destroyed following Maryland state regulations for the destruction of medical records. Two microfilm copies are made, with one copy kept in a bank vault several blocks away to safeguard the study in case of fire or vandalism.

In addition to the backup system for the study forms, there is a backup of the data stored on the magnetic disks. Every month, the information on the disks is copied onto magnetic tapes which are taken to a bank vault several blocks away for safe keeping. Also, at the same time the study forms are microfilmed, the corresponding punch cards are read onto tape. The tapes are stored in a bank vault and the cards are destroyed.

In the effort to maximize clinic adherence to the protocol and good performance with respect to drug adherence and dropouts, the Coordinating Center periodically distributes reports to the Steering Committee and to the clinics in which the following statistics are given, by clinic: (a) percentage of patients on reduced dosage, (b) percentages of dropouts and missed visits, (c) numbers of delinquent forms and ECG's, and (d) percentage of error-free forms received by the Coordinating Center during a specified period. In addition, the clinics are periodically sent lists of patients for whom there is laboratory evidence of poor adherence, so that efforts may be made to improve adherence in these patients.

2.15 Monitoring of the Treatments for Adverse and Beneficial Effects

The primary objective of the CDP, as has been stated, is to evaluate the efficacy of the drugs under study in the long-term treatment of coronary heart disease. The study has a clear ethical obligation to provide a mechanism for effective monitoring of the data for evidence of beneficial or adverse drug effects throughout the course of the study. For this purpose the CDP Data and Safety Monitoring Committee was created early in the course of the study. The committee consists of experts in the fields of cardiology, clinical medicine, biostatistics, epidemiology, and biochemistry (see preface for list of members). Every six months this committee meets in order to review an extensive data report prepared by the Coordinating Center. This report contains data on total mortality, cause-specific mortality, nonfatal cardiovascular events, ECG findings, side effects, laboratory findings possibly related to drug toxicity, lipid responses, drug adherence, dropouts and missed visits, and quality control of the laboratory determinations and ECG readings.

In addition to the semiannual reports, from two to four interim reports are prepared each year by the Coordinating Center and circulated to the Data and Safety Monitoring Committee for review and response. These reports summarize the major mortality and cardiovascular event findings to date

by treatment group. Any member who has a concern about the findings in such a report is at liberty to call an interim meeting of the committee to discuss those findings and to request additional analyses.

No physicians responsible for the clinical care of CDP patients are members of the Data and Safety Monitoring Committee, nor are any CDP physicians apprised of treatment-specific results except when a decision is made to discontinue a treatment group. This withholding of treatment results is done in order to minimize physician biases in the treatment and observation of the CDP patients.

Recommendations for protocol changes involving the discontinuation of one or more treatment groups or a subgroup of patients within a treatment group are made by the Data and Safety Monitoring Committee to the Policy Board. The decisions reached by the Policy Board are subsequently ratified by the Steering Committee and Technical Group.

2.16 Natural History Investigations

As stated earlier, the second major objective of the CDP is to obtain information on the natural history and clinical course of CHD. A Natural History Committee has been created for the purpose of planning analyses and reviewing CDP data on this topic (see preface for membership of this committee). A particular interest of this committee is the investigation of the prognostic significance of the many demographic, clinical, biochemical, and electrocardiographic variables observed at baseline on patients in the placebo group. Three papers have been published, and others are in preparation for publication which present results of these natural history investigations in the CDP.[25-29]

2.17 Methodological Investigations

In accordance with the third major objective of the CDP, a significant amount of effort is going into the investigation of new methodology for the design and conduct of long-term clinical trials. These investigations have included the following topics: (1) external surveillance programs for the Central Laboratory, ECG Reading Center, Drug Procurement and Distribution Center, and Coordinating Center; (2) aspects of study form design; (3) optimum structure of the magnetic disk data files; (4) procedures for electronic editing of the study forms; (5) new statistical procedures for determining the required sample size; (6) statistical methods for monitoring the study over time for adverse and beneficial treatment effects; (7) a system for defining significant ECG worsening over time when abnormal ECG patterns are present at baseline.

2.18 Ancillary Studies

Investigators participating in the CDP are encouraged to carry out ancillary studies with patients in their clinic. It is felt that such ancillary studies may greatly enhance the value of the CDP and insure the continued long-term interest and enthusiasm of investigators and patients.

All proposed ancillary studies must have the approval of the Steering Committee and Policy Board. Every proposal is carefully reviewed in order to make sure that the ancillary study meets human experimentation ethical criteria and will not lead to unblinding of the study drugs or adversely affect patient cooperation.

For those ancillary studies requiring analyses by treatment group, there must be a person not directly involved in the CDP designated as a data repository. If it is desired to analyze the study results by treatment group, such analyses are performed under the supervision of the data repository, with treatment decoding provided by the CDP Coordinating Center. Only summary data (means, standard errors, etc.) for each treatment group are made available to the clinic investigators. In some cases treatment-specific data may be forwarded to an investigator in coded form, without revealing the indentity of each specific treatment if the leadership of the study deems it appropriate in terms of the over-all good of the study.

It is the policy of the CDP that if treatment-specific results from ancillary studies are to be published or presented at a scientific meeting, only those results for discontinued treatment groups and the placebo group may be published or presented prior to the conclusion of the CDP.

2.19 Meetings of Study Personnel

Meetings of the Technical Group are held twice a year. Each meeting is hosted by one of the clinics or one of the other functional units of the CDP. These meetings consist of reports from the Steering Committee, Data and Safety Monitoring Committee, and other CDP committees; reports on clinic performance with respect to adherence to protocol; presentation of CDP baseline findings and natural history results (the clinic investigators are kept blind to treatment-specific data from the CDP except in the case of protocol changes); scientific presentations by researchers in the cardiovascular

field; and question and answer sessions relating to CDP procedures and policies.

The Steering Committee meets twice a year, in conjunction with the Technical Group meetings, to formulate, discuss, and act upon additions and changes in the study protocol; to review ancillary studies and reports on the performances of the clinics, Coordinating Center, Central Laboratory, and ECG Reading Center; and to carry out any other necessary business. In major matters of policy, the Steering Committee makes recommendations to the Policy Board for final decision.

The Data and Safety Monitoring Committee and the Natural History Committee also meet twice a year to carry out their functions as described in sections 2.2, 2.15, and 2.16. Other CDP committees meet periodically.

In addition to the meetings already described, yearly training and refresher sessions are held for the benefit of clinic administrators, secretaries, and laboratory technicians.

Each year visits are made by members of the Steering Committee to eight or ten of the clinics in order to discuss clinic problems and review CDP procedures.

2.20 Newsletters

In an attempt to keep all study personnel apprised of what is going on in the various units of the CDP, a newsletter is prepared twice a year by the Coordinating Center and distributed to every person involved in the operation of the CDP. These newsletters contain announcements of meetings, reports of past meetings, reports on clinic performance, advice on how to answer certain items on the study forms under special circumstances, and announcements of additions and changes in study forms and procedures.

Newsletters are also prepared centrally for all participating patients in the CDP. A special Newsletter Committee consisting of project investigators and administrators has been established with the responsibility of preparing such newsletters periodically. In addition, several of the clinics regularly prepare local newsletters for distribution to their study patients.

3. Baseline Results

The CDP patient population is not a random sample from the general population of men with CHD. It is a selected group of men who are sufficiently motivated to be involved for five years or more and who have satisfied a comprehensive set

THE CORONARY DRUG PROJECT   I-21

of medical admissibility criteria. The distributions of baseline variables given in this section will serve to describe in some detail the characteristics of the group of men selected for study.

Section 3.1 consists of a detailed description of the baseline characteristics of the study population, and section 3.2 describes a number of interrelationships among the variables which are of special interest. With the exception of the qualifying ECG (that ECG which documented the patient's MI prior to entry), all of the variables discussed and tabulated in sections 3.1 and 3.2 were observed or measured at the time of or within a maximum of four months prior to the initiation of the patient's assigned study medication. In each case the number of patients for whom the observation was obtained is given. Missing values occurred as a result of technical problems (such as thawed serum specimens), failure to follow the protocol (including baseline ECG's not taken within the permissible time limits), lack of recollection (in the case of certain historical items), and interference from other variables (such as the inability to obtain accurate bilirubin and SGOT determinations in the presence of certain types of hyperlipidemia).

In sections 3.1 and 3.2 the results are given for all treatment groups combined—a total of 8341 patients. Distributions of many of these variables by treatment group are given in section 4. Such distributions are useful in assessing the comparability of the six treatment groups at baseline when analyzing treatment effects.

3.1 Description of the Population

The variables included in this description are grouped into the following categories: (1) demographic characteristics, (2) CHD historical and clinical variables, (3) ECG characteristics, (4) CHD risk factors, (5) other laboratory and clinical measurements, (6) other clinical and X-ray findings, and (7) usage of various medications at time of entry.

Table 4 gives distributions of baseline demographic characteristics. The mean age of CDP participants at the time of entry was 52 years. Over 93% of the patients were of the white race.

Prior to assignment to treatment, the patients were classified according to risk group. Table 5 shows that 66% of the patients fell into Risk 1, that is, had a single uncomplicated MI prior to entry, while the remaining 34% were in Risk 2. Less than 20% of the patients had a history of more than one MI. Table 5, part D, shows that 35% of the patients

Table 4

Distributions of Baseline Demographic Characteristics

	No. of patients	% of patients
A. Age at entry		
30–34	76	0.9
35–39	310	3.7
40–44	846	10.1
45–49	1571	18.8
50–54	1923	23.1
55–59	2042	24.5
60–64	1573	18.9
Total	8341	
Median = 53.6		
Mean = 52.4		
Standard deviation (SD) = 7.1		
B. Race		
White	7788	93.4
Black	407	4.9
Other	146	1.8
Total	8341	
C. Marital status		
Never married	330	4.0
Married	7420	89.0
Divorced	282	3.4
Widowed	175	2.1
Separated	134	1.6
Total	8341	
D. Occupation		
Professional	1145	13.7
Manager	1428	17.1
Craftsman	945	11.3
Clerical	494	5.9
Sales	645	7.7
Operative	510	6.1
Service worker	616	7.4
Laborer	305	3.7
Farmer	102	1.2
Unemployed or retired	2149	25.8
Total	8339	
E. Type of clinic		
Private hospitals and group practice clinics (27 clinics)	4231	50.7
VA, USPHS hospitals (10 clinics)	1475	17.7
University and general city hospitals (16 clinics)	2635	31.6
Total	8341	
F. Geographic region		
West (10 clinics: Cal., Hawaii, N.M., Ore., Utah)	1674	20.1
Midwest (11 clinics: Ia., Ill., Ind., Minn., Neb., Wisc.)	1693	20.3
Mideast (11 clinics: Md., Mich., Ohio, Pa., W.Va.)	1700	20.4
New England (11 clinics: Mass., N.H., N.Y.)	1645	19.7
South (10 clinics: Fla., Ga., La., Miss., P.R., S.C., Tex.)	1629	19.5
Total	8341	

Table 5

Distributions of Variables Relating to History and Status of CHD at Baseline

	No. of patients	% of patients
A. Risk group		
Risk 1	5498	65.9
Risk 2	2843	34.1
Total	8341	
B. Number of previous MI's		
One	6743	80.8
Two	1316	15.8
Three or more	282	3.4
Total	8341	
C. Complications with MI		
Arrhythmia	681	8.2
Shock	427	5.1
Congestive heart failure	652	7.8
Extension of infarct	285	3.4
Pericardial friction rub	278	3.3
Thromboembolism	111	1.3
One or more complications	1719	20.6
No complications	6620	79.4
Number of patients	8339	
D. Time (in months) from last MI to entry		
< 6	1160	14.2
6–11	1396	17.1
12–35	2730	33.5
36–59	1262	15.5
60–119	1282	15.7
≥ 120	320	3.9
Total	8150	
Median = 22.9		
Mean = 35.7		
SD = 36.5		
E. New York Heart Association functional class		
Class I (no limitation of ordinary physical activity)	3834	46.0
Class II (slight limitation)	4507	54.0
Total	8341	
F. Physical nature of work		
Sedentary	1650	19.8
Light physical work	2912	34.9
Moderate physical work	1436	17.2
Heavy physical work	193	2.3
Unemployed or retired	2149	25.8
Total	8340	
G. Degree of physical activity apart from employment		
Light	5830	69.9
Moderate	2316	27.8
Vigorous	194	2.3
Total	8340	

	No. of patients	% of patients
H. Age at time of first MI		
< 30	53	0.7
30–34	248	3.1
35–39	787	9.7
40–44	1472	18.2
45–49	1932	23.9
50–54	1825	22.5
55–59	1333	16.4
60–64	450	5.5
Total	8100	
Median = 48.9		
Mean = 48.6		
SD = 7.5		
I. History of cardiovascular events		
Acute coronary insufficiency		
Negative	6916	82.9
Suspect	396	4.7
Definite	1028	12.3
Angina pectoris		
Negative	3462	41.5
Suspect	973	11.7
Definite	3906	46.8
Congestive heart failure		
Negative	7039	84.4
Suspect	483	5.8
Definite	819	9.8
Intermittent cerebral ischemic attacks (ICIA)		
Negative	8016	96.1
Suspect	228	2.7
Definite	97	1.2
Stroke		
Negative	8166	97.9
Suspect	39	0.5
Definite	136	1.6
Intermittent claudication		
Negative	7649	91.7
Suspect	239	2.9
Definite	453	5.4
Peripheral arterial occlusion		
Negative	8152	97.7
Suspect	64	0.8
Definite	125	1.5
J. Pulse rate (beats/min)		
<50	30	0.4
50–59	333	4.0
60–69	2106	25.3
70–79	3204	38.4
80–89	2168	26.0
90–99	371	4.4
≥100	126	1.5
Total	8338	
Median = 73.6		
Mean = 74.0		
SD = 9.9		
K. Cardiomegaly (baseline X-ray)		
Negative	6880	82.5
Suspect	691	8.3
Definite	770	9.2
Total	8341	

had their last MI more than three years prior to entry, and for 4% of them the MI had occurred at least ten years prior to entry. Nearly 1100 of the CDP patients (13%) had their first MI before reaching the age of 40 (table 5-H).

Part I of table 5 gives the percentage of patients having a history of various cardiovascular events. About 58% of the patients had a history of suspect or definite angina pectoris, 16% had congestive heart failure, and 8% had intermittent claudication at some time prior to entry. Relatively few patients had problems of the cerebrovascular circulation prior to entry.

Table 5-J gives the baseline distribution of pulse rate. Comparing these results with those in table 6-M for ECG heart rate, we see that the pulse rate averages about five beats per minute higher than the heart rate measured from the ECG. This, no doubt, is due in part to the patient being in a supine position and a more rested condition for the ECG heart rate measurement than for the pulse measurement.

While over 80% of the patients showed major or moderate Q/QS patterns on the qualifying ECG, only 43% showed such patterns on the baseline ECG, as seen in table 6, once again confirming that a patient's ECG may revert back to or toward normal after an MI. Part L of this table indicates that almost 7% of the patients showed no codable ECG abnormalities whatsoever on the baseline ECG.

In the early stages of the CDP, only patients showing Q wave evidence of a previous MI were admitted. In the summer of 1966, in order to improve the patient recruitment rate, the study was opened to patients for whom there was no available Q wave evidence of a previous MI, but who had an ECG with ST-T or T wave evidence of myocardial ischemia or infarction plus an elevated SGOT plus a clinical history compatible with the diagnosis of MI. Part A of table 7 shows that 18% of the patients fell into this category on the basis of the clinics' readings of the qualifying ECG.

The qualifying ECG's were also coded by the ECG Reading Center. The results of the central coding of these records are given in part B of Table 7. Almost 2% of the records read centrally showed no codable findings, and a total of 8% failed to show either Q/QS, ST, or T wave findings. There are many possible reasons for the discrepancy in clinical interpretation and the objective coding of ECG's. There is a natural clinical bias toward sensitivity of reading Q waves and other wave forms when one knows a patient and his history. This bias is not shared by technicians using calibrated measuring instruments and applying unambiguous criteria. In addition, a certain conservatism is built into the objective criteria of the Minnesota Code and in the procedural rules for coding which involve, for example, the choice of lower, less severe classifications in borderline cases. None of these facts mitigates the effectiveness of objective coding in characterizing the qualifying ECG's, nor do they invalidate over-all the clinical decisions made concerning inclusion of subjects in the study.

Another reason for the discrepancy may relate to the fact that the decision to collect and read centrally the qualifying ECG's was not made until 1967, over a year after the beginning of patient recruitment. The clinics were not required to obtain file copies of the qualifying ECG's for the early patients. When the decision was made to start collecting qualifying ECG's, the clinics often found it difficult to go back and obtain the ECG's from other institutions and thus were frequently forced to substitute more recent, less abnormal ECG's.

Part C of Table 7 shows that a total of 34 patients out of the 8341 enrolled had no codable ECG findings on both the qualifying and the baseline ECG. Another nine patients had no codable findings on one of the two ECG's, with the other ECG not available for reading.

Distributions of some commonly regarded predisposing factors for CHD are given in table 8. On the basis of life insurance actuarial tables of desirable weight for given heights,[30] 32% of the patients had an actual body weight at least 20% greater than desirable weight at the time of entry. Over 62% of the patients were not cigarette smokers at the time of entry, while approximately 14% had never been cigarette smokers.

About 9% of the population had a baseline systolic blood pressure of 160 or higher, and 12% had a diastolic pressure of 95 or higher (table 8). While not shown in table 8, it might be noted also that about 16% of the patients had either a systolic blood pressure of 160 or higher or a diastolic blood pressure of 95 or higher at entry into the study; 5% of the patients had elevations of both systolic and diastolic blood pressure (160 or higher and 95 or higher, respectively) at entry.

Approximately half of the patients had serum cholesterol levels of 250 mg/dl or higher, and 3% were 350 mg/dl or higher. The percentages of patients with plasma fasting glucose levels of 110 mg/dl or higher and with plasma one-hour glucose levels of 220 mg/dl or higher were 17% and 16%, respectively (table 8).

I-24

Table 6

Distributions of Baseline ECG Characteristics*

	No. of patients	% of patients
A. Q/QS patterns†		
Major (1.1.1 to 1.1.9)	1899	23.0
Moderate (1.2.1 to 1.2.7)	1662	20.2
Minor (1.2.8 to 1.3.6)	1458	17.7
None	3227	39.1
Total	8246	
B. T wave findings†		
Major (5.1)	150	1.8
Moderate (5.2)	2500	30.3
Minor (5.3)	1127	13.7
Borderline (5.4)	264	3.2
None	4205	51.0
Total	8246	
C. ST depression†		
Major (4.1)	250	3.0
Moderate (4.2)	576	7.0
Minor (4.3)	1224	14.8
ST junction depr. (4.4)	28	0.3
None	6168	74.8
Total	8246	
D. ST elevation†		
Yes (9.2)	329	4.0
No	7917	96.0
Total	8246	
E. A-V conduction defects		
Complete A-V block (6.1)	0	0.0
Partial A-V block (6.2)	5	0.1
Prolonged P-R interval (6.3)	156	1.9
WPW syndrome (6.4)	5	0.1
Short P-R interval (6.5)	171	2.1
None	7909	95.9
Total	8246	
F. Ventricular conduction defects		
Complete LBBB (7.1)	61	0.7
Complete RBBB (7.2)	105	1.3
Incomplete RBBB (7.3)	223	2.7
Intraventricular block (7.4)	174	2.1
R-R' patterns (7.5)	202	2.5
Incomplete LBBB (7.6)	1	0.0
None	7480	90.7
Total	8246	
G. Frequent premature beats (PB's) (≥ 1 per 10 beats)		
Supraventricular PB's (8.1.1)	63	0.8
Ventricular PB's (8.1.2)	240	2.9
Supraventricular and ventricular PB's (8.1.3)‡	22	0.3
None	7921	96.1
Total	8246	

	No. of patients	% of patients
H. Other arrhythmias		
Ventricular tachycardia (8.2)	1	0.0
Atrial fibrillation (8.3)	48	0.6
Supraventricular tachycardia (8.4)	1	0.0
Ventricular rhythm (8.5)	0	0.0
Nodal rhythm (8.6)	8	0.1
None	8188	99.3
Total	8246	
I. Sinus arrhythmias		
Sinus tachycardia (8.7)	83	1.0
Sinus bradycardia (8.8)	205	2.5
None	7958	96.5
Total	8246	
J. QRS axis deviation		
Left axis deviation (2.1)	905	11.0
Right axis deviation (2.2)	27	0.3
Slight R axis deviation (2.3)	114	1.4
Extreme axis deviation (2.4)	31	0.4
Intermediate axis deviation (2.5)	6	0.1
None	7163	86.9
Total	8246	
K. High amplitude R waves		
Left high R (3.1)	355	4.3
Right high R (3.2)	27	0.3
Left high R (optional code) (3.3)	209	2.5
None	7655	92.8
Total	8246	
L. Any ECG findings		
One or more codable findings	7674	93.1
No codable findings	572	6.9
Total	8246	
M. ECG heart rate (beats/min)		
< 50	225	2.7
50– 59	1399	17.0
60– 69	2924	35.5
70– 79	2272	27.6
80– 89	1022	12.4
90– 99	290	3.5
≥ 100	114	1.4
Total	8246	
Median = 68.0		
Mean = 68.9		
SD = 11.4		

*Minnesota codes are given in parentheses. Definitions of these codes are given in Appendix D.

†Most severe findings of three anatomical sites — antero-lateral, anteroseptal, and posterior (inferior). See Appendix D.

‡Individual frequencies < 1 per 10 beats; sum ≥ 1 per 10 beats.

Distributions of various other biochemical, hematological, and clinical measurements at baseline are given in table 9.

The prevalence of various findings from the baseline physical examination are given in table 10, and the usage of various medications at the time of entry is summarized in table 11. This latter table indicates that some 15% of patients were taking digitalis at the time of entry, 14% were taking diuretics, and 44% had nitroglycerin prescribed. None of the patients was taking insulin, in accordance with the admissibility criteria, and just over 5% were taking oral hypoglycemic agents. While the protocol requires that patients not be on anticoagulant medication at the time of entry, that

Table 7

*Distributions of Qualifying ECG Findings and Combined Baseline and Qualifying ECG Results**

	No. of patients	% of patients
A. Qualifying ECG (clinic readings)		
Class 1 Q waves†	4072	48.8
Class 2 Q waves	2807	33.7
ST or T waves, SGOT, and history	1460	17.5
Total	8339	
B. Qualifying ECG (central readings)		
Q/QS patterns (1.1.1 to 1.3.6)	5800	70.4
ST or T wave findings (4.1 to 4.4, 5.1 to 5.4, 9.2)	1813	22.0
Other codable ECG findings (2.1 to 2.5, 3.1 to 3.3, 6.1 to 6.5, 7.1 to 7.6, 8.1 to 8.8, 9.1 to 9.5)	485	5.9
No codable ECG findings	135	1.6
ECG not available for reading	108	
Total	8341	
C. Combined qualifying and baseline ECG results (central readings)		
Q/QS patterns on either Qual. or BL ECG	6478	77.7
Other codable ECG findings (ST or T wave findings, conduction defects, arrhythmias, etc.) but not Q/QS patterns on BL or Qual. ECG	1814	21.8
No codable ECG findings:		
— on both Qual. and BL ECG	34	0.4
— on Qual. ECG; no BL ECG‡	1	0.0
— on BL ECG; no Qual. ECG‡	8	0.1
No Qual. or BL ECG‡	6	
Total	8341	

*Minnesota codes are given in parentheses. Definitions of these codes are given in Appendix D.

†Class 1 and class 2 Q waves are defined as items A to H and I to Q, respectively, of item 20, CDP Form 01 (Appendix I).

‡Central reading not done due to BL ECG taken outside permissible time period, inability to obtain Qual. ECG from other hospital, or loss of ECG.

is, at the time of initiation of the assigned study medication, table 11 shows that three patients taking anticoagulants were erroneously admitted into the study.

3.2 Interrelationships Among Baseline Variables

This section consists of an overview of some of the interrelationships which are found among the baseline variables observed in the CDP.

In Appendix G are given the correlations among 52 baseline characteristics. These include demographic characteristics, variables relating to the history and baseline status of the patient's CHD,

ECG variables, CHD risk factors, other laboratory and clinical measurements, and medication usage. Appendix H gives the codes used in the calculation of the correlations. While Appendix G is useful for reference purposes, it is difficult to read through the 2604 numbers to find the more important correlations. Table 12 provides a summary of the appendix by naming every pair of baseline variables having a correlation of 0.150 or higher or a correlation of −0.150 or less. The choice of the number 0.150 was arbitrary, designed to focus on the 75 or so largest correlations. With a sample size of 8341 patients, a correlation as small as 0.028 is statistically significant at the 0.01 level of significance. Such a correlation, while statistically significant, has little practical significance since only 0.1% (i.e., 0.028^2) of the variation of one of the variables is explained by the other variable. A correlation coefficient of +0.150 or −0.150 is very highly statistically significant (Student's $t = 13.9$) but may be in some cases of only borderline practical significance. Even in this case it should be noted that the one variable still explains only 2.25% of the variation in the other variable.

Table 12 contains a number of large correlations which would be expected as a result of the nature or definitions of the two variables. Such correlations include the following: white blood count and absolute neutrophil count (0.878); ECG heart rate and pulse rate (0.597); risk group and number of MI's (0.606); total and direct bilirubin (0.531); absolute body weight and height (0.515); cholesterol and triglyceride (0.349); intermittent claudication and peripheral arterial occlusion (0.332); angina and nitroglycerin usage (0.427); congestive heart failure and digitalis usage (0.537); T wave and ST depression (0.611); the three pairwise combinations of systolic blood pressure, diastolic blood pressure, and antihypertensive medication (0.227 to 0.720); and the six pairwise combinations of fasting, one-hour, and urine glucose and oral hypoglycemic medication (0.213 to 0.596).

Some of the other correlations in table 12 are now described. Of the biochemical, hematological, and clinical variables measured at baseline on CDP patients, plasma urea nitrogen shows the highest correlation (0.194) with age at entry. Systolic blood pressure is close behind with a correlation of 0.185 with age.

None of the 52 variables is highly correlated with race. As seen in Appendix G, the variable most highly correlated with race is ST elevation (0.112).

Table 8

Distributions of CHD Risk Factors

	No. of patients	% of patients
A. Relative body weight*		
< 0.80	24	0.3
0.80–0.89	207	2.5
0.90–0.99	794	9.6
1.00–1.09	2193	26.4
1.10–1.19	2420	29.1
1.20–1.29	1605	19.3
1.30–1.39	679	8.2
1.40–1.49	244	2.9
1.50–1.59	82	1.0
≥ 1.60	60	0.7
Total	8308	
Median = 1.13		
Mean = 1.15		
SD = 0.15		
B. Number of cigarettes smoked per day at entry		
None	5225	62.6
1–10	889	10.8
11–20	1296	15.5
21–30	553	6.6
31–40	266	1.2
> 40	102	1.2
Total	8341	
C. Cigarette smoking history prior to entry		
Nonsmoker	1028	13.5
Smoker	6579	86.5
Total	7607	
D. Systolic blood pressure (mm Hg)		
< 100	122	1.5
100–109	588	7.0
110–119	1485	17.8
120–129	1888	22.6
130–139	1627	19.5
140–149	1260	15.1
150–159	630	7.6
160–169	382	4.6
170–179	189	2.3
≥180	170	2.0
Total	8341	
Median = 129.6		
Mean = 129.9		
SD = 18.8		
E. Diastolic blood pressure (mm Hg)		
< 65	374	4.5
65– 69	215	2.6
70– 74	1559	18.7
75– 79	712	8.5
80– 84	2429	29.1
85– 89	738	8.8
90– 94	1308	15.7
95– 99	284	3.4
100–104	470	5.6
≥105	252	3.0
Total	8341	
Median = 80.3		
Mean = 81.9		
SD = 10.9		

	No. of patients	% of patients
F. Serum cholesterol (mg/dl)		
< 150	43	0.5
150–174	250	3.0
175–199	775	9.3
200–224	1431	17.2
225–249	1871	22.4
250–274	1658	19.9
275–299	1170	14.0
300–324	604	7.2
325–349	272	3.3
350–374	139	1.7
375–399	65	0.8
≥ 400	63	0.8
Total	8341	
Median = 246.9		
Mean = 250.8		
SD = 48.0		
G. Serum triglyceride (mEq/L)		
< 2.0	90	1.1
2.0– 2.9	872	10.5
3.0– 3.9	1607	19.3
4.0– 4.9	1596	19.1
5.0– 5.9	1225	14.7
6.0– 6.9	861	10.3
7.0– 7.9	564	6.8
8.0– 8.9	426	5.1
9.0– 9.9	289	3.5
10.0–19.9	678	8.1
20.0–29.9	82	1.0
≥ 30.0	50	0.6
Total	8340	
Median = 5.00		
Mean = 6.10		
SD = 4.79		
H. Serum uric acid (mg/dl)		
< 4.0	88	1.1
4.0– 4.9	523	6.3
5.0– 5.9	1744	20.9
6.0– 6.9	2377	28.5
7.0– 7.9	1934	23.2
8.0– 8.9	1001	12.0
9.0– 9.9	390	4.7
10.0–10.9	184	2.2
11.0–11.9	61	0.7
≥ 12.0	37	0.4
Total	8339	
Median = 6.75		
Mean = 6.88		
SD = 1.49		

Systolic and diastolic blood pressures have correlations of only 0.047 and 0.065, respectively, with race (that is, nonwhites with MI tend to have slightly higher blood pressures than whites with MI).

The New York Heart Association functional class is most highly correlated with a history of angina pectoris (0.416). To a lesser degree it is correlated with light physical activity of leisure (0.205) and history of congestive heart failure (0.192).

Supplement 1 to Circulation, Vols. XLVII and XLVIII, March 1973

	No. of patients	% of patients
I. Fasting plasma glucose (mg/dl)		
< 80	112	1.3
80- 89	1328	15.9
90- 99	3383	40.6
100-109	2085	25.0
110-119	696	8.3
120-129	280	3.4
130-149	210	2.5
150-199	161	1.9
200-249	54	0.6
≥ 250	28	0.3
Total	8337	
Median = 97.9		
Mean = 102.3		
SD = 22.1		
J. One-hour plasma glucose (mg/dl)		
< 80	76	0.9
80- 99	371	4.5
100-119	708	8.5
120-139	1130	13.6
140-159	1393	16.7
160-179	1374	16.5
180-199	1115	13.4
200-219	804	9.7
220-239	575	6.9
240-259	316	3.8
260-279	183	2.2
280-299	89	1.1
300-349	113	1.4
≥ 350	74	0.9
Total	8321	
Median = 167.0		
Mean = 172.7		
SD = 54.0		

*Actual body weight divided by Metropolitan Life Insurance Co. desirable weight.

Cardiomegaly, as found on the baseline chest X-ray, is associated with three of the ECG findings, Q/QS patterns (0.152), T wave findings (0.167), and ST depression (0.187). It is also correlated with usage of digitalis (0.219) and diuretics (0.188) and history of congestive heart failure (0.217).

The negative correlation between T wave findings and ventricular conduction defect is an artifact of coding. T wave findings (and likewise ST depression) are not coded in the presence of ventricular conduction defects.

Heart rate, as measured on the baseline ECG, cigarette smoking status, white blood count, and absolute neutrophil count are all correlated with one another. The highest of these correlations, apart from that between WBC and ANC, are between cigarettes and WBC (0.331) and cigarettes and

ANC (0.300). Heart rate is also correlated with fasting and one hour glucose (0.154 and 0.168, respectively). Cigarette smoking status is also correlated with hematocrit (0.190) and is negatively correlated with plasma urea nitrogen (−0.152), that is, the more that is smoked, the lower the urea nitrogen.

A number of biochemical and clinical measurement variables are positively correlated with relative body weight. These include uric acid (0.238), triglyceride (0.189), fasting glucose (0.167), and systolic and diastolic blood pressure (0.179 and 0.214, respectively).

Detailed analyses of these various correlations are not within the scope of this paper. Further investigations of many of these findings are certainly warranted, including partial correlation analyses, cross tabulations, and graphic displays.

4. Comparability of Treatment Groups at Baseline

When analyzing data from clinical trials such as the CDP, it is always important to investigate whether any observed drug-placebo differences for a particular response variable, or the lack of any such differences, might be due to differences in the drug and placebo patient populations at entry into the study. Such investigations were done, for example, when the CDP Data and Safety Monitoring Committee was evaluating the apparent adverse effects of the 5.0-mg dose of estrogen[9] and of the dextrothyroxine regimen.[9, 16]

Table 13 gives, by treatment group, the percentage of patients with specified baseline findings for 43 different variables. The final variable (number 44) in this table is a combination of five risk factors which have been found to be particularly prognostic of mortality in the CDP.[29] For dichotomous (yes-no) variables the percentage of patients with one of the two possible characteristics is given. For continuous variables or discrete variables with three or more classes, two or three different cutting points are used. Thus, in case of age, for example, table 13 gives the percentage of patients age 40 or more, 55 or more, and 60 or more at entry. By subtracting the percentages in the first line from 100, one can obviously obtain the percentage of patients who were less than 40 years at the time of entry.

By means of conventional chi-square calculations, each drug percentage was compared with the placebo percentage for every line in table 13. Drug-placebo differences for which the P value (based on the chi-square distribution) is less than 0.05 and less than 0.01 are denoted in the table by asterisks.

Table 9

Distributions of Other Laboratory and Clinical Measurements

	No. of patients	% of patients
A. Serum total bilirubin (mg/dl)		
< 0.40	2196	26.8
0.40–0.59	3308	40.3
0.60–0.79	1734	21.1
0.80–0.99	595	7.2
≥ 1.00	374	4.6
Total	8207	
Median = 0.50		
Mean = 0.55		
SD = 0.24		
B. Serum direct bilirubin (mg/dl)		
< 0.20	2340	28.5
0.20–0.29	3637	44.3
0.30–0.39	1513	18.4
0.40–0.49	459	5.6
≥ 0.50	256	3.1
Total	8205	
Median = 0.24		
Mean = 0.26		
SD = 0.18		
C. SGOT (Henry units)		
< 20	1177	14.3
20–29	4625	56.3
30–39	1766	21.5
40–49	382	4.7
≥ 50	258	3.1
Total	8208	
Median = 26.0		
Mean = 27.9		
SD = 12.6		
D. Serum alkaline phosphatase (King-Armstrong units)		
< 6.0	1810	21.7
6.0– 7.9	3202	38.4
8.0– 9.9	2112	25.4
10.0–11.9	824	9.9
≥ 12.0	381	4.6
Total	8329	
Median = 7.4		
Mean = 7.8		
SD = 2.7		
E. Plasma urea nitrogen (mg/dl)		
< 12.0	976	11.7
12.0–15.9	2995	35.9
16.0–19.9	2773	33.3
20.0–23.9	1190	14.3
≥ 24.0	402	4.8
Total	8336	
Median = 16.1		
Mean = 16.4		
SD = 4.2		
F. Serum protein-bound iodine (μg/dl)		
< 4.0	141	1.7
4.0–5.9	3807	46.3
6.0–7.9	3772	45.9
8.0–9.9	348	4.2
≥ 10.0	158	1.9
Total	8226	
Median = 6.0		
Mean = 6.2		
SD = 2.0		

	No. of patients	% of patients
G. Hematocrit (%)		
< 38	66	0.8
38–42	1078	12.9
43–47	4282	51.3
48–52	2584	31.0
≥ 53	331	4.0
Total	8341	
Median = 46.1		
Mean = 46.2		
SD = 3.5		
H. White blood count (cells/mm³)		
< 5000	568	6.8
5000– 6999	3181	38.1
7000– 8999	2874	34.5
9000–10999	1132	13.6
≥ 11000	586	7.0
Total	8341	
Median = 7199		
Mean = 7506		
SD = 2134		
I. Absolute neutrophil count (cells/mm³)		
< 3000	1137	13.6
3000–3900	2206	26.5
4000–4900	2185	26.2
5000–5900	1354	16.2
≥ 6000	1457	17.5
Total	8339	
Median = 4361		
Mean = 4619		
SD = 1677		
J. Urine fasting glucose (Clinistix)		
Negative	8190	98.2
Positive	149	1.8
Total	8339	
K. Urine protein (Clinistix)		
Negative	6981	83.7
Trace	1017	12.2
1+	210	2.5
2+, 3+, or 4+	131	1.6
Total	8339	
L. Body weight (lb)		
< 150	1427	17.1
150–174	3309	39.7
175–199	2502	30.0
220–224	857	10.3
≥ 225	240	2.9
Total	8335	
Median = 170.5		
Mean = 172.2		
SD = 25.0		
M. Height (inches)		
< 64	397	4.8
64–67	3021	36.2
68–71	3928	47.1
≥ 72	992	11.9
Total	8338	
Median = 68.1		
Mean = 68.2		
SD = 2.4		

Since there is a total of 420 separate drug-placebo comparisons given in table 13, we would expect to find about 21 of the differences to be significant at

Table 10

Prevalence of Various Clinical Findings at Baseline

Clinical findings	Total no. of patients	No. with findings	% with findings
Pleural effusion (chest X-ray)	8341	25	0.3
Pulmonary congestion (chest X-ray)	8341	160	1.9
Ventricular diastolic gallop	8076	146	1.8
Rales (dry or moist)	8075	286	3.5
Peripheral edema	8076	128	1.6
Palpable spleen	8341	43	0.5
Enlarged liver	8341	277	3.3
Firm liver	8341	543	6.5
Tender liver	8341	54	0.6
Icterus of sclera and/or skin	8341	9	0.1
Vascular spiders	8341	83	1.0
Visible collateral veins on abdomen or chest	8341	29	0.3
Abnormal thyroid	8341	107	1.3
Exophthalmia	8341	24	0.3
Marked finger tremor	8341	79	0.9
Warm, moist skin	8341	44	0.5
Gynecomastia	8341	180	2.2
Breast masses	8341	15	0.2
Ichthyosis	8341	32	0.4
Acanthosis nigricans	8341	12	0.1
Hyperpigmentation	8341	134	1.6
Abnormal or surgically removed prostate	7457	1420	19.0
Abnormal testes	8336	586	7.0
Any abnormality of:			
Gastrointestinal system	8341	420	5.0
Genitourinary system	8341	293	3.5
Nervous system	8341	256	3.1
Musculoskeletal system	8341	349	4.2
Dermal system	8341	206	2.5
Bronchopulmonary system	8341	291	3.5

the 0.05 level and about four of these 21 to be significant at the 0.01 level if there were truly no drug-placebo differences in any of the lines. There are actually 22 differences in table 13 which are significant at the 0.05 level, two of which are significant at the 0.01 level. Thus, on the basis of 43 variables taken one at a time and one combination of five variables, there is no evidence of lack of comparability of the treatment groups at baseline.

5. Summary

The Coronary Drug Project is a collaborative clinical trial supported by the National Heart and Lung Institute. The three main objectives of the CDP are (1) to evaluate the efficacy of several lipid influencing drugs in the long-term therapy of CHD in men of ages 30 through 64 with evidence of previous myocardial infarction; (2) to obtain information on the natural history and clinical course of CHD; and (3) to develop more advanced methodology for the design and conduct of long-

Supplement 1 to Circulation, Vols. XLVII and XLVIII, March 1973

term, large, collaborative clinical trials which can be applied to other such studies.

Table 11

Usage of Various Medications at Time of Entry

Drug or class of drugs	No. of patients	% of patients
Insulin	0	0.0
Oral hypoglycemic agents	434	5.2
Digitalis	1215	14.6
Antiarrhythmic agents	343	4.1
Diuretics	1144	13.7
Antihypertensive agents other than diuretics	551	6.6
Nitroglycerin or other coronary dilators	3633	43.6
Gout medication	224	2.7
Anticoagulants	3	0.0
Cholesterol lowering agents	0	0.0
Other drugs (analgesics, tranquilizers, antibiotics, etc.)	3143	37.7
Number of patients	8341	

I-30   THE CORONARY DRUG PROJECT

Table 12

Baseline Variables with Correlation Coefficients 0.150 or Greater or −0.150 or Less*

		Correlation coefficient
1.	Age by:	
	a. Urea N	0.194
	b. Syst. BP	0.185
	c. ST depr.	0.153
2.	Race†	
3.	Risk by:	
	a. No. of MI's	0.606
	b. CHF	0.303
	c. Digitalis	0.244
	d. T wave	0.169
	e. Q/QS	0.151
4.	No. of MI's by:	
	a. Risk	0.606
	b. Angina	0.194
	c. ACI	0.175
	d. CHF	0.154
	e. NYHA class	0.153
5.	Time to last MI†	
6.	NYHA class by:	
	a. Angina	0.416
	b. Nitroglycerin	0.286
	c. Physical activity	0.205
	d. CHF	0.192
	e. Digitalis	0.187
	f. No. of MI's	0.153
7.	Physical activity by:	
	a. NYHA class	0.205
8.	ACI by:	
	a. Angina	0.263
	b. No. MI's	0.175
9.	Angina by:	
	a. Nitroglycerin	0.427
	b. NYHA class	0.416
	c. ACI	0.263
	d. No. of MI's	0.194
	e. CHF	0.164
10.	CHF by:	
	a. Digitalis	0.537
	b. Diuretics	0.319
	c. Risk	0.303
	d. Cardiomegaly	0.217
	e. NYHA class	0.192
	f. ST depr.	0.181
	g. Angina	0.164
	h. No. of MI's	0.154
11.	ICIA by:	
	a. Stroke	0.220
12.	Stroke by:	
	a. ICIA	0.220
13.	Int. claud. by:	
	a. Periph. art. occl.	0.332
14.	Periph. art. occl. by:	
	a. Int. claud.	0.332
15.	Pulse rate by:	
	a. ECG heart rate	0.597
	b. Cigarettes	0.178

		Correlation coefficient
16.	Cardiomegaly by:	
	a. Digitalis	0.219
	b. CHF	0.217
	c. Diuretics	0.188
	d. ST depr.	0.187
	e. T wave	0.167
	f. Q/QS	0.152
17.	Q/QS by:	
	a. T wave	0.345
	b. ST depr.	0.158
	c. Cardiomegaly	0.152
	d. Risk	0.151
18.	T Wave by:	
	a. ST depr.	0.611
	b. Q/QS	0.345
	c. Vent. cond. def.	−0.186
	d. Digitalis	0.175
	e. Risk	0.169
	f. Cardiomegaly	0.167
19.	ST depression by:	
	a. T wave	0.611
	b. Digitalis	0.254
	c. Cardiomegaly	0.187
	d. CHF	0.181
	e. Q/QS	0.158
	f. Diuretics	0.157
	g. Age	0.153
20.	ST elevation†	
21.	AV cond. def.†	
22.	Vent. cond. def. by:	
	a. T wave	−0.186
23.	VPB's†	
24.	ECG heart rate by:	
	a. Pulse rate	0.597
	b. Cigarettes	0.209
	c. ANC	0.191
	d. WBC	0.189
	e. 1-hr glucose	0.168
	f. Fast. glucose	0.154
25.	Rel. body wt. by:	
	a. Body wt.	0.844
	b. Uric acid	0.238
	c. Dias. BP	0.214
	d. Triglyceride	0.189
	e. Syst. BP	0.179
	f. Fast. glucose	0.167
26.	Cigarettes by:	
	a. WBC	0.331
	b. ANC	0.300
	c. ECG heart rate	0.209
	d. Hematocrit	0.190
	e. Pulse rate	0.178
	f. Urea N	−0.152
27.	Syst. BP by:	
	a. Dias. BP	0.720
	b. Antihypertensives	0.247
	c. Age	0.185
	d. Rel. body wt.	0.179

The following six treatment regimens were included for study in the CDP: (1) equine estrogens 2.5 mg per day, (2) equine estrogens 5.0 mg

THE CORONARY DRUG PROJECT I-31

			Correlation coefficient
28.	Dias. BP by:		
	a.	Syst. BP	0.720
	b.	Antihypertensives	0.227
	c.	Rel. body wt.	0.214
	d.	Body wt.	0.205
29.	Cholesterol by:		
	a.	Triglyceride	0.349
30.	Triglyceride by:		
	a.	Cholesterol	0.349
	b.	Rel. body wt.	0.189
	c.	Body wt.	0.170
	d.	1-hr glucose	0.160
	e.	Uric acid	0.155
31.	Uric acid by:		
	a.	Diuretics	0.242
	b.	Rel. body wt.	0.238
	c.	Body wt.	0.211
	d.	Urea N	0.158
	e.	Triglyceride	0.155
32.	Fast. glucose by:		
	a.	1-hr glucose	0.596
	b.	Oral hypoglycem.	0.450
	c.	Urine glucose	0.339
	d.	Rel. body wt.	0.167
	e.	ECG heart rate	0.154
33.	1-hr glucose by:		
	a.	Fast. glucose	0.596
	b.	Oral hypoglycem.	0.397
	c.	Urine glucose	0.260
	d.	ECG heart rate	0.168
	e.	Triglyceride	0.160
34.	Total bilirubin by:		
	a.	Direct bilirubin	0.531
35.	Direct bilirubin by:		
	a.	Total bilirubin	0.531
36.	SGOT†		
37.	Alk. phosphatase†		
38.	Urea N by:		
	a.	Age	0.194
	b.	Uric acid	0.158
	c.	Cigarettes	−0.152
39.	PBI†		
40.	Hematocrit by:		
	a.	Cigarettes	0.190
	b.	WBC	0.161
41.	White blood count (WBC) by:		
	a.	ANC	0.878
	b.	Cigarettes	0.331
	c.	ECG heart rate	0.189
	d.	Hematocrit	0.161
42.	Abs. neut. count (ANC) by:		
	a.	WBC	0.878
	b.	Cigarettes	0.300
	c.	ECG heart rate	0.191
43.	Urine glucose by:		
	a.	Fast. glucose	0.339
	b.	1-hr glucose	0.260
	c.	Oral hypoglycem.	0.213
44.	Urine protein†		
45.	Body wt. by:		

			Correlation coefficient
	a.	Rel. body wt.	0.844
	b.	Height	0.515
	c.	Uric acid	0.211
	d.	Dias. BP	0.205
	e.	Triglyceride	0.170
46.	Height by:		
	a.	Body wt.	0.515
47.	Oral hypoglycemics by:		
	a.	Fast. glucose	0.450
	b.	1-hr glucose	0.397
	c.	Urine glucose	0.213
48.	Digitalis by:		
	a.	CHF	0.537
	b.	Diuretics	0.324
	c.	ST depr.	0.254
	d.	Risk	0.244
	e.	Cardiomegaly	0.219
	f.	NYHA class	0.187
	g.	T wave	0.175
49.	Antiarrhythmics†		
50.	Diuretics by:		
	a.	Digitalis	0.324
	b.	CHF	0.319
	c.	Antihypertensives	0.318
	d.	Uric acid	0.242
	e.	Cardiomegaly	0.188
	f.	ST depr.	0.157
51.	Antihypertensives by:		
	a.	Diuretics	0.318
	b.	Syst. BP	0.247
	c.	Dias. BP	0.227
52.	Nitroglycerin by:		
	a.	Angina	0.427
	b.	NYHA class	0.286

*See Appendix G for complete table of correlations among the 52 variables and Appendix H for codes used in the correlation analysis.

†No correlations ≥ 0.150 or ≤ -0.150.

per day, (3) clofibrate 1.8 g per day, (4) dextro-thyroxine 6.0 mg per day, (5) nicotinic acid 3.0 g per day, and (6) lactose placebo 3.8 g per day.

There are 53 clinics participating in the CDP. Patient recruitment started in March, 1966 and was completed in October, 1969. A total of 8341 patients were enrolled with approximately 1100 patients allocated to each of the five drug groups and 2789 allocated to the placebo group.

The following admission criteria had to be satisfied in order for a patient to be enrolled in the CDP:

1. Male, between 30 and 64 years of age at time of entry in the study.

2. ECG-documented MI at least three months prior to entry.

Table 13

Percentage of Patients with Selected Baseline Findings, by Treatment

	ESG1	ESG2	CPIB	Treatment* D-T4	NICA	PLBO	All
1. Age at entry							
≥ 45	84.1	85.2	85.2	84.6	87.2	85.2	85.2
≥ 55	42.3	44.9	43.5	41.9	45.0	43.0	43.3
≥ 60	16.3†	20.6	18.7	16.6†	20.6	19.5	18.9
2. Race − nonwhite	6.6	6.4	6.5	6.1	7.1	6.8	6.6
3. Risk group 2	33.8	33.9	33.8	34.1	34.1	34.3	34.1
4. Number of previous MI's							
≥ 2	20.1	17.8	18.0	19.4	18.7	19.9	19.2
≥ 3	3.2	2.3†	3.4	4.1	3.4	3.6	3.4
5. Months from last MI to entry							
≥ 12	86.3	86.8	85.3	83.7	85.8	86.1	85.8
≥ 36	35.7	34.0	34.0	33.3	36.7	35.9	35.1
≥ 72	14.6	13.0	13.4	13.5	14.4	14.2	13.9
6. NYHA class II	55.9	54.0	55.9	53.8	51.9	53.5	54.0
7. Qualifying ECG							
Class 1 or 2 Q waves	83.3	81.7	83.6	81.4	80.6†	83.3	82.5
Class 1 Q waves	49.5	49.1	51.5	46.8	46.6	49.1	48.8
8. Physical activity of leisure							
Moderate or light	97.5	97.3	97.6	97.6	97.5	98.0	97.7
Light	69.1	70.0	72.1	68.8	69.9	69.8	69.9
9. Acute coronary insufficiency							
Suspect or definite	17.3	17.2	16.2	17.9	18.3	16.4	17.1
Definite	12.0	12.3	11.2	13.8	13.0	12.0	12.3
10. Angina pectoris							
Suspect or definite	57.8	57.7	58.9	59.7	60.1	57.8	58.5
Definite	46.0	45.2	47.1	47.1	49.3	46.5	46.8
11. Congestive heart failure							
Suspect or definite	14.2	17.3	17.1	15.1	13.3	16.0	15.6
Definite	8.4	11.2	11.2	9.8	8.8	9.8	9.8
12. Intermittent cerebral ischemic attacks							
Suspect or definite	3.5	5.2†	3.9	4.3	3.9	3.3	3.9
Definite	0.9	1.5	1.1	1.3	1.5	1.0	1.2
13. Stroke							
Suspect or definite	2.0	2.7	2.2	2.1	1.9	2.0	2.1
Definite	1.5	2.1	1.8	1.6	1.3	1.6	1.6
14. Intermittent claudication							
Suspect or definite	7.5	8.8	7.6	7.6	8.8	8.7	8.3
Definite	4.6	5.5	4.8	5.1	6.1	5.8	5.4
15. Peripheral arterial occlusion							
Suspect or definite	1.2†	2.2	2.0	2.7	2.9	2.4	2.3
Definite	0.8	1.7	1.3	1.3	2.1	1.6	1.5
16. Cardiomegaly							
Suspect or definite	19.1	17.9	17.8	15.4†	15.7	18.2	17.5
Definite	10.4	9.2	9.4	7.8	8.6	9.5	9.2
17. Q/QS patterns							
Any Q/QS	60.0	58.8†	63.5	59.5	59.4	62.2	60.9
Major Q/QS	22.9	23.4	23.7	22.1	21.4	23.7	23.0
18. T wave findings							
Any T	46.6	51.6	50.7	48.4	46.5	49.5	49.0
Major T	1.5	3.1‡	1.6	1.4	1.9	1.7	1.8
19. ST depression							
Any STD	24.5	26.4	24.8	26.4	24.1	25.1	25.2
Major or moderate STD	10.7	12.1†	10.2	8.6	10.2	9.4	10.0
20. ST elevation	3.3	3.3	3.9	4.5	4.2	4.2	4.0
21. A-V conduction defects	4.6	4.6	4.7	4.2	3.8	3.5	4.1
22. Ventricular conduction defects	8.7	9.9	8.2	9.6	10.0	9.3	9.3
23. Frequent premature beats	4.0	4.2	4.4	3.4	4.6	3.6	3.9
24. Sinus arrhythmias	3.0	3.5	3.0	3.8	3.0	3.9	3.5

	ESG1	ESG2	CPIB	Treatment* D-T4	NICA	PLBO	All
25. QRS axis deviation	13.7	14.2	12.6	13.2	10.9†	13.6	13.1
26. High amplitude R waves	6.3	7.9	7.4	8.0	6.4	7.0	7.2
27. One or more codable							
ECG findings	92.5	93.1	94.0	91.3‡	92.7	93.8	93.1
28. ECG heart rate (beats/min)							
≥ 50	97.5	97.1	97.5	97.5	97.4	97.0	97.3
≥ 70	45.7	42.4	45.5	46.7	43.7	45.0	44.8
≥ 90	5.4	4.3	4.8	5.4	3.8	5.2	4.9
29. Relative body weight							
≥ 1.00	87.4	87.6	87.9	89.0	85.9	87.9	87.7
≥ 1.15	45.7	42.8†	43.6	47.8	44.4	46.4	45.4
≥ 1.30	11.2†	12.4	12.7	11.7†	12.6	14.3	12.8
30. Number of cigarettes/day							
≥ 1	39.2	36.5	39.0	34.1†	36.6	37.9	37.4
≥ 21	12.2	10.2	10.6	10.6	11.2	11.2	11.0
31. Systolic blood pressure (mm Hg)							
≥ 110	91.3	91.2	92.7	91.8	91.5	91.1	91.5
≥ 130	49.2	50.0	52.8	49.3	52.9	51.5	51.0
≥ 150	14.1	16.1	18.9	15.7	17.6	16.3	16.4
32. Diastolic blood pressure (mm Hg)							
≥ 70	92.2	93.6	92.7	92.7	93.2	93.0	92.9
≥ 85	36.1	34.9	39.1	35.1	37.4	36.7	36.6
≥ 100	7.2	9.6	9.3	10.0	8.7	8.1	8.7
33. Serum cholesterol (mg/dl)							
≥ 200	87.1	88.9	85.9	88.2	86.8	86.8	87.2
≥ 250	48.2	48.1	47.9	47.7	48.3	46.7	47.6
≥ 300	13.4	13.5	13.7	12.3	14.1	14.3	13.7
34. Serum triglyceride (mg/dl)							
≥ 3.0	88.9	88.3	87.8	87.7	89.1	88.6	88.5
≥ 5.0	50.6	49.8	50.1	46.8	52.6	50.2	50.1
≥ 8.0	16.6	18.1	18.9	17.5	18.9	18.9	18.3
35. Serum uric acid (mg/dl)							
≥ 5.0	92.9	92.5	92.4	92.9	91.7	93.1	92.7
≥ 7.0	41.8	44.1	44.6	41.7	42.6	43.8	43.3
≥ 9.0	8.1	8.1	9.5	7.7	7.3	7.9	8.1
36. Fasting plasma glucose (mg/dl)							
≥ 90	82.6	81.4	83.3	81.9	82.9	83.3	82.7
≥ 100	41.7	42.8	43.1	42.1	41.2	42.1	42.1
≥ 110	17.6	18.6	19.3†	17.2	15.0	16.3	17.1
37. One-hour plasma glucose (mg/dl)							
≥ 140	72.3	73.2	72.8	71.9	73.2	72.2	72.5
≥ 180	39.4	38.9	40.1	39.7	38.5	39.2	39.3
≥ 220	16.0	16.0	18.1	15.9	16.3	15.8	16.2
38. Oral hypoglycemic agents	5.0	5.4	5.9	3.8†	5.5	5.4	5.2
39. Digitalis	12.1†	16.4	15.3	14.5	13.5	15.0	14.6
40. Antiarrhythmic agents	4.0	5.1†	3.7	4.6	4.5	3.6	4.1
41. Diuretics	11.5†	13.3	15.8	13.6	13.4	14.1	13.7
42. Antihypertensive agents	6.4	7.2	7.7	5.7	5.2†	6.9	6.6
43. Nitroglycerin	43.1	44.0	45.5	43.3	44.7	42.5	43.6
44. Combination of five risk factors: any ST depression, susp. or def. cardiomegaly, susp. or def. intermittent claudication, usage of diuretics, cholesterol ≥ 250							
One or more of the five	72.1	72.0	73.2	71.1	71.9	70.7	71.6
Two or more of the five	27.1	29.3	30.4	28.8	29.1	29.8	29.2
Three or more of the five	9.3	10.5	10.6	9.0	7.6	9.8	9.3
Four or more of the five	1.6	2.4	2.5	1.6	2.6	2.1	1.9

*ESG1 = estrogen, 2.5 mg per day; ESG2 = estrogen, 5.0 mg per day; CPIB = clofibrate; D-T4 = dextrothyroxine; NICA = nicotinic acid; PLBO = placebo.

†$P < 0.05$ for DRUG-PLBO difference.

‡$P < 0.01$ for DRUG-PLBO difference.

3. New York Heart Association functional class I or II.

4. No previous surgery for coronary artery disease.

5. Freedom from life-limiting disease other than coronary heart disease, freedom from diseases or conditions which might affect long-term follow-up, and freedom from conditions which would contra-indicate the use of any of the CDP drugs.

6. Not on anticoagulant therapy, lipid influencing drugs, or insulin at time of entry.

7. Willingness and ability of patient to partici-pate in the study.

All patients were randomly assigned to one of the six treatment groups in a double blind fashion, that is, with neither the patient nor the clinic personnel informed as to which drug the patient would be taking. All patients will be followed for a minimum of five years, and some patients will be followed for as long as 8½ years. A set of three baseline examinations was performed for each patient, and follow-up examinations are given at four-month intervals after the patient's time of entry into the study. The annual follow-up examination consists of a complete physical examination, interval medical history, resting electrocardiogram, chest X-ray, and an extensive battery of biochemical and hematologi-cal determinations. Assessment of drug adherence is made at every follow-up visit.

The primary response variable in the CDP is total mortality. Other major response variables include cause-specific mortality and nonfatal cardiovascular events such as MI, ACI, development of angina pectoris, stroke, arrhythmias, congestive heart fail-ure, pulmonary embolism, and others.

All completed study forms, ECG's, laboratory determinations, and ECG readings are sent to the Coordinating Center for editing, analysis, and storage. The CDP data are reviewed periodically by a Data and Safety Monitoring Committee for evidence of adverse and beneficial treatment effects.

The following are highlights of the baseline demographic, clinical, and laboratory findings:

1. The mean age of CDP participants at the time of entry was 52 years, and 7% of the patients are nonwhite.

2. About 66% of the patients are in Risk Group 1, that is, had a single uncomplicated MI prior to entry.

3. About 53% of the patients had a history of suspected or definite angina pectoris at entry.

4. Over 37% of the patients were cigarette smokers at the time of entry.

5. About half of the patients had serum choles-terol levels over 250 mg/dl, and 3% were over 350 mg/dl.

On the basis of 43 baseline variables taken one at a time and one combination of five variables, there is no evidence of lack of comparability of the six treatment groups at baseline.

Two papers have been published elsewhere giving findings in the 5.0 mg per day estrogen group, the dextrothyroxine group, and the placebo group.[9, 16] Additional papers dealing with aspects of the natural history of CHD have been published or are being prepared for publication.[25–29]

References

1. KEYS A, ed: Coronary heart disease in seven countries. Circulation 41 and 42 (suppl I), 1970

2. EPSTEIN FJ, OSTRANDER LD, JOHNSON BC, PAYNE MW, HAYNER NS, KELLER JB, FRANCIS T: Epidemiological studies of cardiovascular disease in a total community—Tecumseh, Michigan. Ann Intern Med 62: 1170, 1965

3. KANNEL WB, DAWBER TR, KAGAN A, REVOTSKIE N, STOKES J: Factors of risk in the development of coronary heart disease—six year follow-up experi-ence, the Framingham Study. Ann Intern Med 55: 33, 1961

4. KEYS A, KIMURA N, KUSUKAWA A, BRONTE-STEWART B, LARSEN N, KEYS MH: Lessons from serum cholester-ol studies in Japan, Hawaii and Los Angeles. Ann Intern Med 48: 83, 1958

5. STAMLER J, LINDBERG HA, BERKSON DM, SHAFFER A, MILLER B, POINDEXTER A: Prevalence and incidence of coronary heart disease in strata of the labor force of a Chicago industrial corporation. J Chronic Dis 11: 405, 1960

6. STAMLER J: Lectures on Preventive Cardiology. New York, Grune and Stratton, 1967

7. STAMLER J, PICK R, KATZ L, PICK A, KAPLAN BM, BERKSON DM, CENTURY D: Effectiveness of estrogens for therapy of myocardial infarction in middle-age men. JAMA 183: 632, 1963

8. MARMORSTON J, MOORE FJ, HOPKINS CE, KUZMA OT, WEINER J: Clinical studies of long-term estrogen therapy in men with myocardial infarction. Proc Soc Exp Biol Med 110: 400, 1962

9. Coronary Drug Project Research Group: The Coronary Drug Project: Initial findings leading to modifications of its research protocol. JAMA 214: 1303, 1970

10. HELLMAN L, ZUMOFF B, KESSLER G, KARA E, RUBIN IL, ROSENFELD RS: Reduction of cholesterol and lipids in man by ethyl p-chlorophenoxyisobuty-rate on serum lipid levels. J Atheroscler Res 3: 427, 1963

11. BEST MM, DUNCAN CH: Reduction of serum triglycer-ides and cholesterol by ethyl p-chlorophenoxyisobuty-rate (CPIB). Amer J Cardiol 15: 230, 1965

THE CORONARY DRUG PROJECT I-35

12. Label copy specifications for Choloxin. Flint Laboratories, Morton Grove, Ill, 1965
13. BOYD GS, OLIVER MF: Effects of certain thyroxin analogs on the serum lipids in human subjects. J Endocr 21: 33, 1960
14. BEST MM, DUNCAN CH: Comparative effects of thyroxin analogs as hypocholesterolemic agents. Circulation 24: 58, 1961
15. SEARCY RL, CARLUCCI JS, BERGQUIST LM: Hypolipemic effects of D-thyroxine in coronary patients. Circulation 24: 1103, 1961
16. Coronary Drug Project Research Group: The Coronary Drug Project: Findings leading to further modifications of its protocol with respect to dextrothyroxine. JAMA 220: 996, 1972
17. BERGE KG, ACHOR RWP, CHRISTENSEN NA, MASON HL, BARKER NW: Hypercholesterolemia and nicotinic acid: Long term study. Amer J Med 31: 24, 1961
18. ALTSCHUL R, HOFFER A, STEPHEN JD: Influence of nicotinic acid on serum cholesterol in man. Arch Biochem 54: 558, 1955
19. MAHL M, LANGE K: Long term study of the effect of nicotinic acid medication on hypercholesterolemia. Amer J Med Sci 246: 673, 1963
20. PARSONS WB, FLINN JH: Reduction of serum cholesterol and beta-lipoprotein cholesterol levels by nicotinic acid. Arch Intern Med (Chicago) 103: 783, 1959
21. Criteria Committee of New York Heart Association: Diseases of the Heart and Blood Vessels: Nomenclature and Criteria for Diagnosis, 6th ed. Boston, Little Brown & Co, 1964
22. DUNNETT CW: Multiple comparison procedure for comparing several treatments with a control. J Amer Statistical Ass 50: 1096, 1955
23. ROSE GA, BLACKBURN H: Cardiovascular Survey Methods. Geneva, WHO, 1968
24. HAINLINE A JR: Quality Assurance for the Automated Laboratory, 1970 Technicon International Congress, vol 1. Miami, Thurman Associates, 1971
25. Coronary Drug Project Research Group: Control of hyperlipidemia: IV. Progress in drug trials of secondary prevention, with particular reference to the Coronary Drug Project. In Atherosclerosis: Second International Symposium, edited by RJ Jones. New York, Springer-Verlag, 1970, p 586
26. Coronary Drug Project Research Group: Natural history of myocardial infarction in the Coronary Drug Project: Prognostic indicators following infarction. In Preventive Cardiology, edited by G Tibblin, A Keys, L Werko. Stockholm, Almqvist & Wiksell, p 54
27. Coronary Drug Project Research Group: Prognostic importance of the electrocardiogram following myocardial infarction; experience in the Coronary Drug Project. Ann Intern Med 77: 677, 1972
28. Coronary Drug Project Research Group: Prognostic importance of premature beats following myocardial infarction; experience in the Coronary Drug Project. JAMA, in press
29. Coronary Drug Project Research Group: Natural history of myocardial infarction in the Coronary Drug Project: I. Relationship of entry characteristics to long-term mortality. In preparation.

30. New Weight Standards for Men and Women. Statistical Bull Metropolitan Life Insurance Co 40: 1, 1959
31. KING EJ, ARMSTRONG AR: Convenient method for determining serum and bile phosphatase activity. Canad Med Ass J 31: 376, 1934
32. POWELL MEA, SMITH JJH: Determination of serum acid and alkaline phosphatase activity with 4-aminoantipyrine. J Clin Path 7: 245, 1954
33. KIND PRN, KING EJ: Estimation of plasma phosphatase by determination of hydrolyzed phenol with aminopyrine. J Clin Path 7: 322, 1954
34. GAMBINO SR, DI RE J: Manual on Bilirubin Assay. Chicago, American Society of Clinical Pathologists, 1968
35. JENDRASSIK L, GROF P: Vereinfachte photometrische Methoden zur Bestimmung des Blutbilirubins. Biochem Z 297: 81, 1938
36. BOUTWELL JH JR: Estimation of bilirubin using acetamide. Clin Chem 10: 197, 1964
37. ZLATKIS A, ZAK B, BOYLE AJ: New method for the direct determination of serum cholesterol. J Lab Clin Med 41: 486, 1953
38. AutoAnalyzer method for determination of total cholesterol in serum, Technicon Method N-24. Tarrytown, New York, Technicon Instruments Corp, 1964
39. ABELL LL, LEVY BB, BRODIE BB, KENDALL FE: Simplified method for the estimation of total cholesterol in serum and demonstration of its specificity. J Biol Chem 195: 357, 1952
40. SIEGEL AL, COHEN PS: Automated determination of creatine phosphokinase. 1966 Technicon Symposium "Automation in Analytical Chemistry," vol 1. White Plains, New York, Mediac Inc, 1967, p 474
41. HOFFMAN WS: Rapid photoelectric method for the determination of glucose in blood and urine. J Biol Chem 120: 51, 1937
42. AutoAnalyzer method for glucose, Technicon Method N-2a. Tarrytown, New York, Technicon Instruments Corp, 1963
43. SAX SM, MOORE JJ: Determination of glutamic oxalacetic transaminase activity by coupling of oxalacetate with diozonium salts. Clin Chem 13: 175, 1967
44. MORGANSTERN S, KAUFMAN JH, KLEIN B: Automated determination of serum glutamic oxalacetic transaminase II: Procedure for robot chemist. Clin Chem 13: 270, 1967
45. HENRY RJ, CHAIMORI N, GOLUM PJ, BERKMAN S: Revised spectrophotometric methods for the determination of glutamic oxalacetic transaminase, glutamic-pyruvic transaminase and lactic acid dehydrogenase. Amer J Clin Path 34: 381, 1960
46. PRICE JM: Determination of N-methyl-2-pyridone-5-carboxamide in human urine. J Biol Chem 211: 117, 1954
47. RILEY M, COCHMAN N: Fully automated method for the determination of serum protein-bound iodine. Technicon Corp Bulletin 62. Tarrytown, New York, Technicon Instruments Corp, 1964
48. CARLSON LA: Determination of triglycerides. J Atheroscler Res 3: 334, 1963

49. VAN HANDEL E, ZILVERSMIT DB: Micromethod for the direct determination of serum triglycerides. J Lab Clin Med 50: 152, 1957

50. LOFLAND HB JR: Semiautomated procedure for the determination of triglycerides in serum. Anal Biochem 9: 393, 1964

51. MATHER A, ROLAND D: Automated thiosemicarbazide-diacetyl monoxime method for plasma urea. Clin Chem 15: 393, 1969

52. BROWN H: Determination of uric acid in human blood. J Biol Chem 158: 601, 1945

53. Serum uric acid by AutoAnalyzer, Technicon Method N-13b. Tarrytown, New York, Technicon Instruments Corp, 1965

Role of the Low Density Lipoprotein Receptor in Regulating the Content of Free and Esterified Cholesterol in Human Fibroblasts

MICHAEL S. BROWN, JERRY R. FAUST, and JOSEPH L. GOLDSTEIN

From the Department of Internal Medicine, University of Texas Health Science Center at Dallas, Dallas, Texas 75235

A B S T R A C T The transfer of normal human fibroblasts from medium containing whole serum to medium devoid of lipoproteins produced a 90% decrease in the cellular content of cholesteryl esters and a 30% decrease in the free cholesterol content. When these lipoprotein-deprived cells were subsequently incubated with human low density lipoprotein (LDL), there was a 7-fold increase in the cellular content of esterified cholesterol and a 1.6-fold increase in the cellular content of free cholesterol. The concentration at which LDL produced its half-maximal effect in elevating cellular sterol content (30 µg/ml of LDL-cholesterol) was similar to the half-maximal concentration previously reported for high affinity binding of LDL to its cell surface receptor. High density lipoprotein (HDL) and whole serum from a patient with abetalipoproteinemia (neither of which contains a component that binds to the LDL receptor) did not produce a significant increase in the content of either cholesterol or cholesteryl esters in normal cells. Furthermore, in fibroblasts from patients with the homozygous form of familial hypercholesterolemia, which lack functional LDL receptors, LDL had no effect in raising the cellular content of either free or esterified cholesterol even when present in the medium at concentrations as high as 450 µg sterol/ml. It is concluded that LDL-receptor interactions constitute an important biochemical mechanism for the regulation of the cholesterol content of normal human fibroblasts. Moreover, when considered in light of current concepts of LDL metabolism in intact mammals, the present data suggest that a major function of plasma LDL may be to transport cholesterol from its site of synthesis in liver and intestine to its site of uptake in peripheral tissues.

INTRODUCTION

In cultured human fibroblasts, cellular cholesterol synthesis is controlled by a negative feedback system in which the activity of the rate-controlling enzyme in cholesterol biosynthesis, 3-hydroxy-3-methylglutaryl-CoA reductase (HMG-CoA reductase),[1] is inversely related to the content of extracellular low density lipoprotein (LDL) (1, 2). LDL, the major cholesterol-carrying lipoprotein in human plasma, suppresses the activity of HMG-CoA reductase by binding to specific, high affinity receptor sites located on the cell surface (3-5). Although the precise biochemical mechanism by which binding leads to enzyme suppression is not yet known, it has been shown that the binding of LDL leads to at least two other related enzymatic events: (*a*) the protein component of the lipoprotein is proteolytically degraded to its constituent amino acids (4), and (*b*) cholesteryl ester formation within the cell is markedly stimulated (6). High density lipoprotein (HDL), the other major cholesterol-carrying lipoprotein in plasma, does not bind to the LDL receptor and neither suppresses HMG-CoA reductase activity (1, 2) nor stimulates cellular cholesterol esterification (6).

Analysis of the multiple actions of the LDL receptor has been simplified by studies of cultured cells obtained from subjects with the homozygous form of familial hypercholesterolemia. These mutant cells manifest a

Dr. Brown is an Established Investigator of The American Heart Association and Dr. Goldstein is the recipient of a U. S. Public Health Service Research Career Development Award (GM 70, 277).

Received for publication 4 October 1974 and in revised form 9 December 1974.

[1] *Abbreviations used in this paper:* FCS, fetal calf serum; GLC, gas-liquid chromatography; HDL, high density lipoprotein; HMG-CoA reductase, 3-hydroxy-3-methylglutaryl-CoA reductase; LDL, low density lipoprotein; LPDS, lipoprotein-deficient serum; PBS, phosphate-buffered saline.

primary deficiency in the number of functional LDL receptors and hence are resistant to all of the known biochemical events mediated by this lipoprotein. In the homozygotes' cells, LDL does not bind with high affinity (3–5); the lipoprotein is not degraded at a normal rate (4); cellular cholesterol esterification is not stimulated (6); HMG-CoA reductase activity is not suppressed (2, 7); and cholesterol is overproduced (7, 8).

Recent studies have shown that incubation of normal cells with nonlipoprotein cholesterol can reproduce two of the events observed when LDL binds to its receptor —namely, suppression of HMG-CoA reductase activity (2, 9) and stimulation of cellular cholesteryl ester formation (6). Moreover, nonlipoprotein cholesterol elicits a normal response in the homozygotes' cells even though they do not respond to LDL (2, 6, 9). These observations have raised the possibility that LDL-mediated suppression of HMG-CoA reductase activity and stimulation of cholesteryl ester formation result from an action of the LDL receptor in permitting the net transfer of cholesterol from extracellular LDL to a site within the cell. If the cellular accumulation of cholesterol from LDL does indeed require the LDL receptor, this formulation would explain why nonlipoprotein cholesterol and other related sterols that can enter cells in the absence of the LDL receptor (10) are able to exert similar effects in normal and homozygotes' cells.

The present studies were designed to test the validity of the above hypothesis. Direct measurements have been made of the cellular content of free and esterified cholesterol in normal and mutant fibroblasts incubated in the presence and absence of plasma lipoproteins. The results indicate: (a) that LDL but not HDL produces a net increase in the cellular content of free and esterified cholesterol in normal cells, and (b) that this accumulation of cholesterol is markedly impaired in cells that lack the LDL receptor.

METHODS

Materials. [1,2-³H]Cholesterol (56 Ci/mmol), cholesteryl oleate ([1-¹⁴C]oleate) (50 mCi/mmol), [1-¹⁴C]oleic acid (51.8 mCi/mmol), and D,L-3-hydroxy-3-methyl[3-¹⁴C]glutaryl-CoA (7.67 mCi/mmol) were purchased from New England Nuclear (Boston, Mass.). Na ¹²⁵I (carrier free in 0.05 N NaOH) was obtained from Schwarz/Mann Div. (Becton, Dickinson & Co., Orangeburg, N. Y.). Sodium oleate, cholesterol, and stigmasterol were obtained from Applied Science Labs., Inc. (State College, Pa.). 7-Ketocholesterol was purchased from Steraloids, Inc. (Pawling, N.Y.). All sterols were greater than 99% pure as measured by gas-liquid chromatography (GLC). Silicic acid (100 mesh) was obtained from Mallinckrodt Chemical Works (St. Louis, Mo.). Celite was obtained from Johns-Manville Products Corp. (Denver, Colo.). 3% OV-17 on 100/120 mesh Gas-Chrom Q was obtained from Applied Science

Labs, Inc. All other materials were obtained as previously described (9).

Cells. Skin biopsies were obtained with informed consent, and fibroblast cultures were established in our laboratory as previously described (1, 11). In all experiments except those in Fig. 2, the normal cells were derived either from the foreskin of a healthy newborn or from the nongenital skin of a healthy 10-yr-old boy, and the mutant hypercholesterolemic cell line was obtained from the nongenital skin of J. P., a 12-yr-old female subject with the homozygous form of familial hypercholesterolemia (7). All normal and mutant cell lines used in the present studies have been shown in previous studies to possess the typical phenotypic characteristics of the indicated genotype, as determined by measurements of LDL-mediated suppression of HMG-CoA reductase activity (2), [¹²⁵I]LDL binding and degradation (5), and LDL-dependent cholesteryl ester formation (6). All cells were grown in monolayer and were used between the 5th and 15th passage. Cell lines were maintained in a humidified incubator (5% CO_2) at 37°C in 75-cm² stock flasks containing 10 ml of growth medium consisting of Eagle's minimum essential medium (Grand Island Biological Co., Grand Island, N. Y.) supplemented with penicillin (100 U/ml); streptomycin (100 μg/ml); 20 mM Tricine, pH 7.4; 24 mM $NaHCO_3$; 1% (vol/vol) nonessential amino acids; and 10% (vol/vol) fetal calf serum (FCS). All experiments were carried out using a similar format: confluent monolayers of cells from the stock flasks were dissociated with 0.05% trypsin-0.05% EDTA solution (day 0), and an indicated inoculum of cells was seeded into a series of petri dishes containing growth medium with 10% FCS. Fresh growth medium with 10% FCS was added at intervals of 2–3 days as indicated in the figure legends. When the cells were in the late logarithmic phase of growth, each cellular monolayer was washed with phosphate-buffered saline (PBS), and various lipoprotein additions and incubations were made as indicated in the figure legends.

Measurement of cellular sterol content. To remove all nonspecifically bound extracellular lipoproteins, each cell monolayer was washed five times at 4°C as previously described (3, 4). Each of the first five washes was carried out with either 3- (60-mm dishes) or 5-ml (100-mm dishes) aliquots of buffer containing 50 mM Tris-Cl, pH 7.4; 0.15 M NaCl; and 2 mg/ml of bovine albumin stock solution, followed by one final wash with either 3 or 5 ml of buffer containing 50 mM Tris-Cl, pH 7.4 and 0.15 M NaCl. The washed cells were scraped with a rubber policeman, centrifuged (900 *g*, 3 min, 4°C), and resuspended in 1 ml of 0.15 M NaCl. After a 50-μl aliquot was removed for protein determination (12), the cell suspension was recentrifuged (900 *g*, 3 min, 24°C). To the cell pellet was added 2 ml of chloroform: methanol (2:1) containing as an internal standard for recovery tracer amounts (< 80 ng of sterol) of [1,2-³H]cholesterol (2×10^5 cpm) and cholesteryl oleate ([1-¹⁴C]oleate) (2×10^4 cpm). The mixture was then agitated for 30 s and allowed to stand at 24°C (or in some experiments at 50°C) for 30 min. To separate the phases, 0.5 ml of H_2O was added (13), and each tube was agitated for 30 s and then centrifuged (900 *g*, 5 min, 24°C). The bottom phase was washed once with 1.5 ml of pure upperphase solvent consisting of chloroform: methanol: H_2O (15:240:235) (13), followed by recentrifugation and removal of the upper aqueous phase.

The bottom phase was evaporated to dryness under nitrogen, and the lipids were resuspended in 150 μl of benzene and applied to a column (100× 5 mm) packed with silicic acid:Celite (wt:wt, 2:1) equilibrated in benzene (14).

The cholesteryl esters were first eluted with a total of 3.3 ml of benzene. The free cholesterol was then eluted with a total of 2 ml of ethyl acetate. For the purposes of GLC, a second internal standard consisting of 7.5 µg of stigmasterol was added to each of the two fractions obtained from the silicic acid: Celite column.

The cholesterol fraction was evaporated to dryness under nitrogen, the residue was resuspended in 100 µl of benzene, and a 5-µl aliquot was removed for liquid scintillation counting of the [³H]cholesterol. At this stage, the recovery of free cholesterol averaged 74%. Double-label counting indicated that there was no contamination with [¹⁴C]cholesteryl oleate. The cholesterol fraction was then evaporated to dryness, resuspended in 15 µl of choloroform, and 2-µl aliquots were subjected to GLC for measurement of cholesterol content.

The cholesteryl ester fraction from the silicic acid: Celite column was evaporated to dryness and resuspended in 100 µl of benzene, and a 5-µl aliquot was removed for liquid scintillation counting of the [¹⁴C]cholesteryl oleate. At this stage, the recovery of cholesteryl oleate averaged 67%. Double-label counting indicated that there was no contamination with [³H]cholesterol. 400 µl of 0.625 N ethanolic potassium hydroxide was added to the remaining 95 µl of benzene solution containing the cholesteryl esters. The alkaline hydrolysis mixture was heated at 80°C for 30 min, the hydrolysis solution was then evaporated under nitrogen, and the residue was resuspended in 500 µl of H₂O. The free cholesterol was extracted by addition of 2 ml of choloroform: methanol (2:1), followed by centrifugation to separate the two phases, and removal of the upper aqueous phase. The lower phase was washed three times with 1.5 ml of pure upper-phase solvent (13) and then evaporated under nitrogen, and the residue was resuspended in 15 µl of chloroform. 2-µl aliquots were subjected to GLC for measurement of the hydrolyzed cholesterol content.

GLC was performed using the internal standard-area ratio technique employing stigmasterol as the internal standard. A Hewlett-Packard model 5750 research chromatograph with flame ionization detector and Hewlett-Packard model 3370 B integrator (Hewlett-Packard Co., Avondale, Pa.) were used in these analyses. The sterols were separated at 260°C on a 6-foot (2 mm ID) glass column packed with 3% OV-17 on 100/120 mesh Gas-Chrom Q. The flow rate of the nitrogen carrier gas was 45 ml/min. The flame ionization detector operated at hydrogen and air flow rates of 62 and 222 ml/min, respectively. Average elution times for cholesterol and stigmasterol were 243 and 338 s, respectively. Since the detector and integrator gave the same response (area of peak) to equal masses of cholesterol and stigmasterol, the amount of cholesterol in each sample was calculated by multiplying the peak area ratio (cholesterol: stigmasterol) by the amount of stigmasterol added to each sample (7.5 µg). Each microgram value was then divided by the fractional recovery of cholesterol and cholesteryl esters as determined by the scintillation counting procedure as described above. The final value, which represented the micrograms of cholesterol present as either free cholesterol or cholesteryl esters in the original sample, was then expressed as micrograms of sterol per milligram of total cell protein.

Other assays. The activity of HMG-CoA reductase in cell-free extracts (2), the specific high affinity binding and degradation of [¹²⁵I]LDL by cell monolayers (4), and the rate of [1-¹⁴C]oleate incorporation into cholesteryl esters by cell monolayers (6) were measured exactly as described in the cited references. For the experiments in Figs. 8 and 9, the sodium oleate-albumin solutions were prepared by a modification (6) of the method described by Van Harken, Dixon, and Heimberg (15).

Lipoproteins. Human LDL (d 1.019-1.063 g/ml), HDL (d 1.063-1.215 g/ml), and lipoprotein-deficient serum (LPDS, d > 1.215 g/ml) were prepared from single 500-ml units of blood collected in 0.1% EDTA from healthy subjects who had been fasted for 15 h (2). Lipoproteins were fractionated by sequential flotation in a Beckman preparative ultracentrifuge (Beckman Instruments, Inc., Spinco Div., Palo Alto, Calif.) at 214,000 g (average) and 4-10°C for 16-24 h according to standard techniques (16) using solid KBr for density adjustment (17). The lipoprotein-deficient fraction of FCS, which was used only in the growth studies in Fig. 7, was prepared by a single centrifugation of FCS at 214,000 g for 48 h at 4-10°C after density adjustment to 1.215 using solid KBr (9). The isolated human and calf fractions were dialyzed at least 36 h at 4°C against three changes of at least 50 vol of buffer containing 10 mM Tris-Cl, pH 7.4; 0.15 M NaCl; and 0.3 mM sodium EDTA. After dialysis, the human LPDS was defibrinated with thrombin as previously described (2), sterilized by Millipore filtration (Millipore Corp., Bedford, Mass.), adjusted to a protein concentration of 50 mg/ml using the dialysis buffer, and stored at 4°C. After dialysis, the volume of the lipoprotein-deficient fraction of FCS was adjusted so as to equal that of the starting FCS (9). HDL and LDL each migrated as a homogeneous peak on lipoprotein electrophoresis (18). For the experiment in Fig. 5, blood samples from a patient with abetalipoproteinemia and from a healthy subject were collected in tubes without anticoagulants and allowed to clot at 24°C. The resulting whole serum was heated at 56°C for 20 min before addition to the growth medium to inactivate complement. The cholesterol content of sera and lipoprotein fractions was measured either by a modification of the method of Zak (19) or by GLC (see above). The protein content of the lipoprotein fractions was determined by the method of Lowry, Rosebrough, Farr, and Randall (12) using bovine serum albumin as a standard.

RESULTS

The content of free and esterified cholesterol in normal human fibroblasts varied according to the lipoprotein content of the culture medium (Fig. 1). In normal fibroblasts grown continuously in 10% FCS, nearly 40% of the total cholesterol was in an esterified form (Fig. 1A). When the FCS was removed from the medium and the cells incubated for 48 h in medium containing either no serum or the lipoprotein-deficient fraction of human serum, there was an 80-90% decline in the content of cholesteryl esters but only a 30% drop in the content of free cholesterol. The addition of human LDL to the medium at the time of removal of FCS largely prevented the decline in cholesteryl esters. When compared with normal fibroblasts, cells from a homozygote with familial hypercholesterolemia grown in 10% FCS contained a lower level of cholesteryl esters, and there was little change when the fetal calf lipoproteins were removed (Fig. 1B). Moreover, in contrast to the normal cells, the mutant cells did not show a significantly increased cholesteryl ester content in the presence of LDL.

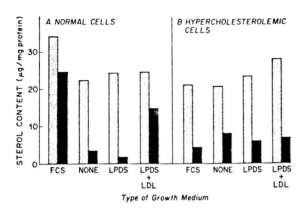

FIGURE 1 Content of free and esterified cholesterol in normal (A) and hypercholesterolemic (B) fibroblasts incubated in the presence and absence of serum lipoproteins. Cells were plated (day 0) at a concentration of 1.5×10^5 cells/100-mm petri dish in 7 ml of growth medium containing 10% FCS. On day 2, the medium was replaced with 7 ml of fresh growth medium containing 10% FCS. On day 4, each cell monolayer was washed with 5 ml of PBS, after which 5 ml of one of the following types of growth medium was added: 10% (vol/vol) FCS (8 mg protein/ml); no serum; 10% (vol/vol) human LPDS (5 mg protein/ml); or 10% (vol/vol) human LPDS (5 mg protein/ml) plus 85 μg/ml of LDL-cholesterol. After incubation at 37°C for 48 h (day 6), each cell monolayer was washed and harvested for measurement of sterol content as described in Methods. Each bar represents the mean value of duplicate dishes. The stippled bars refer to free cholesterol, and the solid bars refer to esterified cholesterol.

To document further the difference in cholesteryl ester content in normal and hypercholesterolemic [2] cells and to obviate a variability that was associated with different batches of FCS,[3] the free and esterified cholesterol content in cell lines from five normal subjects and five homozygotes with familial hypercholesterolemia was compared in the presence and absence of a high concentration of LDL (Fig. 2). When grown in the lipoprotein-deficient fraction of human serum for 48 h, both the normal and mutant cells exhibited a low cholesteryl ester content. However, whereas the addition of LDL to the medium during the last 24 h raised the cholesteryl ester content in each of the normal cell lines, it had little effect on the hypercholesterolemic cells (Fig. 2A and B). As a result, in the presence of LDL the mean cholesteryl ester content of the normal cells was about sevenfold higher than in the hyper-

[2] For the sake of convenience, the term "hypercholesterolemic cells" is used to designate the mutant cell lines derived from subjects with the homozygous form of familial hypercholesterolemia.

[3] In the course of these studies, it was observed that the cholesteryl ester content of normal fibroblasts grown in 10% FCS varied from 10 to 25 μg sterol/mg protein, depending on the batch of FCS used.

cholesterolemic cells with no overlap between the two groups. In the same experiment, LDL consistently caused a 1.6-fold increase in the free cholesterol content of each of the normal cell lines, whereas it had no consistent elevating effect in the hypercholesterolemic cells (Fig. 2C and D).

The diminished LDL response in the homozygotes' cells suggested that in normal cells the accumulation of sterols in the presence of LDL required the action of the LDL receptor. This conclusion was supported by

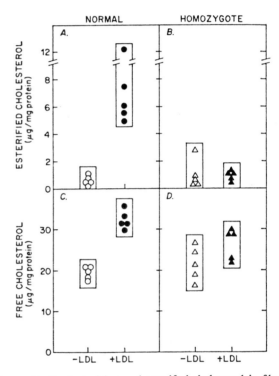

FIGURE 2 Content of free and esterified cholesterol in fibroblasts from five normal subjects (O, ●) and five homozygotes with familial hypercholesterolemia (△, ▲) incubated in the presence and absence of LDL. Each of the normal and mutant cell lines used in these studies has been previously characterized biochemically and was shown to have a phenotype consistent with the indicated genotype (5). The 5 mutant cell lines are the same as those reported previously (5, 6), and the 5 normal cell lines were chosen at random from among the 13 normal cell lines previously characterized (5). Cells were plated (day 0) at a concentration of 3×10^5 cells/100-mm petri dish in 7 ml of growth medium containing 10% FCS. On day 4, the medium was changed to fresh medium containing 10% FCS. On day 6, all of the cell monolayers were washed with 5 ml of PBS, after which 5 ml of fresh growth medium containing 5% human LPDS (2.5 mg protein/ml) was added. After 24 h (day 7), 375 μg of LDL-cholesterol was added in a volume of 10 μl to half of the dishes for each cell line. After a further incubation for 24 h at 37°C, each cell monolayer was washed and harvested for measurement of sterol content as described in Methods. Each point represents the mean value of duplicate dishes.

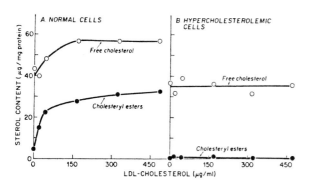

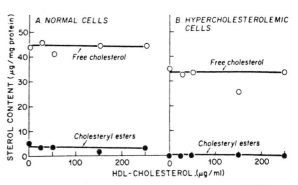

FIGURE 3 Effect of increasing concentrations of LDL on the content of free (O) and esterified (●) cholesterol in normal (A) and hypercholesterolemic (B) fibroblasts. Cells were plated (day 0) at a concentration of 1×10^5 cells/60-mm petri dish in 3 ml of growth medium containing 10% FCS. On day 4, the medium was replaced with fresh growth medium containing 10% FCS. On day 7, each cell monolayer was washed with 3 ml of PBS, after which 2 ml of fresh growth medium containing 5% human LPDS (2.5 mg protein/ml) was added. After 24 h (day 8), the medium was replaced with 2 ml of fresh growth medium containing 5% human LPDS and the indicated concentration of LDL-cholesterol added in a volume of 1–30 μl. After a further 24 h, each cell monolayer was washed and harvested. For each data point the cells from three dishes were pooled for measurement of sterol content as described in Methods.

a study of the relation between cellular cholesterol content and the concentration of the lipoprotein in the medium (Fig. 3). When incubated in the presence of increasing concentrations of LDL for 24 h, the content of free and esterified cholesterol in normal cells reached a maximum at an LDL level of about 100 μg/ml of LDL-cholesterol.[4] Half-maximal accumulation of sterol occurred at an LDL-cholesterol concentration in the range of 30 μg/ml (equivalent to 20 μg/ml of LDL-protein). This value is similar to the previously reported concentration for half-maximal binding of LDL to its receptor (i.e., 10–15 μg/ml of LDL-protein [4]). In the hypercholesterolemic cells, which are deficient in functional LDL receptors, no significant increase in the cellular content of free or esterified cholesterol was observed at LDL-cholesterol levels up to 450 μg/ml (Fig. 3B).

In contrast to the LDL effect, HDL, when added to the medium to give cholesterol concentrations up to 250 μg/ml, did not produce a significant change in the cellular content of free or esterified cholesterol in either the normal or hypercholesterolemic fibroblasts (Fig. 4). Similarly, whereas normal human serum raised the cholesteryl ester content of normal cells, serum from a

---

[4] In the LDL used in these studies, the ratio between total cholesterol content (micrograms) and the total protein content (micrograms) was 1.6. 72% of the total cholesterol in this LDL preparation was in an esterified form.

FIGURE 4 Effect of increasing concentrations of HDL on the content of free (O) and esterified (●) cholesterol in normal (A) and hypercholesterolemic (B) fibroblasts. Cells were grown exactly as described in the legend to Fig. 3 except that on day 8 the medium contained the indicated concentrations of HDL-cholesterol rather than LDL-cholesterol. Cells were incubated for 24 h, washed, harvested, and pooled for measurement of sterol content as described in the legend to Fig. 3.

patient with abetalipoproteinemia, which is devoid of LDL (20), had no such effect, even when added to the medium at cholesterol concentrations much higher than those at which normal serum was effective (Fig. 5). Considered together, the data in Figs. 3–5 suggest that

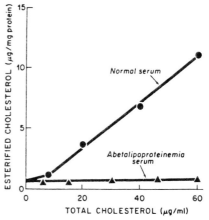

FIGURE 5 Failure of abetalipoproteinemic serum to increase the cholesteryl ester content of normal fibroblasts. Cells were grown exactly as described in the legend to Fig. 2 except that on day 7 the medium was replaced with 5 ml of fresh growth medium containing either normal serum (●) or abetalipoproteinemic serum (▲) to give the indicated final concentration of total cholesterol on the medium. After incubation at 37°C for 24 h, each cell monolayer was washed and harvested for measurement of esterified cholesterol content as described in Methods. To obtain comparable total cholesterol values for the two sera, the normal whole serum was diluted fivefold with human LPDS before addition to the medium. The concentration of free and esterified cholesterol in the undiluted normal serum was 52 and 148 mg/dl, respectively, and in the abetalipoproteinemic serum these respective values were 12.5 and 18 mg/dl. Each point represents the data from a single dish.

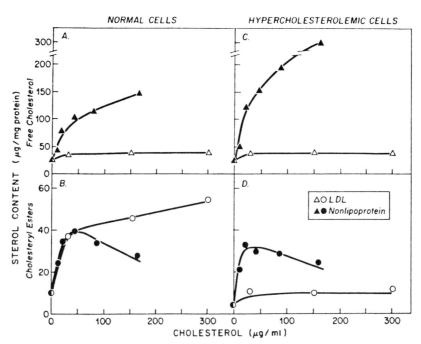

FIGURE 6 Comparison of the effect of increasing concentrations of LDL-cholesterol (△, ○) and nonlipoprotein cholesterol (▲, ●) on the content on free (△, ▲) and esterified (○, ●) cholesterol in normal (A, B) and hypercholesterolemic (C, D) fibroblasts. Cells were grown exactly as described in the legend to Fig. 3 except that on day 8 the medium contained 30 μl of ethanol and the indicated concentration of cholesterol added either as LDL or non-lipoprotein sterol dissolved in ethanol. Cells were incubated for 24 h, washed, harvested, and pooled for measurement of sterol content as described in the legend to Fig. 3.

the net transfer of cholesterol from human lipoproteins to cultured fibroblasts requires the presence of both apolipoprotein B and the LDL receptor. These requirements for cholesterol accumulation by cells are the same as those previously demonstrated for lipoprotein-mediated suppression of HMG-CoA reductase activity (2) and stimulation of cellular cholesteryl ester formation (6).

The requirement for LDL and its receptor for suppression of HMG-CoA reductase activity and stimulation of cellular cholesteryl ester formation can be obviated by the addition to the medium of free cholesterol in a nonlipoprotein form (2, 6, 9). Similarly, the data in Fig. 6 show that nonlipoprotein cholesterol can elevate the cellular content of free and esterified cholesterol in both normal and hypercholesterolemic cells. In normal cells at sterol concentrations up to 50 μg/ml, nonlipoprotein cholesterol was equally as effective as LDL-cholesterol in raising the cellular cholesteryl ester content (Fig. 6B). This occurred despite the fact that more than two-thirds of the LDL-cholesterol in the medium was already in an esterified form. Despite the similar increase in cholesteryl ester content, the free cholesterol content rose to a much greater extent in the presence of nonlipoprotein cholesterol as compared with LDL-cholesterol (Fig. 6A and B). Whereas LDL-

cholesterol had no effect in the hypercholesterolemic cells, nonlipoprotein cholesterol produced an increase in cholesteryl esters similar to that in the normal cells (Fig. 6D), confirming that these mutant cells have no basic defect in the mechanism for esterifying cholesterol provided the sterol becomes available to the cell (6).

The physiological significance of the observation that LDL rather than HDL functions to deliver cholesterol from plasma to cells is indicated by the results of the growth experiment in Fig. 7. When normal fibroblasts are cultured in the presence of 7-ketocholesterol but in the absence of a source of exogenous cholesterol, the suppression of endogenous cholesterol synthesis by 7-ketocholesterol, a sterol that specifically reduces HMG-CoA reductase activity, is so marked that cell growth ceases (9). This inhibition of cell growth could be effectively prevented by the addition to the medium of either nonlipoprotein cholesterol or LDL (Fig. 7). On the other hand, HDL, when added at a cholesterol concentration equivalent to that of LDL, was unable to sustain a normal rate of growth, presumably because it, unlike LDL, was unable to cause a net transfer of its cholesterol into the cells. However, the fact that cell number did not decline in the presence of HDL, as it did with 7-ketocholesterol alone, suggests that this

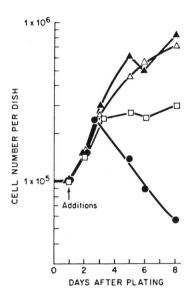

FIGURE 7 Effect of LDL,· HDL, and nonlipoprotein cholesterol on the growth of normal fibroblasts cultured in the presence of 7-ketocholesterol. Cells were initially plated (day 0) at a concentration of 1×10^5 cells/dish in 3 ml of growth medium containing 10% lipoprotein-deficient FCS. 24 h after plating (day 1), the medium was changed to 3 ml of growth medium containing 10% lipoprotein-deficient FCS, 4.8 μg of 7-ketocholesterol added in 2 μl of ethanol, and one of the following additions: ▲, 45 μg of cholesterol added in 2 μl of ethanol; △, 20 μg of LDL-cholesterol and 2 μl of ethanol; □, 21 μg of HDL-cholesterol and 2 μl of ethanol; or ●, 2 μl of ethanol. Fresh medium containing lipoprotein-deficient FCS, 7-ketocholesterol, and the indicated addition was added on days 3 and 6 after plating. Cell number was determined at the indicated time by counting trypsinized cells using a hemocytometer. Each value represents the mean of duplicate counts of duplicate dishes.

lipoprotein may play some undefined role in preserving the integrity of cells depleted of cholesterol.

We have previously shown that in normal cells the addition of LDL to the medium produces a 40-fold increase in the ability of the cells to incorporate [¹⁴C]-oleate into the fatty acid portion of cholesteryl esters (6). To determine whether the availability of long-chain fatty acids is an important limiting factor in the ability of cells to form cholesteryl esters, normal fibroblasts were incubated with increasing concentrations of oleate in the presence and absence of LDL (Fig. 8). At zero oleate concentration, the addition of LDL caused the expected sixfold increase in cholesteryl esters. The addition of increasing amounts of oleate caused only an additional 1.5-fold increase in cholesteryl ester content, a rise that was similar both in the presence and absence of LDL. Thus, the availability of exogenous free fatty acids does not appear to be a major limiting factor in the ability of normal cells to accumulate cholesteryl esters.

The relation between the time courses of the LDL-dependent accumulation of cholesterol and the other known functions of the LDL receptor in normal cells was examined in the experiments shown in Fig. 9. At each of the two different concentrations of LDL, high affinity LDL binding to its receptor reached a maximum between 2 and 4 h after addition of the lipoprotein (Fig. 9A). On the other hand, the degradation of the protein component of LDL was linear with time up to 8 h after an initial lag (Fig. 9B). The major suppression of HMG-CoA reductase activity occurred between 2 and 6 h (Fig. 9C). The ability of the cells to incorporate oleate into the fatty acid portion of cellular cholesteryl esters, as determined by repeated pulse labeling, increased progressively after a brief lag (Fig. 9D). The free and esterified cholesterol content of the cells showed little change at the lower LDL level, but both increased with time at the higher LDL level (Fig. 9E and F). The data in Fig. 9 show that at the lower level of LDL marked suppression of HMG-CoA reductase occurred without any significant rise in the total cellular content of free or esterified cholesterol. Whereas these data do not exclude the possibility that enzyme suppression results from an increase in either free or esterified cholesterol contained in a small pool, they do indicate that large increases in cellular sterol content are not necessary to bring about suppression of HMG-CoA reductase activity.

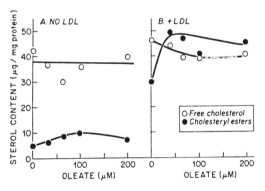

FIGURE 8 Effect of increasing concentrations of oleate on the content of free (○) and esterified (●) cholesterol in normal fibroblasts incubated in the absence (A) and presence (B) of LDL. Cells were grown exactly as described in the legend to Fig. 3 except that on day 8 the medium was replaced with 2 ml of fresh growth medium containing 5% human LPDS (2.5 mg protein/ml), 75 μg/ml of LDL-cholesterol as indicated, and the indicated concentration of oleate-albumin solution added in a volume of 5–30 μl. After a further 24 h, each cell monolayer was washed and harvested. For each data point, the cells from three dishes were pooled for measurement of sterol content as described in Methods.

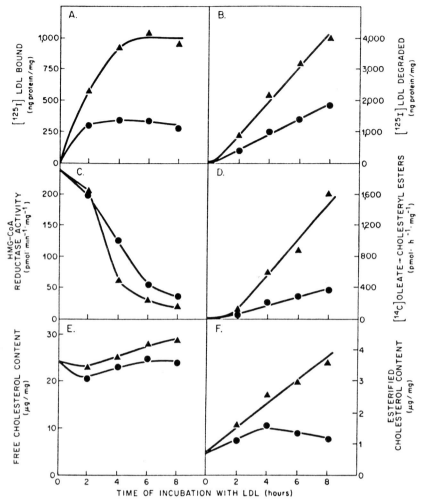

FIGURE 9 Manifestations of LDL-receptor interactions in normal fibroblasts incubated with LDL at 5 (●) and 25 (▲) μg protein/ml for varying time intervals. Cells from one normal subject were plated (day 0) into 94 petri dishes (60 mm) at a concentration of 1×10^{6} cells/dish in 3 ml of growth medium containing 10% FCS. Cells were grown exactly as described in the legend to Fig. 3 except that on day 8 the medium was replaced with 2 ml of fresh growth medium containing 5% human LPDS and either [^{125}I]LDL (120 cpm/ng protein, exps. A and B) or unlabeled LDL (exps. C–F) at a concentration of either 5 (●) or 25 (▲) μg protein/ml. After incubation at 37°C for the indicated time, the following determinations were made. High affinity [^{125}I]LDL binding (A) and degradation (B): The medium was removed, its content of ^{125}I-labeled, trichloroacetic acid-soluble degradative products was measured (4), and the amount of ^{125}I radioactivity bound to the cells was determined (4). High affinity binding and degradation were calculated by subtracting the amount of radioactivity bound or degraded in the presence of 395 μg protein/ml of unlabeled LDL from that bound or degraded in its absence (4). At both concentrations of LDL, the high affinity binding and degradation (plotted above) accounted for more than 80% of the total radioactivity bound or degraded in the absence of the unlabeled LDL. HMG-CoA reductase activity (C): Cells were harvested, cell-free extracts were prepared, and HMG-CoA reductase activity was determined as described (2). [1-^{14}C]oleate incorporation into cholesteryl esters (D): 30 min before each indicated time point, cell monolayers were pulse-labeled with [1-^{14}C]-oleate (56 cpm/pmol) bound to albumin (6) at a final oleate concentration of 0.1 mM. After 30 min, the cells were harvested and the content of [^{14}C]cholesteryl esters was determined (6). Cellular content of free (E) and esterified (F) cholesterol: Cells from two dishes were washed, harvested, pooled, and the content of free and esterified cholesterol was determined as described in Methods. In all experiments (A-F), each data point represents the mean of duplicate determinations.

790 *M. S. Brown, J. R. Faust, and J. L. Goldstein*

DISCUSSION

As a result of the previous studies of Bailey and co-workers (21) and Rothblat, Hartzell, Mialhe, and Kritchevsky (22, 23), it is known that mammalian cells cultured in the presence of animal serum synthesize little cholesterol, but are able to take up exogenous cholesterol contained in the serum lipoproteins of the medium. The present studies indicate that in human fibroblasts the exogenous cholesterol that enters these cells in the presence of serum is derived mainly from LDL and that this transfer requires the action of the LDL receptor. Evidence for the specific involvement of LDL and its receptor in this process rests on the following observations: (a) the hyperbolic relation between the cellular accumulation of free and esterified cholesterol and the concentration of LDL in the medium resembles the previously reported saturation curve for LDL binding to its receptor (4); (b) HDL, which does not bind to the LDL receptor (3), does not cause a net increase in the cellular content of either free or esterified cholesterol under conditions in which LDL causes an increase in both forms of the sterol; (c) cells from homozygotes with familial hypercholesterolemia, which lack the LDL receptor, do not shown an increase in cellular free or esterified cholesterol when incubated with LDL; (d) serum from a patient with abetalipoproteinemia, which is devoid of LDL (20), does not raise the content of free and esterified cholesterol in normal cells; and (c) cells in which endogenous sterol synthesis is suppressed by 7-ketocholesterol are able to derive enough exogenous sterol from LDL to grow normally, whereas their growth ceases in the presence of HDL.

In the present studies, we have measured directly the levels of cellular cholesterol in the presence of various plasma lipoproteins. At any given time, this sterol content reflects the end result of several opposing events: (a) a balance between the rates of cellular influx and efflux of sterols; (b) a balance between the rates of hydrolysis of cholesteryl esters and esterification of free cholesterol; and (c) the rate of endogenous synthesis of cholesterol. Although the method of direct measurement of cellular sterol levels has two advantages over experiments using radioisotopes (it permits an assessment of the end result of a complex physiologic process, and it avoids the problems of pool size and isotope exchange), this direct method has a major limitation in that it does not permit separate examination of the rates of cellular influx and efflux of cholesterol. Nevertheless, the close correlation between the net cellular accumulation of total cholesterol from LDL and the observed rate of degradation of the protein component of LDL suggests that this LDL receptor-mediated process produces a unidirectional flux of sterol

into the cell. Moreover, the fact that sterol accumulates in the normal cells in the presence of LDL at a time when endogenous cholesterol synthesis is suppressed indicates that the increased cellular cholesterol is derived from LDL (6).

In addition to the specific LDL receptor-mediated process for sterol uptake described in this paper, we have observed a different type of uptake process in which radiolabeled free cholesterol of lipoproteins exchanges with cellular cholesterol apparently on a molecule-for-molecule basis.[5] In contrast to the LDL receptor-mediated process, this exchange process does not lead to a change in cellular sterol content, it can involve the cholesterol of HDL as well as LDL, and it can be observed in both hypercholesterolemic and normal fibroblasts [5] as well as in erythrocyte ghosts (24). This exchange process appears to resemble that previously reported by Bailey and Butler, who measured the uptake of [^{3}H]cholesterol from HDL by cultured cells (25). Because in our experiments this exchange process produces no net change in cellular cholesterol content and because it does not exhibit a clear-cut requirement for either a specific lipoprotein or a specific membrane receptor, its physiological function has been difficult to define.

Assuming that the LDL receptor-mediated process produces a net influx of cholesterol into normal cells, it would seem likely that some other process exists to permit the net efflux of sterols from cells. In this regard, Stein and Stein (26) and Bates and Rothblat (27) have presented data in other mammalian cell culture systems to suggest that HDL under some circumstances may selectively enhance the efflux of cellular sterol. Although such an HDL effect was not observed in the present study (Fig. 4), our experiments were carried out under conditions in which the cellular cholesterol content was already low due to prior growth of the cells in LPDS. Additional studies are in progress to determine whether a specific mechanism exists for eliciting net efflux of sterols in human fibroblasts.

A consideration of the present data, in light of current concepts of LDL metabolism in mammals, suggests that an important function of LDL may be to transport cholesterol from its site of synthesis in liver and intestine to its site of uptake in peripheral tissues. Liver and intestine, which are the only two tissues known to synthesize the protein component of LDL (28, 29), also have a much higher rate of cholesterol synthesis than do other tissues and are thought to be the ultimate source of at least 80% of the cholesterol in plasma (30). Unlike liver and intestine, peripheral tissues in the body (such as skin, adipose tissue, and muscle) resemble cultured fibroblasts in that they have much

[5] Unpublished observations.

lower rates of cholesterol synthesis (31, 32) and appear to derived a significant fraction of their steady-state content of cholesterol from plasma lipoproteins (33).

If the LDL receptor functions in the body as it does in cultured cells, all of its known actions—namely, binding and degradation of the lipoprotein, transfer of its cholesterol into the cell, suppression of HMG-CoA reductase activity, and stimulation of cellular cholesterol ester formation—would constitute a major biochemical mechanism by which nonhepatic and nonintestinal cells preferentially take up exogenous LDL-cholesterol and suppress endogenous cholesterol synthesis. Since liver and intestine synthesize and secrete large amounts of cholesterol despite levels of plasma LDL that are sufficient to suppress cholesterogenesis in peripheral tissues, it would seem likely that these two secretory tissues possess control mechanisms other than LDL-receptor interactions. Indeed, it is known that in liver, cholesterogenesis is suppressed primarily by dietary cholesterol carried in chylomicrons (30), and in intestine, cholesterogenesis is suppressed mainly by bile acids (30).

ACKNOWLEDGMENTS

Jean Helgeson and Helen Bohmfalk provided excellent assistance with the cell culture studies. We thank Dr. Charles E. Mize for allowing us to obtain blood from his patient with abetalipoproteinemia.

This research was supported by grants from the American Heart Association (72 629 and 74 983), the National Institutes of Health (HL 16024 and GM 19258), and the Harry S. Moss Heart Fund.

REFERENCES

1. Brown, M. S., S. E. Dana, and J. L. Goldstein. 1973. Regulation of 3-hydroxy-3-methylglutaryl coenzyme A reductase activity in human fibroblasts by lipoproteins. *Proc. Natl. Acad. Sci. U. S. A.* **70**: 2162–2166.
2. Brown, M. S., S. E. Dana, and J. L. Goldstein. 1974. Regulation of 3-hydroxy-3-methylglutaryl coenzyme A reductase activity in cultured human fibroblasts: comparison of cells from a normal subject and from a patient with homozygous familial hypercholesterolemia. *J. Biol. Chem.* **249**: 789–796.
3. Brown, M. S., and J. L. Goldstein. 1974. Familial hypercholesterolemia: Defective binding of lipoproteins to cultured fibroblasts associated with impaired regulation of 3-hydroxy-3-methylglutaryl coenzyme A reductase activity. *Proc. Natl. Acad. Sci. U. S. A.* **71**: 788–792.
4. Goldstein, J. L., and M. S. Brown. 1974. Binding and degradation of low density lipoproteins by cultured human fibroblasts: comparison of cells from a normal subject and from a patient with homozygous familial hypercholesterolemia. *J. Biol. Chem.* **249**: 5153–5162.
5. Brown, M. S., and J. L. Goldstein. 1974. Expression of the familial hypercholesterolemia gene in heterozygotes: Mechanism for a dominant disorder in man. *Science (Wash. D. C.).* **185**: 61–63.
6. Goldstein, J. L., S. E. Dana, and M. S. Brown. 1974. Esterification of low density lipoprotein cholesterol in human fibroblasts and its absence in homozygous familial hypercholesterolemia. *Proc. Natl. Acad. Sci. U. S. A.* **71**: 4288–4292.
7. Goldstein, J. L., and M. S. Brown. 1973. Familial hypercholesterolemia: identification of a defect in the regulation of 3-hydroxy-3-methylglutaryl coenzyme A reductase activity associated with overproduction of cholesterol. *Proc. Natl. Acad. Sci. U. S. A.* **70**: 2804–2808.
8. Khachadurian, A. K., and F. S. Kawahara. 1974. Cholesterol synthesis by cultured fibroblasts: Decreased feedback inhibition in familial hypercholesterolemia. *J. Lab. Clin. Med.* **83**: 7–15.
9. Brown, M. S., and J. L. Goldstein. 1974. Suppression of 3-hydroxy-3-methylglutaryl coenzyme A reductase activity and inhibition of growth of human fibroblasts by 7-ketocholesterol. *J. Biol. Chem.* **249**: 7306–7314.
10. Goldstein, J. L., J. R. Faust, G. Y. Brunschede, and M. S. Brown. 1974. Steroid structural requirements for suppression of 3-hydroxy-3-methylglutaryl coenzyme A reductase activity in cultured human fibroblasts. *Adv. Exp. Med. Biol.* In press.
11. Goldstein, J. L., M. J. E. Harrod, and M. S. Brown. 1974. Homozygous familial hypercholesterolemia: specificity of the biochemical defect in cultured cells and feasibility of prenatal detection. *Am. J. Hum. Genet.* **26**: 199–206.
12. Lowry, O. H., N. J. Rosebrough, A. L. Farr, and R. J. Randall. 1951. Protein measurement with the folin phenol reagent. *J. Biol. Chem.* **193**: 265–275.
13. Folch, J., I. Ascoli, M. Lees, J. A. Meath, and F. N. LeBaron. 1951. Preparation of lipide extracts from brain tissue. *J. Biol. Chem.* **191**: 833–841.
14. Frantz, I. D., Jr., E. Dulit, and A. G. Davidson. 1957. The state of esterification of the sterols of rat skin. *J. Biol. Chem.* **226**: 139–144.
15. Van Harken, D. R., C. W. Dixon, and M. Heimberg. 1969. Hepatic lipid metabolism in experimental diabetes. V. The effect of concentration of oleate on metabolism of triglycerides and on ketogenesis. *J. Biol. Chem.* **244**: 2278–2285.
16. Havel, R. J., H. A. Eder, and J. H. Bragdon. 1955. The distribution and chemical composition of ultracentrifugally separated lipoproteins in human serum. *J. Clin. Invest.* **34**: 1345–1353.
17. Radding, C. M., and D. Steinberg. 1960. Studies on the synthesis and secretion of serum lipoproteins by rat liver slices. *J. Clin. Invest.* **39**: 1560–1569.
18. Noble, R. P. 1968. Electrophoretic separation of plasma lipoproteins in agarose gel. *J. Lipid Res.* **9**: 693–700.
19. Zak, B. 1957. Simple rapid microtechnic for serum total cholesterol. *Am. J. Clin. Pathol.* **27**: 583–588.
20. Fredrickson, D. S., A. M. Gotto, and R. I. Levy. 1972. Familial lipoprotein deficiency. *In* The Metabolic Basis of Inherited Diseases. J. B. Stanbury, J. B. Wyngaarden, and D. S. Fredrickson, editors. McGraw-Hill Book Co., New York. 3rd edition. 493–530.
21. Bailey, J. M. 1973. Regulation of cell cholesterol content. *In* Atherogenesis: Initiating Factors. *CIBA Found. Symp.* **12**: 63–92.
22. Rothblat, G. H., R. Hartzell, H. Mialhe, and D. Kritchevsky. 1967. Cholesterol metabolism in tissue culture cells. *In* Lipid Metabolism in Tissue Culture. G. H. Rothblat and D. Kritchevsky, editors. Wistar Press, Philadelphia. 129–146.

23. Rothblat, G. H. 1972. Cellular sterol metabolism. *In* Growth, Nutrition, and Metabolism of Cells in Culture. G. H. Rothblat and V. J. Cristofalo, editors. Academic Press, Inc., New York. I: 297–325.

24. Bruckdorfer, K. R., and C. Green. 1967. The exchange of unesterified cholesterol between human low-density lipoproteins and rat erythrocyte 'ghosts'. *Biochem. J.* **104**: 270–277.

25. Bailey, J. M., and J. Butler. 1973. Cholesterol uptake from doubly-labeled α-lipoproteins by cells in tissue culture. *Arch. Biochem. Biophys.* **159**: 580–581.

26. Stein, O., and Y. Stein. 1973. The removal of cholesterol from Landschütz ascites cells by high-density apolipoprotein. *Biochim. Biophys. Acta.* **326**: 232–244.

27. Bates, S. R., and G. H. Rothblat. 1974. Regulation of cellular sterol flux and synthesis by human serum lipoproteins. *Biochim. Biophys. Acta.* **360**: 38–55.

28. Roheim, P. S., L. I. Gidez, and H. A. Eder. 1966. Extrahapetic synthesis of lipoproteins of plasma and chyle. Role of the intestine. *J. Clin. Invest.* **45**: 297–300.

29. Windmueller, H. G., and R. I. Levy. 1968. Production of β-lipoprotein by intestine in the rat. *J. Biol. Chem.* **243**: 4878–4884.

30. Dietschy, J. M., and J. D. Wilson. 1970. Regulation of cholesterol metabolism. *N. Engl. J. Med.* **282**: 1128–1138, 1179–1183, and 1241–1249.

31. Dietschy, J. M., and M. D. Siperstein. 1967. Effect of cholesterol feeding and fasting on sterol synthesis in seventeen tissues of the rat. *J. Lipid Res.* **8**: 97–104.

32. Dietschy, J. M., and J. D. Wilson. 1968. Cholesterol synthesis in the squirrel monkey. Relative rates of synthesis in various tissues and mechanisms of control. *J. Clin. Invest.* **47**: 166–174.

33. Wilson, J. D. 1970. The measurement of the exchangeable pools of cholesterol in the baboon. *J. Clin. Invest.* **49**: 655–665.

THE LANCET, JANUARY 4, 1975

PLASMA-HIGH-DENSITY-LIPOPROTEIN CONCENTRATION AND DEVELOPMENT OF ISCHÆMIC HEART-DISEASE

G. J. MILLER

Medical Research Council Pneumoconiosis Unit, Llandough Hospital, Penarth, South Wales

N. E. MILLER

Department of Cardiology and Lipid Research Laboratory, Royal Infirmary, Edinburgh, Scotland

Summary The body cholesterol pool increases with decreasing plasma-high-density-lipoprotein (H.D.L.), but is unrelated to the plasma concentrations of total cholesterol and other lipoproteins. This finding supports existing evidence that H.D.L. facilitates the uptake of cholesterol from peripheral tissues and its transport to the liver for catabolism and excretion. Plasma-H.D.L. is reduced in several conditions associated with an increased risk of future ischæmic heart-disease (I.H.D.), namely hypercholesterolæmia, hypertriglyceridæmia, male sex, obesity, and diabetes mellitus, while subjects with existing clinical I.H.D. have lower levels of H.D.L. than healthy subjects within the same community. It is proposed that a reduction of plasma-H.D.L. concentration may accelerate the development of atherosclerosis, and hence I.H.D., by impairing the clearance of cholesterol from the arterial wall.

INTRODUCTION

CORONARY atherosclerosis, the major cause of ischæmic heart-disease (I.H.D.), is characterised histologically by the accumulation of lipid, predominantly cholesterol, in the arterial wall together with a local connective-tissue reaction.[1] However, the origin of the cholesterol and the cause of its accumulation remain uncertain. Although there is evidence that this may be due, at least in part, to the filtration into the arterial intima of cholesterol-rich low-density lipoprotein (L.D.L.) from plasma,[2] the possible contributions of local synthesis and of impaired clearance of cholesterol from the arterial wall have not been resolved. It has been suggested that the transport of cholesterol from peripheral tissues to the liver, for subsequent catabolism and excretion, may be a function of plasma-high-density-lipoprotein (H.D.L.).[3] We present new evidence for the regulation of tissue-cholesterol pools by H.D.L., and draw attention to the association of low plasma-H.D.L. concentrations with clinical I.H.D. and with several coronary risk factors. It is suggested that a reduction in plasma-H.D.L. may impair the normal clearance of cholesterol from the arterial wall and thereby accelerate the development of atherosclerosis.

H.D.L. AND TISSUE CHOLESTEROL

Tissue cholesterol pools, measured indirectly by isotope dilution [4-9] or directly by chemical analysis,[10,11] have been reported to be unrelated or only weakly related to the plasma concentration of total cholesterol in man. However, the possibility that tissue cholesterol might be correlated with the concentration of individual plasma-lipoproteins has not been explored. The opportunity to examine this question was recently presented by the

THE LANCET, JANUARY 4, 1975 17

parallel study of plasma-lipoprotein concentrations and cholesterol metabolism in eight middle-aged patients with hypercholesterolæmia. The details of these investigations are presented elsewhere.[6,12] In brief, body cholesterol pools and turnover were estimated by 2-pool analysis of the plasma-cholesterol specific activity-time curve after the intravenous infusion of radiolabelled cholesterol.[6] With this technique body exchangeable cholesterol is conceived as behaving as two pools, one which equilibrates rapidly with plasma-cholesterol (pool A) and another which equilibrates slowly (pool B). Pool A comprises most of the cholesterol within erythrocytes, liver, spleen, and ileum, while that within other tissues, including adipose tissue, muscle, xanthomata, and arterial wall, belongs predominantly to pool B.[13,14] In each subject the cholesterol and triglyceride within plasma-very-low-density-lipoprotein (V.L.D.L.), L.D.L., and H.D.L. were measured on 4 or more days during the turnover study, using a combined technique involving preparative ultracentrifugation and lipoprotein precipitation.[15]

Cholesterol pool size was unrelated to the mean plasma concentration of total cholesterol, total triglyceride, V.L.D.L., or L.D.L. However, both pool A and pool B showed a strong negative correlation with the plasma-H.D.L. cholesterol. The values for pool A excluded the contribution made by plasma[5] and were corrected to a standard body-weight of 70 kg.,[6] while those for pool B were the minimum estimates of that pool[5] corrected for the known effect of excess body fat.[5,16] The relations were: pool A = 38 − 0.43 (H.D.L. cholesterol); $r = -0.93$, P < 0.001; and pool B = 77 − 0.85 (H.D.L. cholesterol); $r = -0.84$, P < 0.01, where pool size and H.D.L. cholesterol are expressed in grammes and mg. per 100 mL., respectively.

H.D.L. AND CORONARY RISK FACTORS

Epidemiological studies have shown that certain conditions (coronary risk factors)[17] are associated statistically with an increased risk of subsequent I.H.D. However, the relevance of these factors to the pathogenesis of the disease is not fully understood. Examination of published reports has revealed that many of these conditions are associated with a reduced concentration of H.D.L.

Hypercholesterolæmia

The risk of developing future I.H.D. increases with

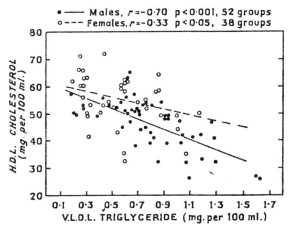

Fig. 2—Relation between plasma concentrations of V.L.D.L. triglyceride and H.D.L. cholesterol reported for single groups of healthy subjects in seven countries.[12,20−31,33]

Each point represents the mean values for one group. When necessary, lipid concentrations have been calculated from total lipoprotein concentrations using published data on lipoprotein composition.[20] V.L.D.L. = density < 1.006 g. per ml.

---

increasing plasma cholesterol.[18,19] Most of the cholesterol within plasma exists as a component of L.D.L.[20] An inverse correlation between plasma L.D.L. and H.D.L. concentrations was noted in American men and women,[20] and a similar relation is apparent in the data presented by Nikkilä[21] for adult males in Finland ($r = -0.34$, n = 58, P < 0.01). We have examined the average lipoprotein concentrations reported for groups of healthy men and women in six developed countries.[12,20−31] The data for L.D.L. and H.D.L. cholesterol are summarised in fig. 1, in which each point represents the average values reported for a single group of subjects. These results confirm the inverse correlation between L.D.L. and H.D.L., and also suggest that separate relations apply for males and females across the range of populations studied. In accordance with these observations, patients with familial hypercholesterolæmia (primary type-II hyperlipoproteinæmia[29]) tend to have somewhat lower H.D.L. levels than healthy controls, especially in the homozygote for this condition.[15,32] However, the Eskimos of rural Greenland differ from these technologically advanced communities in having high average plasma concentrations of both L.D.L. and H.D.L. cholesterol.[25]

Hypertriglyceridæmia

Carlson and Böttiger[19] found that the risk of developing I.H.D. also increased with increasing fasting plasma-triglyceride concentration. In the fasting state plasma-triglyceride exists predominantly as a component of V.L.D.L.,[20] and a negative correlation between the plasma concentrations of V.L.D.L. and H.D.L. has been reported from the U.S.A.[20] and Sweden.[22] In fig. 2 we have summarised the average concentrations of V.L.D.L. triglyceride and H.D.L. cholesterol reported for individual groups of healthy subjects in seven countries.[12,20−31,33] The inverse relation between plasma H.D.L. and V.L.D.L. again differs between the sexes, but within each sex applies across the range of communities examined. In accordance with this relation, low plasma-H.D.L. concentrations are associated with increased V.L.D.L. in primary hyperlipoproteinæmia of types IV and V.[15,29,32]

Other Risk Factors

Obesity,[34] diabetes mellitus,[35] physical inactivity,[36] and male sex[37,38] have also been reported to be risk factors for subsequent I.H.D. Obesity[39] and diabetes mellitus[28,40]

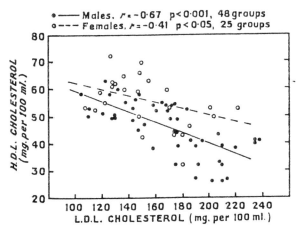

Fig. 1—Relation between plasma concentrations of L.D.L. cholesterol and H.D.L. cholesterol reported for single groups of healthy subjects in six countries.[12,20−31]

Each point represents the mean values for one group. When necessary, lipid concentrations have been calculated from total lipoprotein concentrations using published data on lipoprotein composition.[20] L.D.L. = density 1.006−1.063 g. per ml.; H.D.L. = density > 1.063 g. per ml.

18   THE LANCET, JANUARY 4, 1975

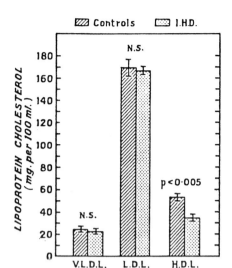

Fig. 3—Lipoprotein cholesterol concentrations in eight patients with I.H.D. but normal plasma-total-cholesterol concentration (< 250 mg. per 100 ml.) and fourteen healthy controls.[21]

Ages: I.H.D. 54±1 years; controls 51±2 years (mean±S.E.M.).

are commonly associated with a reduced plasma-H.D.L., and in Sweden lower H.D.L. concentrations were reported in the general male population [23] than in male skiers with high levels of physical activity.[37] Many studies have confirmed that men have lower plasma-H.D.L. concentrations than women.[20–22,24,28–30,32]

H.D.L. AND CLINICAL I.H.D.

Patients with clinical I.H.D. as a group have significantly lower plasma-H.D.L. concentrations than healthy subjects within the same community.[21,41–45] Data drawn from a study by Nikkilä [21] (fig. 3) show that this remained true even for those patients with I.H.D. whose concentrations of total plasma-cholesterol were within the normal range (<250 mg. per 100 ml.), and whose average V.L.D.L. and L.D.L. concentrations were similar to those of the control group.

Little information is available on plasma-lipoprotein concentrations in communities with low mortality-rates from I.H.D. However, Eskimos in rural Greenland have considerably higher H.D.L. levels and a lower I.H.D. mortality than men in Denmark.[25]

DISCUSSION

The foregoing associations raise the possibility that low plasma concentrations of H.D.L. may be involved in the pathogenesis of coronary atherosclerosis. Evidence has been presented by other investigators that H.D.L. may be important for the normal clearance of cholesterol from tissues, which has been shown by kinetic studies to be a major determinant of the size of the body cholesterol pool.[5] Although cholesterol is synthesised in most tissues of the body,[46] including arterial wall and atheromatous tissue,[47,48] it can be catabolised and excreted in quantitatively important amounts only by the liver.[49] Cholesterol must therefore be transported from these tissues to the liver during cholesterol turnover. Cholesterol exists within the body in esterified and unesterified forms, but only the latter can exchange readily between plasma-lipoproteins and tissues.[8] The activity of the plasma-cholesterol esterifying enzyme, lecithin/cholesterol acyltransferase (L.C.A.T.), has been shown in vitro to

promote the transfer of cholesterol from erythrocytes to plasma by maintaining a shift in the equilibrium between plasma and cell-membrane unesterified cholesterol.[50] This process has been reported to be accelerated by the addition to the incubation medium of H.D.L.,[51] the unesterified cholesterol of which is the preferred substrate for L.C.A.T. activity.[52] More recently, cholesterol efflux from ascites tumour cells has been demonstrated using H.D.L. apoprotein as the receptor.[53] By contrast, in Tangier disease, in which there is a near absence of H.D.L., cholesterol accumulates in many tissues, including the blood-vessel walls.[54] This evidence for a role of H.D.L. in tissue-cholesterol clearance is now strengthened by the demonstration of an inverse relation between plasma-H.D.L. concentration and the size of the body cholesterol pool, suggesting that the concentration of H.D.L. may be rate-limiting for this process.

The cholesterol of atheroma seems to be derived more from that of plasma than from local synthesis,[55] and its accumulation must therefore represent an imbalance between the addition of lipoprotein cholesterol to the arterial wall and its subsequent removal. The feeding of high-cholesterol diets to laboratory animals has been shown to promote the development of atherosclerosis,[1] while evidence has been presented in man for the filtration of L.D.L. into the arterial intima in proportion to its plasma concentration.[2,56] For these reasons emphasis has been placed on the possible importance of an increase in cholesterol influx during atherogenesis, rather than a decrease in its removal. However, on the basis of the foregoing observations, it is now suggested that the development of atherosclerosis may also be accelerated by a decreased clearance of cholesterol from the arterial wall secondary to a reduction in the plasma concentration of H.D.L. Unlike previous proposals, this hypothesis offers a single explanation for the association of an increased risk of future I.H.D. not only with hypercholesterolæmia but also with hypertriglyceridæmia, obesity, diabetes mellitus, and perhaps also physical inactivity, while also accounting for the higher frequency of I.H.D. in men than in women. The biochemical mechanisms underlying the reduction in H.D.L. concentration in these situations are not known, but may be related to competition between lipoproteins for common structural components [20,39] and to hormonal effects on lipoprotein metabolism.[57]

In accordance with this hypothesis, it is further proposed that the development of atherosclerosis might be more successfully prevented by increasing plasma-H.D.L., and hence the clearance of cholesterol from the arterial wall, than by conventional attempts to reduce the plasma cholesterol and other lipoproteins alone. The low incidence of clinical I.H.D. in the Eskimos of rural Greenland, despite their having high average plasma L.D.L., is consistent with such a protective effect of increased H.D.L.[25] The proposal is further strengthened by the differing effects of clofibrate and cholestyramine in patients with familial hypercholesterolæmia. Although cholestyramine and similar resins are usually more potent than clofibrate in reducing plasma cholesterol and L.D.L. concentrations [58–62] in such patients, clofibrate seems to be much more effective in mobilising and reducing tissue

THE LANCET, JANUARY 4, 1975

cholesterol pools,[4,6,9,63-65] and may do so even in the absence of a fall in plasma-cholesterol.[63] These findings may be explained by the ability of clofibrate,[59,61] but not of cholestyramine,[12,66] to increase plasma-H.D.L. The demonstration that the in-vitro efflux of cholesterol from atheromatous tissue is promoted by the addition of H.D.L. to the incubation medium provides additional support for the possible value of increasing the plasma concentration of · this lipoprotein.[67]

REFERENCES

1. Adams, C. W. M. *J. clin. Path.* 1973, **26**, suppl. 5, 38.
2. Walton, K. W., Williamson, N. *J. Atheroscler. Res.* 1968, **8**, 599.
3. Glomset, J. A. *J. Lipid Res.* 1968, **9**, 15.
4. Goodman, De W. S., Noble, R. P. *J. clin. Invest.* 1968, **47**, 231.
5. Nestel, P. J., Whyte, H. M., Goodman, De W. S. *ibid.* 1969, **48**, 982.
6. Miller, N. E., Clifton-Bligh, P., Nestel, P. J. *J. Lab. clin. Med.* 1973, **82**, 876.
7. Samuel, P., Perl, W. *J. clin. Invest.* 1970, **49**, 346.
8. Samuel, P., Lieberman, S. *J. Lipid Res.* 1973, **14**, 189.
9. Goodman, De W. S., Noble, R. P., Dell, R. B. *ibid.* 1973, **52**, 2646.
10. Insull, W. M., Hsi, B., Hoshimura, S. *J. Lab. clin. Med.* 1968, **72**, 885.
11. Schreibman, P. H. *Clin. Res.* 1973, **21**, 638.
12. Clifton-Bligh, P., Miller, N. E., Nestel, P. J. *Clin. Sci.* (in the press).
13. Chobanian, A. V., Hollander, W. *J. clin. Invest.* 1962, **41**, 1732.
14. Samuel, P., Perl, W., Holtzman, C. M., Rochman, N. D., Lieberman, S. *ibid.* 1972, **51**, 266.
15. Fredrickson, D. S., Levy, R. I., Lindgren, F. T. *ibid.* 1968, **47**, 2446.
16. Nestel, P. J., Schreibman, P. H., Ahrens, E. H. *ibid.* 1973, **52**, 2389.
17. Simborg, D. W. *J. chron. Dis.* 1970, **22**, 515.
18. Kannel, W. B., Castelli, W. P., Gordon, T., McNamara, P. M. *Ann. intern. Med.* 1971, **74**, 1.
19. Carlson, L. A., Böttiger, L. E. *Lancet*, 1972, i, 865.
20. Nichols, A. V. *Adv. biol. med. Phys.* 1967, **11**, 109.
21. Nikkilä, E. *Scand. J. clin. Lab. Invest.* 1953, **5**, suppl. 8.
22. Carlson, L. A. *J. clin. Path.* 1973, **26**, suppl. 5, 32.
23. Carlson, L. A. *ibid.* p. 43.
24. Lewis, B., Chait, A., Wootton, I. D. P., Oakley, C. M., Krikler, D. M., Sigurdsson, G., February, A., Maurer, B., Birkhead, J. *Lancet*, 1974, i, 141.
25. Bang, H. O., Dyerberg, J., Nielsen, A. B. *ibid.* 1971, i, 1143.
26. Mills, G. L., Wilkinson, P. A. *Br. Heart J.* 1966, **28**, 638.
27. Carlson, L. A., Mossfeldt, F. *Acta physiol. scand.* 1964, **62**, 51.
28. Furman, R. H., Howard, R. P., Lakshmi, K., Norcia, L. N. *Am. J. clin. Nutr.* 1961, **9**, 73.
29. Fredrickson, D. S., Levy, R. I., Lees, R. S. *New Engl. J. Med.* 1967, **276**, 148.
30. Fredrickson, D. S., Levy, R. I., Lindgren, F. T. *J. clin. Invest,* 1968, **47**, 2446.
31. Miller, N. E., Nestel, P. J. *Eur. J. clin. Invest.* (in the press).
32. Fredrickson, D. S., Levy, R. I. in Metabolic Basis of Inherited Disease (edited by J. B. Stanbury, J. B. Wyngaarden, and D. S. Fredrickson); p. 545. New York, 1972.
33. Dyerberg, J., Hjorne, N. *Scand. J. clin. Lab. Invest.* 1973, **31**, 473.
34. Keys, A., Aravanis, C., Blackburn, H., Van Buchem, F. S. P., Buzina, R., Djordjevic, B. S., Fidanza, F., Karvonen, M. J., Menotti, A., Puddu, V., Taylor, H. L. *Ann. intern. Med.* 1972, **77**, 15.
35. Entmacher, P. S., Marks, H. H. *Diabetes*, 1965, **14**, 212.
36. Morris, J. N., Chave, S. P. W., Adam, C., Sirey, C., Epstein, L. *Lancet*, 1973, i, 333.
37. Kannel, W. B., Kagan, A., Dawber, T. R., Revotskie, N. *Geriatrics*, 1962, **17**, 675.
38. Slack, J. *Lancet*, 1969, ii, 1380.
39. Wilson, D. E., Lees, R. S. *J. clin. Invest.* 1972, **51**, 1051.
40. Cornwell, D. G., Kruger, F. A., Hamiri, G. J., Brown, J. B. *Am. J. clin. Nutr.* 1961, **9**, 41.
41. Brunner, D., Lobl, K. *Ann. intern. Med.* 1958, **49**, 732.
42. Keys, A., Fidanza, F. *Circulation*, 1960, **22**, 1091.
43. Barr, D. P., Russ, E. M., Eder, H. A. *Am. J. Med.* 1957, **11**, 480.
44. Carlson, L. A. *Acta med. scand.* 1960, **167**, 399.
45. Jencks, W. P., Hyatt, M. R., Jetton, M. R., Mattingly, T. W., Durrum, E. L. *J. clin. Invest.* 1956, **9**, 980.
46. Dietschy, J. M., Wilson, J. D. *ibid.* 1968, **47**, 166.
47. Bjørkerud, S. in Atherosclerosis (edited by R. J. Jones); p. 126. Berlin, 1970.
48. Day, A. J., Wilkinson, G. K. *Circulation Res.* 1967, **21**, 593.
49. Nestel, P. J. *Adv. Lipid Res.* 1970, **8**, 1.
50. Murphy, J. *J. Lab. clin. Med.* 1962, **60**, 86.
51. Glomset, J. A. *Am. J. clin. Nutr.* 1970, **23**, 1129.
52. Akanuma, Y., Glomset, J. *J. Lipid Res.* 1968, **9**, 620.
53. Stein, O., Stein, Y. *Biochim. biophys. Acta*, 1973, **326**, 232.

References continued at foot of next column

DR G. J. MILLER AND DR N. E. MILLER : REFERENCES—*continued*

54. Fredrickson, D. S., Gotto, A. M., Levy, R. I. in Metabolic Basis of Inherited Disease (edited by J. B. Stanbury, J. B. Wyngaarden, and D. S. Fredrickson); p. 493. New York, 1972.
55. Zilversmit, D. B. *Ann. N.Y. Acad. Sci.* 1968, **149**, 710.
56. Smith, E. B., Slater, R. S. *Lancet*, 1972, i, 463.
57. Scanu, A. M. *Adv. Lipid Res.* 1965, **3**, 63.
58. Levy, R. I., Quarfordt, S. H., Brown, W. V. *Adv. exp. Med. Biol.* 1969, **4**, 377.
59. Levy, R. I. *Ann. intern. Med.* 1972, **77**, 267.
60. Hashim, S. A., Van Itallie, T. B. *J. Am. med. Ass.* 1965, **192**, 289.
61. Strisower, E. H., Adamson, G., Strisower, B. *Am. J. Med.* 1968, **45**, 488.
62. Hunninghake, D. B., Tucker, D. R., Azarhoff, D. L. *Circulation*, 1969, **39**, 675.
63. Grundy, S. M., Ahrens, E. H., Salen, G., Nestel, P. J. *J. Lipid Res.* 1972, **13**, 531.
64. Sodhi, H. S., Kudchodkar, B. J., Horlick, L. *Atherosclerosis*, 1973, **17**, 1.
65. Kudchodkar, B. J., Sodhi, H. S., Horlick, L. *Clin. Res.* 1972, **20**, 944.
66. Jones, R. J., Dobrilovic, L. *J. Lab. clin. Med.* 1970, **75**, 953.
67. Bondjers, G., Bjørkerud, S. *Proc. Eur. Soc. clin. Invest.* 1974, **8**, 123.

Volume 56, number 2   FEBS LETTERS   August 1975

FAMILIAL HYPERLIPOPROTEINEMIA TYPE III: DEFICIENCY OF A SPECIFIC APOLIPOPROTEIN (APO E-III) IN THE VERY-LOW-DENSITY LIPOPROTEINS

G. UTERMANN, M. JAESCHKE and J. MENZEL

Institut für Humangenetik der Universität 3550 Marburg/Lahn, Bahnhofstrasse 7 A, BRD

Received 13 June 1975

1. Introduction

Familial hyperlipoproteinemia type III is a primary disorder of lipid metabolism characterized by an elevation of cholesterol and triglycerides in plasma and by the occurrence of an atypical lipoprotein in the VLDL fraction of affected individuals. This lipoprotein has β- instead of pre-β-mobility in electrophoresis [1] and is rich in cholesterol [2] and in an arginine-rich apolipoprotein [3]. There is evidence that this lipoprotein is an intermediate in the catabolism of triglyceride-rich lipoproteins which accumulate in hyperlipoproteinemia type III [3].

The disease is associated with premature arteriosclerosis, but is usually not expressed before the age of twenty. The primary biochemical lesion in the familial disorder is not known and there is uncertainty on its mode of inheritance [1,4,5].

In the present study we have shown that one protein component of mol. wt ~ 39 000 is deficient in the VLDL from patients with hyperlipoproteinemia type III. This most likely is the underlying defect in the hereditary dyslipoproteinemia.

2. Materials and methods

Fasting plasma was obtained from eight patients with hyperlipoproteinemia type III, five first degree

Abbreviations: VLDL: Very-low-density lipoproteins (d < 1.006 g/ml). LDL-1: Low-density-lipoproteins-1 (d = 1.006–1.019 g/ml). LDL-2: Low-density-lipoproteins-2 (d = 1.019–1.063 g/ml). HDL: High-density-lipoproteins (d = 1.063–1.21 g/ml). PAGE: Polyacrylamide gel electrophoresis. SDS: Sodium dodecyl suphate.

relatives of type III probands, who had type IV or type II hyperlipoproteinemia, sixteen normolipidemic blood donors, twenty patients with type IV and one with type V hyperlipoproteinemia. The diagnosis of type III hyperlipoproteinemia was established by demonstration of primary hyperlipidemia, β-migrating VLDL and a cholesterol: triglyceride ratio in VLDL considerably higher than 0.2 (between 0.53 and 0.77 in all the patients studied here) [6,7]. The eight type III patients were all from different families. A detailed description of these patients and their relatives will be published elsewhere [8]. Two of the type III patients have already been documented in previous publications (E. M. = III, 19 in [9] and E. R. in [10]) and familial involvement has been verified in both [8,10].

Lipoprotein fractions VLDL, LDL-1, LDL-2 and HDL were isolated by sequential ultracentrifugation in a Spinco model L2-65 B preparative centrifuge according to standard procedures [11] with minor modifications [12]. Electrophoretic analysis of lipoproteins in agarose gels was done as described by van Melsen et al. [13]. Soluble lipoproteins were delipidated by five successive extractions with 50 volumes of acetonethanol 1:1 (v/v) at −15°C and finally dried with nitrogen [14]. The arginine-rich apolipoprotein E and the C apoproteins were isolated from apo VLDL by preparative SDS-PAGE in the discontinous system of acetone-ethanol 1:1 (v/v) at −15°C and finally dried Analytical SDS-PAGE was performed according to Weber and Osborne [16] using a 10% monomer concentration. Analytical isoelectric focusing of the urea soluble apo VLDL polypeptides was done by an adaption [12] of the method of Wrigley [17]. Scanning densitometry of the focusing gels was performed after staining with Coomassie brillant blue in a Vitatron

North-Holland Publishing Company – Amsterdam

Volume 56, number 2   FEBS LETTERS   August 1975

TLD. Standard curves for quantitative determinations of Apo C and Apo E in the urea soluble fraction of apo VLDL were established by running known amounts of pure apolipoproteins in parallel gels. Protein was determined according to Lowry et al. [18] with 0.1% SDS in the reaction mixture, cholesterol by the procedure of Roeschlau et al. [19] and triglycerides by the method of Eggstein and Kreutz [20].

3. Results and discussion

In a search for the primary metabolic defect in familial hyperlipoproteinemia type III, we have studied the polypeptide composition of VLDL in patients with hyperlipoproteinemia type III, first degree relatives of type III probands with and without other phenotypic expressions of dyslipoproteinemia and for comparison a control group comprising of normolipidaemic volunteers and of patients with type IV and V hyperlipoproteinemia.

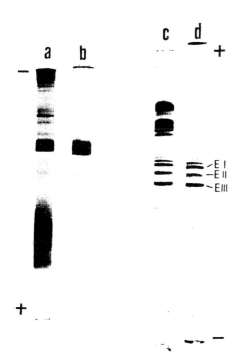

Fig.1. (Left) SDS-PAGE of apo VLDL (a) and purified Apo E (b). (Right) Analytical isoelectric focusing of urea soluble apo VLDL in polyacrylamide gels at pH 3.5–10 (c) and the same apo E preparation as in gel b (d).

The characteristic polypeptide composition of VLDL as demonstrated by SDS-PAGE is shown in fig.1. There are three main components in this fraction: Apo B, Apo C and an arginine-rich protein we have designated Apo E [14]. The latter protein, which has an apparent mol. wt of ~39 000 in SDS-PAGE, is heterogenous and shows three major components in analytical isoelectric focusing in the presence of 6 M urea (fig.1, [14]).

The three Apo E polypeptides were demonstrated in a ratio of roughly 2:1:2 in the apo VLDL of all the thirty-seven controls. Quantitatively Apo E represented 18% of the urea soluble fraction of normolipidaemic subjects (table 1) and about 10% of the total apo VLDL [14]. On the other hand, none of type III patients demonstrated this normal apo VLDL focusing pattern. Two deviations from normal were evaluated by inspection and standardizing scanning densitometry of the stained gels (fig.2, table 1). First the percentage of apo E in the urea soluble apo VLDL was on the average 57% which is considerably higher than in the controls. This finding is in general agreement with previous results of Havel and Kane [3]. Despite the predominance of the arginine-rich Apo E in this fraction, none of the eight type III probands showed significant amounts of a protein preliminary designated Apo E-III ([14] fig.1,2) which was present in all the controls.

Apo E-III could not be detected in any of the other lipoprotein fractions of the patients and seems thus to be deficient in their lipoprotein system. Only traces of Apo E were detected in the HDL and LDL-2 of the type III patients by SDS-PAGE or isoelectric focusing. Their LDL-1, however, contained particles of β-mobility which were extremely rich in total Apo E, but the specific Apo E-III was also deficient in this fraction (fig.3).

The catabolism of triglyceride-rich lipoproteins proceeds through different steps [21]. One of these is apparently impaired in familial type III hyperlipoproteinemia, resulting in the accumulation of the intermediate β-VLDL [3]. Recent evidence along with that presented here suggests that Apo E is intimately associated with the conversion of triglyceride-rich to cholesterol ester-rich lipoproteins and is primarily involved in the transport and metabolism of cholesterol [3,8,22–24]. The specific function of the arginine-rich Apo E in this process is not yet

Volume 56, number 2   FEBS LETTERS   August 1975

Table 1
Characteristics of VLDL fractions from patients with primary hyperlipoproteinemia type III

Patient	Phenotype	C/TG	Mobility prae-β · β		Urea soluble apoproteins (weight %) Apo C	Apo E	Apo E (% of densitometric area) E-I	E-II	E-III
H. Sch.	III	0.53	+	+	60	40	42	58	–
E. R.	III	0.53	+	+	27	73	41	59	–
E. M.	III	0.66	+	+	44	56	42	58	–
Ch. J.	III	0.55	+	+	41	59	51	49	–
S. J.	III	0.77	+	+	45	55	42	58	–
Mean ± SD		0.63 ± 0.09			43 ± 12	57 ± 12	43.6 ± 4.4	56.4 ± 4.4	–
Control[a]	N	0.24	+	–	82	18	38	23	39

C/TG = Cholesterol/Triglyceride ratio
[a]VLDL isolated from a pool of 12 normolipidemic blood donors.

understood. The data known on the metabolic role of Apo E, however, is compatible with the hypothesis that a defect in the regulation or structure of Apo E-III is responsible for the hereditary human disease hyperlipoproteinemia type III.

The data presented here suggest that Apo E-III deficiency is a genuine marker for familial broad-β-disease. This marker may help to establish the diagnosis in uncertain cases and allows to differentiate secondary forms [8].

Apo E-III was not deficient in the apo VLDL from first degree relatives of type III probands, who had

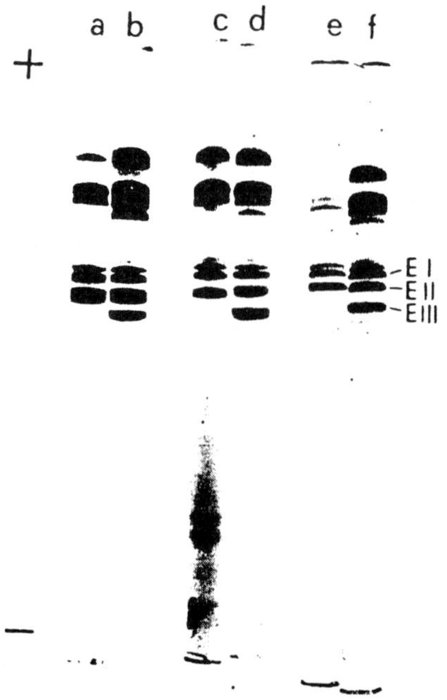

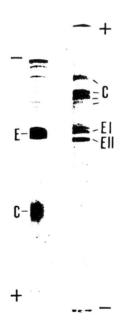

Fig.2. Analytical isoelectric focusing in polyacrylamide gels at pH 3.5–10 of apo VLDL from patients E. M. (a), H.Sch. (c) and E. R. (e) with familial hyperlipoproteinemia type III, the son O. M. of proband E. M. who had a type IV pattern (b) and controls (d,f).

Fig.3. SDS-PAGE (left) and analytical isoelectric focusing at pH 3.5–10 (right) of urea-soluble apo LDL-1 proteins from patient E. M. with hyperlipoproteinemia type III.

Volume 56, number 2 FEBS LETTERS August 1975

other phenotypic forms of hyperlipidemia (fig.2), and in both parents of one type III proband (E. R.). The genetical aspects of these observations and a family study which is in progress in our laboratory will be discussed elsewhere in detail [8]. The preliminary results from the family study indicate that the deficiency of Apo E-III is transmitted by an autosomal recessive mode of inheritance and that patients with type III are homozygous for this defect.

Acknowledgments

We thank Miss Annegret Knauf and Miss Lucie Theus for skillful technical assistance. We are indepted to Professor Canzler (Hannover), Professor Kaffarnik, Drs G. and O. Mühlfellner, Dr J. Schneider (Marburg/ Lahn), Dr W. Schoenborn (Starnberg) and Dr K. H. Vogelberg (Düsseldorf) for providing plasma from their hyperlipidaemic patients.

This work was supported by a grant from the Deutsche Forschungsgemeinschaft.

References

[1] Fredrickson, D. S. and Levy, R. J. (1972) in: The Metabolic Basis of Inherited Disease, (Stanbury, J. B., Wyngaarden, J. B. and Fredrickson, D. S., eds.) pp. 545–614, McGraw-Hill, Inc. New York.

[2] Quarfordt, S., Levy, R. J. and Fredrickson, D. S. (1971) J. Clin. Invest. 50, 754–761.

[3] Havel, R. J. and Kane, J. P. (1973) Proc. Natl. Acad. Sci. USA 70, 2015–2019.

[4] Morganroth, J., Levy, R. J. and Fredrickson, D. S. (1975) Annals of Internal Medicine 82, 158–174.

[5] Hazzard, W. R., O'Donnell, T. F. and Lee, Y. L. (1975) Annals of Internal Medicine 82, 141–149.

[6] Hazzard, W. R., Porte, D. and Bierman, E. L. (1972) Metabolism 21, 1009–1021.

[7] Fredrickson, D. S., Morganroth, J. and Levy, R. J. (1975) Annals of Internal Medicine 82, 150–157.

[8] Utermann, G., Jaeschke, M., Vogelberg, K. H. and Menzel, J. In Preparation.

[9] Fuhrmann, W., Schoenborn, W., Huth, H. and Reimers, J. (1971) XIII. International Congress of Pediatrics, Wien, Austria, 2–42, 199–204.

[10] Schneider, J., Maurer, A. and Kaffarnik, H. (1974) Klin. Wschr. 52, 941–942.

[11] Havel, R. J., Eder, H. A. and Bragdon, J. H. (1955) J. Clin. Invest. 34, 1345.

[12] Utermann, G., Menzel, H. J. and Schoenborn, W. (1975) Clin. Genet. in press.

[13] Van Melsen, A., De Greve, Y., Vanderveiken, F., Vastesaeger, M., Blaton, V. and Paeters, H. (1974) Clin. Chim. Acta 55, 225–234.

[14] Utermann, G. (1975) Hoppe Seyler's Zeitschr. Physiol. Chem. in press.

[15] Neville, D. M. Jr. (1971) J. Biol. Chem. 246, 6328–6334.

[16] Weber, K. and Osborne, M. (1969) J. Biol. Chem. 244, 4406–4412.

[17] Wrigley, C. (1968) Sci. Tools 15, 17.

[18] Lowry, O. H., Rosebrough, N. J., Farr, A. L. and Randall, R. J. (1951) J. Biol. Chem. 193, 265–275.

[19] Roeschlau, P. (1974) Z. Klin. Chem. Klin. Biochem. 12, 226.

[20] Eggstein, M. and Kreutz, F. H. (1966) Klin. Wschr. 44, 262.

[21] Eisenberg, S., Bilheimer, D. W., Levy, R. J. and Lindgren, F. T. (1973) Biochim. Biophys. Acta 326, 361–377.

[22] Shore, B., Shore, V., Solel, A., Mason, D. and Zelis, R. (1974) Biochem. Biophys. Res. Comm. 58, 1–7.

[23] Shore, V. G., Shore, B. and Hart, R. G. (1974) Biochemistry 13, 1579–1585.

[24] Utermann, G., Menzel, H. J., Langer, K. H. and Dieker, P. (1975) Humangenetik 27, 185–197.

Volume 72, number 2   FEBS LETTERS   December 1976

COMPETITIVE INHIBITION OF 3-HYDROXY-3-METHYLGLUTARYL COENZYME A REDUCTASE BY ML-236A AND ML-236B FUNGAL METABOLITES, HAVING HYPOCHOLESTEROLEMIC ACTIVITY

Akira ENDO, Masao KURODA and Kazuhiko TANZAWA

Fermentation Research Laboratories, Sankyo Co., Ltd., 1-2-58 Hiromachi, Shinagawa-ku, Tokyo 140, Japan

Received 15 November 1976

1. Introduction

Fungal metabolites, ML-236A and ML-236B (fig.1), have been isolated from cultures of *Penicillium citrinum* as potent inhibitors of cholesterol synthesis in vitro in this laboratory [1].

These metabolites (LD_{50} for mice > 2 g, per os) cause a marked decrease in serum cholesterol levels in rats [1], and in hens and dogs (Kitano, Tsujita and Endo, in preparation). The experiments reported in this paper demonstrate that ML-236A and ML-236B inhibit specifically 3-hydroxy-3-methylglutaryl (HMG)-CoA reductase (EC 1.1.1.34), the rate-limiting enzyme in cholesterol synthetic pathway, without affecting the rest of the enzymes involved in this pathway, and that the inhibition is competitive with respect to the substrate HMG-CoA.

2. Materials and methods

[$1\text{-}^{14}C$]Acetate (59.5 mCi/mmol) and D,L-[$2\text{-}^{14}C$] mevalonolactone (27.3 mCi/mmol) were obtained from Radiochemical Centre. [$1\text{-}^{14}C$]Acetyl-CoA (49.8 mCi/mmol) and D,L-[$3\text{-}^{14}C$]HMG-CoA (26.2 mCi/mmol) were purchased from New England Nuclear. Lactone forms of ML-236A and ML-236B were prepared as previously described [1]. Acid forms (sodium salts) (fig.1) of these compounds were prepared by saponification of their respective lactone forms in 0.1 N NaOH at 50°C for 2 h. Other chemicals were of the best grade commercially available.

2.1. Incorporation experiments

Rat liver microsomes and cytosolic enzyme fraction were isolated as described previously [2]. The reaction mixture (0.2 ml) contained: 1 mM ATP, 10 mM glucose-1-phosphate, 6 mM glutathione, 6 mM $MgCl_2$, 40 μM CoA, 0.25 mM NAD, 0.25 mM NADP, 100 mM potassium phosphate buffer (pH 7.4) 0.15 mg protein of microsomes, 1.5 mg protein of cytosolic enzyme fraction and 1 mM [$1\text{-}^{14}C$]acetate (1.5 mCi/mmol). Where indicated, [$1\text{-}^{14}C$]acetate was replaced by 0.15 mM [$1\text{-}^{14}C$]acetyl-CoA (1.0 mCi/mmol), 0.13 mM D,L-[$3\text{-}^{14}C$]HMG-CoA (7.3 mCi/mmol) or 0.52 mM D,L-[$2\text{-}^{14}C$]mevalonate (1.26 mCi/mmol). After incubation at 37°C for 60 min, the reaction was terminated by addition of 1 ml 15% alcoholic KOH. The synthesized nonsaponifiable lipids and fatty acid were measured as described previously [2]. Under these conditions, the incorporations of radiolabeled substrates were proportional to time up to 120 min.

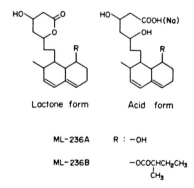

Fig.1. Structures of ML-236A and ML-236B.

North-Holland Publishing Company – Amsterdam

Volume 72, number 2   FEBS LETTERS   December 1976

2.2. HMG-CoA reductase assay

Rat liver microsomes were obtained as described previously [2], from which HMG-CoA reductase was solubilized by the method of Heller and Gould [3] and partially purified by fractionation with ammonium sulfate. The fraction precipitated by 35–50% saturation was used after dialysis for 3 h against 40 mM potassium phosphate buffer, pH 7.2, containing 100 mM sucrose, 50 mM KCl, 30 mM EDTA and 1 mM dithiothreitol. The reaction mixture (50 μl) contained: 100 mM potassium phosphate buffer (pH 7.4) 10 mM EDTA, 10 mM dithiothreitol, 5 mM NADPH, 0.11 mM D,L-[3-^{14}C]HMG-CoA (1.6 mCi/mmol) and 1–2 μg of enzyme protein. After incubation at 37°C for 20 min, the reaction was terminated by addition of 20 μl of 2 N HCl, and the mevalonolactone formed was isolated and counted as described previously [2]. The specific activity of the enzyme used was 10–17 nmol of mevalonate formed/min/mg protein under standard conditions.

Protein was determined by the method of Lowry et al. [4].

3. Results

3.1. Incorporation of radiolabeled substrates into lipids

As reported in a previous paper [1], ML-236B lactone is far more inhibitory in the [1-^{14}C]acetate incorporation into nonsaponifiable lipids than ML-236A lactone. The inhibitory potency was approximately doubled by the conversion of lactone forms to their respective acid forms (sodium salts). Of the four derivatives tested, ML-236B sodium salt was the most inhibitory. Concentrations required for 50% inhibition of nonsaponifiable lipid synthesis were: ML-236A 0.85 μM, ML-236A sodium salt 0.35 μM, ML-236B lactone 0.026 μM, ML-236B sodium salt 0.014 μM (0.006 μg/ml). None of these compounds had significant effects on the fatty acid synthesis from [^{14}C]acetate at concentrations which caused 50% or more reduction in the nonsaponifiable lipid synthesis.

Table 1 shows the effects of ML-236B sodium salt on the incorporation of various radiolabeled substrates into nonsaponifiable lipids. As indicated, conversions

Table 1
Inhibitory effects of ML-236B sodium salt on the incorporation of various
radiolabeled substrates into nonsaponifiable lipids

Substrate	ML-236B sodium salt (nM)	Incorporation dpm/mg[a]	% of control
[1-^{14}C]Acetate	None	13 770	
	5.0	10 080	73.2
	50	4120	29.9
[1-^{14}C]Acetyl-CoA	None	8270	
	5.0	6020	72.8
	50	2410	29.2
D,L-[3-^{14}C]HMG-CoA	None	1050	
	5.0	570	53.7
	50	270	26.0
D,L-[2-^{14}C]Mevalonate	None	35 870	
	5.0	34 940	97.4
	50	34 180	95.3

[a] Counts incorporated/mg protein/60 min. The values for [1-^{14}C]acetate and [1-^{14}C]acetyl-CoA were calculated on the assumption that 33% of the radioactivity in these substrates were converted into CO_2 during their incorporation into nonsaponifiable lipids.

Experimental conditions are described in Materials and methods. The results are the average of duplicate incubations.

Volume 72, number 2   FEBS LETTERS   December 1976

of [^{14}C]acetate, [^{14}C]acetyl-CoA and D,L-[^{14}C]HMG-CoA were inhibited to similar extent at two concentrations of the agent, 5 nM and 50 nM. On the other hand, D,L-[^{14}C]mevalonate conversion into non-saponifiable lipids was not affected by ML-236B sodium salt at concentrations up to 50 nM, indicating that this compound inhibited specifically the enzymatic step for the conversion of HMG-CoA to mevalonate catalyzed by HMG-CoA reductase.

3.2. *Inhibition of HMG-CoA reductase*

As shown in fig.2, all the four compounds were inhibitory to HMG-CoA reductase. The acid forms (sodium salts) of both ML-236A and ML-236B were more effective in inhibiting the reductase than their respective lactone forms, and the two forms of ML-236B were more potent inhibitors than those of ML-236A. Concentrations required for 50% inhibition were: ML-236A lactone 3.4 μM, ML-236A sodium salt 1.2 μM, ML-236B lactone 0.10 μM, ML 236B sodium salt 0.023 μM. The data correlated well with the results obtained for the inhibition of nonsaponifiable lipid synthesis from [^{14}C]acetate, although higher concentrations of the compounds were required for inhibition of the reductase.

The inhibition of HMG-CoA reductase by these

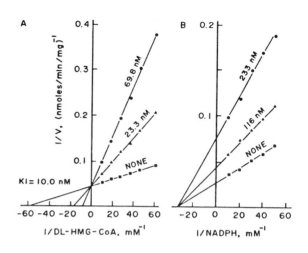

Fig.3. Double reciprocal plots of the inhibition of HMG-CoA reductase by ML-236B sodium salt. Experiments were carried out as described in Materials and methods, except that concentrations of HMG-CoA (A) and NADPH (B) were varied as indicated.

compounds was competitive with respect to HMG-CoA and noncompetitive with respect to NADPH (fig.3). The K_i values were: ML-236A sodium salt 0.22 μM, ML-236B sodium salt 0.010 μM. Under these conditions, K_m values for the two substrates were: D,L-HMG-CoA 33 μM, NADPH 40 μM.

4. Discussion

The α-methylbutyrate residue of ML-236B (fig.1) appears to play a significant role in the inhibition of HMG-CoA reductase activity, since both lactone and acid forms of ML-236A, lacking such a residue in their structure, are far less inhibitory than ML-236B analogs. The acid forms of both ML-236A and ML-236B contain a portion having a chemical structure very similar to that of 3-hydroxy-3-methyl-glutarate (fig.1). This is compatible with the fact that these compounds are competitive inhibitors of HMG-CoA reductase (competitive against HMG-CoA) and further that the acid forms are more potent than the corresponding lactone forms. The present results, considered together with those given in the previous paper [1], provide good evidence that a specific inhibitor of HMG-CoA reductase is effective in reducing cholesterol synthesis in vivo, and thereby in lowering cholesterol levels in blood.

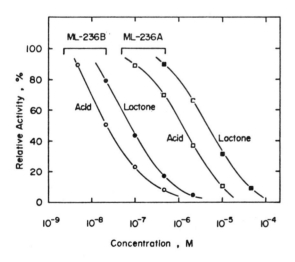

Fig.2. Inhibition of HMG-CoA reductase by ML-236A and ML-236B. Experiments were carried out as described in Materials and methods. The results are expressed as % of control (without inhibitor). The value for control was 16.5 nmol/min/mg protein.

References

[1] Endo, A., Kuroda, M. and Tsujita, Y. (1976) J. Antibiotics in the press.

[2] Kuroda, M. and Endo, A. (1976) Biochim. Biophys. Acta 486, 70–81.

[3] Heller, R. A. and Gould, R. G. (1973) Biochem. Biophys. Res. Commun. 50, 859–865.

[4] Lowry, O. H., Rosebrough, N. J., Farr, A. L. and Randall, R. J. (1951) J. Biol. Chem. 193, 265–275.

Proc. Natl. Acad. Sci. USA
Vol. 77, No. 1, pp. 225–229, January 1980
Biochemistry

Inhibition of receptor-mediated clearance of lysine and arginine-modified lipoproteins from the plasma of rats and monkeys

(lipoprotein catabolism/protein modification/cell receptors/protein turnover)

ROBERT W. MAHLEY*, KARL H. WEISGRABER*, GEORGE W. MELCHIOR[†], THOMAS L. INNERARITY*, AND KATHLEEN S. HOLCOMBE[†]

[†]Laboratory of Experimental Atherosclerosis, National Heart, Lung, and Blood Institute, National Institutes of Health, Bethesda, Maryland 20205; and
*Gladstone Foundation Laboratories for Cardiovascular Disease, University of California, San Francisco, California 94110

Communicated by Donald S. Fredrickson, October 9, 1979

ABSTRACT   Reductive methylation of at least 30% of the lysine residues or 1,2-cyclohexanedione modification of 45% of the arginine residues prevented low density lipoproteins (LDL) from binding to cell surface receptors of fibroblasts in vitro, without significantly altering other physical or chemical properties of the LDL. When rat or human LDL with more than 30% of the lysine residues methylated were injected intravenously into rats, the clearance of these lipoproteins from the plasma was slowed considerably. The half-life of the reductively methylated LDL was approximately twice that obtained for control (unmodified) LDL, and the value for the fractional catabolic rate was approximately half that of the control. Furthermore, when human LDL modified by reductive methylation were injected into rhesus monkeys, the rate of clearance was similarly retarded, and the value for the fractional catabolic rate was reduced by approximately 50% as compared with the value for control LDL. A dual isotope labeling technique (^{125}I and ^{131}I) was used to compare the disappearance of the control and modified LDL in the same animal. It was demonstrated that not only modification of lysine residues but also modification of the arginine residues with 1,2-cyclohexanedione retarded the plasma clearance of the rat LDL. However, the cyclohexanedione modification was spontaneously reversible at 37°C, whereas reductive methylation of the lysine residues was stable. It is concluded that the selective chemical modification of lysine or arginine residues of LDL interferes with the normal uptake of these lipoproteins in vivo as well as by fibroblasts in vitro. These data provide an estimation of the level of receptor-mediated clearance of LDL from the plasma, a value that may be as high as 50% in rats and monkeys.

The protein moieties of certain plasma lipoproteins have been shown to be involved in the control of various aspects of lipoprotein metabolism. It has been reported that the recognition site on lipoproteins responsible for their binding to the cell surface receptors of cultured fibroblasts resides with specific apoproteins (1–4). The B apoprotein of low-density lipoproteins (LDL) and the E apoprotein of certain high-density lipoproteins (HDL$_1$, HDL$_c$) react with the same receptors on the cell surface (1, 3). The modification of a limited number of arginine and lysine residues has been shown to prevent these lipoproteins from reacting with the apo-B,E receptor sites (5, 6).

Arginine residues were selectively modified with 1,2-cyclohexanedione by a mild procedure that did not otherwise significantly alter the physical or chemical properties of the LDL (5). The lysine residues were modified by acetoacetylation and reductive methylation (6). Both procedures were shown to be selective and mild. An important difference between the two procedures used for lysine modification was that acetoacetylation neutralized the positive charge on the ε-amino group, whereas reductive methylation did not alter the charge.

Because modification of the arginine or lysine residues abolished the ability of LDL to react with the cell surface receptors, it was postulated that if these modified lipoproteins were injected intravenously, they would be removed slowly from the plasma. This would demonstrate that the modification had interfered with receptor-mediated uptake in vivo. On the contrary, however, after injection into dogs or rats, acetoacetylated LDL were rapidly cleared from the plasma (7, 8). It has been shown that acetoacetylation triggers the rapid removal of LDL by Kupffer cells in the liver (7), and that these modified lipoproteins are also avidly taken up and degraded by macrophages in culture (8). Similar results with macrophages have been reported for acetylated LDL (9). It appears that the alteration in charge resulting from acetoacetylation may be a stimulus for the rapid clearance. Moreover, as will be shown in this paper, reductive methylation, which does not alter the charge on the ε-amino group of lysine, does not activate the Kupffer cell removal system. Thus it is possible to obtain data that will estimate the peripheral cell component of LDL clearance from the plasma by comparing the difference in clearance of control and reductively methylated LDL.

MATERIALS AND METHODS

Isolation and Iodination of Lipoproteins. Human LDL (ρ = 1.02–1.05 g/ml) were obtained from the plasma of a fasted male subject by sequential ultracentrifugation at 59,000 rpm in a 60 Ti rotor (Beckman). The LDL were obtained after 18 hr of centrifugation and washed at ρ = 1.050 g/ml with an additional centrifugation. Rat LDL were isolated by ultracentrifugation (ρ = 1.006–1.063 g/ml) of plasma from fasted rats and purified by Geon-Pevikon block electrophoresis as described (10). Human and rat LDL were iodinated by the iodine monochloride method (11). Lipid labeling of the iodinated LDL accounted for less than 2% of the total activity. Greater than 90% of the radioactivity in the dose and in the plasma at all time intervals was trichloroacetic acid precipitable. Sodium [^{131}I]- and [^{125}I]iodide (carrier free) were purchased from Amersham. The specific activities of the ^{125}I-LDL and ^{131}I-LDL ranged from 30 to 225 and 120 to 300 cpm/ng of protein, respectively. The purity of the LDL preparations was monitored by paper electrophoresis, sodium dodecyl sulfate/polyacrylamide gel electrophoresis, and negative staining electron microscopy, as described (12, 13). Dual isotope counting was accomplished with a Beckman model 8000 counter.

Abbreviations: LDL, low-density lipoproteins; HDL$_1$ and HDL$_c$, high-density plasma lipoproteins in dogs, rats, and swine that are distinguished from typical HDL by the presence of the E apoprotein and ability to react with the fibroblast receptors; FCR, fractional catabolic rate; $t_{1/2}$, half-life of the lipoprotein in the plasma compartment.

226   Biochemistry: Mahley *et al.*

Proc. Natl. Acad. Sci. USA 77 (1980)

Reductive Methylation of LDL. Reductive methylation of radiolabeled LDL (protein at ≈ 2 mg/ml) in 0.15 M NaCl/0.01% EDTA, pH 7.0, was performed at 0°C by the addition of 1 mg of sodium borohydride followed by six additions over 30 min of 1 μl of 37% (wt/vol) aqueous formaldehyde. Additions of formaldehyde were made at zero time, 6, 12, 18, 24, and 30 min. The sequence was repeated for more extensive modification. The methodology has been described in detail (6). The level of modification (% of the total lysine residues) was determined by the trinitrobenzenesulfonic acid colorimetric assay. Previously, it was shown that the colorimetric assay gave results that were in good agreement with amino acid analysis (6).

Cyclohexanedione Modification of LDL. The effective conditions for this modification procedure have been described fully (5). Lipoprotein protein (2–5 mg) in 1 ml of 0.15 M NaCl/0.01% EDTA was mixed with 2 ml of 0.15 M 1,2-cyclohexanedione in 0.2 M sodium borate buffer (pH 8.1) and incubated at 35°C for 2 hr. The sample was then dialyzed for 16 hr against 0.15 M NaCl/0.01% EDTA at 4°C. This procedure, under the conditions described, consistently resulted in the modification of 50% of the arginine residues of LDL (5).

Assays for Binding, Internalization, and Degradation. The binding and degradation assays were performed with human fibroblasts by the methods of Goldstein and Brown (14) with minor modifications as described (3, 15).

***In Vivo* Studies.** Male Sprague-Dawley rats (200–250 g) were lightly anesthetized with ether and injected via an exposed saphenous vein with the ^{131}I- and ^{125}I-labeled lipoproteins at a dose of 40–100 μg of protein. Each rat used in the study was weighed just prior to injection, and the plasma volume of each rat was estimated as 4% of the body weight. At specified time intervals after lipoprotein injection, the rats were exsanguinated through the abdominal aorta.

Rhesus monkeys (5 to 10 kg) of both sexes were immobilized with ketamine hydrochloride (Vetalor, Parke Davis) and injected intravenously with 500 μg of human LDL protein (control ^{131}I-LDL and modified ^{125}I-LDL). Blood samples were obtained through the saphenous vein from awake animals in restraining chairs. The animals were accustomed to the chairs. Each animal was weighed, and a plasma volume of 4% of the body weight was used for the calculations. The value was determined experimentally in three monkeys by the Evans blue dye method (16). All data were plotted as a percentage of the total injected dose that remained in the plasma at each time interval. The curves were analyzed by the standard curve-peeling technique, and the fractional catabolic rate was calculated by using the slopes and intercepts of the two exponentials as described by Matthews (17). The values for the half-life $t_{1/2}$ are reported for the second exponential.

Reversibility of the Modification of Lysine and Arginine Residues. Seventy-nine percent of the lysine residues were reductively methylated with [^{14}C]formaldehyde. [^{14}C]Cyclohexanedione was used to label the arginine residues; approximately 60% of the arginine residues were modified (LDL incubated with cyclohexanedione for 2.5 hr). Both preparations were incapable of displacing ^{125}I-LDL from the cell receptors of fibroblasts in binding assays conducted at 4°C. In one study the modified LDL were incubated with whole human serum or 0.1 M phosphate buffer, pH 7.4, for 24 hr at 37°C. After the incubation, the modified LDL were dialyzed against 0.15 M NaCl/0.01% EDTA for 24 hr at 4°C to remove the labeled reactants that were liberated by the incubation. Reversibility was determined by liquid scintillation counting of the activity associated with the modified LDL prior to the serum or buffer incubation. Values are reported as a percentage of the original activity that was present after the final dialysis.

In an additional study, the reductively methylated and cyclohexanedione-modified human LDL were incubated at 37°C for various time intervals with human $\rho > 1.21$ g/ml ultracentrifugal fraction (lipoprotein-deficient serum). At the specified times, aliquots were taken and their abilities to compete with control ^{125}I-LDL were compared in the competitive binding assay conducted with human fibroblasts at 4°C as described (3).

RESULTS

Previously, we observed that reductive methylation of 30% or more of the lysine residues of LDL totally prevented the binding of these lipoproteins to the high-affinity cell surface receptors of fibroblasts in culture (5). We now report that reductive methylation of the lysine residues of rat or human LDL resulted in a marked retardation in the clearance of these lipoproteins from the plasma of rats after intravenous injection. As shown in Fig. 1 for a representative experiment using rat lipoproteins, the control (unmodified) ^{131}I-LDL were cleared from the plasma more rapidly than were the reductively methylated ^{125}I-LDL. At each time interval, the activities (^{125}I and ^{131}I) in the plasma were obtained in three individual rats by dual isotope counting. The $t_{1/2}$ of the second exponential and the fractional catabolic rate (FCR) for the control and modified LDL are compiled in Table 1.

Rat LDL, equivalent to human LDL, were isolated from the

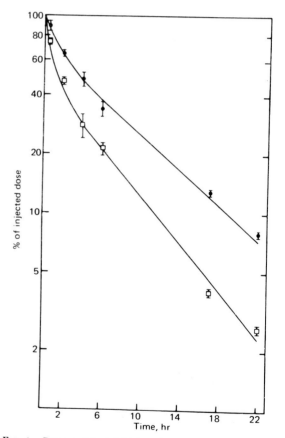

FIG. 1.   Percent of the total injected dose of control rat ^{131}I-LDL (□) and reductively methylated rat ^{125}I-LDL (●) that remained in the plasma as a function of time after intravenous injection into rats. The mean ± SD (bar) represents values obtained in three rats by dual isotope counting at each time point. Each rat received 20 μg of control and methylated LDL protein. The reductively methylated LDL had 95% of the lysine residues modified.

Biochemistry: Mahley *et al.*

Proc. Natl. Acad. Sci. USA 77 (1980)   227

Table 1.   Simultaneous injection of control ¹³¹I-LDL and methylated ¹²⁵I-LDL into rats

LDL	Rat LDL injected		Human LDL injected	
	$t_{1/2}$, hr	FCR	$t_{1/2}$, hr	FCR
Control	4.7*	0.256*	7.3	0.113
Methylated	7.0	0.133	10.0	0.069

* In an additional study, a different preparation of control rat ¹²⁵I-LDL had a $t_{1/2}$ of 5.0 hr and an FCR of 0.230. These results confirm the values in the table.

$\rho = 1.006$–1.063 g/ml ultracentrifugal fraction and purified by preparative Geon-Pevikon block electrophoresis. Previously, we reported that this ultracentrifugal fraction was composed of two distinctly different lipoproteins, which could occur in approximately equal concentrations. These were the apo-B-containing LDL and the apo-E-containing lipoprotein referred to as HDL₁ (10, 18). The purified rat LDL used in the above studies were enriched in apo-B (approximately 80–85% of the protein as estimated from stained sodium dodecyl sulfate/polyacrylamide gels), but also invariably contained some low molecular weight (apo-C) apoproteins. To avoid the complication of the presence of C apoproteins, we investigated the possibility of using human LDL (greater than 95% apo-B). We previously used rat and human LDL in rats with qualitatively similar results (7). As described above with rat LDL, modification of 30% or more of the lysine residues of human LDL resulted in a retardation of the clearance of the LDL from the plasma of rats (Fig. 2). Although the absolute values for the $t_{1/2}$ of rat and human LDL were different, the FCRs were similarly decreased by 40 to 50% after modification of the lysine residues by reductive methylation (Table 1).

In six separate experiments with human LDL injected into rats, we observed a similar retardation in clearance of LDL in every case in which more than 30% of the lysine residues were reductively methylated. As shown in Fig. 3, the rates of plasma

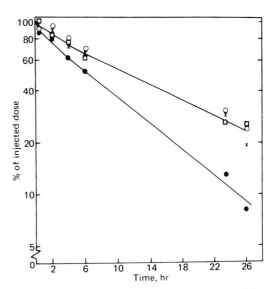

FIG. 3.   Percent of the total injected dose of control human ¹²⁵I-LDL (●) and methylated human ¹²⁵I-LDL [35% (X), 62% (○), and 91% (□) of the lysine residues modified] that remained in the plasma of the rats. Each point represents the value obtained in a single rat (100 μg of lipoprotein protein injected per rat).

clearance of LDL with 35, 62, and 91% of their lysine residues modified were essentially identical. All preparations of the modified LDL used in this study were incapable of interacting with the cell surface receptors of fibroblasts in culture.

To establish that decreased clearance of LDL after reductive methylation was not peculiar to metabolism in the rat, we injected rhesus monkeys with control and modified human LDL. As shown in Fig. 4, modification of the lysine residues retarded the clearance of intravenously injected LDL from the plasma

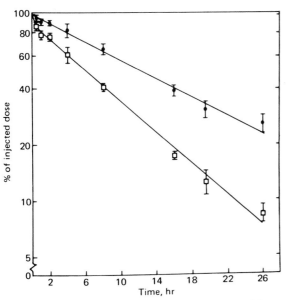

FIG. 2.   Percent of the total injected dose of normal human ¹³¹I-LDL (□) and reductively methylated human ¹²⁵I-LDL (●) that remained in the plasma as a function of time after intravenous injection into rats. Three rats were used at each point, and each rat received 50 μg of each lipoprotein. The methylated LDL had 90% of the lysine residues modified. Similar results were obtained in a separate study in which the labeled lipoproteins were reversed (normal human ¹²⁵I-LDL and methylated ¹³¹I-LDL).

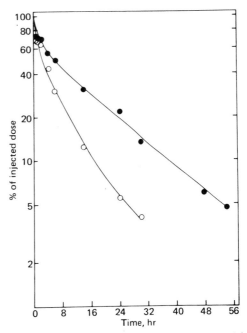

FIG. 4.   Percent of the total injected dose of control human ¹³¹I-LDL (○) and methylated human ¹²⁵I-LDL (●) that remained in the plasma of a rhesus monkey after 500 μg of each lipoprotein had been simultaneously injected. The methylated LDL had 90% of the total lysine residues modified. A 5-kg normal rhesus female was the recipient.

228   Biochemistry: Mahley *et al.*   *Proc. Natl. Acad. Sci. USA* 77 (1980)

Table 2.   Simultaneous injection of control human ^{131}I-LDL and methylated human ^{125}I-LDL into rhesus monkeys

		Control LDL		Methylated LDL		
Exp.	Sex	$t_{1/2}$, hr	FCR	$t_{1/2}$, hr	FCR	Lysines modified, %
I*	♂	9.2	0.086	21.3	0.041	77
II*	♂	6.5	0.123	13.5	0.068	85
III*	♀	6.8	0.135	13.3	0.056	90
Mean		7.5	0.115	16.0	0.055	
±SD		±1.5	±0.026	±4.6	±0.014	

* Three different monkeys and three different preparations of LDL were used.

of a monkey ($t_{1/2}$ of second exponential: control, 6.8 hr; modified, 13.3 hr). This observation was confirmed in additional studies and the results are compiled in Table 2. The modified LDL had a longer $t_{1/2}$ (approximately twice that of control LDL; calculated from the second exponential) and a smaller FCR ($\approx$50% less).

Because we had previously demonstrated that binding of LDL to the cell surface receptors of fibroblasts could also be prevented by modification of arginine residues (5), studies were conducted *in vivo* with control LDL and LDL modified by treatment with 1,2-cyclohexanedione. As shown in Fig. 5, modification of approximately 50% of the arginine residues of rat LDL caused a retardation in their clearance from the plasma of rats. However, it has been reported (19) that the formation of the cyclohexanedione derivative of arginine is spontaneously reversible at 37°C.

To determine the stability of both the arginine modification with cyclohexanedione and the lysine modification with reductive methylation, [^{14}C]cyclohexanedione and [^{14}C]methyl derivatives of LDL were prepared, and the reversals with time were determined in serum or phosphate buffer. Methylation of the lysine residues was found to be a stable modification. After a 24-hr incubation at 37°C with whole serum, >95% of the label was still associated with the LDL. However, only 67% of the label was associated with the LDL after [^{14}C]cyclohex-

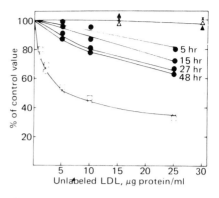

FIG. 6.   Competitive displacement of human ^{125}I-LDL from the cell surface receptors of human fibroblasts by various control and modified lipoproteins. □, Control LDL; ○, control LDL incubated for 48 hr in $\rho > 1.21$ g/ml lipoprotein-deficient sera at 37°C; △, methylated LDL kept at 4°C for 48 hr; ▲, methylated LDL incubated in $\rho > 1.21$ g/ml sera at 37°C for 48 hr; X, cyclohexanedione-modified LDL kept at 4°C for 48 hr; and ●, cyclohexanedione-modified LDL incubated in $\rho > 1.21$ g/ml sera at 37°C for 5, 15, 27, or 48 hr as indicated. The binding study was performed at 4°C for 2 hr (2 μg of ^{125}I-LDL protein, 123 cpm/ng of protein). Percent of control value determined by binding in the absence of added lipoprotein (maximal binding 40 ng of ^{125}I-LDL per dish).

anedione-modified LDL were incubated in serum for 24 hr at 37°C. Furthermore, the modification was 53% reversible when [^{14}C]cyclohexanedione-modified LDL were incubated in phosphate for 24 hr at 37°C. This spontaneous reversibility of the cyclohexanedione modification of the LDL arginine residues was found to be progressive with increasing incubation time in $\rho > 1.21$ g/ml lipoprotein-deficient sera at 37°C. The regeneration of the arginine residues was determined by measuring the abilities of the various lipoprotein preparations incubated for different times to compete with control ^{125}I-LDL for receptor binding activity in fibroblasts. As shown in Fig. 6, cyclohexanedione-modified LDL that were not incubated at 37°C prior to the experiment were incapable of displacing the ^{125}I-LDL from the receptors. However, there was a progressive restoration of binding activity with time from 5 to 48 hr of incubation. By contrast, incubation of reductively methylated LDL for 48 hr in the $\rho > 1.21$ g/ml lipoprotein-deficient sera at 37°C did not restore binding activity to these lipoproteins (Fig. 6).

DISCUSSION

The observation that the modification of a limited number of lysine or arginine residues of the B apoprotein of LDL prevented their binding to the cell surface receptors of fibroblasts *in vitro* (5, 6) led to the postulate that the plasma clearance of these chemically modified lipoproteins would be retarded. If LDL are at least partially metabolized via a receptor-mediated uptake process by peripheral cells, such as fibroblasts, *in vivo*, as is strongly supported by the studies of Goldstein, Brown, and coworkers (20, 21), the rate of disappearance of the modified LDL, as compared with control LDL, would serve as an approximation of the magnitude of this process. However, interpretation of these data should be made with some reservation. The value obtained for the peripheral cell component of LDL plasma clearance could represent an overestimate, because the liver might also remove LDL by an uptake process that could also be blocked by the chemical modification of the lipoproteins. Nevertheless, studies with chemically modified lipoproteins are useful to probe the mechanisms and cell types responsible for lipoprotein catabolism.

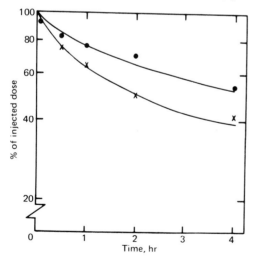

FIG. 5.   Percent of the total injected dose of control rat ^{125}I-LDL (X) and cyclohexanedione-modified rat ^{125}I-LDL (●) that remained in the plasma as a function of time. Each point represents the value obtained from an individual rat (100 μg of lipoprotein protein injected). The extent of the level of modification of the arginine residues by cyclohexanedione is estimated at 50%, on the basis of previous experience (5). The modified LDL lacked the ability to bind to the cell receptors of cultured fibroblasts.

Biochemistry: Mahley *et al.*   *Proc. Natl. Acad. Sci. USA 77 (1980)*   229

When 30% or more of the lysine residues of LDL were modified by reductive methylation, the plasma clearance was markedly reduced, as determined by following the plasma activity of control and modified LDL. This was observed with both rat and human LDL injected intravenously into rats and with human LDL injected into rhesus monkeys. The values for the FCR were reduced by 40–50% in the rat and by 50% in the monkey by comparison with the values obtained for control LDL. The retardation in clearance of the lysine-modified LDL is compatible with the interpretation that methylation prevents LDL from interacting with receptor-mediated uptake processes in the whole animal. On the basis of the turnover data for LDL obtained by Simons *et al.* (22) and Bilheimer *et al.* (23), it has been speculated that two-thirds of the LDL degraded daily in man are degraded by the receptor-mediated pathway (21). Data from the present study for rats and monkeys would indicate that approximately half of the plasma clearance of LDL is mediated by the receptor process.

It was also demonstrated that modification of the arginine residues of the B apoprotein of LDL with cyclohexanedione retarded plasma clearance of these lipoproteins. However, the cyclohexanedione modification of the arginine residues was not stable at 37°C and was slowly reversed over a period of a few hours. The spontaneous reversibility has been reported previously (19). Modification of the lysine residues by reductive methylation was stable at 37°C.

In conclusion, it has been shown that selective chemical modification of specific amino acid residues of LDL resulted in an altered metabolism *in vivo*. The changes suggest a role *in vivo* for cell surface receptors previously described for cells grown in culture.

We thank Ms. C. Groff for typing the manuscript. Portions of this work were performed under a National Heart, Lung, and Blood Institute contract with Meloy Laboratories.

1. Mahley, R. W. & Innerarity, T. L. (1978) in *Sixth International Symposium on Drugs Affecting Lipid Metabolism*, eds. Kritchevsky, D., Paoletti, R. & Holmes, W. L. (Plenum, New York), pp. 99–127.
2. Bersot, T. P., Mahley, R. W., Brown, M. S. & Goldstein, J. L. (1976) *J. Biol. Chem.* **251**, 2395–2398.
3. Innerarity, T. L. & Mahley, R. W. (1978) *Biochemistry* **17**, 1440–1447.
4. Pitas, R. E., Innerarity, T. L., Arnold, K. S. & Mahley, R. W. (1979) *Proc. Natl. Acad. Sci. USA* **76**, 2311–2315.
5. Mahley, R. W., Innerarity, T. L., Pitas, R. E., Weisgraber, K. H., Brown, J. H. & Gross, E. (1977) *J. Biol. Chem.* **252**, 7279–7287.
6. Weisgraber, K. H., Innerarity, T. L. & Mahley, R. W. (1978) *J. Biol. Chem.* **253**, 9053–9062.
7. Mahley, R. W., Weisgraber, K. H., Innerarity, T. L. & Windmueller, H. G. (1979) *Proc. Natl. Acad. Sci. USA* **76**, 1746–1750.
8. Mahley, R. W., Innerarity, T. L., Weisgraber, K. H. & Oh, S. Y. (1979) *J. Clin. Invest.*, in press.
9. Goldstein, J. L., Ho, Y. K., Basu, S. K. & Brown, M. S. (1979) *Proc. Natl. Acad. Sci. USA* **76**, 333–337.
10. Weisgraber, K. H., Mahley, R. W. & Assmann, G. (1977) *Atherosclerosis* **28**, 121–140.
11. Bilheimer, D. W., Eisenberg, S. & Levy, R. I. (1972) *Biochim. Biophys. Acta* **260**, 212–221.
12. Mahley, R. W., Weisgraber, K. H. & Innerarity, T. L. (1974) *Circ. Res.* **35**, 722–733.
13. Mahley, R. W., Weisgraber, K. H., Innerarity, T., Brewer, H. B., Jr. & Assmann, G. (1975) *Biochemistry* **14**, 2817–2823.
14. Goldstein, J. L. & Brown, M. S. (1974) *J. Biol. Chem.* **249**, 5153–5162.
15. Mahley, R. W. & Innerarity, T. L. (1977) *J. Biol. Chem.* **252**, 3980–3986.
16. Gregersen, M. I. & Rawson, R. A. (1959) *Physiol. Rev.* **39**, 307–342.
17. Matthews, C. M. E. (1957) *Phys. Med. Biol.* **2**, 36–53.
18. Mahley, R. W. (1978) in *Disturbances in Lipid and Lipoprotein Metabolism*, eds. Dietschy, J. M., Gotto, A. M., Jr. & Ontko, J. A. (American Physiological Society, Bethesda, MD), pp. 181–197.
19. Patthy, L. & Smith, E. L. (1975) *J. Biol. Chem.* **250**, 557–564.
20. Goldstein, J. L. & Brown, M. S. (1977) *Annu. Rev. Biochem.* **46**, 897–930.
21. Brown, M. S. & Goldstein, J. L. (1979) *Harvey Lect.* **73**, 163–201.
22. Simons, L. A., Reichl, D., Myant, N. B. & Mancini, M. (1975) *Atherosclerosis* **21**, 283–298.
23. Bilheimer, D. W., Goldstein, J. L., Grundy, S. M. & Brown, M. S. (1975) *J. Clin. Invest.* **56**, 1420–1430.

BRITISH MEDICAL JOURNAL   VOLUME 282   6 JUNE 1981   1847

MEDICAL PRACTICE

Occasional Review

Strategy of prevention: lessons from cardiovascular disease

GEOFFREY ROSE

If an obstetrician had a case of eclampsia he would ask, "What went wrong?" The occurrence of a preventable disaster is a threat to his professional reputation, for an obstetrician accepts prevention as an integral part of his normal professional responsibilities. Antenatal care is in fact largely preventive, and the integration of prevention with treatment has led to an excellent fall in maternal and perinatal mortality rates. In paediatrics too there are no demarcation disputes between prevention and treatment; and a similar trend is now also appearing in general practice. If a stroke occurs in an untreated or badly treated hypertensive patient, a good general practitioner asks, "What went wrong?" For, in middle age at least, strokes are largely preventable. When one occurs it suggests a possible failure of practice organisation.

Clinician and prevention

Unfortunately, in other branches of medicine there is a continuing and regrettable separation of the therapeutic and the preventive roles, and doctors generally continue to see the care of the sick as their whole responsibility.

CORONARY HEART DISEASE IS PREVENTABLE

Figure 1 shows the recent trends in mortality from coronary heart disease in various countries of the world. In Japan the rates have throughout this period been extremely low. In

Based on the Adolf Streicher memorial lecture given at the North Stafford-shire Medical Institute, Stoke-on-Trent, on 13 November 1980, which will be published in full later this year in the *Journal of the North Staffordshire Medical Institute.*

Department of Medical Statistics and Epidemiology, London School of Hygiene and Tropical Medicine, London WC1
GEOFFREY ROSE, DM, FRCP, professor of epidemiology

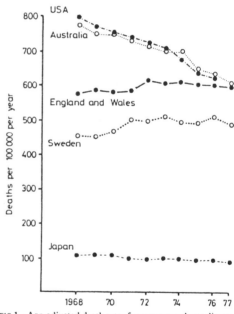

FIG 1—Age-adjusted death rates from coronary heart disease (ICD, 8th revision, 410-14) among men aged 35-74 in various countries.

Australia and the United States at the start of the period they were high, but they have fallen by some 25%. In England and Wales they started a little short of the American and Australian rates and have shown little change. The Japanese owe their low rates not to their genes but to their way of life: when they move to America they rather quickly acquire American rates. The large recent declines in Australia and the United States must surely be due largely to a declining incidence of disease, since

1848

BRITISH MEDICAL JOURNAL   VOLUME 282   6 JUNE 1981

only a limited part of that large decline can be attributed to therapeutic advances. These patterns show that coronary heart disease is largely preventable.

In Britain, then, we are failing to prevent a preventable disease. If we had shared in the Australian and American decline each year in England and Wales there would be upwards of 25 000 fewer coronary deaths. One can imagine the outcry if some shortcoming in therapeutic services were to cause even a tiny fraction of this number of unnecessary deaths. Why then, one may ask, do we not as a profession evince a corresponding alarm at a failure of prevention ? Why do we not feel that it is our fault ? Why is so large a part of our research devoted to the "mechanics of dying," and so little to the scientific, social, and economic basis of prevention ?

The answers to these questions are satisfactorily complex. We do not know why the Australians and the Americans have done well in their control of coronary heart disease, or whether (if we did know) we could have shared their good fortune. Yet surely, as a profession, we should at least feel deeply disturbed by the problem and involved in it. We have a professional responsibility for prevention, both in research and in medical practice. When ordinary doctors do not accept that responsibility then prevention is taken over (if at all) by uncritical propagandists, by cranks, and by battling commercial interests.

"High-risk" strategy

As doctors we are trained to feel responsible for patients— that is, to care for the sick; and from that position accepting responsibility for those with major risk factors is not too difficult a transition. They are almost patients. A general practitioner, say, makes a routine measurement of a man's blood pressure and finds it raised. Thereafter both the man and the doctor will say that he "suffers" from high blood pressure. He walked in a healthy man but he walks out a patient, and his new-found status is confirmed by the giving and receiving of tablets. An inappropriate label has been accepted because both public and profession feel that if the man were not a patient the doctor would have no business treating him. In reality the care of the symptomless hypertensive person is preventive medicine, not therapeutics.

ABSOLUTE AND RELATIVE RISK

Life insurance experts concerned with charging the right premiums taught us that "high risk" meant "high relative risk," and in this until recently they have been abetted by the epidemiologists. Figure 2(a), taken from life insurance data,[1] shows for each of four age groups the relation of blood pressure to the relative risk of death, taking the risk for the whole of each age group as 100. The relative risk is seen to increase with increasing pressure, but the gradient gets a little less steep as age advances. That is perhaps not surprising, because a systolic pressure of 160 mm Hg is common in older men, and we would not expect it to be so unpleasant as at younger ages, when it is rare.

In figure 2(b) the same data are shown but with a scale of absolute instead of relative risk. The pattern now appears quite different. In particular, the absolute excess risk associated with raised pressure is far greater in the older men. A systolic pressure of 160 mm Hg may be common at these ages, but common does not mean good. To identify risk in relative units rather than absolute units may be misleading.

To take another example, at any given age a woman taking oral contraceptives has a risk of cardiovascular death about 2·8 times that of her contemporary who is not taking the pill. This relative risk is more or less independent of age, and it is the same in smokers and non-smokers.[2] But although relative risk does not change, the absolute excess or *attributable risk* is profoundly different (table I). We are nowadays discouraging

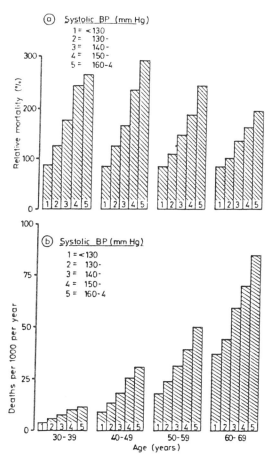

FIG 2—Age-specific mortality in men according to blood pressure and age, from life insurance data: (*a*) relative risk, and (*b*) absolute risk.

TABLE I—*Cardiovascular risk in users of oral contraceptive*[2]

	Age (yr)	
	30–9	40–4
Relative risk	2·8	2·8
Attributable risk (per 100 000 a year)	3·5	20·0

the use of oral contraceptives in older women, especially those with any coronary risk factor, because we recognise that advice must relate to absolute not relative risk.

ABSOLUTE AND RELATIVE BENEFIT

The same argument applies in assessing the benefits of preventive action. In the Veterans Administration trial of antihypertensive treatment[3] the effectiveness of treatment expressed in relative terms was around 50-60% regardless of age or the presence of cardiovascular-renal abnormality (table II). The final column of the table, however, expresses treatment effectiveness in absolute units; and again we now see a quite different pattern. The absolute benefit received from this form of preventive action is nearly five times greater in the older age group with risk factors than in the younger age group without risk factors. To express the results of trials only in terms of percentage effectiveness is to conceal what the user really needs to know.

BRITISH MEDICAL JOURNAL   VOLUME 282   6 JUNE 1981   1849

TABLE II—*Relative and absolute benefits from the treatment of hypertension, according to age and the presence of cardiovascular-renal abnormality*[3]

Age (yr)	Cardiovascular-renal abnormality	Treatment effectiveness (%)	Lives saved per 100 treated
< 50	–	59	6
	+	62	14
> 50	–	50	15
	+	60	29

POPULATION RISK

If we are to take decisions, then, we need to measure risks and benefits in absolute rather than relative terms. Nevertheless, although such measures will describe the situation for individuals they tell us next to nothing about the effects on the whole community of a strategy based on identifying and caring for high-risk individuals. Unfortunately the effects of a "high-risk strategy" may be more limited than we imagine, for the community benefit depends not only on the benefit that each individual receives but also on the prevalence of the risk factor. If a large benefit is conferred on only a few people then the community as a whole is not much better off. In familial hypercholesterolaemia affected men have a risk of premature coronary death or more than 50%; but fortunately it is rare. Consequently, serious though the disease is for affected individuals, the deaths resulting from it make up less than 1% of all coronary deaths. What we may call *population attributable risk*—the excess risk associated with a factor in the population as a whole—depends on the product of the individual attributable risk (the excess risk in individuals with that factor) and the prevalence of the factor in the population.

Figure 3 illustrates the relation in the Framingham Study[4] between coronary mortality and the concentration of serum cholesterol when men entered the study. The risk rises fairly

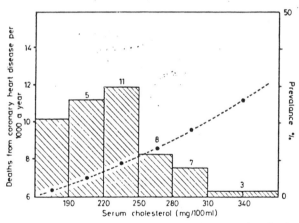

FIG 3—Prevalence distribution of serum cholesterol concentration related to coronary heart disease mortality (- - - -) in men aged 55-64. Number above each bar represents estimate of attributable deaths per 1000 population per 10 years. (Based on Framingham Study.[4])

Conversion: SI to traditional units—Cholesterol: 1 mmol/l ≈ 38·6 mg/100 ml.

steeply with increasing cholesterol concentration; but out on the right, where the risk to affected individuals is high, the prevalence is fortunately low. If we want to ask, "How many excess coronary deaths is the cholesterol-related risk responsible for in this population?," we simply multiply the excess risk at each concentration by the number of people with that concentration who are exposed to that risk. In fig 3 these attributable deaths are shown as the numbers on top of the bars. They add up to 34 extra deaths per 1000 of this population over a 10-year

period, of which only three arise at concentrations at or above 310 mg/100 ml (8 mmol/l)—which would be called high ("outside the normal range") by conventional clinical standards. The rest (90%) arise from the many people in the middle part of the distribution who are exposed to a small risk.

This illustrates a fundamental principle in the strategy of prevention. A large number of people exposed to a low risk is likely to produce more cases than a small number of people exposed to a high risk. In business the same principle underlies the mass market: profits are larger when small amounts are taken from the masses than when large amounts are taken from the few rich people; and this principle of the mass market applies to many community health hazards.

In our Whitehall Study[5] we examined some 20 000 middle-aged male civil servants in London, noting among other things their blood pressures. Follow-up shows that mortality rises rather steeply with increasing pressure. One may calculate (just as with the Framingham cholesterol data) the numbers of deaths attributable to the different levels of raised blood pressure (table III). Two-thirds of the attributable coronary

TABLE III—*Population attributable mortality from coronary heart disease and stroke arising at different levels of blood pressure*[5]

Diastolic BP (mm Hg)	Cumulative % of excess deaths attributable to hypertension	
	Coronary heart disease	Stroke
< 80	(0)	(0)
< 90	21	14
< 100	47	25
< 110	67	73
≥ 110	100	100

deaths and three-quarters of the attributable deaths from stroke occur in men with diastolic pressures below 110 mm Hg, and about half the attributable coronary deaths and a quarter of the attributable deaths from stroke occur below 100 mm Hg.

In the "high-risk" preventive strategy we go out and identify those at the top end of the distribution and give them some preventive care—for example, control of hypertension or hyperlipidaemia. But this "high-risk" strategy, however successful it may be for individuals, cannot influence that large proportion of deaths occurring among the many people with slightly raised blood pressure and a small risk. Hypertension clinics, lipid clinics, diabetic clinics—excellent though they may be for the individuals who receive their benefits—offer only a limited answer to the community problem of heart disease.

Mass strategy

We are therefore driven to consider mass approaches, of which the simplest is the endeavour to lower the whole distribution of the risk variable by some measure in which all participate. Supposing that some dietary measure, such as moderation of salt intake, were able to lower the whole blood pressure distribution, we may estimate how the potential benefits might compare with what is currently achieved by the "high-risk" strategy of detecting and treating hypertension. From the Whitehall study data one can consider two strategies whose effects might be expected to be equivalent. The first predicates a 100%-effective treatment for high blood pressure given to and accepted by everyone with a diastolic (phase 4) pressure of 105 mm Hg or more. We can estimate how many lives that would save, assuming a commensurate fall in risk. On the same assumption, a similar benefit might follow a mass lowering of the whole blood pressure distribution of the population by 7-8 mm Hg. In practice, however, treatment is

1850   BRITISH MEDICAL JOURNAL   VOLUME 282   6 JUNE 1981

not completely effective, all cases are not detected, and the people who are detected will often not take our treatment. Making allowance for these shortcomings, we may estimate that all the life-saving benefits achieved by current antihypertensive treatment might be equalled by a downward shift of the whole blood pressure distribution in the population by a mere 2-3 mm Hg. The benefits from a mass approach in which everybody receives a small benefit may be unexpectedly large.

THE INDIVIDUAL GAINS LITTLE

The mass approach is inherently the only ultimate answer to the problem of a mass disease. But, however much it may offer to the community as a whole, it offers little to each participating individual. When mass diphtheria immunisation was introduced in Britain 40 years ago, even then roughly 600 children had to be immunised in order that one life would be saved—599 "wasted" immunisations for the one that was effective. If all male British doctors wore their car seat belts on every journey throughout their working lives, then for one life thereby saved there would be about 400 who always take that preventive precaution: 399 would have worn a seat belt every day for 40 years without benefit to their survival. This is the kind of ratio that one has to accept in mass preventive medicine. A measure applied to many will actually benefit few.

Table IV presents some estimates made from the Framingham data.[3] If we supposed that throughout their adult life, up to the

TABLE IV—Estimated proportion of men and women who might avoid clinical coronary heart disease before age 55 if they had reduced their serum cholesterol concentration by 0·65 mmol/l (25 mg/100 ml) throughout adult life, based on Framingham estimates of risk[4]

	Men	Women
Average risk*	1 in 50	1 in 400
High risk†	1 in 25	1 in 150

*Serum cholesterol 6·1 mmol/l (235 mg/100 ml), systolic BP 120 mm Hg, non-smoker.
†Serum cholesterol 6·7 mmol/l (260 mg/100 ml), systolic BP 150 mm Hg, smoker.

age of 55, Framingham men were to modify their diet in such a way as to reduce their cholesterol levels by 10%, then among men of average coronary risk about one in 50 could expect that through this preventive precaution he would avoid a heart attack (if change in a risk factor leads to commensurate reduction in risk): 49 out of 50 would eat differently every day for 40 years and perhaps get nothing from it. For the same preventive measure in a higher-risk group (those with a little hypertension and a slightly raised cholesterol concentration and smoking cigarettes), the ratio rises to one in 25. For women the prospects for individual benefit from this preventive measure are much smaller.

THE "PREVENTION PARADOX"

We arrive at what we might call the prevention paradox— "a measure that brings large benefits to the community offers little to each participating individual." It implies that we should not expect too much from individual health education. People will not be motivated to any great extent to take our advice, because there is little in it for each of them, particularly in the short and medium term. Change in behaviour has to be for some the larger and more immediate reward.

SOCIAL MOTIVATION

There has been a gratifying decline in smoking by male doctors in Britain in the past 20 years. In most cases the motivation has probably not been the intellectual argument that in the end some will obtain health benefits; it has been social pressure. Being a smoking doctor is uncomfortable these days for your colleagues either pity you or despise you. Not smoking may be easier. Social pressure brings immediate rewards for those who conform.

Few doctors are optimistic about their ability to achieve weight reduction in obese patients and to maintain it. But many young women make strenuous, sustained, and successful efforts to control their weight, not for medical reasons but because thinness is socially acceptable and obesity is not. So in health education our aim should perhaps be to create social pressure that makes "healthy behaviour" easier and more acceptable, thereby bringing immediate social rewards for those who conform.

Another major determinant of behaviour is the force of economics and convenience. In the United States and Australia, and more latterly in Britain, there has been a large market shift away from butter and towards soft margarine. Though the medical argument has helped, the main reason has probably been the price, and the fact that butter when kept in the refrigerator goes hard and soft margarine does not. Thus the friends of butter, quite apart from the bad scientific basis for their case, have little chance of making much headway. To influence mass behaviour we must look to its mass determinants, which are largely economic and social.

SAFETY IS PARAMOUNT

The recent World Health Organisation controlled trial of clofibrate produced disturbing results.[6] In the treated group non-fatal myocardial infarction was reduced by 26% (about the effect predicted from the fall in cholesterol concentrations). Mortality from non-cardiac causes, however, increased by one-third, an effect rather unlikely to be due to chance. This finding is important to the strategy of prevention. Clofibrate has been in use for many years and has been given to enormous numbers of patients. Until the results of this trial appeared there was no suspicion that it might kill. Indeed, by clinical standards it can still be called a relatively safe drug, since the estimate of excess mortality works out at only about one death per 1000 patient-years. In patients with severe hyperlipoproteinaemia we would be prepared to take such a risk if it was thought that the drug might reduce their very high death rate.

Intervention for prevention where the risk is low is totally different. I suggested earlier that a large number of people exposed to a small risk might yield more cases in the community than a small number exposed to a big risk. There is a counterpart to that in regard to intervention. If a preventive measure exposes many people to a small risk, then the harm it does may readily—as in the case of clofibrate—outweigh the benefits, since these are received by relatively few. Unfortunately we cannot have many trials as large as the clofibrate study, nor are we able to keep such trials going for longer than a few years, usually five at the most. We may thus be unable to identify that small level of harm to individuals from long-term intervention that would be sufficient to make that line of prevention unprofitable or even harmful. Consequently we cannot accept long-term mass preventive medication.

Conclusions

In chronic diseases the clinician's first contact with the patient comes late in the natural history of the disease, usually after a catastrophe or major complication and when there is already much irreversible pathological change. Indeed, in some 20% of

BRITISH MEDICAL JOURNAL   VOLUME 282   6 JUNE 1981   1851

cases of coronary heart disease there is no contact with physicians at all, the first recognised occurrence being sudden death. It follows inexorably that prevention is essential. With coronary heart disease, the recent experience of Australia and the United States shows also that prevention is possible, at least in part.

The preventive strategy that concentrates on high-risk individuals may be appropriate for those individuals, as well as being a wise and efficient use of limited medical resources; but its ability to reduce the burden of disease in the whole community tends to be disappointingly small. Potentially far more effective, and ultimately the only acceptable answer, is the mass strategy, whose aim is to shift the whole population's distribution of the risk variable. Here, however, our first concern must be that such mass advice is safe.

ADDITION AND REMOVAL

We may usefully distinguish two types of preventive measure. The first consists of the removal of an unnatural factor and the restoration of "biological normality"—that is, of the conditions to which presumably we are genetically adapted. For coronary heart disease such measures would include a substantial reduction in our intake of saturated fat, giving up cigarettes, avoiding severe obesity and a state of permanent physical inactivity, maybe *some* increase in the intake of polyunsaturated fat, and maybe avoidance of those occupational and social conditions that are conducive to so-called "type A" behaviour. Such normalising measures may be presumed to be safe, and therefore we should be prepared to advocate them on the basis of a reasonable presumption of benefit.

The second type of mass preventive measure is quite different. It consists not in removing a supposed cause of disease but in adding some other unnatural factor, in the hope of conferring protection. The end result is to increase biological abnormality by an even further removal from those conditions to which we are genetically adapted. For coronary heart disease such measures include a *high* intake of polyunsaturates and all forms of long-term medication. Long-term safety cannot be assured, and quite possibly harm may outweigh benefit. For such measures as these the required level of evidence, both of benefit and (particularly) of safety, must be far more stringent.

References

[1] Society of Actuaries. *Build and blood pressure study 1959.* Chicago Illinois: Society of Actuaries, 1959-60.
[2] Mann JI. Oral contraceptives and the cardiovascular risk. In: Oliver MF, ed. *Coronary heart disease in young women.* Edinburgh: Churchill Livingstone, 1978:184-94.
[3] Veterans Administration Cooperative Study Group on Antihypertensive Agents. Effects of treatment on morbidity in hypertension. *Circulation* 1972;45:991-1004.
[4] Kannel WB, Gordon T, eds. Section 26. *Some characteristics related to the incidence of cardiovascular disease and death: Framingham Study, 16-year follow-up.* Washington, DC: US Govt Printing Office, 1970.
[5] Reid DD, Hamilton PJS, McCartney P, Rose G, Jarrett RJ, Keen H. Smoking and other risk factors for coronary heart-disease in British civil servants. *Lancet* 1976;ii:979-84.
[6] Committee of Principal Investigators. A co-operative trial in the primary prevention of ischaemic heart disease using clofibrate. *Br Heart J* 1978; 40:1069-1118.

(*Accepted 30 March 1981*)

The Lancet · Saturday 17 September 1983

TREATMENT OF HYPERLIPIDAEMIA RETARDS PROGRESSION OF SYMPTOMATIC FEMORAL ATHEROSCLEROSIS
A Randomised Controlled Trial

R. G. M. Duffield   B. Lewis
N. E. Miller   C. W. Jamieson
J. N. H. Brunt   A. C. F. Colchester

Departments of Surgery and Chemical Pathology and Metabolic Disorders, St Thomas' Hospital, London; Department of Medical Biophysics, University of Manchester; and Department of Neurology Atkinson Morley's Hospital, London

Summary The effect of plasma lipid reduction on the progression of femoral atherosclerosis was studied in hyperlipidaemic patients with stable intermittent claudication. 24 patients were randomly assigned to treatment and usual-care groups, the former receiving dietary advice and cholestyramine, nicotinic acid, or clofibrate depending on their lipoprotein phenotype. Biplanar arteriography was performed when the study began and after a mean period of 19 months. Angiograms were assessed visually, with blinding, and by computerised image analysis. Therapy reduced mean plasma total cholesterol by 25%, mean low density lipoprotein (LDL) cholesterol by 28%, and mean plasma triglycerides by 45%. Significantly fewer arterial segments showed detectable progression of atherosclerosis in the treatment group. The mean increase in plaque area (mm^2/segment/year) in the treatment group was only one third of that in the usual-care group. The mean increase in edge irregularity index (a measure of the severity of disease) in the treatment group was only 40% of that in the usual care group. Twice as many arterial segments showed improvement in the treatment group. In both groups changes in edge irregularity index were directly related to plasma LDL cholesterol concentration. This study, the first randomised controlled trial of its type, provides evidence that effective treatment of hyperlipidaemia favourably influences the natural history of symptomatic peripheral atherosclerosis.

Introduction

MOST trials of plasma lipid reduction in the primary prevention of coronary heart disease (CHD) have produced beneficial results[1-4] but in some there has been little benefit.[5,6] The design and execution of such trials is difficult, and the statistical need for a large sample size conflicts with the requirement for close supervision to ensure full compliance, hence to obtain a substantial reduction in plasma lipids. Advances in arteriography[7,8] have made it possible to assess the evolution of atherosclerosis directly. This approach was pioneered by Barndt et al[9] in an uncontrolled open trial the results of which suggested that early atheroma in the femoral artery of hyperlipidaemic patients more often regressed in those who responded with a large fall in plasma lipids to lipid-lowering therapy than in those whose plasma lipids showed little change. Other uncontrolled studies[10,11] produced similar results. There are many reports of regression of atherosclerosis during the treatment of hyperlipidaemia.[12] While atherosclerosis is generally progressive, it may regress even in the absence of intervention;[13-15] therefore a control group is essential in studying the effects of risk factor reduction.

In 1977 we started a randomised controlled trial of the effect of treatment of hyperlipidaemia on symptomatic femoral atherosclerosis. Features of the design included the requirement that plasma lipid levels be substantially reduced, with normal levels being achieved in most of the intervention group. Serial arteriograms were assessed blindly by computerised image analysis and manual measurements.

Patients and Methods

Patients were recruited from the Peripheral Vascular Clinics at St. Thomas' and Hammersmith Hospitals. Men and women presenting with a history of at least 6 months of stable intermittent claudication caused by femoro-popliteal disease were eligible for recruitment if serum total cholesterol exceeded 6·5 mmol/l and/or triglyceride exceeded 1·8 mmol/l on two occasions in the fasted state. Femoro-popliteal disease was confirmed by exercise Doppler pressure measurements. Patients with functionally important aorto-iliac disease were not studied; progression of such lesions was likely to have led to withdrawal from the study for surgery, and might have invalidated observations on the femoral artery. Predetermined exclusion criteria were evidence of arteritis, diabetes mellitus (British Diabetic Association criteria), diastolic blood pressure >100 mm Hg, age >65 years at presentation, major organ disease, malignant disease, causes of secondary hyperlipidaemia, endocrine disease, rest pain, or the presence of indications for surgical treatment. Two patients with evidence of Buerger's disease, six hypertensives, and eight diabetics were excluded.

Informed written consent was obtained. After full clinical examination, biochemistry, haematology, 12-lead electrocardiograph (ECG), and chest X-ray, 25 patients were randomly allocated

TABLE I—BASELINE CHARACTERISTICS

Characteristic	Treatment	Usual-care
Mean age (yr)	54·8	56·1
Males (n)	10	11
Females (n)	2	1
Mean duration of symptoms (months)	14	12
Edge irregularity index (mean±SEM)	0·153±0·01	0·141±0·04
Hyperlipoproteinaemia:		
IIa, IIb	8	8
III	3	1
IV	1	3
Plasma lipids (mmol/l; mean± SEM):		
Cholesterol	8·05±0·41	7·72±0·26
Triglyceride	3·25±0·80	3·10±0·50
HDL cholesterol	1·23±0·12	1·20±0·07
LDL cholesterol	5·41±0·39	5·19±0·39
VLDL cholesterol	1·41±0·23	1·33±0·11
Cigarettes/day:		
0	4	4
1–10	2	4
11–20	3	2
>20	3	2
Blood pressure (mm Hg):		
Mean systolic	151±15	148±22
Mean diastolic	89±11	84±9
Fibrinogen (g/l)	4·5±0·23	4·3±0·25
PCV (%)	44±4	43±2

PCV = packed cell volume.

to intervention and usual-care groups. These were closely matched by age, risk factor status, duration of symptoms, and severity of atherosclerosis (table I). None of the differences between groups was statistically significant.

Arteriography

Biplanar transfemoral arteriography was performed at entry to the study and after 15–24 months (means: treatment group 20; usual-care 18 months). To ensure precisely repeatable orientation the limb was positioned in a specially designed frame. We took many measurements from bony landmarks to ensure reproducible positioning. A single X-ray machine was used throughout the study, with standard intensifying screens, 0·6 mm focal spot diameter, maximum focus-film distance (135 mm), and short film-limb distance. The film used was 'Curix' RPI (Agfa-G), developed in an X-oMat automatic developer. Nicotinic acid and other lipid-lowering drugs were not administered in the 18 hours before arteriography.

All patients were premedicated with pethidine, and under local anaesthesia an 18 gauge Paul New arteriogram needle was introduced into the common femoral artery immediately distal to the inguinal ligament. A preliminary bolus injection of 60% w/v meglumine iothalamate under image intensification was used to time the main run, which consisted of slow injection of 30 ml of warmed contrast at standardised constant pressure. The 20 msec exposure was timed—by linking it with the R wave of the ECG through a delay circuit—to occur late in diastole to avoid the effect of the pulse-wave on the arteriogram.

We used a Joyce Loebl 'Magiscan 2' programmable image analyser to quantify paired sequential femoral arteriograms. Input was by a high performance (CCIR standard) 625-line video camera. The signal was digitised by a high speed analogue-to-digital converter with a 6-bit resolution giving 64 grey levels and it was logarithmically transformed before being stored in an image memory. The digital signal represents a raster scan of the image with a resolution of 256×256 points at a magnification of 10 pixels per mm. To compare individual segments 25 mm lengths of artery were analysed. Calibration for the concentration of intraluminal contrast was achieved by reference to branch vessels, assuming these to be circular in cross-section and disease-free. Selected contrast-filled arterial segments were scanned at 0·8 mm intervals and transverse density profiles perpendicular to the axial line of the vessel were constructed.[16] The area under each profile was directly

proportional to the cross-sectional area of the vessel at that site, whether circular or irregular. All artery displayed between the profunda femoris and the popliteal bifurcation was assessed, excluding sites where crossing branches or underlying dense bone made quantitative study impossible.

As a measure of disease progression or regression we used an index of edge irregularity, based on pathological studies that showed a strong correlation between edge irregularity and arterial disease.[17] The index was calculated in the present study as the standard deviation of the multiple cross-sectional area measurements for each segment on the sequential arteriograms, normalised by dividing by the mean area of the appropriate segment.

For visual assessment, diameters were measured perpendicular to the axial line, by means of ×2 magnification and Vernier callipers accurate to 0·01 mm. Cross-sectional areas of atheromatous plaques were assessed by plotting a smoothed line from regions not obviously diseased, inside which plaque height was measured every 1 mm. To ensure that the same segments were assessed in the two arteriograms careful measurements were made from the points of origin of branch vessels, and also from bony landmarks.

The films were masked by a colleague not participating in the study to conceal their identity and sequence; the code number was randomly allocated and the code was broken after all measurements were recorded. The two observers agreed on which segments to exclude from evaluation. We used the means of their independent measurements to evaluate the results. Inter-observer error (coefficient of variation of duplicate measurements) was 4·2%; and the mean intra-observer error was 2·3%.

The study was approved by the Research Ethical Committee of St Thomas' Hospital.

Lipid Measurements

Blood was drawn with minimal stasis after a 12–14 h overnight fast; analyses were started on the same day. Plasma lipoprotein cholesterol and triglyceride concentrations were measured enzymatically (Boehringer-Mannheim nos. 187313 and 166448, respectively). Very low density lipoprotein (VLDL; d<1·006 g/ml) was isolated by preparative ultracentrifugation;[18] high density lipoprotein (HDL) was isolated by precipitation of other lipoproteins with heparin-manganese chloride.[19] Low density lipoprotein cholesterol (LDL) concentration was calculated by difference. Types IIa, IV, and IIb hyperlipoproteinaemia were defined by concentrations of LDL-cholesterol, VLDL-triglyceride, or both exceeding the 95th centile of a London population.[20] Type III hyperlipoproteinaemia was defined electrophoretically, and by the presence of combined hyperlipidaemia caused by a rise in VLDL lipids in which the molar ratio of VLDL cholesterol to triglyceride was >1·0. Two baseline measurements were made before randomisation.

Management

Patients in both groups received repeated anti-smoking advice and a weight-reducing diet as appropriate. Those in the intervention group were instructed in a fat-modified diet in which total fat provided 30% energy, with a polyunsaturated fatty acid: saturated fatty acid ratio of 1·0 and cholesterol content of <250 mg per day. All patients in this group received one or two lipid-lowering drugs appropriate for the type of hyperlipidaemia. Type II hyperlipidaemia was treated with cholestyramine 12–24 g, per day, supplemented with nicotinic acid 3–6 g per day in 5 of the patients. Type III hyperlipidaemia was treated with clofibrate 1·5 or 2 g per day, and type IV was treated with nicotinic acid. Intervention group patients were seen initially every four weeks and, when adequate control of hyperlipidaemia had been achieved, every three months. Usual-care group patients were seen every three months. All participants received routine care as given to patients with claudication attending the vascular clinics. Full examination, ECG, and chest X-ray were repeated at the time of the second arteriogram. One member of the intervention group declined a second arteriogram and was withdrawn.

Results

During the trial, plasma cholesterol and triglyceride concentrations were respectively 19% and 37% lower in the treated group than in the usual-care group. LDL-cholesterol levels were 24% lower in the intervention group, whilst mean HDL-cholesterol was 41% higher. Only minor lipoprotein changes occurred in the usual-care group (table II).

There were no significant differences between the two groups for trends in blood pressure and weight during the course of the study. There was a slight reduction in cigarette use in both groups, but the mean number of cigarettes smoked per day during the study did not significantly differ between the two groups (table II). The changes in

TABLE II—RISK FACTOR STATUS DURING TRIAL (MEANS±SEM)

Factor	Treatment	Usual care
Cholesterol (mmol/l)	6·06±0·32	7·48±0·25†
Triglyceride (mmol/l)	1·80±0·20	2·87±0·48*
HDL cholesterol (mmol/l)	1·55±0·08	1·10±0·09*
LDL cholesterol (mmol/l)	3·91±0·32	5·13±0·38†
VLDL cholesterol (mmol/l)	0·60±0·09	1·26±0·19†
Fibrinogen (g/l)	4·1 ±0·17	4·2 ±0·14
PCV (%)	45±3	42±2
Cigarettes per day	16±2·7	14±3·2
Systolic BP (mm Hg)	145±19	150±22
Diastolic BP (mm Hg)	87±8	86±9

*$p < 0·05$.
†$p < 0·01$.

arteriographic appearances in the treatment and usual-care groups are shown in table III. Visual assessment indicated that the proportion of 1 cm segments showing progression of atherosclerosis was reduced by 60% compared with the usual-care group ($p < 0·01$, χ^2). In the intervention group the visually measured rate of increase in plaque cross-sectional area was one-third of that in the usual-care group ($p = 0·06$, Mann Whitney U test). The change in edge irregularity index, calculated from computerised analysis of the digitised arteriogram, was 2·5-fold greater in the usual-care group than in the treatment group ($p < 0·05$, Mann Whitney U test). This latter technique demonstrated progression of disease in most arterial segments examined. However, 15 of 46 segments in the treatment group, and 7 of 46 in the usual-care group showed a decrease in edge irregularity index during the study ($p = 0·05$, χ^2).

In both groups and in the pooled data there were positive correlations between mean LDL cholesterol concentration during the trial and the rate of progression of disease (table IV). A weak negative correlation was evident between HDL

TABLE III—VISUAL ASSESSMENT AND IMAGE ANALYSIS OF ARTERIOGRAMS

—	Treatment	Usual care
Visual assessment		
Number of assessed segments	144	156
Segments showing progression (n)	10	27*
% segments showing progression	6·9	17·3
Mean increase in plaque area (mm² per year per segment) (range)	0·58 (0–12)	1·72† (0–14)
Computerised image analysis		
Change in edge irregularity index		
Mean	0·019	0·047‡
Range	−0·180 to 0·116	−0·144 to 0·183
% of segments showing decrease in edge irregularity	33	15§

*$p < 0·01$ ($\chi^2 = 7·44$).
†$p = 0·06$ (Mann-Whitney U test).
‡$p < 0·05$ (Mann-Whitney U test).
§$p = 0·05$ ($\chi^2 = 3·82$).

TABLE IV—RELATION BETWEEN MEAN LIPID AND LIPOPROTEIN CONCENTRATIONS AND CHANGES IN EDGE IRREGULARITY INDEX DURING STUDY

	Treatment	Usual care	Pooled data
Cholesterol	0·38	0·40	0·48
Triglyceride	0·05	−0·20	0·02
HDL cholesterol	−0·20	−0·20	−0·32
LDL cholesterol	0·51	0·58†	0·59†
LDL/HDL cholesterol	0·57*	0·50	0·54

*$p = 0·06$.
†$p < 0·05$.

cholesterol and disease progression, but this did not achieve statistical significance.

Discussion

The study has demonstrated the feasibility of randomised controlled trials of lipid-lowering therapy in which angiographic assessment of atherosclerosis is used as an end-point, and has provided data on which power calculations for future larger trials may be based. Randomisation produced successful matching of the two groups. Good patient compliance with hypolipidaemic treatment was achieved, and there were no untoward effects of the treatment or of the radiological procedure. The various criteria used for assessing the angiograms provided consistent results.

A feature of the study design was to produce a large difference between the intervention and control groups in lipoprotein concentrations. This was achieved by use of individual treatment regimens to provide optimum therapy for the lipoprotein disorder,[21] and by modification of such therapy as required during the course of the study. Hence, the clinicians were aware of the treatment given. However, when they read the arteriograms they did not know the treatment category and sequence of films. Benefit cannot be attributed to any single therapeutic measure; our hypothesis was that reduction of raised plasma lipids would favourably influence the natural history of atherosclerosis.

The study is the first randomised controlled trial of lipid-lowering therapy on the course of femoral atherosclerosis, as directly assessed by angiography in hyperlipidaemic subjects. The rate of progression of disease was reduced by approximately 60% by hypolipidaemic treatment. Within the relatively short period of the trial only a minority of arterial segments showed radiological improvement; but this occurred in twice as many segments in the treatment group as in the usual-care group. Our study provides the first longitudinal evidence that the rate of progression 'of atherosclerosis in hyperlipidaemic patients is significantly related to the ambient LDL concentrations, previous evidence having been provided by cross-sectional studies only.[22]

The results of the study suggest that effective hypolipidaemic treatment favourably influences the natural history of symptomatic peripheral atherosclerosis in patients with hyperlipoproteinaemia. A more extensive trial over a longer period is being planned to answer further questions: what is the effect of treatment on earlier asymptomatic lesions? Does atherosclerosis in arteries other than the femoral respond similarly to risk factor reduction?

R. G. M. D. was supported by a grant from Bristol Myers Laboratories.

Correspondence should be addressed to B. L., Department of Chemical Pathology and Metabolic Disorders, St Thomas' Hospital Medical School, London SE1 7EH.

References overleaf

R. G. M. DUFFIELD AND OTHERS: REFERENCES

1. Miettinen M, Turpeinen O, Karvonen MJ, Elosuo R, Paavilainen E. Effect of cholesterol-lowering diet on mortality from coronary heart disease and other causes. *Lancet* 1972; ii: 835–38.

2. Dayton S, Pearce ML, Goldman H, et al. Controlled trial of a diet high in unsaturated fat for prevention of atherosclerotic complications. *Lancet* 1968; ii: 1060–62.

3. Committee of Principal Investigators. A cooperative trial in the primary prevention of ischaemic heart disease using clofibrate. *Br Heart J* 1978; **40**: 1069–1118.

4. Hjermann I, Velve Byre K, Holme I, Leren P. Effect of diet and smoking intervention on the incidence of coronary heart disease. *Lancet* 1981; ii: 1303–10.

5. WHO European Collaborative Group. Multifactorial trial in the prevention of coronary heart disease: 3. Incidence and mortality results. *Eur Heart J* 1983; **4**: 141–47.

6. MRFIT Research Group. Multiple risk factor intervention trial: risk factor changes and mortality results. *JAMA* 1982; **248**: 1465–77.

7. Crawford DW, Brooks SH, Selzer SH, Barndt R, Beckenbach S. Computer densitometry for angiographic assessment of arterial cholesterol content and gross pathology in human atherosclerosis. *J Lab Clin Med* 1977; **89**: 378–92.

8. Erikson U, Helmius G, Hemmingsson A, Olsson AG, Ruhn G. Evaluation of atherosclerosis by arteriography and microdensitometry. *Ann Radiol* (in press).

9. Barndt R, Blankenhorn DH, Crawford DW, Brooks SH. Regression and progression of early femoral atherosclerosis in treated hyperlipoproteinemic patients. *Ann Intern Med* 1977; **86**: 139–46.

10. Nikkila EA, Vinkinkoski P, Valle M. Effect of lipid lowering treatment on progression of coronary atherosclerosis assessed by angiography. *Circulation* 1978; **58** (suppl II): 50 (abstr).

11. Olsson AG, Carlson LA, Erikson U, Helmius G, Hemmingsson A, Ruhn G. Regression of computer estimated femoral atherosclerosis after pronounced serum lipid lowering in patients with asymptomatic hyperlipidaemia. *Lancet* 1982; i: 1311.

12. Malinow MR. Regression of atherosclerosis in humans: fact or myth? *Circulation* 1981; **64**: 1–3.

13. Chivers AG, Lea Thomas M, Browse NL. The progression of arteriosclerosis. A radiological study. *Circulation* 1974; **50**: 402–08.

14. Gensini GG, Esente P, Kelly A. Natural history of coronary disease in patients with and without coronary bypass graft surgery. *Circulation* 1974; 50-II: 98–102.

15. Bruschke AVG, Proudfit WL, Sones FM. Progress study of 590 consecutive non-surgical cases of coronary disease followed 5–9 years. *Circulation* 1973; **47**: 1154–63.

16. Colchester A, Brunt J. Measurement of vessel calibre and volume blood flow by dynamic quantitative digital angiography. *J Cereb Flow Metab* 1983; **3**: S640–41.

17. Dejdar R, Roubkova H, Cachovan M, Kruml J, Linhart J. Vergleich postmortaler Angiogramme mit makro-und mikroskopischen Befunden an A femoralis und A. poplitea. *Arch Kreislaufforsch* 1967; **54**: 309–35.

18. Havel RJ, Eder HS, Bragdon JH. The distribution and chemical composition of ultracentrifugally separated lipoproteins in human serum. *J Clin Invest* 1955; **34**: 1345–53.

19. Warnick GR, Albers JJ. HDL cholesterol quantitation: comparison of six precipitation methods and ultracentrifugation. In: Lippel K, ed. Report of HDL Methodology Workshop. US Department of Health Education and Welfare. Bethesda: NIH, 1979.

20. Lewis B, Chait A, Wootton IDP et al. Frequency of risk factors for ischaemic heart disease in a healthy British population with particular reference to serum lipoprotein levels. *Lancet* 1974; i: 141–46.

21. Lewis B. The hyperlipidaemias: clinical and laboratory practice. ch 16. Oxford: Blackwell Scientific, 1976..

22. Miller NE, Hammett F, Saltissi S, Rao S, Van Zeller H, Coltart J, Lewis B. Relationship of angiographically defined coronary artery disease to plasma lipoprotein subfractions and apolipoproteins. *Br Med J* 1981; **282**: 1741–44.

Original Contributions

The Lipid Research Clinics Coronary Primary Prevention Trial Results

I. Reduction in Incidence of Coronary Heart Disease

Lipid Research Clinics Program

● The Lipid Research Clinics Coronary Primary Prevention Trial (LRC-CPPT), a multicenter, randomized, double-blind study, tested the efficacy of cholesterol lowering in reducing risk of coronary heart disease (CHD) in 3,806 asymptomatic middle-aged men with primary hypercholesterolemia (type II hyperlipoproteinemia). The treatment group received the bile acid sequestrant cholestyramine resin and the control group received a placebo for an average of 7.4 years. Both groups followed a moderate cholesterol-lowering diet. The cholestyramine group experienced average plasma total and low-density lipoprotein cholesterol (LDL-C) reductions of 13.4% and 20.3%, respectively, which were 8.5% and 12.6% greater reductions than those obtained in the placebo group. The cholestyramine group experienced a 19% reduction in risk ($P<.05$) of the primary end point—definite CHD death and/or definite nonfatal myocardial infarction—reflecting a 24% reduction in definite CHD death and a 19% reduction in nonfatal myocardial infarction. The cumulative seven-year incidence of the primary end point was 7% in the cholestyramine group v 8.6% in the placebo group. In addition, the incidence rates for new positive exercise tests, angina, and coronary bypass surgery were reduced by 25%, 20%, and 21%, respectively, in the cholestyramine group. The risk of death from all causes was only slightly and not significantly reduced in the cholestyramine group. The magnitude of this decrease (7%) was less than for CHD end points because of a greater number of violent and accidental deaths in the cholestyramine group. The LRC-CPPT findings show that reducing total cholesterol by lowering LDL-C levels can diminish the incidence of CHD morbidity and mortality in men at high risk for CHD because of raised LDL-C levels. This clinical trial provides strong evidence for a causal role for these lipids in the pathogenesis of CHD.

(*JAMA* 1984;251:351-364)

CORONARY heart disease (CHD) remains the major cause of death and disability in the United States and in other industrialized countries despite recent declines in CHD mortality rates. It accounts for more deaths annually than any other disease, including all forms of cancer combined.[1] Nationally, more than 1 million heart attacks occur each year and more than a half million people still die as a result. Coronary heart disease ranks first in terms of social security disability, second only to all forms of arthritis for limitation of activity and all forms of cancer combined for total hospital bed days. In direct health care costs, lost wages, and productivity, CHD costs the United States more than $60 billion a year.

This enormous toll has focused attention on the possible prevention of CHD by various means, especially through lowering of the plasma cholesterol level. Observational epidemiologic studies have established that the higher the plasma total or low-density lipoprotein cholesterol (LDL-C) level, the greater the risk that CHD will develop.[2] The view that LDL-C is intimately involved in atherogenesis, the basic pathophysiologic process responsible for most CHD, is sustained by reports from other epidemiologic studies as well as many animal experiments, pathological observations, clinical investigations, and metabolic ward studies.[3]

Plasma total and LDL-C levels may be reduced by diets and drugs. However, before such treatment can be advocated with confidence and before it can be concluded that cholesterol plays a causal role in the pathogenesis of CHD, it is desirable to show that reducing cholesterol levels safely reduces the risk of CHD in man. Many clinical trials of cholesterol lowering have been conducted, but their results, although often encouraging, have been inconclusive.

The most appropriate clinical trial of the efficacy of cholesterol lowering would be a dietary study, because of the links between diets high in saturated fat and cholesterol typical of most industrialized populations, high plasma total and LDL-C levels, and a

From the Lipid Metabolism-Atherogenesis Branch, National Heart, Lung, and Blood Institute, Bethesda, Md.

Reprint requests to Lipid Metabolism-Atherogenesis Branch, National Heart, Lung, and Blood Institute, Federal 401, Bethesda, MD 20205 (Basil M. Rifkind, MD).

high incidence of CHD. However, the 1971 National Heart and Lung Institute Task Force on Arteriosclerosis recommended against conducting a large-scale, national diet-heart trial in the general population because of concern regarding the blinding of such a study, the large sample size, and the prohibitive cost, then estimated to range from $500 million to more than $1 billion.[4] Accordingly, the Lipid Research Clinics Coronary Primary Prevention Trial (LRC-CPPT) was initiated in 1973 as an alternative test of the efficacy of reducing cholesterol levels. The choice of hypercholesterolemic men at high risk of CHD events developing reduced the necessary sample size to a feasible level; in this regard, women were not recruited because of their lower risk of CHD.

The use of the drug cholestyramine resin permitted a double-blind design. This drug, previously approved for general use by the Food and Drug Administration, was selected on account of its known effectiveness in reducing total cholesterol and LDL-C levels,[5] the availability of a suitable placebo, its nonabsorbability from the gastrointestinal (GI) tract, its few systemic effects, and its low level of significant toxicity.

Reported herein is the outcome of the study with respect to its major response variables, definite CHD death and/or definite nonfatal myocardial infarction, and related data.

PARTICIPANTS AND METHODS

The design of the LRC-CPPT has been described in detail.[6] Briefly, the LRC-CPPT was a double-blind, placebo-controlled clinical trial that tested the efficacy of lowering cholesterol levels for primary prevention of CHD. Twelve participating Lipid Research Clinics (LRCs) recruited 3,806 middle-aged men with primary hypercholesterolemia (type II hyperlipoproteinemia) free of, but at high risk for, CHD because of elevated LDL-C levels. The men were randomized into two groups that were similar in baseline characteristics. The treatment group received the bile acid sequestrant cholestyramine resin, and the control group received a placebo; both groups followed a moderate cholesterol-lowering diet. To ensure comparability of all data across the 12 clinics over a ten-year period, a common protocol documenting all procedures in detail was strictly adhered to by clinical personnel, who were trained and certified in stan-

dardized procedures.[7] All aspects of the conduct of the study were carefully monitored by the Central Patient Registry and Coordinating Center and by the Program Office. The progress of the trial and the possibility of serious side effects were reviewed twice a year by a Safety and Data Monitoring Board. Any protocol violations that were identified were brought to the attention of this board; none were regarded by them to put the trial into jeopardy.

Selection of Participants

The LRCs recruited men aged 35 to 59 years with a plasma cholesterol level of 265 mg/dL or greater (the 95th percentile for 1,364 men aged 40 to 49 years who participated in a previous LRC pilot study) and with an LDL-C level of 190 mg/dL or greater. Men with triglyceride levels averaging greater than 300 mg/dL or with type III hyperlipoproteinemia were excluded.

The numerous sources of the volunteer participants and the techniques of their recruitment have been described.[8,9] Of the approximately 480,000 age-eligible men screened between July 1973 and July 1976, 3,810 were eventually entered into the trial.[10] Four, two in each treatment group, were subsequently removed when they were found to have type III hyperlipoproteinemia, and the results reported are for the 3,806 type II participants. The participants were preponderantly college- or high school–educated whites. Their mean age was 47.8 years. Informed consent was obtained from each participant randomized into the study.

Participants were also excluded if they had any of the following clinical manifestations of CHD: (1) history of definite or suspect myocardial infarction; (2) angina pectoris, as determined by Rose Questionnaire; (3) angina pectoris during exercise electrocardiography; (4) various ECG abnormalities, according to the Minnesota code—left bundle-branch block, tertiary or secondary heart block, two or more consecutive ventricular premature beats, left ventricular hypertrophy, R-on-T-type ventricular premature beats, or atrial flutter or fibrillation; or (5) congestive heart failure. Men with a positive exercise test result in the absence of other manifestations of CHD were not excluded. Only men in good health and free of conditions associated with secondary hyperlipoproteinemia, such as diabetes mellitus, hypothyroidism, nephrotic syndrome, hepatic disease, hyperuricemia, and notable obesity, were selected. Men were excluded if they had hypertension or were receiving antihypertensive medication or had life-limiting or comorbid conditions such as cancer or nonatherosclerotic cardiovascular disease. Men who required long-term

use of certain other medications were also excluded.

Screening (Prerandomization) Visits

The accrual phase consisted of four screening visits at monthly intervals. Physical examinations, lipid and lipoprotein level determinations, clinical chemistry measurements, medical history ascertainment, and resting and graded exercise ECGs were performed. At the second screening visit, a moderate cholesterol-lowering diet, which aimed to provide 400 mg of cholesterol per day and a polyunsaturated-to-saturated fat ratio of approximately 0.8 and which was designed to lower cholesterol levels 3% to 5%, was prescribed for all potential participants.[6]

A cholesterol-lowering diet was offered to potential participants because, when the LRC-CPPT began, it was the practice of many physicians to recommend such a diet to hypercholesterolemic patients. Although the cholesterol lowering expected from the diet given to both study groups had the potential to diminish the statistical power of the trial by reducing the subsequent incidence of CHD, it was hoped that such a diet, along with a nutritional counseling program, would facilitate recruitment of participants. Moreover, since the diet was introduced before randomization, it was possible to exclude men whose plasma cholesterol levels were highly sensitive to diet. Thus, men whose LDL-C levels fell below 175 mg/dL at the third or fourth screening visit were excluded. The maintenance of both treatment groups on the diet after randomization minimized the opportunity for confounding of the study because of differential dietary intakes. Dietary intake was assessed semiannually by means of a 24-hour dietary recall.[11]

Randomization

At the fifth visit to the clinic, eligible participants were randomly divided by the permuted block method into two treatment groups within eight prognostic strata at each of the 12 clinics. The strata were based on high and low risk of CHD with respect to LDL-C level ($\geq$ or <215 mg/dL), ST-segment depression during exercise testing, and a logistic risk function of age, cigarette smoking, and diastolic blood pressure.

Only five of 83 variables compared at baseline showed statistically significant differences (height, weight, and two-hour postchallenge glucose, SGOT, and albumin levels).[10] Because the observed differences were small and the number of statistically significant differences is that expected by chance in comparisons involving a large number of variables, the randomization and stratification process was found to produce two almost identical groups.

Study Medication

Participants were prescribed either the bile acid sequestrant cholestyramine resin at 24 g/day (six packets per day, divided into two to four equal doses) or an equivalent amount of placebo, dispensed in identical sealed packets. Those unable to tolerate six packets per day were prescribed a reduced dosage. Rigorous steps such as unique marking of individual packets and boxes and continuous external auditing of medications were followed to ensure proper drug-allocation assignment. Medication adherence was monitored by means of a packet count (packets issued minus packets returned, divided by the number of days elapsed since the packets were issued).

Postrandomization Visits

Participants attended clinics every two months, at which time the study medication was dispensed, dietary and drug counseling was given, and end points and possible drug side effects, as well as possible confounding variables such as blood pressure and weight, were evaluated. Intervention by LRC-CPPT staff was restricted to prescription of the study medication and the diet. At annual and/or semiannual visits, resting and graded exercise ECGs, 24-hour dietary recalls, and complete physical examinations and medical histories were obtained. All participants initially entered were followed up to the completion of the trial irrespective of their levels of adherence and the frequency of their visits.

Lipid Measurements

Lipid levels were determined with high precision and accuracy. Comparability of the measurements of the 12 LRC laboratories was ensured by a rigorous quality control program especially designed for the LRC Program and maintained by the Lipid Standardization Laboratory. The lipid levels at the second screening (prediet) visit were used as the baseline to calculate the changes in levels of total cholesterol and LDL-C and triglyceride observed at subsequent visits. Since the measurement of HDL-cholesterol (HDL-C) levels at the second screening visit was not performed according to protocol at several clinics, the levels at the first screening visit were used as the baseline to calculate change in HDL-C levels.

End Points

The primary end point for evaluating the treatment was the combination of definite CHD death and/or definite nonfatal myocardial infarction. Appendix A gives the detailed definitions of these events as well as the definition of suspect CHD death and suspect nonfatal myocar-

dial infarction. Other end points included all-cause mortality, the development of an ischemic ECG response to exercise (positive exercise test result), angina pectoris as determined by Rose Questionnaire, atherothrombotic brain infarction, arterial peripheral vascular disease (intermittent claudication as determined by Rose Questionnaire), and transient cerebral ischemic attack. Detailed definitions of these nonprimary end points have been published elsewhere.[6]

The classification of cause of death was based on the examination of death certificates, hospital records, and interviews with physicians, witnesses of the death, and next of kin. The diagnosis of nonfatal myocardial infarction was based on ECGs, blood enzyme levels, and history of chest pain at the time of the clinical event. A physician at the clinic at which the potential end point occurred classified the end point. In addition, each potential end point was classified independently by two members of a blinded verification panel. If the three reviewers agreed, the diagnosis was accepted. If there was disagreement, the case was submitted for definitive classification to the LRC-CPPT Cardiovascular Endpoints Committee.[6] Classification of deaths not caused by CHD was also performed by a blinded panel.

An intraoperative event was classified on the basis of ECG changes occurring during coronary bypass surgery or other cardiac surgery or during the recovery period extending from the time of surgery until discharge from the hospital.

Statistical Methods

The hypothesis of the LRC-CPPT was that lowering cholesterol (or LDL-C) levels would reduce the incidence of end points, and, hence, a one-sided test was used for the main hypothesis. The statistic reported is a stratified (using the eight baseline risk strata) log rank (Mantel-Haenszel) statistic.[12] This statistic compares the life-table survival (or failure) curves in the two groups rather than the proportion of failures. In view of the necessity for periodic review, the data were analyzed many times, and conventional methods of computing statistical significance no longer applied. Several statistical methods were used to monitor the trial. These methods included a modification of the method of O'Brien and Fleming,[13] the two-dimensional rank statistic of Majundar and Sen,[14] and a modification of the method of Breslow and Haug.[15] All of these methods essentially gave the same result, and, in view of its ease of presentation, the modified O'Brien and Fleming method was used for this article. As formulated by O'Brien and Fleming, the data are analyzed k times after an equal number of end points. In

practice, the data for this trial were analyzed at 15 equal time intervals, and strictly speaking, the method of determining the critical value proposed by O'Brien and Fleming does not hold. The distribution of the statistic taking into account the actual times when the analyses were conducted was determined by simulation and the critical z value for a one-sided test with $\alpha = 0.05$ was found to be 1.87, as compared with the O'Brien-Fleming value of 1.83. The simulated critical value 1.87 is used in this report.

This method for determining significance was used for the primary end point of the study. Other statistical tests reported use the nominal level of significance. The reader is cautioned that interpretation of these nominal P values should include the possibility that some may be significant by chance because of the many comparisons made.

The Kaplan-Meier method was used for construction of the life-table plots.[12] The percentage reduction of end points is reported as $(1-RR) \times 100$, where RR is the estimated relative risk of an event in the cholestyramine group, compared with the placebo group. For end points where time of occurrence could be obtained precisely, the relative risk was estimated from the life tables. Where the actual time of occurrence (eg, the onset of angina) could not be precisely determined, the relative risk was estimated from the 2×2 table defined by treatment and the occurrence of an end point. All relative risks were estimated, taking into account the baseline risk strata, unless otherwise noted.

To conform with the one-sided test of the main hypothesis, 90% confidence intervals for the estimated reduction in risk are reported. The Cox proportional hazards model[12] was used to adjust the treatment comparisons for other variables, such as blood pressure. Tests of interaction in the proportional hazards model were accomplished by including cross-product terms in the model.

Homogeneity of treatment effect over risk strata was assessed by an efficient scores test based on the proportional hazards model and included parameters for treatment and strata.[16] Homogeneity of effect over clinic was similarly assessed.

RESULTS
Follow-up

All men were followed up for a minimum of seven and up to ten years. The average period of follow-up was 7.4 years. Between May 15 and Aug 27, 1983, contact was made with all of the men who were still living, including any who discontinued visits during the course of the trial. Thus, the vital status is known for all men

Table 1.—Median Daily Dietary Intake

| | Placebo | | | | Cholestyramine Resin | | | |
| | Pre-entry | | Postentry | | Pre-entry | | Postentry | |
Dietary Variable	Prediet	On-Diet	1st Year	7th Year	Prediet	On-Diet	1st Year	7th Year
Total calories	2,264	2,023	2,056	2,060	2,278	2,027	2,058	2,086
Cholesterol, mg	309	248	255	284	308	243	261	288
Total fat, g	95	79	83	87	97	80	82	89
Saturated fat, g	33	24	26	28	34	24	26	29
P/S* ratio	0.48	0.73	0.69	0.67	0.47	0.72	0.67	0.66

*Ratio of polyunsaturated fats to saturated fats.

Table 2.—Mean Plasma Lipid and Lipoprotein Cholesterol Concentrations

| | Placebo | | | | Cholestyramine Resin | | | |
| | Pre-entry | | Postentry | | Pre-entry | | Postentry | |
Lipid	Prediet	On-Diet	1st Year	7th Year	Prediet	On-Diet	1st Year	7th Year
Total cholesterol, mg/dL	291.8	279.2	275.4	277.3	291.5	280.4	238.6	257.1
LDL* cholesterol, mg/dL	216.2	204.5	198.8	197.6	216.6	205.3	159.4	175.9
HDL* cholesterol, mg/dL	45.1	44.4	44.5	45.5	45.0	44.4	45.6	46.6
HDL cholesterol/total cholesterol	0.16	0.16	0.16	0.17	0.16	0.16	0.20	0.19
Triglycerides, mg/dL	158.4	153.2	162.0	173.5	159.8	156.3	172.2	182.9

*LDL indicates low-density lipoprotein; HDL, high-density lipoprotein.

originally entered into the study. In addition, every man or a close relative was questioned before and at the end of the study regarding previous hospitalizations for CHD or other reasons.

Adherence to Treatment

During the first year, the mean daily packet count for participants attending clinic was 4.2 in the cholestyramine and 4.9 in the placebo group, falling to 3.8 and 4.6, respectively, by the seventh year. Adherence to the diet as determined by a 24-hour dietary recall conducted at six-month intervals showed no important differences between the two treatment groups (Table 1). A rise of 2 kg in body weight occurred in each group during the seven years of the study.

Maintenance of Blind

No cases of medical emergency required the unblinding of participants or staff and no one asked to be told his treatment assignment.

Lipids and Lipoproteins

When the LRC-CPPT diet was introduced, total cholesterol levels fell 11.1 ± 0.65 (mean $\pm$ SE) mg/dL in the cholestyramine group and 12.6 ± 0.67 mg/dL in the placebo group

(Table 2). Corresponding falls of 10.3 ± 0.61 and 11.7 ± 0.63 mg/dL occurred in LDL-C levels. During the first year of follow-up, there were additional falls of 41.8 ± 0.81 mg/dL and 45.9 ± 0.82 mg/dL in total and LDL-C levels in the cholestyramine group and 3.8 ± 0.51 mg/dL and 5.7 ± 0.48 mg/dL in the placebo group. By seven years, the total and LDL-C levels had fallen, from the pre-entry postdiet levels, 23.3 ± 0.99 mg/dL and 30.4 ± 0.99 mg/dL in the cholestyramine group and 1.9 ± 0.75 mg/dL and 6.9 ± 0.70 mg/dL in the placebo group. Almost all of the change in total cholesterol was in the LDL-C fraction. During treatment, the cholestyramine group experienced average plasma total cholesterol and LDL-C reductions of 13.4% and 20.3%, respectively, which were 8.5% and 12.6% greater ($P<.001$) than those obtained in the placebo group. (It should be noted that these percentage changes were computed for each individual and then averaged.) There was a 1.6 ± 0.19-mg/dL increase in HDL-C levels and a larger increase in triglyceride levels attributable to cholestyramine therapy. There also was a rise in triglyceride levels in the placebo group, although not as great as in the cholestyramine group. Additional details are provided in the companion article.[17]

Primary End Point

The cholestyramine group experienced 155 definite CHD deaths and/or definite nonfatal myocardial infarctions, whereas the placebo group had 187 such events (Table 3). When the stratified log rank test was used to take into account the stratification of participants at entry and their differing lengths of follow-up, the incidence rate of CHD was estimated to be 19% lower in the cholestyramine than in the placebo group. The z score for this difference was 1.92 with $P<.05$, after adjustment for multiple looks at the data. Both the fatal and nonfatal categories of the primary end points showed corresponding reductions. Thirty CHD deaths occurred in the cholestyramine group as compared with 38 CHD deaths in the placebo group, representing a reduction in risk of 24%. The cholestyramine group experienced 130 definite nonfatal myocardial infarctions, compared with 158 in the placebo group, with a 19% reduction in risk. The inclusion of the categories of suspect CHD death and suspect nonfatal myocardial infarction resulted in an overall reduction in risk of 15%, with a 30% reduction for fatal events and a 15% reduction for nonfatal events. The z score for this comparison exceeded the nominal 5% threshold (1.65) for statistical significance and

Table 3.—Definite or Suspect Primary End Points and All-Cause Mortality								
End Point	**Placebo (N=1,900)**		**Cholestyramine Resin (N=1,906)**		**% Reduction In Risk***	**90% Confidence Interval for % Reduction In Risk**		**z Score**
	No.	%	No.	%				
Definite coronary heart disease (CHD) death and/or definite nonfatal myocardial infarction	187†	9.8	155†	8.1	19	+3	+32	1.92‡
Definite CHD death	38	2.0	30	1.6	24	...	...	...
Definite nonfatal myocardial infarction	158	8.3	130	6.8	19	...	...	...
Definite or suspect CHD death or nonfatal myocardial infarction	256†	13.5	222†	11.6	15	+1	+27	1.80
Definite or suspect CHD death	44	2.3	32	1.7	30	...	...	...
Definite or suspect nonfatal myocardial infarction	225	11.8	195	10.2	15	...	...	...
All-cause mortality	71	3.7	68	3.6	7	−23	+30	0.42

*Percent reduction in risk is defined as $(1-RR)\times100\%$, where RR is the incidence rate ratio of an event in the cholestyramine group compared with the placebo. Percent reduction in risk and z score are adjusted for follow-up time and stratification.
†A subject experiencing a myocardial infarction and CHD death is counted once in this category. Hence, this line is not the sum of the following two lines.
‡The .05-level, one-sided critical value of the z score adjusted for multiple looks at the data is 1.87.

was close to the modified O'Brien-Fleming threshold of 1.87 (see "Participants and Methods" section). Thus, the conclusion that treatment was beneficial is not essentially altered by the inclusion of suspect events. The separate category of intraoperative myocardial infarction (Table 4) also showed more cases in the placebo group (7 *v* 5), although the difference is not statistically significant. (One of the four type III participants excluded after the randomization experienced a nonfatal myocardial infarction; he was in the placebo group.)

The life-table failure rates in the two groups are plotted in the Figure. Very early in the follow-up period, the number of CHD events was higher in the cholestyramine group, but by two years the two curves were identical. Thereafter, there was a steady divergence of the two sets of event rates, and at seven years of follow-up the event rate was 8.6% in the placebo group and 7.0% in the cholestyramine group, a reduction of 19%.

The primary end points were examined within the risk strata defined at randomization. The hypothesis of homogeneity of effect across these strata was not rejected. Thus, although differences were observed in the estimated relative risk among the strata, there was insufficient statistical evidence to claim that the treatment was more beneficial in one stratum than in another. The cholestyramine-treated group at seven clinics had at least 18% fewer primary

Table 4.—Other Cardiovascular Events*					
End Point	**Placebo (N=1,900)**		**Cholestyramine Resin (N=1,906)**		**% Reduction In Risk**
	No.	%	No.	%	
Coronary disease					
Positive exercise test	345	19.8†	260	14.9†	25‡
Angina (Rose Questionnaire)	287	15.1†	235	12.4†	20‡
Coronary bypass surgery	112	5.9	93	4.9	21‡
Congestive heart failure	11	0.6	8	0.4	28
Intraoperative myocardial infarction	7	0.4	5	0.3	29
Resuscitated coronary collapse	5	0.3	3	0.2	40
Cerebrovascular disease					
Definite or suspect transient cerebral ischemic attack	22	1.2	18	0.9	18
Definite or suspect atherothrombotic brain infarction	14	0.7	17	0.9	−21
Peripheral vascular disease					
Intermittent claudication (Rose Questionnaire)	84	4.4†	72	3.8†	15‡

*Counts all events for each individual, including events occurring after a nonfatal myocardial infarction.
†Percent of those without condition at baseline.
‡Percent reduction in risk is adjusted for stratification.

end points than placebo-treated men. At four clinics there was essentially no treatment difference; only one clinic showed an excess of events in the drug group. The statistical hypothesis of homogeneity of effect among clinics also was not rejected; thus, the benefit of cholestyramine resin treatment cannot be attributed to effects in only a small number of clinics.

This stratified analysis provided an estimate of treatment benefit adjusted for baseline strata of what were considered to be the most important CHD risk factors when the study began. Adjustment for a more extensive list of baseline characteristics, including LDL-C, HDL-C, triglycer-

ide, age, cigarette smoking, and systolic blood pressure, each considered as a continuous variable, as well as exercise test outcome, was performed by Cox proportional hazards analysis. The adjusted estimates of treatment effect (20.0% risk reduction) and z score (2.05) were slightly greater than those obtained in the stratified analysis. There was no significant interaction of the treatment effect with any of the seven baseline characteristics. Thus, the proportional hazards and stratified analyses both indicate that it is highly unlikely that the treatment benefit could have arisen from inequality of the two treatment groups with respect to CHD risk at baseline or from a par-

Coronary Heart Disease—Lipid Research Clinics Program

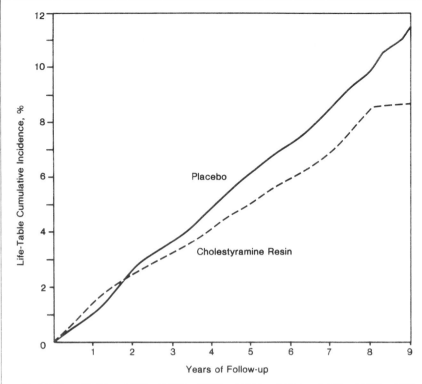

N=3,806   3,753   3,701   3,659   3,615   3,564   3,520   3,466   1,816   302

Life-table cumulative incidence of primary end point (definite coronary heart disease death and/or definite nonfatal myocardial infarction) in treatment groups, computed by Kaplan-Meier method. N equals total number of Lipid Research Clinics Coronary Primary Prevention Trial participants at risk for their first primary end point, followed at each time point.

ticular subgroup of LRC-CPPT participants.

Other Cardiovascular End Points

The frequency of other cardiovascular end points in the two treatment groups is reported in Table 4. Each of the CHD categories having a large number of events showed a reduction in incidence similar to the 19% reduction in the primary end point. Thus, the cholestyramine group showed reductions of 20% (P<.01) in the incidence of the development of angina ascertained by the Rose Questionnaire, 25% (P<.001) in the development of a new positive exercise test result, and 21% (P=.06) in incidence of coronary bypass surgery. The two cerebrovascular disease categories did not provide a consistent or significant pattern of benefit, but the numbers were small. For peripheral vascular disease there was a 15% (P>.1) reduction in new intermittent claudication in the cholestyramine group. None of the other differences in Table 4 were statistically significant, possibly because of the small numbers.

All-Cause Mortality

Although the incidence of definite and of definite and suspect CHD death was reduced by 24% and 30%, respectively, in the cholestyramine group, that of all-cause mortality was reduced by only 7% (Table 3), reflecting an increase in deaths not caused by CHD. Table 5, patterned after a similar table reported in the World Health Organization Clofibrate Trial,[18] breaks down the all-cause mortality into major categories. None of the differences are statistically significant. More details are provided in Appendix B. The only noteworthy difference (P=.08) was 11 deaths from accidents and violence in the cholestyramine group, compared with four in the placebo group. Of these, five in the cholestyramine and two in the placebo group were homicides or suicides, and six in the cholestyramine and two in the placebo group were accidents, mainly automobile. Each of the other major categories, including malignant neoplasms, differed only by one or two cases.

The possibility that a CHD event

could have been the underlying cause of a violent or accidental death was examined. All of these deaths had been evaluated by the Cardiovascular Endpoints Committee without knowledge of treatment group, and none had met the study criteria of a CHD death. Furthermore, none had any clinical evidence suggestive of myocardial ischemia. Subsequent to the conclusion of the study, all of these deaths were carefully scrutinized for the possibility of a CHD event. Seven were due to homicide or suicide, and in none of these was there any reason to doubt the diagnosis. Autopsy information was available for seven of the eight accidental deaths; seven of these deaths were due to automobile or motorcycle accidents. None showed evidence of new coronary thrombosis or acute myocardial infarction. Half had high blood alcohol levels. In four, this information and the circumstances of death made it virtually certain that CHD was not an underlying cause of death. In the other four, although the circumstances of death did not completely rule it out, a CHD episode was regarded as highly unlikely.

Possible Confounders

The results described previously show that the cholestyramine-treated group had a reduced rate of CHD. If during the course of the LRC-CPPT there were changes in CHD risk factors other than total cholesterol or LDL-C levels that were not the same in the two groups, this could pose an alternative explanation of the observed treatment benefit. Table 6 gives the pre-entry, first-year, and seventh-year mean values for selected variables that include the major known risk factors for CHD. For all of these major risk factors, the change from baseline was similar in the two groups, and, thus, they do not explain the treatment benefit. In addition, very similar percentages of participants in both groups (eg, placebo, 37%, v cholestyramine, 38%, at year 7) reported taking at least one aspirin in the previous week. Slightly more placebo- than cholestyramine-treated participants reported the use of β-blockers at the end of the trial.

Side Effects and Toxicity

Many possible side effects to treatment were monitored throughout the

Table 5.—Deaths in the Lipid Research Clinics Coronary Primary Prevention Trial

Cause of Death	Placebo	Cholestyramine Resin
Coronary heart disease (CHD)	44	32
Other vascular	3	5
Malignant neoplasm	15	16
Other medical causes	5	4
Accidents and violence	4	11
Total, all causes other than CHD	27	36
All causes other than CHD, other vascular, and accidents and violence	20	20
Total, all causes	71	68

Table 6.—Selected Variables Before and During Treatment

Variable	Placebo			Cholestyramine Resin		
	Pre-entry	1st Year	7th Year	Pre-entry	1st Year	7th Year
Mean systolic blood pressure, mm Hg	121	120	122	121	120	122
Mean diastolic blood pressure, mm Hg	80	79	78	80	78	78
Mean Quetelet index, g/sq cm	2.6	2.6	2.7	2.6	2.6	2.7
Mean weight, kg	81	81	83	80	80	82
% current smokers	37	35	26	38	36	27
Mean cigarettes per day for current smokers	25	24	25	26	25	26
% regular exercisers	30	...*	27	31	...*	28
Median alcohol consumption, g/wk	61	58	51	64	57	53

*No assessment of exercise was done in the first year.

trial. There were no noteworthy differences in non-GI side effects between the groups. Gastrointestinal side effects occurred frequently in the placebo- and cholestyramine-treated participants, especially the latter (Table 7). In the first year, 68% of the cholestyramine group experienced at least one GI side effect, compared with 43% of the placebo group. These diminished in frequency so that by the seventh year, approximately equal percentages of cholestyramine and placebo participants (29% v 26%) were so affected. Constipation and heartburn, especially, were more frequent in the cholestyramine group, which also reported more abdominal pain, belching or bloating, gas, and nausea. The side effects were usually not severe and could be dealt with by standard clinical means.

Little or no differences were seen between the two treatment groups for most of the clinical chemical tests monitored during the study (Appendix C). During the first year, serum alkaline phosphatase levels, iron binding capacity, SGOT levels, and the WBC count were higher in the cholestyramine group, while carotene

and uric acid levels were lower (Table 8). These differences were generally less apparent by the seventh year; none was associated with clinically apparent disease.

The number of participants hospitalized for conditions other than CHD was monitored. The hospitalizations were classified, using the H-ICDA code, eighth revision,[19] according to the primary diagnosis on the hospital discharge form. In particular, hospitalizations for GI tract disease were monitored (Appendix D). Of the many categories, the only difference with nominal statistical significance, using a test of comparison of proportions, was the primary diagnosis of deviated nasal septum, with more (16 v 6) cases in the cholestyramine group. Similar monitoring of all noncardiac operations or procedures was conducted. The only significant difference was a greater number in the cholestyramine group (40 v 23) of operations or procedures involving the nervous system. This excess mainly reflected more operations or procedures in the cholestyramine group for spinal disease (23 v 10), especially lumbar (19 v 9), and for decompres-

sion of the carpal tunnel (7 v 1).

Diagnoses and procedures involving the gallbladder were scrutinized in view of the ability of certain lipid-lowering drugs to produce gallstones and gallbladder disease. A few more hospitalized participants in the cholestyramine group had, as their main diagnosis, gallstones (16 v 11) and more cholestyramine-treated participants had an operation involving the gallbladder (36 v 25), but the differences were not significant. Gallstones, not necessarily as the main diagnosis, were reported in the cholestyramine group slightly more frequently than in the placebo group (31 v 30), as were other gallbladder and biliary tract diseases (28 v 23). No death attributable to gallbladder disease was recorded.

Appendix E indicates that the numbers of incident and fatal cases of malignant neoplasms were similar in the two groups: 57 incident cases in the placebo group, of which 15 were fatal; and 57 incident cases in the cholestyramine group, of which 16 were fatal. The cholestyramine group had a few more malignant neoplasms in some categories (eg, buccal cavity and pharynx) and less in others (eg, respiratory system) than the placebo group, but the numbers were small. When the various categories of GI tract cancers (buccal cavity-pharynx, esophagus, stomach, colon, rectum, and pancreas) were considered together, there were 11 incident cases and one fatal case in the placebo group and 21 incident and eight fatal cases in the cholestyramine group. The total number of incident colon cancers was identical.

COMMENT
Previous Trials of Cholesterol Lowering

The LRC-CPPT demonstrated that treatment with cholestyramine resin reduced the incidence of CHD. This result is in agreement with those of previous clinical trials of cholesterol lowering, which have shown a general trend of efficacy for selected CHD end points. However, the earlier trials have not been regarded as conclusive because of such factors as inadequate sample size, absence of a double-blind, failure to achieve identical treatment groups, inadequate cholesterol lowering, or questionable statis-

Table 7.—Percent of Participants Reporting Moderate or Severe Side Effects

Side Effect	Placebo			Cholestyramine Resin		
	Pre-entry	1st Year	7th Year	Pre-entry	1st Year	7th Year
Abdominal pain	5	11	7	5	15	7
Belching or bloating	10	16	6	10	27	9
Constipation	3	10	4	4	39	8
Diarrhea	6	11	8	5	10	4
Gas	22	26	12	22	32	12
Heartburn	10	10	7	10	27	12
Nausea	4	8	4	3	16	3
Vomiting	2	5	3	2	6	2
At least 1 gastrointestinal side effect	34	43	26	34	68	29

Table 8.—Mean Laboratory Values Influenced by Cholestyramine Resin

Laboratory Value	Placebo			Cholestyramine Resin		
	Pre-entry	1st Year	7th Year	Pre-entry	1st Year	7th Year
Alkaline phosphatase, IU/L of serum	71	70	71	71	82	74
Carotene, µg/dL of serum	150	146	149	149	111	132
Iron-binding capacity, µg/dL of serum	355	355	324	357	371	334
SGOT, units/L of serum	30	31	35	30	34	36
Uric acid, mg/dL of serum	6.3	6.1	6.3	6.2	5.8	6.1
WBC count, per cu mm	6,205	6,178	6,043	6,327	6,443	6,299

tical procedures.[20,21]

Several major primary prevention trials of diet have reported encouraging, although not always significant, reductions in CHD incidence. They include the New York Anti-Coronary Club Study,[22] the Los Angeles Veterans Administration Study,[23] and the Finnish Mental Hospital Study.[24] The interpretation of the results of these studies, as well as secondary prevention studies using diet, is clouded by the ascertainment bias that may result from a nonblinded design. Because of this and other shortcomings, these trials have also been regarded as inconclusive.[21] Primary prevention of CHD by diet has been evaluated during concurrent reduction of other CHD risk factors. A 47% lower CHD incidence was observed in the hypercholesterolemic participants in the Oslo Study who were treated with a cholesterol-lowering diet and counseled to reduce their cigarette smoking.[25] The investigators attributed most of the lower CHD incidence to the cholesterol reduction. The Multiple Risk Factor Intervention Trial (MRFIT) achieved too small an overall difference (2%) between the cholesterol levels of its two treatment groups to assess the effect of choles-

terol lowering.[26]

One major primary prevention trial of a lipid-lowering drug has been reported: the WHO Clofibrate Study obtained a 9% fall in serum cholesterol levels and a significant 20% reduction in the overall incidence of major ischemic heart disease events, similar in magnitude to the LRC-CPPT findings.[18] However, unlike the LRC-CPPT, this decline was confined to nonfatal myocardial infarction, whereas the incidence of fatal heart attack was similar in both treatment and control groups. Of concern in this study was the increased incidence in all-cause mortality in the clofibrate group, which became more significant during a four-year posttrial follow-up.[18,27]

The Coronary Drug Project (CDP) was a major secondary prevention trial of several lipid-lowering drugs. Three of its groups (high-dose estrogen, low-dose estrogen, and d-thyroxine) had to be discontinued prematurely because of evidence of toxicity.[28-30] The nicotinic acid group, in which a 9.9% fall in cholesterol levels occurred, showed a 27% lower incidence of nonfatal myocardial infarction but little difference in fatal CHD.[31] The clofibrate group, in which

a 6.5% reduction in cholesterol levels occurred, had a 9% lower incidence of fatal and nonfatal CHD, but statistical significance was not attained.[31] Two trials of clofibrate, the Newcastle Study[32] and the Scottish Society of Physicians Study,[33] had previously reported a suggestion of benefit, especially in subjects with pre-existing angina, but the post hoc use of subgroups and discordance in placebo group events has led to questioning of the conclusions from these two studies.[34]

The results of these various studies of lipid-lowering drugs for the prevention of CHD indicate that even though some evidence of reduction of CHD has attended their use, noteworthy and sometimes serious toxicity has occurred for each drug.

Side Effects and Clinical Chemistry Analyses

The use of cholestyramine resin resulted in several GI side effects, although these were also common in the placebo group. They were most evident in the initial stages of the study and could usually be handled by symptom-specific treatment, but sometimes they were the basis for cessation of, or reduction in, the drug dose. These side effects, which have been previously noted for cholestyramine resin, reflect the properties of a drug that is not metabolized in, or absorbed from, the GI tract. The monitoring of hospitalizations showed that the two treatment groups were similar for almost all of the large number of primary diagnoses and procedures. Of special interest is the absence of a significant increase in gallstones or cholecystectomy. This contrasts with clofibrate, which, unlike cholestyramine resin, is known to alter the lithogenicity of bile and has been associated in the WHO and CDP trials with an increased incidence of gallbladder disease.[18,31] The results of a systematic radiological study for gallstones in participants at two LRCs before and after the LRC-CPPT will be published.

A greater incidence of respiratory system hospitalizations and of operations and procedures on the nervous system was observed in the cholestyramine group. However, examination of the individual diagnoses or procedures within these categories failed to reveal any disorder for which there was a plausible explanation of an effect that could be attributed to cholestyramine resin. In view of the more than 60 diagnoses and procedures assessed, the two categories in which significant differences were found may represent chance occurrences.

Cholestyramine treatment altered results of several clinical chemistry studies, especially alkaline phosphatase, SGOT, and carotene. Such changes have been previously reported for cholestyramine use and, as in the present study, have not been associated with clinical disease.[5]

Malignant Neoplasms

The total incidence of fatal and nonfatal malignant neoplasms was similar in both treatment groups. When the many different categories are examined, various GI tract cancers were somewhat more prevalent in the cholestyramine group. Other cancers (eg, lung and prostate) were more frequent in the placebo group. The small numbers and the multiple categories prevent conclusions being drawn. However, in view of the fact that cholestyramine resin is confined to the GI tract and not absorbed and of animal experiments in which cholestyramine resin has been found to be a promoter of colon cancer when a cancer-inducing agent was also fed orally,[35] further follow-up of the LRC-CPPT participants is planned for cause-specific mortality and cancer morbidity.

CHD End Points

The LRC-CPPT shows that treatment with cholestyramine resin results in a significantly lower incidence of CHD as measured by the primary end point of the study. The benefit of treatment was not concentrated in any one subgroup or in a few clinics but was widespread. Inspection of the life-table curves shows that benefit became apparent two years after initial treatment. This benefit was reflected in both categories of primary end points. The findings were not essentially altered when the men classified as having a "suspect" primary event were added to the definite CHD category, nor were they altered by the inclusion of

the small number of intraoperative events in the primary end-point category. The possibility was considered that some deaths attributed to violence or accidents were precipitated by a CHD event, especially since more of them occurred in the cholestyramine group. As described, an extensive review of autopsy and clinical evidence was convincing that it was extremely unlikely that an underlying CHD event had occurred in any of the accidental or violent deaths.

The evidence of reduction of CHD incidence is further strongly supported by the analysis of other CHD end points for which a sufficient number occurred. Other studies have reported that angina and a positive exercise test result identify subjects at increased risk for CHD. In the LRC-CPPT, angina at entry was an exclusion. A positive exercise test result at entry, in the absence of chest pain, was a significant independent predictor of a subsequent primary end point, using proportional hazards analysis (to be published). Thus, the development of angina or new positive exercise test results, although not primary study end points, seem to be valid indicators of CHD risk status. Incident cases of the development of angina or of a new positive exercise test result were substantially lower by 20% and 25%, respectively, in the cholestyramine group. A corresponding 21% reduction was observed in the number of participants progressing to coronary bypass surgery. Also of interest is the 15% reduction in intermittent claudication.

All-Cause Mortality

There was only a 7% reduction of all-cause mortality in the cholestyramine group, reflecting a larger number of violent and accidental deaths. Several other primary prevention trials have reported higher noncardiovascular mortality in their active treatment groups, resulting from a variety of medical causes.[36] Excess mortality in the LRC-CPPT cholestyramine group was confined to violent and accidental deaths. Since no plausible connection could be established between cholestyramine treatment and violent or accidental death, it is difficult to conclude that this could be anything but a chance occurrence.

Confounding

The lower incidence in CHD events seen in the cholestyramine group does not seem to be attributable to changes in CHD risk factors other than cholesterol. The use of randomization and stratification procedures produced two treatment groups that, at entry, were similar with respect to all the major CHD risk factors, other minor or possible risk factors, and a variety of other measurements. The levels of CHD risk factors such as cigarette smoking, systolic and diastolic blood pressure, body weight, and reported levels of physical activity continued to be similar throughout the study. Both groups reported similar nutrient intakes and alcohol consumption.

Maintenance of Double-Blind

Many steps were taken to ensure that neither participants nor clinic staff knew to which treatment group participants had been assigned.[7] No need arose during the study to identify a participant's treatment group to him or to clinical staff. The higher incidence of GI effects in the cholestyramine group, mainly in the first year, made it possible that some loss of the double-blind might have occurred, although the high prevalence of such side effects in the placebo group makes this less likely. A survey at the end of the study showed that approximately equal numbers of participants (cholestyramine group, 56.0% v placebo group, 54.6%) or clinic staff (cholestyramine group, 55.2% v placebo group, 52.9%) could correctly identify treatment assignments.

Implementation of Study Design

The extent to which the LRC-CPPT was able to implement its original design objectives[6] is noteworthy (Table 9). The study exceeded its original sample size goal of 3,550 and successfully randomized 3,806 participants into two similar treatment groups. Participants were followed up for an average of 7.4 years. Consistent with the initial study parameters, a 4.8% reduction in plasma total cholesterol levels attributed to diet was obtained in the placebo group. In the seventh year, men taking cholestyramine resin maintained a mean plasma total cholesterol level reduction of 13.9%, attributable to the combination of drug and diet. Thus, the additional reduction in cholesterol levels attributable to cholestyramine resin was only 9.1%, well below the desired 24%. Although the 27% of participants who were taking no drug by seven years was lower than the predicted 35%, a number of participants were not taking the full dose of six packets. Difficulties in adherence related to the bulk, texture, and side effects of the drug seem to explain much of the shortfall in cholesterol lowering. It can be effectively argued that additional deterrents to taking the drug were the participants' lack of knowledge, for seven to ten years, as to which treatment group they were in as well as of their cholesterol levels during treatment. Better cholesterol lowering with cholestyramine resin could be expected when it is used in a routine clinical context. In addition, knowledge that treatment with cholestyramine resin prevents CHD can be expected to motivate adherence.

The seven-year incidence of the combined primary end points in the LRC-CPPT placebo group, 8.6%, was almost identical to the 8.7% predicted in the original study design based on data derived from the Framingham Study.[37] However, the actual incidence of definite CHD death was well below the predicted rate, whereas the rate of definite nonfatal myocardial infarction was increased above the predicted rate. A lower-than-predicted CHD death rate has been a feature of several clinical trials, including the recent MRFIT study.[26] Possible explanations include the stringent selection processes employed, resulting in an atypically healthier study population, better health monitoring and management during the course of the study, and the concurrent national decline in CHD mortality.

Implications of the LRC-CPPT

Caution should be exercised before extrapolating the CPPT findings to cholesterol-lowering drugs other than bile acid sequestrants. It has been shown that bile acid sequestration leads to a substantial reduction in plasma total and LDL-C levels by increasing the removal of LDL from the blood through increased activity

of specific cell-surface LDL receptors.[38] This mode of action is conceptually attractive inasmuch as it represents the enhancement of a physiological mechanism for the control of LDL levels. The mode of action, cholesterol-lowering potency, and possible toxicity of other cholesterol-lowering drugs must be taken into account before their use is advocated for the prevention of CHD.

The LRC-CPPT was not designed to assess directly whether cholesterol lowering by diet prevents CHD. Nevertheless, its findings, taken in conjunction with the large volume of evidence relating diet, plasma cholesterol levels, and CHD, support the view that cholesterol lowering by diet also would be beneficial. The findings of the LRC-CPPT take on additional significance if it is acknowledged that it is unlikely that a conclusive study of dietary-induced cholesterol lowering for the prevention of CHD can be designed or implemented.

The consistency of the reductions in CHD manifestations observed with cholestyramine resin in this controlled trial, which extend from the softer end points of angina, a positive exercise test result, and coronary bypass surgery to the hard end points of nonfatal myocardial infarction and CHD death, leaves little doubt of the benefit of cholestyramine therapy. These results could be narrowly interpreted to apply only to the use of bile acid sequestrants in middle-aged men with cholesterol levels above 265 mg/ dL (perhaps 1 to 2 million Americans). The trial's implications, however, could and should be extended to other age groups and women and, since cholesterol levels and CHD risk are continuous variables, to others

with more modest elevations of cholesterol levels. The benefits that could be expected from cholestyramine treatment are considerable. In the LRC-CPPT, treatment was associated with an average cholesterol fall of 8.5% beyond diet, and an average 19% reduction in CHD risk. Moreover, a companion article[17] that looks at cholesterol reduction and CHD more closely indicates that a 49% reduction in CHD incidence would be predicted for subjects who obtained a 25% fall in plasma cholesterol levels or a 35% fall in LDL-C levels, which are typical responses to 24 g of cholestyramine resin daily.

Funding for the study came from the following National Heart, Lung, and Blood Institute contracts and interagency agreements: N01-HV1-2156-L, N01-HV1-2160-L, N01-HV2-2914-L, N01-HV3-2931-L, Y01-HV3-0010-L, N01-HV2-2913-L, N01-HV1-2158-L, N01-HV1-2161-L, N01-HV2-2915-L, N01-HV2-2932-L, N01-HV2-2917-L, N01-HV2-2916-L, N01-HV1-2157-L, N01-HV1-2243-L, N01-HV1-2159-L, N01-HV3-2961-L, and N01-HV6-2941-L.

The Lipid Research Clinics Program acknowledges the long-term commitment of the volunteer participants in this clinical trial.

Lipid Research Clinics Coronary Primary Prevention Trial sites and key personnel are listed as follows.

Lipid Research Clinics

Baylor College of Medicine, Houston
Principal investigator: William Insull, MD; associate director (former principal investigator): Antonio M. Gotto, MD, PhD; CPPT director: Jeffrey Probstfield, MD; former CPPT directors: O. David Taunton, MD, Ellison Wittels, MD; key personnel: Susan Andrews, MA, Mohammed Attar, MD, Katherine Canizares, Janice Henske, MPH, RD, Tsai-Lien Lin, MS, Wolfgang Patsch, MD, Georgia White, RN.
University of Cincinnati Medical Center
Principal investigator: Charles J. Glueck, MD; CPPT director: Jane Third, MD; former CPPT directors: Ronald Fallat, MD, Moti Kashyap, MD, Evan Stein, MD; key personnel: Robert Adolph, MD, W. Fraser Bremner, MD, Jack Friedel, PhD, Rhea Larsen, RD, Susan McNeeley, MS, Paula Steiner, MS.

Table 9.—Comparison of LRC-CPPT* Design Goals and Actual Experience

Design Feature	Goal	Experience
Sample size	3,550	3,806†
Duration of follow-up, yr	7	7.1
Lost to follow-up	0	0
Reduction of plasma total cholesterol levels in placebo group	4%	4.8%
Nonadherers‡ at yr 7	35%	27%
Reduction of plasma total cholesterol levels in men adhering‡ to cholestyramine resin treatment	28%	13.9%§
7-yr incidence of primary end point in placebo group	8.7%	8.6%
Reduction in primary end point	36%	19%

*LRC-CPPT indicates Lipid Research Clinics Coronary Primary Prevention Trial.
†After removal of four type III participants.
‡A nonadherer is someone averaging less than half a packet of cholestyramine resin per day.
§Computed for seventh year.

George Washington University Medical Center, Washington, DC
Principal investigator: John C. LaRosa, MD; CPPT director: Valery Miller, MD; former clinical trials director: Marilyn Bassford-McKeown, RN; key personnel: Donna Embersit, Agnes Gordon Fry, RD, Richard Muesing, PhD, Diane Stoy, RN.

University of Iowa Hospitals, Iowa City
Co-principal investigators: Francois Abboud, MD, Helmut Schrott, MD; former principal investigator: William E. Connor, MD; CPPT director: Helmut Schrott, MD; key personnel: Erling Anderson, PhD, Paul King, Nancy Merideth, RN, Karen Smith, MS, RD, Linda Snetselaar, PhD, RD, Marlys Svare, RN, Lori Ziegenhorn, PAC.

Johns Hopkins Hospital, Baltimore
Principal investigator: Peter O. Kwiterovich, MD; CPPT director: Angeliki Georgopoulos, MD; former CPPT directors: William Benedict, MD, Michael Ezekowitz, MD, Lindsay Wyndham, MD; key personnel: Stephen Achuff, MD, Paul Bachorik, PhD, Frank A. Franklin, PhD, Katherine Salz, RD, MS, Thomas Weber, MS.

University of Minnesota, Minneapolis
Co-principal investigators: Ivan D. Frantz, Jr, MD, Donald B. Hunninghake, MD; CPPT director: Donald B. Hunninghake, MD; key personnel: Elizabeth Brewer, RD, Florine Campbell, RN, Kanta Kuba, MS, Monica LaDouceur, Lynn Lau, Arthur Leon, MD.

Oklahoma Medical Research Foundation, Oklahoma City
Principal investigator: Reagan H. Bradford, MD, PhD; former CPPT director: Thomas F. Whayne, MD, PhD; key personnel: Betty Edge, RD, Gerald First, MD, Hans Kloer, MD, Arlene Meier, RN, Katherine Moore, RD, Carl Rubenstein, MD.

Washington University School of Medicine, St Louis
Principal investigator: Gustave Schonfeld, MD; CPPT director: Anne Goldberg, MD; former CPPT directors: Boas Gonen, MD, Joseph Witztum, MD; key personnel: Thomas Cole, PhD, Wolfgang Patsch, MD, Joseph Ruwitch, MD, Stuart Weidman, PhD.

University of California at San Diego, La Jolla
Principal investigator: Fred H. Mattson, MD; former principal investigators: W. Virgil Brown, MD, Daniel Steinberg, MD, PhD; CPPT codirectors: Joseph Witztum, MD, Richard C. Gross, MD; key personnel: Joe Juliano, Jackie Sooter-Bochenek, MS, RD, Helen Stalmer, Eileen Taylor, RD, Edward Wade, MS, Magdalen Wong.

University of Washington, Seattle
Principal investigator: Robert H. Knopp, MD; former principal investigators: William R. Hazzard, MD, Edwin L. Bierman, MD; CPPT director: James T. Ogilvie, MD; former CPPT director: Robert H. Knopp, MD; key personnel: John J. Albers, PhD, Elizabeth R. Burrows, RD, MS, Margaret R. Poole, RN, Gene B. Trobaugh, MD, G. Russell Warnick, MS.

Stanford University, Stanford, Calif
Principal investigator: John W. Farquhar, MD; CPPT director: Daniel E. Feldman, PhD; former CPPT directors: Thomas Maneatis, MD, Michael Stern, MD; key personnel: Denise Desmond, Judy Halloran, William L. Haskell, PhD, Lillian O'Toole, Anne Schlagenhaft, Stephen Sidney, MD, H. Robert Superko, MD, Phyllis Ullman, RD, Sharon Vanden Bossche, Peter D. Wood, DSc.

Universities of Toronto and McMaster, Toronto and Hamilton, Ontario, Canada
Principal investigator: J. Alick Little, MD, CPPT coordinator: Josephine Bird, MD; CPPT directors: Randolph Lee, MD, David Stinson, MD, Maurice Mishkel, MD; former CPPT director: George Steiner, MD; key personnel: Carl Breckenridge, PhD, Gary Kakis, PhD, Norma Mishkel, Valerie McGuire, RPD, Joan McLaughlin, RPD, J. K. Wilson, MD.

Central Patient Registry and Coordinating Center, University of North Carolina, Chapel Hill
Principal investigator: O. Dale Williams, PhD; former principal investigator: James E. Grizzle, PhD; director, CPPT division: C. E. Davis, PhD; assistant director, CPPT division: Melvin Jackson, MSPH; key personnel: Bruce Allen, MS, Carol Bittinger, MSPH, Lars-Goran Ekelund, MD, Karen Graves, PhD, Carol Hazard, MS, James Hosking, PhD, Sandra Irving, MS, John Karon, PhD, James Knoke, PhD, Kenneth Kral, MS, Joanne Kucharski, Robert McMahan, J. J. Nelson, MSPH, Patricia Scott, Ratna Thomas, MS, Mary Williams.

Central Electrocardiographic Laboratory, University of Alabama, Birmingham
Principal investigator: L. Thomas Sheffield, MD; codirector: David Roitman, MD; key personnel: Carol Troxell.

Lipid Standardization Laboratory, Centers for Disease Control, Atlanta
Director: Gerald R. Cooper, MD, PhD; codirector: Adrian Hainline, PhD; key personnel: Barbara L. Botero, Myron Kuchmak, PhD, Linnard Taylor, Carole Winn.

Central Clinical Chemistry Laboratory, BioScience Laboratory, Van Nuys, Calif
Principal investigator: James Demetriou, PhD; former principal investigator: Frank Ibbott, PhD.

Nutrition Coding Center, University of Minnesota, Minneapolis
Principal investigator: Marilyn Buzzard, PhD,

RD; associate director: Joyce Wenz, MS, RD; former principal investigator: Victor Grambsch.

Drug Supply and Distribution Center, Mead-Johnson, Evansville, Ind
Key personnel: John Boegnik, PhD.

Recruitment and Adherence Consultants, Stanford University, Calif
Director: Stewart Agras, MD; former directors: Albert Stunkard, MD, Steven M. Zifferblatt, PhD; deputy director: Jacqueline Dunbar, PhD; key personnel: Melbourne Hovell, PhD, Gary Marshall, PhD, Barbara Newman, MA, Mary Southam, PhD.

Program Office: Lipid Metabolism-Atherogenesis Branch, Division of Heart and Vascular Diseases, National Heart, Lung, and Blood Institute, Bethesda, Md.
Chief: Basil M. Rifkind, MD; former chief: Robert I. Levy, MD; CPPT coordinator: Ronald S. Goor, MPH, PhD; former CPPT coordinator: Richard Havlik, MD; medical officer: David Gordon, MD, PhD; key personnel: Conrad Blum, MD, Virginia Keating, RD, MS, Kenneth Lippel, PhD, Gail Morrison, MD, Marjorie Myrianthopoulos, RD, Beverly Neal, Gary J. Nelson, PhD, Beth Schucker, MA, Alan Seplowitz, MD.

Safety and Data Monitoring Board
Chairman: Basil M. Rifkind, MD; former chairman: Robert I. Levy, MD; members: James Dalen, MD, Harold Fallon, MD, William Friedewald, MD, PhD, James Grizzle, PhD, Proctor Harvey, MD, Robert I. Levy, MD, Caroline S. Lurie, Henry McGill, Jr, MD, William F. Taylor, PhD, Herman A. Tyroler, MD; former member: Steven M. Zifferblatt, PhD.

Cardiovascular Endpoints Committee
Stephen Achuff, MD, Robert Adolph, MD, Edward Atwood, MD, Fraser Bremner MD, Dennis Costello, MD, Robert DeBusk, MD, Brian Gaffney, MD, David Gordon, MD, PhD, Patrick Gorman, MD, Richard Miller, MD, Jeffrey Probstfield, MD, Barbara Roberts, MD, Donald Romhilt, MD, Douglas Rosing, MD, Carl Rubenstein, MD (chairman), Joseph Ruwitch, MD, Leonard Schwartz, MD, Brian Sealey, MD, Abid Sha, MD, L. Thomas Sheffield, MD, Gene Trobaugh, MD, John Wilson, MD.

The computations for this manuscript were done by David Christiansen, Ronald Parker, Cynthia Nash, Hope Bryan, Dawn Stewart, Gail Olson, Douglas Baber, Judi Connor, Doyle Hawkins, and Joanne Kucharski. Janet Bungay provided editorial assistance. Typing assistance was provided by Edna Wilkerson and Ernestine Bland.

References

1. Levy RI: Review: Declining mortality in coronary heart disease. *Arteriosclerosis* 1981; 1:312-325.

2. Gordon T, Castelli WP, Hjortland MC, et al: The prediction of coronary heart disease by high-density and other lipoproteins: An historical perspective, in Rifkind B, Levy R (eds): *Hyperlipidemia—Diagnosis and Therapy*. New York, Grune & Stratton Inc, 1977, pp 71-78.

3. Stamler J: Population studies, in Levy RI, Rifkind BM, Dennis BH, et al (eds): *Nutrition, Lipids, and Coronary Heart Disease*. New York, Raven Press, 1979, pp 25-88.

4. *Arteriosclerosis: A Report by the National Heart and Lung Institute Task Force on Arteriosclerosis*, Dept of Health, Education, and Welfare publication (NIH) 72-137. Washington, DC, National Institutes of Health, 1971, vol 1.

5. Levy RI, Fredrickson DS, Stone NJ, et al: Cholestyramine in type II hyperlipoproteinemia: A double-blind trial. *Ann Intern Med* 1973; 79:51-58.

6. The Lipid Research Clinics Program: The Coronary Primary Prevention Trial: Design and implementation. *J Chronic Dis* 1979;32:609-631.

7. *Protocol for the Lipid Research Clinics Type II Coronary Primary Prevention Trial.* Chapel Hill, NC, University of North Carolina Department of Biostatistics, 1980.

8. The Lipid Research Clinics Program: Participant recruitment to the Coronary Primary Prevention Trial. *J Chronic Dis* 1983;36:451-465.

9. The Lipid Research Clinics Program: Recruitment for clinical trials: The Lipid Research Clinics Coronary Primary Prevention Trial experience. *Circulation* 1982;66(suppl 4):1-78.

10. The Lipid Research Clinics Program: Pre-entry characteristics of participants in the Lipid Research Clinics Coronary Primary Prevention Trial. *J Chronic Dis* 1983;36:467-479.

11. Dennis B, Ernst N, Hjortland M, et al: The NHLBI nutrition data system. *J Am Diet Assoc* 1980;77:641-647.

12. Kalbfleisch JD, Prentice RL: *The Statisti-cal Analysis of Failure Time Data.* New York, John Wiley & Sons, 1980.

13. O'Brien PC, Fleming TR: A multiple testing procedure for clinical trials. *Biometrics* 1979;35:549-556.

14. Majundar H, Sen PK: Nonparametric testing for simple linear regression under progressive censoring with staggering entry and random withdrawal. *Communication in Statistics—Theory and Methods.* 1978;A7:349-371.

15. Breslow N, Haug C: Sequential comparison of exponential survival curves. *J Am Stat Assoc* 1972;67:691-697.

16. Tsiatis AA: The asymptotic joint distributions of efficient scores test for the proportional hazards model over time. *Biometrika* 1981;68:311-315.

17. Lipid Research Clinics Program: The Lipid Research Clinics Coronary Primary Prevention Trial Results: II. The relationship of reduction in incidence of coronary heart disease to cholesterol lowering. *JAMA* 1984;251:365-374.

18. Committee of Principal Investigators, W.H.O. Clofibrate Trial: A cooperative trial in the primary prevention of ischaemic heart disease using clofibrate, report. *Br Heart J* 1978; 40:1069-1118.

19. *H-ICDA: Hospital Adaptation of ICDA*, ed 2, eighth revision. Ann Arbor, Mich, Commission on Professional and Hospital Activities, 1973, vol 1.

20. Cornfield J, Mitchell S: Selected risk factors in coronary disease: Possible intervention effects. *Arch Environ Health* 1969;19:382-391.

21. Davis CE, Havlik R: Clinical trials of lipid lowering and coronary artery disease prevention, in Rifkind BM, Levy RI (eds): *Hyperlipidemia—Diagnosis and Therapy*. New York, Grune & Stratton Inc, 1977, pp 79-92.

22. Rinzler SH: Primary prevention of coronary heart disease by diet. *Bull NY Acad Med* 1968;44:936-949.

23. Dayton S, Pearce ML, Hashimoto S, et al: A controlled clinical trial of a diet high in unsaturated fat in preventing complications of atherosclerosis. *Circulation* 1969;39-40(suppl 2):1-63.

24. Turpeinen O, Karvonen MJ, Pekkarinen M, et al: Dietary prevention of coronary heart disease: The Finnish Mental Hospital Study. *Int J Epidemiol* 1979;8:99-118.

25. Hjermann I, Velve Byre K, Holme I, et al: Effect of diet and smoking intervention on the incidence of coronary heart disease: Report from the Oslo Study Group of a randomized trial in healthy men. *Lancet* 1981;2:1303-1310.

26. Multiple Risk Factor Intervention Trial Research Group: Multiple Risk Factor Intervention Trial: Risk factor changes and mortality results. *JAMA* 1982;248:1465-1477.

27. Committee of Principal Investigators, W.H.O. Clofibrate Trial: W.H.O. Cooperative Trial on primary prevention of ischaemic heart disease using clofibrate to lower serum cholesterol: Mortality follow-up report. *Lancet* 1980; 2:379-385.

28. Coronary Drug Project Research Group: The Coronary Drug Project: Initial findings leading to modification of its research protocol. *JAMA* 1970;214:1303-1313.

29. Coronary Drug Project Research Group: The Coronary Drug Project: Findings leading to discontinuation of the 2.5 mg/day estrogen group. *JAMA* 1973;226:652-657.

30. Coronary Drug Project Research Group: The Coronary Drug Project: Findings leading to further modifications of its protocol with respect to dextrothyroxine. *JAMA* 1972;220:996-1008.

31. Coronary Drug Project Research Group: The Coronary Drug Project: Clofibrate and niacin in coronary heart disease. *JAMA* 1975; 231:360-381.

32. Group of Physicians of the Newcastle Upon Tyne Region: Trial of clofibrate in the treatment of ischaemic heart disease: Five-year study. *Br Med J* 1971;4:767-775

33. Research Committee of the Scottish Society of Physicians: Ischaemic heart disease: A secondary prevention trial using clofibrate. *Br Med J* 1971;4:775-784.

34. Friedewald WT, Halperin M: Clofibrate in ischemic heart disease. *Ann Intern Med* 1972; 76:821-823.

35. Asano T, Pollard M, Madsen DC: Effects of cholestyramine on 1,2-dimethylhydrazine-induced enteric carcinoma in germfree rats. *Proc Soc Exp Biol Med* 1975;150:780-785.

36. Oliver MF: Serum cholesterol: The knave of hearts and the joker. *Lancet* 1981;2:1090-1095.

37. Kannel WB, Castelli WP, Gordon T, et al: Serum cholesterol, lipoproteins and the risk of coronary heart disease: The Framingham Study. *Ann Intern Med* 1971;74:1-12.

38. Goldstein JL, Kita T, Brown MS: Defective lipoprotein receptors and atherosclerosis: Lessons from an animal counterpart of familial hypercholesterolemia. *N Engl J Med* 1983; 309:288-296.

39. Blackburn H, Keys A, Simonson E, et al: The electrocardiogram in population study. *Circulation* 1960;21:1160-1175.

Appendix A.—Definition of Primary End Points

Primary End Points

I. Definite atherosclerotic coronary heart disease death—either or both of the following categories:

   A. Death certificate with consistent underlying or immediate cause plus either of the following:

      1. Preterminal hospitalization with definite or suspect myocardial infarction (see below).

      2. Previous definite angina or suspect or definite myocardial infarction when no cause other than atherosclerotic coronary heart disease could be ascribed as the cause of death.

   B. Sudden and unexpected death (requires all three characteristics):

      1. Deaths occurring within one hour after the onset of severe symptoms or having last been seen without them.

      2. No known nonatherosclerotic acute or chronic process or event that could have been potentially lethal.

      3. An "unexpected" death occurs only in a person who is not confined to his home, hospital, or other institution because of illness within 24 hours before death.

II. Criteria for definite nonfatal myocardial infarction—any one or more of the following categories using the stated definitions:

   A. Diagnostic ECG at the time of the event.

   B. Ischemic cardiac pain and diagnostic enzymes.

   C. Ischemic cardiac pain and equivocal enzymes and equivocal ECG.

   D. A routine Lipid Research Clinics ECG is diagnostic for myocardial infarction while the previous one was not.

III. Suspect atherosclerotic coronary heart disease death—one or both of the following categories:

   A. Death certificate with consistent underlying or immediate cause but neither adequate preterminal documentation of the event nor previous atherosclerotic coronary heart disease diagnosis.

   B. Rapid and unexpected death (requires all three characteristics):

      1. Death occurring between one and 24 hours after the onset of severe symptoms or having last been seen without them.

      2. No known nonatherosclerotic acute or chronic process or event that could have been potentially lethal.

      3. An "unexpected death" occurs only in a person who is not confined to his home, hospital, or other institution because of illness within 24 hours before death.

IV. Suspect myocardial infarction—any one or more of the following categories using the stated definitions:

   A. Ischemic cardiac pain.

   B. Diagnostic enzymes.

   C. Equivocal ECG and equivocal enzymes.

   D. Equivocal ECG alone, provided that it is not based on ST or T-wave changes only.

(Continued on page 363.)

Appendix A.—Definition of Primary End Points (cont)

Glossary

I. Ischemic cardiac pain—severe substernal pain having a deep or visceral quality and lasting for half an hour or more.

II. ECG (classified by Minnesota Code)[39]
  A. Diagnostic—either of the following must be present:
    1. Unequivocal Q or QS pattern (code 1-1).
    2. Q or QS pattern (codes 1-2-1 to 1-2-7), plus any T-wave item (codes 5-1 to 5-3).
    Only the first criterion applies in the presence of ventricular conduction defects.
  B. Equivocal—any of the following must be present:
    1. Q or QS pattern (codes 1-2-1 to 1-2-7).
    2. ST junction and segment depression (codes 4-1 to 4-3).
    3. T-wave item (codes 5-1 to 5-2).
    4. Left bundle-branch block (code 7-1).

III. Enzymes
  A. Diagnostic enzymes—all of the following conditions:
    1. Creatine kinase, SGOT, or lactic dehydrogenase values determined coexistent with the event.
    2. The upper limit of normal for the local laboratory is recorded.
    3. The determined value for one or more enzymes is at least twice the upper limit of the local laboratory but does not exceed 15 times that value.
  B. Equivocal enzymes—all of the following conditions:
    1. Creatine kinase, SGOT, or lactic dehydrogenase values determined coexistent with the event.
    2. The upper limit of normal for the local laboratory is recorded.
    3. The determined value for one or more enzymes is elevated but does not fulfill criteria for diagnostic enzymes.

Appendix B.—Deaths Not Attributed to Coronary Heart Disease

Cause of Death	Placebo	Cholestyramine Resin
Cardiovascular (non-coronary heart disease)	3	5
Cerebrovascular	2	2
Peripheral vascular with gangrene	0	1
Surgical complications*	1	2
Malignant neoplasm†	15	16
Other illnesses	5	4
Infectious diseases‡	3	2
Chronic obstructive pulmonary disease	1	1
Alcoholism	1	1
Trauma	4	11
Accidents	2	6
Homicide	0	1
Suicide	2	4
Total	27	36

*One placebo participant died while undergoing cardiac catheterization. Two cholestyramine resin participants died of complications ensuing from mitral valve replacement and from carotid endarterectomy.
†Listed by site in Appendix E.
‡Three deaths (two in the placebo group) caused by pneumonia, one placebo death caused by staphylococcal septicemia, and one cholestyramine resin death resulting from an undetermined infectious cause.

Appendix C.—Mean Laboratory Values Not Influenced by Cholestyramine Resin						
	Placebo			Cholestyramine Resin		
Laboratory Value	Pre-entry	1st Year	7th Year	Pre-entry	1st Year	7th Year
Albumin, g/dL of serum	4.3	4.2	4.2	4.3	4.2	4.2
Bilirubin, direct, mg/dL of serum	0.04	0.04	0.04	0.04	0.05	0.04
Bilirubin, total, mg/dL of serum	0.52	0.52	0.61	0.52	0.54	0.62
Calcium, mEq/L of serum	4.8	4.8	4.7	4.9	4.8	4.6
Chloride, mEq/L of serum	103	104	103	103	105	103
Creatinine, mg/dL of serum	1.03	1.02	0.98	1.03	1.01	0.98
Globulin, g/dL of serum	2.9	3.0	3.0	2.9	3.0	3.0
Glucose, mg/dL of serum	98	96	101	98	94	100
Hematocrit, %	46	45	45	46	45	45
Iron, µg/dL of serum	114	113	103	113	114	103
Phosphorus, mg/dL of serum	3.1	3.0	3.0	3.1	3.0	3.0
Potassium, mEq/L of serum	4.5	4.5	4.4	4.5	4.5	4.4
Sodium, mEq/L of serum	140	141	141	140	140	141
Thyroxine, µg of T$_4$/dL of serum	4.1	4.0	4.3	4.1	4.1	4.3
Total protein, g/dL of serum	7.2	7.2	7.3	7.2	7.2	7.3
Vitamin A, IU/dL of serum	228	234	267	229	236	270

Appendix D.—Hospitalizations With a Primary Diagnosis* of Gastrointestinal Tract Disease		
Primary Diagnosis†	Placebo	Cholestyramine Resin
Intestinal infectious diseases	13	9
Neoplasm		
Benign	11	12
Malignant	11	15
Unspecified	0	1
Diseases of esophagus	5	6
Ulcer	20	30
Gastritis	5	12
Functional and other disorders of stomach	3	0
Appendicitis	4	11
Hernia	100	97
Intestinal obstruction	5	4
Enteritis and colitis	2	1
Diverticular disease of intestine	9	10
Anal fissure and fistula	9	5
Abscess of anal and rectal region	5	5
Peritonitis	0	1
Functional and other diseases of intestine	3	6
Liver disease	2	3
Gallstones	11	16
Other gallbladder and biliary tract disease	19	22
Pancreas	0	3
Hemorrhoids	27	29
Signs, symptoms, and ill-defined conditions	23	16

*Participants are counted only once within each category.
†By H-ICDA code, eighth revision, 1973.

Appendix E.—Incident Malignant Neoplasms				
	Placebo (N=1,900)		Cholestyramine Resin (N=1,906)	
Primary Site	All Cases	Deaths*	All Cases	Deaths*
Buccal cavity–pharynx	0	0	6	0
Esophagus	1	0	2	2
Stomach	2	1	0	0
Colon	6	0	6	2
Rectum	2	0	4	1
Pancreas	0	0	3	3
Larynx	3	0	1	0
Lung	10	8	6	3
Leiomyosarcoma	1	1	0	0
Melanoma	5	1	0	0
Other skin	5	0	3	0
Prostate	11	1	7	1
Urinary bladder	3	0	7	0
Kidney	1	0	2	0
Brain	1	1	3	3
Thyroid	1	1	0	0
Thymus	0	0	1	0
Lymphatic tissue	1	0	4	1
Hematopoietic tissue	3	1	2	0
Unknown	1	0	1	0
Total	57	15	57†	16

*Four men with malignant neoplasms (two in each treatment group) died of nonneoplastic causes. They are counted among the incident cases but not among the deaths in this Table.
†One cholestyramine group participant, who survived to the end of the study, had both a prostate carcinoma and a lymphoma; he is counted only once in the total.

The Lipid Research Clinics Coronary Primary Prevention Trial Results

II. The Relationship of Reduction in Incidence of Coronary Heart Disease to Cholesterol Lowering

Lipid Research Clinics Program

● In the Lipid Research Clinics Coronary Primary Prevention Trial (LRC-CPPT), a 19% lower incidence of coronary heart disease (CHD) in cholestyramine-treated men was accompanied by mean falls of 8% and 12% in plasma total (TOTAL-C) and low-density lipoprotein (LDL-C) cholesterol levels relative to levels in placebo-treated men. When the cholestyramine treatment group was analyzed separately, a 19% reduction in CHD risk was also associated with each decrement of 8% in TOTAL-C or 11% in LDL-C levels (P<.001). Moreover, CHD incidence in men sustaining a fall of 25% in TOTAL-C or 35% in LDL-C levels, typical responses to the prescribed dosage (24 g/day) of cholestyramine resin, was half that of men who remained at pretreatment levels. Adherence to medication was associated with reduced incidence of CHD only when accompanied by falls in TOTAL-C and LDL-C levels. Small increases in high-density lipoprotein cholesterol levels, which accompanied cholestyramine treatment, independently accounted for a 2% reduction in CHD risk. Thus, the reduction of CHD incidence in the cholestyramine group seems to have been mediated chiefly by reduction of TOTAL-C and LDL-C levels.

(JAMA 1984;251:365-374)

THE ASSOCIATION of total plasma cholesterol levels (TOTAL-C) with incidence of coronary heart disease (CHD) is well established.[1,2] The low-density lipoprotein cholesterol (LDL-C) subfraction is the main contributor to this relationship, while high-density lipoprotein cholesterol (HDL-C) levels are inversely related to CHD incidence.[3,4] Whether levels of very low-density lipoprotein cholesterol or triglyceride (TG) are independently related to CHD incidence is uncertain.[5]

Although TOTAL-C and LDL-C are potent risk factors for CHD, observational studies cannot prove that lowering these cholesterol levels by diet or drugs or both will reduce the subsequent incidence of CHD. The Lipid Research Clinics Coronary Primary Prevention Trial (LRC-CPPT),[6,7] the results of which are reported in part I,[8] was designed to test this hypothesis. In the LRC-CPPT, despite only a moderate difference in mean TOTAL-C and LDL-C levels between the two treatment groups, the incidence of CHD (defined as definite CHD death and/or definite nonfatal myocardial infarction[6,8]) was 19% lower among men assigned to active treatment (P<.05). Trends toward lower incidence of CHD in treated subjects have also been observed in many other randomized trials,[9-17] al-

though no single one of these studies is convincing.[18-22]

In this article, the LRC-CPPT results are considered critically with respect to the quantitative impact of cholesterol lowering on CHD incidence. Specifically, the wide range of reductions in TOTAL-C and in LDL-C levels attained by persons treated with cholestyramine resin is used to relate the degree of cholesterol reduction to incidence of CHD. The relationship of changes in TG, HDL-C, and HDL-C/TOTAL-C levels to incidence of CHD is also examined. Such analyses, because they are not based on comparison of the randomly assigned treatment groups, may be influenced by extraneous factors related to adherence to medication. Nevertheless, these analyses may complement and illuminate the rigorous demonstration of treatment benefit presented in the accompanying article[8] by addressing the following specific questions: (1) Was CHD incidence within the cholestyramine group related to the degree of reduction in TOTAL-C and LDL-C levels? (2) Did differences in CHD incidence among men with differing degrees of cholesterol reduction arise from an underlying "dose-response" relationship or from self-selection? (3) Might cholestyramine resin also have modified CHD risk by its effect on HDL-C or TG levels? (4) Are the LRC-CPPT results internally consistent? (5) Are the LRC-CPPT results consistent with those of observational studies and other clinical trials of cholesterol lowering?

From the Lipid Metabolism–Atherogenesis Branch, National Heart, Lung, and Blood Institute, Bethesda, Md.

Reprint requests to Lipid Metabolism–Atherogenesis Branch, National Heart, Lung, and Blood Institute, Federal 401, Bethesda, MD 20205 (Basil M. Rifkind, MD).

METHODS
The Study Design

In the LRC-CPPT, the incidence of CHD (definite CHD death and/or definite nonfatal myocardial infarction) in hypercholesterolemic men treated with cholestyramine resin and diet was compared with that in similar men treated with placebo and diet. The trial, its participants, and its main findings are described elsewhere in detail.[6,8]

Estimation of Adherence to Medication

Cholestyramine resin was dispensed in sealed packets, each containing 4 g of the active medication. Placebo was dispensed in similar packets. Adherence to the prescribed dosage (six packets per day) was estimated from the number of packets returned by each participant at bimonthly visits (the packet count).[8]

Measurement of Plasma Lipid and Lipoprotein Levels

Fasting plasma levels of TOTAL-C, TG, and HDL-C were measured at each clinic on a bimonthly basis.[23] Posttreatment levels were expressed as percent changes (%Δ) from the participant's baseline (prediet) level.[8]

Missing Data

Complete bimonthly data were required for packet count, TOTAL-C, LDL-C, HDL-C, and TG for every participant up to the occurrence of a primary end point or the end of follow-up, whichever came first. Because of the occasional failure of participants to attend clinic, return unused packets of medication, or fast for 12 hours, as well as infrequent laboratory problems, this information was sometimes incomplete. Missing values of these variables were, therefore, imputed by methods described in the "Appendix". Because this imputation assumed that protracted absences from clinic implied nonadherence to medication and return to baseline lipid levels, the estimates of mean adherence, %ΔTOTAL-C, %ΔLDL-C, %ΔHDL-C, and %ΔTG reported herein are slightly smaller than those reported in the companion article, in which no imputation was done.[8]

Statistical Methods

Year-by-Year Descriptive Tabulation.— The 155 men in the cholestyramine group who had a primary CHD end point were subdivided into cohorts according to the year of follow-up that included their final scheduled clinic visit before their respective CHD events (see "Appendix"). The mean %ΔLDL-C for each cohort of cases was compared with that of men without a primary CHD end point for the concurrent and each prior follow-up year. For example, first-year cases were compared with noncases only in the first year of follow-up, while seventh-year cases were compared with noncases in each of the first seven years of follow-up. To control for potentially confounding baseline inequalities in CHD risk factors between cases and noncases, the mean %ΔLDL-C for each cohort was covariance adjusted[24] for baseline measures of LDL-C, HDL-C, TG, age, systolic blood pressure, cigarettes smoked daily, and exercise test outcome. Separate computations were performed for each follow-up year.

Proportional Hazards Models.—The proportional hazards model of Cox[25] was used to quantify the parameters relating changes in lipid levels to incidence of CHD within each treatment group. In this method, CHD events are first ordered by the time of occurrence during follow-up. At the time of each successive event, a pre-event characteristic of the CHD case (eg, his %ΔLDL-C) is compared with those of all men in his treatment group known to be free of CHD at the same follow-up time. A standard statistical package was used to fit each model.[26] Adjustment for pretreatment inequalities between men who did and did not have a CHD event was accomplished by including covariance terms for baseline measures of LDL-C, HDL-C, TG, age, systolic blood pressure, cigarettes smoked daily, and exercise test outcome in each model. Since it is unlikely that modifying plasma lipid levels alters CHD risk instantaneously, the models reported in this article were based on averages of %ΔTOTAL-C, %ΔLDL-C, etc, for the two years immediately preceding the CHD event. Similar models, based on averages taken over two months, six months, one year, three years, and five years, gave equivalent results and are not reported herein.

Computation of Percent Risk Reduction for Strata of %ΔLDL-C

To examine the dependence of CHD incidence on the two-year average of %ΔLDL-C without assuming a specific mathematical model, the risk of CHD within strata of %ΔLDL-C was estimated and compared with a common reference level of risk. These strata were based on the distribution for all participants in each treatment group of the two-year average of %ΔLDL-C, evaluated at visits selected at random, one per participant, such that sampling probability was uniform over follow-up time. The distributions were divided into 5% intervals of %ΔLDL-C; the tails of each distribution, defined so as to contain at least 100 men, were each considered as single strata. Cases were placed within these strata according to their %ΔLDL-C averaged over the two years preceding their CHD events. The estimated CHD risk for each %ΔLDL-C stratum (ie, the number of cases divided by the number of men in the stratum) was compared with that of a hypothetical man in the cholestyramine group who experienced no change in LDL-C level. This latter reference level of risk was estimated by multiplying the risk of CHD in the cholestyramine group as a whole (155/1,906) by $\exp(-\beta \times \overline{\%\Delta LDL\text{-}C})$, where β and $\overline{\%\Delta LDL\text{-}C}$ are the proportional hazards coefficient and mean value, respectively, for %ΔLDL-C in the cholestyramine group. Covariance adjustment for baseline measures of LDL-C, HDL-C, TG, age, systolic blood pressure, cigarettes smoked daily, and exercise test outcome was used to eliminate potentially confounding inequalities between CHD cases and other participants.

Comparison With the Results of Other Clinical Trials of Cholesterol Lowering

Since life-table–based statistics were not reported for all studies and individual follow-up times were not available, percent reduction of CHD incidence (CHD death and/or myocardial infarction) in the active treatment group was defined as $100\% \times (1 - ad/bc)$, where a equals the number of incident CHD cases in the actively treated group, b equals the number of actively treated participants remaining free of CHD, c equals the number of incident CHD cases in the control group, and d equals the number of control participants remaining free of CHD. Treatment differentials in cholesterol levels were obtained by averaging annual mean levels in each treatment group over the years of follow-up. Since most studies did not measure lipoprotein levels, only TOTAL-C was considered. No correction was made for selection bias resulting from missing values of TOTAL-C for some participants. Methodological differences in cholesterol determination were also ignored.

RESULTS
Effect of Cholestyramine Resin on Plasma Lipid and Lipoprotein Levels

The response of plasma lipid and lipoprotein levels to treatment is summarized in Fig 1. The initial dietary intervention was associated in both groups with a 3.4% fall in TOTAL-C, a 3.8% fall in LDL-C, a 0.4% fall in HDL-C, and a 1% rise in TG levels as well as a 3.7% rise in HDL-C/TOTAL-C ratio. The introduction of cholestyramine resin was accompanied by additional falls of 14% in TOTAL-C and 21% in LDL-C levels during the first year of follow-

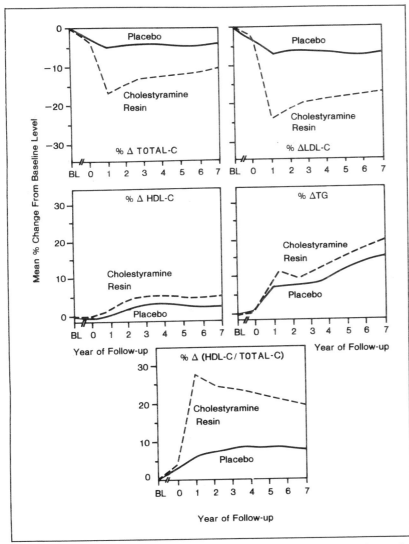

Fig 1.—Mean yearly plasma lipid levels for cholestyramine- and placebo-treated men. On abscissa, BL represents baseline (prediet) period and 0 years represents three-month interval between initiation of Lipid Research Clinics diet and study medication. Year 1 is average of visits 7 through 13, and each year thereafter represents average of six visits (see "Appendix"). Δ indicates change from baseline level; TOTAL-C, plasma total cholesterol levels; LDL-C, low-density lipoprotein cholesterol levels; TG, triglyceride levels; and HDL-C, high-density lipoprotein cholesterol.

up; slight falls were also observed in the placebo group during this year. Mean TOTAL-C and LDL-C levels rose slowly in the actively treated men in succeeding years, and the treatment differential gradually diminished to 6.5% in TOTAL-C and 9.6% in LDL-C by year 7. Mean HDL-C levels were consistently 3% higher in the cholestyramine group than in the placebo group (which also sustained a slight rise). Mean TG levels steadily increased over the course of the trial in both treatment groups and were consistently 2% to 4.5% higher in the cholestyramine group. A similar tendency of cholesty-

ramine resin to raise TG levels has been reported by others.[27] Cholestyramine therapy accounted for a 21% increment in HDL-C/TOTAL-C ratio in the first year of treatment and a 12% increment in the seventh year of treatment. Except in the case of TG, the differences between treatment groups in each year of treatment were significant ($P<.001$). Significant ($P<.05$) differences for TG were seen only for the first and fourth years.

Mean reported packet counts were relatively stable over the course of the trial. During the first year, the average daily packet count was 4.1 in the cholestyramine group and 4.7 in

the placebo group; these values fell to 3.6 and 4.4 packets per day, respectively, in year 7. The relationships of plasma lipid changes to packet count, averaged over seven years, are displayed in Table 1. With the exception of HDL-C, there was a clear dose-response relationship of each lipid and lipoprotein change to reported intake of cholestyramine resin. However, the relationship of %ΔTOTAL-C and %ΔLDL-C to packet count was not constant throughout the study. Men who attended clinic during the first year of treatment and reported an intake of at least 20 g of cholestyramine resin (five packets) daily showed mean falls of 23% in TOTAL-C and 33% in LDL-C levels from their (prediet) baseline levels. The same reported packet count was accompanied on the average by only a 17% fall in TOTAL-C and a 26% fall in LDL-C levels in the seventh year. These trends may indicate either that the drug lost some efficacy over time or that the packet count provided a progressively less reliable measure of drug intake.

Relationship of Lipid Changes and Adherence to CHD Incidence

Descriptive Tabulation.—The cholestyramine and placebo groups differed by 8.2% in mean %ΔTOTAL-C and by 12.0% in mean %ΔLDL-C, averaged over the entire trial. However, many participants in the cholestyramine group, especially those who took five or more packets of medication daily, sustained levels of TOTAL-C and LDL-C at least 25% and 35% below their respective baseline levels, while many others who adhered less well had little or no change. This wide range of decreases in TOTAL-C and LDL-C levels within the cholestyramine group provided an opportunity to study the relation between the degree of cholesterol lowering and the incidence of CHD. Furthermore, analysis of the placebo group, which contained adherent and nonadherent participants who differed little from each other with respect to changes in TOTAL-C and LDL-C levels, made it possible to investigate whether self-selection influenced this relationship.

Since the mean reduction of TOTAL-C and LDL-C levels tended to diminish with time in the cholestyramine group (Fig 1), it was appro-

Table 1.—Dose-Response Relationships of Lipid Level Changes to Packet Count*

Mean Daily Packet Count	N	%ΔTOTAL-C†	%ΔLDL-C†	%ΔHDL-C†	%Δ(HDL-C/TOTAL-C)	%ΔTG†
			Cholestyramine Resin			
0-1	294	−3.9	−6.6	+5.2	+10.8	+10.7
1-2	145	−5.4	−8.7	+2.3	+10.1	+12.7
2-3	135	−8.2	−13.1	+5.5	+17.2	+12.9
3-4	156	−11.1	−16.5	+6.0	+22.3	+14.2
4-5	205	−14.0	−20.9	+3.8	+23.5	+15.5
≥5	965	−19.0	−28.3	+4.3	+32.3	+17.1
			Placebo			
0-1	133	−3.2	−4.8	+2.8	+7.5	+8.9
1-2	79	−1.7	−3.6	+5.4	+8.5	+7.9
2-3	88	−4.0	−6.9	+5.4	+11.3	+9.7
3-4	105	−3.5	−6.3	+3.8	+8.4	+9.0
4-5	214	−4.1	−6.0	+1.8	+7.2	+11.3
≥5	1,274	−5.4	−8.4	+1.2	+8.2	+11.7

*As calculated until the occurrence of (1) death, (2) definite myocardial infarction, or (3) the completion of the seventh year of follow-up. Only those clinic visits at which packet counts and plasma lipid measurements were obtained were included in the computation; there was no imputation of missing data. Six cholestyramine-treated and seven placebo-treated participants did not attend clinic after the first month of follow-up and were not included in this tabulation.

†Δ indicates change from baseline level; TOTAL-C, plasma total cholesterol; LDL-C, low-density lipoprotein cholesterol; HDL-C, high-density lipoprotein cholesterol; and TG, triglyceride.

Table 2.—Mean Percent Change in LDL-C in Cholestyramine Resin–Treated Men With and Without a Primary Coronary Heart Disease (CHD) End Point*

Year of Visit Before CHD Event†	No. of Men	Year of Follow-up							
		1	2	3	4	5	6	7	+8
No CHD event‡	1,751	−24.9	−21.0	−19.9	−18.9	−18.4	−17.9	−16.9	−15.8
Year 1	32	−26.6	...	...	...	...	...	...	...
Year 2	19	−22.7	−16.9	...	...	...	...	...	...
Year 3	14	−14.2	−13.4	−12.9	...	...	...	...	...
Year 4	21	−12.7	−11.3	−7.7	−7.1	...	...	...	...
Year 5	17	−21.8	−14.7	−15.0	−15.7	−12.2	...	...	...
Year 6	12	−27.2	−23.7	−22.1	−19.1	−18.3	−18.5	...	...
Year 7	25	−21.2	−18.5	−17.0	−15.5	−14.6	−14.1	−10.1	...
Year 8+	13	−19.8	−12.0	−10.9	−13.2	−12.4	−10.9	−10.0	−5.8

*Adjusted for low-density lipoprotein cholesterol (LDL-C), high-density lipoprotein cholesterol, triglyceride, age, systolic blood pressure, cigarette smoking, and exercise test outcome at baseline (see "Methods" section).

†Grouped according to follow-up year of final clinic visit before CHD event (see "Methods" section). Two men with primary CHD end points in the first month of follow-up are not included in the tabulation.

‡Men who had no primary CHD event during the trial. Their number diminished slightly in successive follow-up years because of non-CHD death; 1,728 survived to the seventh year. Although the minimum length of follow-up was seven years, 1,437 participants were followed up for longer periods; 13 had CHD events.

priate to compare participants in whom CHD developed only with others who were at risk *at the same point of follow-up.* In Table 2, the 155 cholestyramine-treated men who had a primary CHD end point at some point in the trial were subdivided into cohorts according to the follow-up time at which their end point occurred (see "Methods" section). Each row in the Table (except the first) represents one such cohort. The mean levels of %ΔLDL-C (adjusted for seven baseline CHD risk factors, see "Methods" section) for each cohort during each year of follow-up before their CHD event were then compared with the yearly averages of

%ΔLDL-C for the cohort of men without a primary CHD end point. Note that, with the exception of the first-year and sixth-year cases, the CHD cases showed substantially smaller mean falls in LDL-C levels than did the men without CHD at every point of follow-up. By examining the diagonals of this table (upper left to lower right), one may note that these differences were often greatest during the one to two years immediately preceding each group of events. The absence of any effect for the first-year cases is not surprising, since one would not necessarily expect an immediate reduction of CHD risk when the LDL-C level is lowered. The

similarity of the sixth-year cases to CHD-free men with respect to %ΔLDL-C may be due to chance, since there were only 12 cases in this group. A similar tabulation of %ΔTO-TAL-C (not shown) gave essentially the same results. (This tabulation and similar ones for packet count and other lipids and lipoproteins in both treatment groups are available on request. All were consistent with the more concise analyses of two-year pre-event averages presented in the next section.)

Proportional Hazards Analysis.—To quantify more concisely how these variables are related to CHD and to assess more readily the statistical significance of these relationships, Cox proportional hazards models of two-year averages of packet count, %ΔTOTAL-C, %ΔLDL-C, %ΔHDL-C, %Δ(HDL-C/TOTAL-C), and %ΔTG were computed (Table 3). A positive regression coefficient implies that a decrease in the posttreatment variable is associated with lower CHD incidence; a negative coefficient implies an inverse relationship to CHD incidence. Adherence to cholestyramine resin but not to placebo, as measured by mean daily packet count, was associated with lower incidence of CHD. The relationships of decreases in TOTAL-C and LDL-C levels to reduction of CHD incidence in the cholestyramine group were both significant ($P<.001$). When terms for the two-year average of packet count and either %ΔTOTAL-C or %ΔLDL-C were included simultaneously in the same model, the term for either cholesterol change remained significant ($P<.001$) while the term for packet count was noncontributory ($P>.85$). Thus, there was no evidence for an effect of packet count on CHD incidence in the cholestyramine group other than that from the cholesterol-lowering effect of the drug.

The analysis also showed a relationship ($z=−1.81$) of increases in HDL-C levels to reduced incidence of CHD in the active drug group. When the coefficient for %ΔHDL-C was adjusted by including a term for %ΔLDL-C (or %ΔTOTAL-C) in the same model, neither coefficient changed appreciably. Thus, changes in LDL-C and HDL-C levels were related independently to incidence of CHD in the active drug group.

Reflecting the independent associations of %ΔHDL-C and %ΔTOTAL-C (or %ΔLDL-C) with CHD incidence, increases in HDL-C/TOTAL-C ratio were also strongly predictive of reduced incidence of CHD.

No association of lipid or lipoprotein changes with CHD was demonstrated in the placebo group. This result may reflect the inability of this type of analysis to detect an effect when changes in levels of TOTAL-C, LDL-C, etc, are not distributed over a sufficiently broad range. Although the regression coefficients for these variables in the placebo group were all smaller than their counterparts in the drug group, the differences between the corresponding drug and placebo coefficients were not statistically significant. Thus, there is insufficient evidence to demonstrate that %ΔLDL-C, for example, was related differently to CHD when it was produced by diet alone (placebo group) rather than the combination of diet and cholestyramine resin.

In Fig 2, the reduction in CHD risk estimated for strata based on 5% intervals of %ΔLDL-C (see "Methods" section) is compared with that predicted by the proportional hazards model. In view of the variability of the data points about the line representing the proportional hazards model in the cholestyramine group, the possibility of nonlinear (quadratic or cubic or both) effects was assessed; only the linear effect was significant. This finding tends to confirm the model's assumption of a log-linear relationship between CHD risk and %ΔLDL-C. In the range of %ΔLDL-C where sufficient data were available, similar reductions in CHD risk were observed in both treatment groups. However, since decreases of more than 25% in LDL-C levels were observed in only 3% of the placebo group (v 32% of the cholestyramine group), a linear trend is not readily demonstrable when the placebo group is considered alone. In the cholestyramine group, a 64% reduction in CHD risk was observed in the strata with decreases of more than 25% in LDL-C levels. The proportional hazards model for the cholestyramine group predicts a 49% reduction in CHD risk for a 35% decrease in LDL-C levels.

Application to Comparison of Treatment Groups

One may use the proportional hazards models to compare the observed 18.8% reduction in CHD incidence in the cholestyramine relative to the placebo group,[8] with the reduction one would expect based on the mean difference in TOTAL-C and LDL-C levels between the two treatment groups. In the models for the cholestyramine group, an 18.8% reduction in CHD incidence corresponds to a 7.9% decrease in TOTAL-C and a 10.8% decrease in LDL-C levels. The actual mean differences between the cholestyramine and placebo groups were 7.2% in TOTAL-C and 10.4% in LDL-C levels (based on two-year averages).

One may also use the proportional hazards models to analyze the separate contributions of changes in lipid levels and the lipoprotein cholesterol components to the observed treatment benefit (Table 4). The models for the cholestyramine group predict that the observed treatment differences of 7.2% in %ΔTOTAL-C and 10.4% in %ΔLDL-C should have brought about reductions of 17.1% and 18.1%, respectively, in CHD incidence in the cholestyramine v the placebo group. The 2.8% mean treatment difference in HDL-C levels, con-

Table 3.—Cox Proportional Hazards Models for Incidence of Coronary Heart Disease*

Postrandomization Variable	Cholestyramine Resin (155 Cases)		Placebo (187 Cases)	
	Regression Coefficient	z Score†	Regression Coefficient	z Score†
Mean daily packet count	−0.069	−1.79	−0.021	−0.53
ΔTOTAL-C‡	2.63	3.47	0.67	0.71
ΔLDL-C	1.92	3.37	0.70	0.93
ΔHDL-C	−1.15	−1.81	−0.25	−0.44
Δ(HDL-C/TOTAL-C)	−1.46	−3.64	−0.35	−0.78
ΔTG	0.14	0.63	0.06	0.24

*Each model contains a single postrandomization variable, averaged over the two years preceding each case's coronary heart disease event (see "Appendix"). Lipid changes (Δ) are expressed as proportions of baseline levels. Each model also contained terms for each of the following baseline covariates: low-density lipoprotein cholesterol (LDL-C), high-density lipoprotein cholesterol (HDL-C), triglyceride (TG), age, systolic blood pressure, cigarettes smoked daily, and exercise test outcome.
†The ratio of the regression coefficient and its SE. The one-sided and two-sided thresholds for statistical significance (P<.05) are |z|≥1.65 and 1.96, respectively.
‡TOTAL-C indicates plasma total cholesterol.

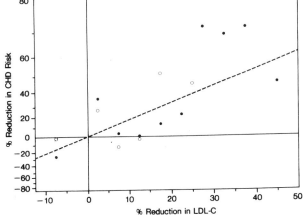

Fig 2.—Relationship of reduction in low-density lipoprotein cholesterol (LDL-C) levels to reduction in coronary heart disease (CHD) risk (logarithmic scale). Risk reduction was estimated by comparing distribution of percent change in LDL-C levels among CHD cases to that among all participants in same treatment group (see "Methods" section). Dashed line represents reduction in CHD risk predicted by proportional hazards model for given decrease in LDL-C level in cholestyramine group. Estimates of percent reduction in CHD risk for men in cholestyramine group (solid circles) and placebo (open circles) group with differing degrees of LDL-C level reduction are compared with this line. Each point (except those at either extreme) is plotted at center of 5% interval of percent change in LDL-C levels that it represents. Points for open-ended strata at extremes are plotted at their approximate median values of percent change in LDL-C levels.

Table 4.—Estimated Risk Reduction Predicted by Cox Proportional Hazards Models for Lipid Level Change

Model	Change From Baseline, %*		Cox Regression Coefficient†	Estimated Risk Reduction, %
	Cholestyramine Resin	Placebo		
	Single Response Variable			
%ΔTOTAL-C‡	−11.0	−3.8	2.63	17.1
%ΔLDL-C‡	−16.4	−6.0	1.92	18.1
%ΔHDL-C‡	+4.0	+1.2	−1.15	3.2
%ΔTG‡	+10.9	+8.8	0.14	−0.3
	Combined Response Variable			
%Δ(HDL-C/TOTAL-C)	+20.1	+6.3	−1.46	18.2
%ΔHDL-C	+4.0	+1.2	−1.07	20.2
%ΔLDL-C	−16.4	−6.0	1.88	

*Means of two-year averages calculated at a single randomly selected visit for each participant.
†For cholestyramine group.
‡Δ indicates change from baseline level; TOTAL-C, plasma total cholesterol; LDL-C, low-density lipoprotein cholesterol; HDL-C, high-density lipoprotein cholesterol; TG, triglyceride.

sidered alone, could explain only a 3.2% reduction in CHD risk in the cholestyramine group. When one examines the incremental effect of changes in HDL-C levels (above that of changes in LDL-C levels) by simultaneously including terms for %ΔHDL-C and %ΔLDL-C in the same model (Table 4, %ΔHDL-C and %ΔLDL-C under "Combined Response Variables"), the estimated reduction in CHD risk is 2.1% greater than when %ΔLDL-C is considered alone. The observed 13.8% treatment difference of %Δ(HDL-C/TOTAL-C) accounted for an 18.2% reduction in CHD incidence, about the same as that accounted for by the 10.4% difference in %ΔLDL-C. The observed 2.1% increase in TG levels in the cholestyramine v the placebo group had no apparent effect on CHD incidence.

COMMENT

The most important finding in this report is the strong and consistent association between intake of cholestyramine resin, lowering of plasma total and LDL cholesterol levels, and reduction of CHD risk. These results extend those that were reported in the companion article[8] by indicating that the reduced incidence of CHD in the cholestyramine group was mediated chiefly by cholesterol lowering.

Influence of Self-selection

Although the LRC-CPPT was a randomized experiment, the results reported herein are based on comparisons of men with differing levels of adherence and response to treatment

within the cholestyramine group. Because these levels were determined by the participant's behavior rather than the experimental design, these analyses could be vulnerable to the biases that may occur in any observational study. In the Coronary Drug Project, for example, a significant inverse relationship between mortality and adherence to placebo was reported.[28] This relationship, which the authors attributed to self-selection, was just as strong as that between mortality and adherence to an active drug (clofibrate) in their study.

Nevertheless, the relationship of changes in TOTAL-C and LDL-C levels to incidence of CHD among cholestyramine-treated men in the LRC-CPPT seems genuine for the following reasons.

1. No significant association was demonstrated between adherence to placebo and incidence of CHD.

2. When terms for packet count and %ΔTOTAL-C or %ΔLDL-C were included in the same proportional hazards model of CHD incidence, the coefficient for packet count was almost zero. This result implies that participants in the cholestyramine group who had high packet counts but little change in TOTAL-C or LDL-C levels had essentially the same incidence of CHD as those who did not take the drug at all.

3. All analyses were adjusted for baseline levels of the known major CHD risk factors. Thus, it is unlikely that the relationship reported herein could have arisen from differences in these risk factors between good and poor adherers that were present

before treatment began.

4. These relationships are quantitatively consistent with the observed difference (18.8%) in incidence of CHD between randomized treatment groups, given the differences that were obtained in TOTAL-C and in LDL-C levels. This latter result cannot be attributed to selection bias, since it was derived by comparing the treatment groups as initially, randomly assigned.

Internal Consistency of LRC-CPPT Results

The internal consistency of the LRC-CPPT results is illustrated by considering three ways of estimating the reduction in CHD risk associated with a 22.3-mg/dL (10.4%) decrement in LDL-C levels, the mean treatment differential (based on two-year averages) actually attained in the LRC-CPPT (Table 5). (1) When the relationship of baseline LDL-C level to subsequent CHD was examined in the placebo group, a 22.3-mg/dL decrement predicted a 16.0% reduction in incidence of CHD. (2) Within the cholestyramine group, a 22.3-mg/dL fall in LDL-C level during treatment was associated with a 17.2% reduction in incidence of CHD. (3) A mean 22.3-mg/dL difference in %ΔLDL-C between the cholestyramine- and placebo-treatment groups was associated with an 18.8% difference in their incidence of CHD.

The consistency of these three distinct estimates is impressive.

External Consistency: Observational Studies

The quantitative estimate of the reduction in CHD incidence for a given decrement in baseline TOTAL-C levels in the LRC-CPPT placebo group is also consistent with the findings of observational studies of men in the same age range. In Table 6, the findings of the five component studies of the Pooling Project examined by the Framingham investigators[29] and of the Seven Countries Study[2] are compared with the LRC-CPPT placebo group. Six of the studies predict an 11% to 19% reduction in CHD incidence for a 20.7-mg/dL decrement in TOTAL-C levels, with the LRC-CPPT, at 15.1%, falling in the middle of this range. Only the results of the two smallest studies, the Chica-

Table 5.—Internal Consistency of Lipid Research Clinics Coronary Primary Prevention Trial (LRC-CPPT) Results

LRC-CPPT Treatment Group	LDL-C* Determination	Study Design	Reduction in CHD* Incidence per 22.3 mg/dL Decrement in LDL-C Levels, %
Placebo	Baseline	Observational	16.0†
Cholestyramine resin	Change from baseline (two-year average)	Observational	17.2†
Both (cholestyramine resin v placebo)	Treatment difference (two-year average)	Experiment (comparison of randomized treatment groups)	18.8‡

*LDL-C indicates low-density lipoprotein cholesterol; CHD, coronary heart disease.
†Based on proportional hazards models containing terms for LDL-C, high-density lipoprotein cholesterol, triglyceride, age, systolic blood pressure, cigarette smoking, and exercise stress test outcome at baseline. The model for cholestyramine resin also contained a term for the two-year average of change (in milligrams per deciliter) of LDL-C from its baseline level.
‡Based on stratified life-table analysis.[8]

Table 6.—Multiple Logistic Coefficients* for a Single Determination of Total Cholesterol as Predictor of First Myocardial Infarction or Coronary Heart Disease (CHD) Death (Males)

Study	N	Mean Years of Follow-up	Age, yr	Mean TOTAL-C	Regression Coefficient	Reduction in CHD Incidence per 20.7-mg/dL Decrement in TOTAL-C, %†
Framingham[29]	1,089	11.5	40-54	226.5	0.0068	13.1
Albany[29]	1,675	9.9	40-54	229.1	0.0080	15.2
Chicago (Gas)[29]	934	9.7	40-54	237.5	0.0048	9.4
Chicago (Western Electric)[29]	1,806	8.5	40-54	247.7	0.0057	11.1
Tecumseh[29]	563	8.0	40-54	230.5	0.0197	33.5
US railroad (Seven Countries)[2]	2,404	5.0	40-59	239.3	0.009	17.0
Europe (Seven Countries)[2]	8,728	5.0	40-59	211.4	0.010	18.7
LRC-CPPT (placebo)	1,900	7.4	35-59	293.7	0.0079	15.1

*The coefficients of all eight studies were covariance adjusted for systolic blood pressure and cigarette smoking. Those for the Seven Countries populations were also adjusted for age and body mass index. The coefficient for the Lipid Research Clinics Coronary Primary Prevention Trial (LRC-CPPT) was based on a proportional hazards rather than a logistic model and was adjusted for age, high-density lipoprotein cholesterol, triglyceride, and exercise test outcome at baseline, as well as smoking and systolic blood pressure.
†The mean difference in plasma total cholesterol (TOTAL-C) levels (two-year average) between the LRC-CPPT cholestyramine and placebo group.

go Gas and Tecumseh studies, fall outside this range.

External Consistency: Other Clinical Trials

Many other trials of cholesterol lowering have been reported since the early 1960s.[9-17] It is difficult to compare or summarize their results because of differences in their design (eg, sample size and composition, primary v secondary prevention, treatment modality, assignment to treatment groups, end point, and length and completeness of follow-up) and in how they reported their findings. However, one can make a meaningful assessment of the consistency of the LRC-CPPT with other studies sharing at least the following features: (1) Subjects were assigned randomly to

either an active treatment or control group. (2) Results for the combined end point CHD death and/or nonfatal myocardial infarction were reported. (3) Posttreatment mean TOTAL-C levels were reported. (4) The study protocol incorporated no co-intervention with respect to potential nonlipid CHD risk factors, such as smoking, blood pressure, exercise, and sex hormone levels. (5) At least 100 subjects were assigned to each treatment group. (6) The study was planned to last at least three years, so as to allow a reasonable time for the hypothesized benefit of lipid lowering to take effect. (7) The CHD status of all (or almost all) randomized subjects was known at the end of the study.

Some important studies that did not meet one or more of these criteria

(given in parentheses for each study) and were therefore excluded from further analysis herein are the estrogen trials of Stamler et al[30] and the Coronary Drug Project[31,32] (No. 3 and 4), the Upjohn colestipol study[33] (No. 6 and 7), the Finnish Mental Hospital study[34] (No. 1), the nicotinic acid–clofibrate combined therapy report of Rosenhamer and Carlson[35] (No. 7), the Oslo study of diet and smoking cessation[36] (No. 4), the Multiple Risk Factor Intervention Trial[37] (No. 2 and 4), and the National Heart, Lung, and Blood Institute (NHLBI) Type II Coronary Intervention Study[38] (No. 2 and 5).

The studies (including the LRC-CPPT) that did meet all seven criteria are summarized in Table 7 (see "Methods" section). Note that eight were secondary prevention studies, while three were essentially primary prevention studies. Seven studies employed cholesterol-lowering drugs, while four used only diet. Two studies included a small proportion (~20%) of women among their participants;[11,12] the remainder were restricted to men. Most of these trials did not report a statistically "significant" treatment benefit with respect to their predefined primary end point. However, the calculated reductions in CHD incidence demonstrate beneficial trends in nine of the 11 studies.

The overall consistency of these studies with respect to the effect of TOTAL-C on incidence of CHD, despite their methodological differences, may be illustrated graphically[21] by adopting the approach of Peto (Fig 3). The results of eight of the 11 studies in Table 7 (including the LRC-CPPT) fit the regression line based on proportional hazards analysis of CHD incidence *within the LRC-CPPT cholestyramine group*. This regression line, in turn, agrees closely with Peto's regression lines, which project 15.3% (for diet) and 20.9% (for drug) reductions in CHD incidence per 10% decrement in TOTAL-C level. Only the dextrothyroxine arm of the Coronary Drug Project,[14] in which the adverse trend was attributed by the investigators to drug-specific cardiotoxic effects; the Newcastle clofibrate trial,[11] in which the incidence of CHD in the placebo group was unusually high; and the London Medical Research Council Low Fat Diet Study,[15] which because of small sample size

Table 7.—Randomized Trials of Cholesterol Lowering and Coronary Heart Disease (CHD)								
			Treatment Group			Control Group		Reduction in CHD Incidence, %§
Trial	Mode of Intervention	Years of Follow-up*	N	Mean TOTAL-C†	No. of CHD Cases‡	N	Mean TOTAL-C†	No. of CHD Cases‡	
Primary prevention									
A. LRC-CPPT*‖	Cholestyramine resin	7	1,906	251	155	1,900	276	187	18.9
B. World Health Organization⁹	Clofibrate	5	5,331	224¶	167	5,296	244¶	208	20.9
C. Los Angeles Veterans Administration¹⁰#	Diet	8	424	195	52	422	226	65	28.2
Secondary prevention									
D. Newcastle¹¹	Clofibrate	5	244	227	54	253	253	85	48.6
E. Edinburgh¹²	Clofibrate	6	350	227	59	367	263	79	26.1
F. Coronary Drug Project (CDP)—clofibrate¹³	Clofibrate	5	1,103	235	309	2,789	251	839	9.5
G. CDP—nicotinic acid¹³	Nicotinic acid	5	1,119	226	287	2,789	251	839	19.8
H. CDP—dextrothyroxine¹⁴	Dextrothyroxine	5	1,083	226	197	2,715	255	449	−12.2
I. London Medical Research Council (MRC) Low-Fat Diet¹⁵	Diet	3	123	219	46	129	240	48	−0.8
J. London MRC—soya bean oil¹⁶	Diet	4	199	224	45	194	258	51	18.1
K. Oslo Diet—heart¹⁷	Diet	5	206	240	61	206	284	81	35.1

*Length of follow-up specified in study design. Because of the finite time required for recruitment, not every surviving participant was followed up for the specified times. Study H was halted after approximately three years, two years before the planned termination, because of evidence that treatment may have had adverse effects. For studies I and J, mean follow-up time is listed since the authors did not state how long they initially intended to follow up their participants.

†Average of annual posttreatment levels for participants attending clinic. TOTAL-C indicates plasma total cholesterol.

‡Definite nonfatal myocardial infarction or CHD death.

§Obtained by subtracting the odds ratio from unity and multiplying by 100% (see "Methods" section).

‖LRC-CPPT indicates Lipid Research Clinics Coronary Primary Prevention Trial.

¶Adjusted to the Edinburgh laboratory by use of conversion factors published by investigators.¹⁴

#Since 7.1% of its subjects had a prior myocardial infarction, this was not a pure primary prevention trial.

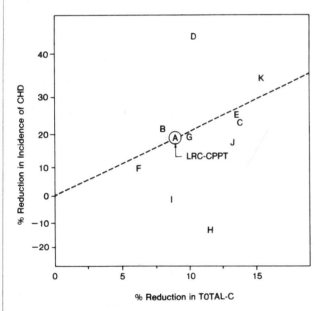

Fig 3.—Comparison of results of 11 cholesterol-lowering trials (indexed in Table 7) with experience of Lipid Research Clinics Coronary Primary Prevention Trial (LRC-CPPT) cholestyramine group. Percent reduction in coronary heart disease (CHD) incidence (logarithmic scale) observed between actively treated and control group in each trial is plotted v mean difference in plasma total cholesterol (TOTAL-C) levels (expressed as percent of mean level for control group) resulting from treatment (see "Methods" section). Reduction in CHD incidence predicted by proportional hazards model for given decrease in TOTAL-C levels within LRC-CPPT cholestyramine group is indicated by dashed line. Slope of this line has been adjusted by factor 7.14/8.99 to compensate for imputation procedure used in computing two-year averages (see "Appendix"). Numerator and denominator of this adjustment factor are mean percent differences in TOTAL-C levels between LRC-CPPT treatment groups estimated with and without imputation, respectively.

and short follow-up time had little statistical power, were outliers. The observed difference in CHD incidence between the two LRC-CPPT treatment groups is in close accord both with the regression line derived for the cholestyramine group (internal consistency) and with the mainstream of the results of comparable studies (external consistency).

Changes in HDL-C and CHD Incidence

Increases in HDL-C levels among cholestyramine-treated participants were associated with an additional reduction of CHD risk beyond that arising from reduction in LDL-C levels. This result is qualitatively similar to the findings of the NHLBI Type

II Coronary Intervention Study, a secondary prevention trial that used the same drug but a somewhat more rigid diet and a different outcome measure (angiographic assessment of change in coronary artery disease) and that also reported a treatment benefit.³⁸ Changes in HDL-C levels seemed to be responsible for a larger portion of the treatment benefit in the latter study than in the LRC-CPPT, wherein the average treatment differential in HDL-C level was less than 3%. However, both studies found that the combination of changes in HDL-C and LDL-C levels, expressed as a ratio of HDL-C to TOTAL-C or LDL-C, was sufficient to explain the observed benefit of cholestyramine treatment.

Clinical Implications

Although the average CHD risk reduction observed in the LRC-CPPT may seem relatively modest, this reduction was attained with a mean treatment differential of only 8% in TOTAL-C and 12% in LDL-C levels. However, LDL-C levels typically fell by 35% in LRC-CPPT participants taking the prescribed 24 g of cholestyramine resin daily. If such a response were sustained, a 49% reduction of CHD incidence would be predicted (Fig 2). The inability of randomized long-term trials, especially those that were blinded, to maintain overall response at such levels over a period of years does not imply that this degree of cholesterol

change cannot be maintained when a patient and his or her physician know posttreatment lipid levels and are able to modify treatment and dosage accordingly. The LRC-CPPT results and those of similar trials thus suggest that the risk of an initial CHD episode in hypercholesterolemic middle-aged men can be reduced by half with currently available appropriate cholesterol-lowering agents and diets.

CONCLUSIONS

The LRC-CPPT results give a clear and consistent picture of the relationship of its primary end point, CHD incidence, to changes in cholesterol levels. Whether one (1) examines baseline data prospectively, (2) relates posttreatment cholesterol change, or (3) compares the cholestyramine and placebo groups as randomly assigned, the result is the same: a decrement of 22.3 mg/dL (10.4%) in LDL-C levels is associated with a 16% to 19% reduction in CHD risk (internal consistency). The results of observational studies and other trials of cholesterol lowering,

including those of secondary as well as primary prevention of CHD and those of diet as well as drugs, are consistent with this finding (external consistency). The predicted and observed CHD incidence in men maintaining a 25% fall in TOTAL-C or a 35% fall in LDL-C levels, responses often achieved by men taking 24 g of cholestyramine resin daily, was about half that of men with no cholesterol lowering. Thus, the benefit of effective cholesterol-lowering therapy in men with type II hyperlipoproteinemia with regard to incidence of CHD is of great potential clinical as well as statistical significance.

Funding for the study came from the following National Heart, Lung, and Blood Institute contracts and interagency agreements: N01-HV1-2156-L, N01-HV1-2160-L, N01-HV2-2914-L, N01-HV3-2931-L, Y01-HV3-0010-L, N01-HV2-2913-L, N01-HV1-2158-L, N01-HV1-2161-L, N01-HV2-2915-L, N01-HV2-2932-L, N01-HV2-2917-L, N01-HV2-2916-L, N01-HV1-2157-L, N01-HV1-2243-L, N01-HV1-2159-L, N01-HV3-2961-L, and N01-HV6-2941-L.

The Lipid Research Clinics Program acknowledges the long-term commitment of the volunteer participants in this clinical trial. The list of key personnel in the Lipid Research Clinics Coronary Primary Prevention Trial appears at the end of part I.

References

1. Pooling Project Research Group: Relationship of blood pressure, serum cholesterol, smoking habit, relative weight, and ECG abnormalities to incidence of major coronary events: Final report of the pooling project. *J Chronic Dis* 1978;31:201-306.
2. Keys A, Aravanis C, Blackburn H, et al: Probability of middle-aged men developing coronary heart disease in five years. *Circulation* 1972;45:815-828.
3. Gordon T, Castelli WP, Hjortland MC, et al: High density lipoprotein as a protective factor against coronary heart disease: The Framingham Study. *Am J Med* 1977;62:707-714.
4. Heiss G, Johnson NJ, Reiland S, et al: The epidemiology of plasma high density lipoprotein cholesterol levels: The Lipid Research Clinics Program Prevalence Study: Summary. *Circulation* 1980;62(suppl 4):116-136.
5. Lippel K, Tyroler HA, Eder H, et al: Meeting summary: Relationship of hypertriglyceridemia to atherosclerosis. *Arteriosclerosis* 1981;1:406-417.
6. The Lipid Research Clinics Program: The Coronary Primary Prevention Trial: Design and implementation. *J Chronic Dis* 1979;32:609-631.
7. The Lipid Research Clinics Program: Pre-entry characteristics of participants in the Lipid Research Clinics Coronary Primary Prevention Trial. *J Chronic Dis* 1983;36:467-479.
8. Lipid Research Clinics Program: The Lipid Research Clinics Coronary Primary Prevention Trial Results: I. Reduction in incidence of coronary heart disease. *JAMA* 1984;251:351-364.
9. Committee of Principal Investigators, WHO Clofibrate Trial: A cooperative trial in the primary prevention of ischaemic heart disease using clofibrate. *Br Heart J* 1978;40:1069-1118.
10. Dayton S, Pearce ML, Hashimoto S, et al: A controlled clinical trial of a diet high in unsaturated fat in preventing complications of

atherosclerosis. *Circulation* 1969;40(suppl 2):1-63.
11. Group of Physicians of the Newcastle Upon Tyne Region: Trial of clofibrate in the treatment of ischaemic heart disease. *Br Med J* 1971;4:767-775.
12. Research Committee of the Scottish Society of Physicians: Ischaemic heart disease: A secondary prevention trial using clofibrate. *Br Med J* 1971;4:775-784.
13. Coronary Drug Project Research Group: Clofibrate and niacin in coronary heart disease. *JAMA* 1975;231:360-381.
14. Coronary Drug Project Research Group: The Coronary Drug Project: Findings leading to further modifications of its protocol with respect to dextrothyroxine. *JAMA* 1972;220:996-1008.
15. Research Committee to the Medical Research Council: Low-fat diet in myocardial infarction—a controlled trial. *Lancet* 1965;2:501-504.
16. Research Committee to the Medical Research Council: Controlled trial of soya-bean oil in myocardial infarction. *Lancet* 1968;2:693-700.
17. Leren P: The Oslo Diet Heart Study: Eleven-year report. *Circulation* 1970;42:935-942.
18. Cornfield J, Mitchell S: Selected risk factors in coronary disease: Possible intervention effects. *Arch Environ Health* 1969;19:382-391.
19. Davis CE, Havlik RJ: Clinical trials of lipid lowering and coronary artery disease prevention, in Rifkind B, Levy R (eds): *Hyperlipidemia—Diagnosis and Therapy*. New York, Grune & Stratton Inc, 1977, pp 79-92.
20. Oliver MF: Coronary heart disease prevention: Trials using drugs to control hyperlipidemia, in Miller NE, Lewis B (eds): *Lipoproteins, Atherosclerosis, and Coronary Heart Disease*. Amsterdam, Elsevier North Holland Biomedical Press, 1981, pp 165-195.
21. Mann JI, Marr JW: Coronary heart disease

prevention: Trials of diets to control hyperlipidemia, in Miller NE, Lewis B (eds): *Lipoproteins, Atherosclerosis, and Coronary Heart Disease*. Amsterdam, Elsevier North Holland Biomedical Press, 1981, pp 197-210.
22. May GS, Eberlein KA, Furberg CD, et al: Secondary prevention after myocardial infarction: A review of long-term trials. *Prog Cardiovasc Dis* 1982;24:331-352.
23. *Manual of Laboratory Operations: Lipid Research Clinics Program: I. Lipid and Lipoprotein Analysis*, Dept of Health, Education, and Welfare publication (NIH) 75-628. National Institutes of Health, 1974.
24. Kleinbaum DG, Kupper LL: *Applied Regression Analysis and Other Multivariate Methods*. North Scituate, Mass, Duxbury Press, 1978, pp 210-213.
25. Cox DR: Regression models and life tables. *J R Stat Soc B* 1972;34:187-220.
26. Dixon WJ (ed): *BMDP Statistical Software*. Los Angeles, University of California Press, 1981, pp 576-594.
27. Levy RI, Fredrickson DS, Stone NJ, et al: Cholestyramine in type II hyperlipoproteinemia: A double blind trial. *Ann Intern Med* 1973; 79:51-58.
28. Coronary Drug Project Research Group: Influence of adherence to treatment and response of cholesterol on mortality in the Coronary Drug Project. *N Engl J Med* 1980; 303:1038-1041.
29. McGee D, Gordon T: The results of the Framingham Study applied to four other U.S.-based epidemiologic studies of cardiovascular disease, in Kannel WB, Gordon T (eds): *The Framingham Study: An Epidemiologic Investigation of Cardiovascular Disease*, Dept of Health, Education, and Welfare publication (NIH) 76-1083. National Institutes of Health, 1976.

30. Stamler J, Pick R, Katz LN, et al: Effectiveness of estrogens for therapy of myocardial infarction in middle-aged men. *JAMA* 1963; 183:632-638.

31. Coronary Drug Project Research Group: The Coronary Drug Project: Initial findings leading to modifications of its research protocol. *JAMA* 1970;214:1303-1313.

32. Coronary Drug Project Research Group: The Coronary Drug Project: Findings leading to discontinuation of the 2.5 mg estrogen group. *JAMA* 1973;226:652-657.

33. Dorr AE, Gundersen K, Schneider JC, et al: Colestipol hydrochloride in hypercholesterolemic patients: Effect on serum cholesterol and mortality. *J Chronic Dis* 1978;31:5-14.

34. Turpeinen O, Karvonen MJ, Pekkarinen M, et al: Dietary prevention of coronary heart disease: The Finnish Mental Hospital Study. *Int J Epidemiol* 1979;8:99-118.

35. Rosenhamer G, Carlson LA: Effect of combined clofibrate nicotinic acid treatment in ischemic heart disease: An interim report. *Atherosclerosis* 1980;37:129-138.

36. Hjermann I, Velve Byre K, Holme I, et al: Effect of diet and smoking intervention on the incidence of coronary heart disease: Report from the Oslo Study Group of a randomized trial in healthy men. *Lancet* 1981;2:1303-1310.

37. Multiple Risk Factor Intervention Trial Research Group: Multiple Risk Factor Intervention Trial: Risk factor changes and mortality results. *JAMA* 1982;248:1465-1477.

38. Levy RI: The influence of cholestyramine-induced lipid changes on coronary artery disease progression: The NHLBI Type II Coronary Intervention Study. *Circulation* 1983;68(suppl 3):188.

APPENDIX

Computation of Posttreatment Averages of Packet Count and Lipid Level Change

Since this article deals specifically with the relation of treatment and its effects on plasma lipid levels to incidence of coronary heart disease (CHD), two issues that are commonly not considered systematically in the descriptions of adherence and lipid levels in most clinical trials required explicit attention: (1) the handling of missing data and (2) the definition of the time frame over which one considers these variables. The mechanisms that were devised to deal with these issues are described as follows.

Missing Data.—After successfully completing five pretreatment evaluations, Lipid Research Clinics Coronary Primary Prevention Trial participants were scheduled for clinic visits at two weeks (visit 6) and four weeks (visit 7) after randomization and at bimonthly intervals thereafter. For a typical bimonthly visit, 80% to 95% of participants attended, returned their unused packets of medication, and had valid plasma lipid measurements performed. Perhaps half of the men with incomplete or missing data for a given visit were chronic absentees who were known not to take the study medication. Others simply missed an occasional visit or forgot to return their unused medication while adhering at their customary level. A small number of participants, who moved some distance away from the nearest lipid research clinic but continued to participate in the study, attended clinic at annual or semiannual intervals. To accommodate these different situations as well as possible, missing packet count and lipid data were imputed as follows.

1. When a sequence of five or fewer missed visits or visits with missing values of a particular variable was followed by a visit in which a measurement of that variable was recorded, that measured value was imputed for the entire sequence of missing values.

2. When a sequence of six or more missed visits or visits with such missing values was followed by a visit with a recorded value, that recorded value was imputed for the last five visits in the sequence. The variable was affixed at its baseline level (zero for packet count) for all previous visits in the sequence.

3. Baseline values were imputed for all open-ended sequences of at least two missed visits. When only the final visit was missed, the value of each variable for the next-to-last visits was imputed.

Thus, packet counts and plasma lipid levels obtained after absences of less than one year were assumed to represent the entire interval since the last clinic visit attended, while longer absences were assumed to contain periods of nonadherence. When this imputation process was complete, every participant had an unbroken sequence of packet counts and plasma lipid and lipoprotein values representing two-month intervals until he died, suffered a myocardial infarction, or completed his close-out visit in mid-1983.

Computation of Averages Over Time.—Although each clinic visit was supposed to occur within a fixed range of follow-up times, visits occasionally were completed well outside their target intervals. Computational considerations required that each clinic visit be specified to occur at exactly the same follow-up time for each participant. The median time was used for each visit—31 days for visit 7, 92 days for visit 8, etc, increasing by 61-day increments for successive visits. This approximation occasionally led to minor incongruities, such as not using visit 8 data for a man who died on day 91 even if he completed visit 8 on day 87 of follow-up. Since the full dosage of medication often was not prescribed immediately, packet count and lipid data obtained at visit 6 (two weeks after randomization) were not used.

Three kinds of averages were computed in this article.

1. For descriptive purposes (Fig 1, Table 2), one-year blocks of data were averaged. The first follow-up year (which actually contained 13 months) consisted of visits 7 through 13; visit 7, which represented only a month of follow-up, was given half weight. All other years contained six equally weighted bimonthly visits. Data for the final (partial) year of follow-up for participants who were followed up for a nonintegral number of years were included in these presentations.

2. In Table 1, averages were computed over a variable length of follow-up beginning with visit 7. All visits in the defined interval were averaged, with visit 7 again given half weight.

3. Elsewhere in this article, averages representing a constant period, usually two years, measured backward in time from a defined point of follow-up, such as the occurrence of a CHD event, were computed. In this averaging process, the three months between the introduction of the lipid research clinic diet and randomization were represented by the average of visits 3 through 5. Prediet baseline levels (see "Methods" section) were used when it was necessary to extrapolate back further than visit 2. For example, a man with TOTAL-C equaling 300 mg/dL at visit 2, 280 mg/dL at visits 3 through 5, and 240 mg/dL at visits 7 through 10, would have a two-year average TOTAL-C=

$$\frac{240 \times 7 + 280 \times 3 + 300 \times 14}{24 \text{ mo}} = 280 \text{ mg/dL}$$

at visit 10. Packet counts before randomization were, of course, affixed at zero.

Total and cardiovascular mortality in relation to cigarette smoking, serum cholesterol concentration, and diastolic blood pressure among black and white males followed up for five years

The Multiple Risk Factor Intervention Trial screening program provided an opportunity (1) to study the association of diastolic blood pressure level, serum cholesterol concentration, and cigarettes per day with all-cause and cause-specific mortality after 5 years among 23,490 black males and (2) to compare these associations with those observed among 325,384 white males. The relationship of serum cholesterol concentration and reported cigarettes per day to all-cause, coronary heart disease (CHD), and cerebrovascular disease mortality was similar for black and white males. Diastolic blood pressure was more positively associated with cerebrovascular disease death among black males than white males (p = 0.047) according to logistic regression analysis. The lower CHD mortality among black males compared to white males was most apparent among hypertensive males (diastolic blood pressure ≥90 mm Hg). The relative risk (black vs white) of CHD death adjusted for age, serum cholesterol concentration, and cigarettes per day was 0.69 for hypertensive males compared to 1.15 for nonhypertensive males (p = 0.012 for difference in relative risk estimates). These findings suggest that the causes of CHD and cerebrovascular disease may be different for black and white males, particularly in regard to how these disease processes relate to blood pressure. (Am Heart J 108:759, 1984.)

James D. Neaton, M.S., Lewis H. Kuller, M.D., D.P.H., Deborah Wentworth, M.P.H., and Nemat O. Borhani, M.D.*
Minneapolis, Minn., Pittsburgh, Pa., and Davis, Calif.

From the Division of Biometry, University of Minnesota School of Public Health, Minneapolis, the Department of Epidemiology, University of Pittsburgh Graduate School of Public Health, Pittsburgh, and the Department of Community Health, School of Medicine, University of California, Davis.

Supported by National Institutes of Health grant No. 1-RO1-HL28715-01.

Reprint requests: James D. Neaton, M.S., 2829 University Ave. S.E., Suite 508, Minneapolis, MN 55414.

*For the Multiple Risk Factor Intervention Trial Research Group.

The relationship of diastolic blood pressure level, serum cholesterol concentration, and cigarette smoking to cardiovascular disease (CVD), coronary heart disease (CHD) death and incidence, and all-cause mortality among white males has been well documented in several large epidemiologic studies both in the United States and internationally.[1-4] The data for black males are less well established,[5-7] and

759

September, 1984
American Heart Journal

therefore any black-white differences in risk factor associations with all-cause and cause-specific mortality are difficult to assess. It is not clear whether the greater CVD mortality among black males in comparison to white males, particularly death from cerebrovascular disease, results from the increased prevalence of hypertension among blacks or whether for a given blood pressure level a black male is at a greater risk of CVD than a white male. Furthermore, a paradoxical situation has been noted in comparisons of CHD mortality for black and white males. Although the prevalence of hypertension is substantially greater among blacks, the CHD death rate is similar to, or actually lower than, the death rate for white males.[8,9] This raises the question of whether the relationship between blood pressure level and subsequent CHD mortality is different for black and white males.

The purpose of this investigation is to examine the association of these risk factors with death from CVD, particularly CHD and cerebrovascular disease, and from all causes after 5 years, in white and black middle-aged males screened for eligibility in the Multiple Risk Factor Intervention Trial (MRFIT).[10] The difference between white and black males in the relationship of each of the risk factors to cause-specific and all-cause mortality is examined, and the extent to which differences in mortality rates between black and white males depend on differences in the distribution of diastolic blood pressure, serum cholesterol concentration, and cigarette smoking is assessed.

METHODS

The study population consisted of 361,662 males initially screened in a national study of CHD prevention, the MRFIT. The data collection and screening methods used have recently been reported[11] and are summarized only briefly here. The purpose of the initial screening visit was to define eligibility for the trial on the basis of three risk factors—diastolic blood pressure level, serum cholesterol concentration, and number of cigarettes smoked per day—and to recognize certain major exclusion criteria. The males screened were 35 to 57 years of age and volunteered for screening examinations in 18 U.S. cities at 22 MRFIT clinical centers. Screening began in November 1973 and ended in November 1975. The clinics began screening at different times, and the screening program at each clinic lasted 18 months on the average. Males were recruited for the initial screening in a variety of ways. Most centers used several methods, including house-to-house canvasing, and screened government or industrial employee populations, civic groups, unions, and church groups.

Blood pressure was measured according to a standardized protocol by certified technicians. The first and fifth Korotkoff phases were recorded as the systolic and diastolic blood pressures. Three readings were taken with a standard mercury sphygmomanometer. The average of the second and third diastolic readings is used in this report. Serum cholesterol concentration was determined at one of 14 local laboratories using an AutoAnalyzer II.[12] A short questionnaire was given to determine the number of cigarettes smoked and to record demographic characteristics such as race (white, black, Oriental, American Indian, other), date of birth, and social security number. Information was also elicited concerning the following three criteria for exclusion: (1) expected movement from the area, (2) previous hospitalization of more than 2 weeks for "heart attack," and (3) prescription of medication for diabetes.

Mortality ascertainment and classification. The mortality status of all males screened through February 28, 1982, the same period of follow-up as that used with the randomized MRFIT group, is currently being ascertained from data provided by the Social Security Administration (SSA). The identification of deaths and the collection of death certificates are ongoing. The preliminary results reported here are derived from a data tape provided by the SSA, which contains information on U.S. deaths since 1962. The data provided on the tape consisted of social security number, last name, and month and year of death. Location of death was not provided. Deaths that occurred since 1974 and that matched MRFIT records of social security number and the first two letters of the last name were identified.

Since the location of death was not known, death certificates have initially been requested only from the state where the participant was screened. The death certificates were abstracted, checked for correct match, and coded by one of two trained nosologists using the ninth revision of the International Classification of Diseases (ICD).[13] Codes 390 to 459 are used to identify CVD deaths; codes 410 to 414 are used to identify deaths from CHD; and codes 430 to 438 are used to identify deaths from cerebrovascular disease.

Statistics. This report is restricted to males who identified themselves as black or white; participants who identified themselves as American Indian (0.1%), Oriental (1.2%), or other (0.4%) were excluded. Risk factor differences between white and black males were summarized by Student's t test for independent samples. A weighted risk factor difference was obtained after determining the black-white difference for each clinical center and weighting the difference inversely proportionally to its variance.[14]

The mortality data are presented as 5-year rates. When data are not presented for a specific age group, the direct method of standardization[15] is used to adjust for differences in the age distribution of the subgroups. The rates have been standardized to the age distribution of the total group of males screened. Cerebrovascular, CHD, and all-cause mortality rates are presented by quintile of serum cholesterol and diastolic blood pressure level. The approximate quintiles are determined with the use of the entire screened population and are presented from lowest (I) to highest (V). For the study of the association of cigarette smoking with all-cause and cause-specific mortality, participants are categorized as nonsmokers or as cigarette smokers using 1-15, 16-25, 26-35, or greater than 35 cigarettes per day.

Logistic regression analysis was used to study the joint relationship of age, serum cholesterol concentration, diastolic blood pressure level, and cigarettes smoked per day to CVD, CHD, cerebrovascular, and all-cause mortality for white and black males. This particular model was chosen for simplicity of comparison of black and white males and because of the large body of data demonstrating that this model fits endpoint data, such as those considered here, reasonably well. Other factors that might have been considered as candidates for confounding variables were not collected at the initial screening visit. Maximum likelihood estimates of the regression coefficients were obtained by discriminant function analysis for the initial estimates,[16] followed by Gauss-Newton iteration. The regression coefficients presented are unstandardized coefficients. To study whether the association of these risk factors with the mortality endpoints is similar for white and black males, we compared the regression coefficients from the prediction equations for white and black males. The test statistic used for this comparison is the difference between the regression coefficients divided by the standard error of the difference, that is, the square root of the sum of the variance estimates for the coefficients. For each endpoint the comparison is made for all black and white males, as well as for black and white males who reported at screening that they did not take medication for diabetes and had not been previously hospitalized for a heart attack. This restriction excluded 4.5% of black males and 2.9% of white males.

Comparisons of the 5-year rates for black and white males are summarized by relative risk estimates. Relative risk estimates are given as the risk of a black male's dying relative to (i.e., divided by) the risk of a white male's dying. The relative risk is estimated with the use of the crude 5-year rates (1) after adjustment for age, diastolic blood pressure, serum cholesterol concentration, and cigarettes smoked per day by the multiple logistic model with an indicator variable for race and (2) after adjustment for the aforementioned factors and clinical center by the Mantel-Haenzel method.[17] These latter two methods actually yield estimates of adjusted relative-odds ratios. The Mantel-Haenzel method gives a pooled-odds ratio that is a weighted estimate of the relative odds over the 352 2 × 2 tables that arise from the subclassification of participants into two categories each by age, serum cholesterol concentration, diastolic blood pressure, and cigarettes per day and into one of 22 clinics.

RESULTS

Completeness of mortality ascertainment and classification. To estimate the completeness of the death ascertainment, we compared the known mortality rate of the 12,866 males who participated in the

Table I. Risk factor levels by race for males screened in MRFIT (35 to 37 years of age)

	Black[*]		White[†]		Difference (weighted)
	Mean	SD	Mean	SD	
Age (yr)	45.4	6.3	46.1	6.4	−0.7 (−0.6)
Diastolic BP (mm Hg)	87.3	12.5	83.7	10.5	3.6 (3.3)
Serum cholesterol (mg/dl)	210.1	42.4	214.9	39.3	−4.8 (−3.9)
Percent smokers	50.0	—	35.9	—	14.1 (12.9)
Cigarettes per day (smokers)	18.5	10.6	26.9	13.3	−8.4 (−8.6)

SD = Standard deviation; BP = blood pressure.
[*]n = 23,490.
[†]n = 325,384.

clinical trial to that derived from the SSA data. Of 409 known deaths that occurred between 1974 and 1980, the SSA search correctly identified 359 (87.8%). Characteristics of the deaths identified by the SSA are compared to those not identified in an analysis performed by Wentworth et al.[18] Deaths among married males were more likely to be identified than deaths among nonmarried males. The percentage of deaths identified by the SSA increased steadily by year of death, with a range of 60.0% in 1974 to 95.4% in 1980. The differential ascertainment by marital status and year of death has been attributed to characteristics of the SSA files used. No differences in identification rates were found by age, race, diastolic blood pressure, serum cholesterol concentration, or number of cigarettes smoked. Alvey and Aziz[19] noted that on the basis of SSA data, the completeness of death reporting during 1975 was lower for black males (67%) than white males (82%). The difference between that investigation and the MRFIT experience may be due to the predominant use of employed populations for screening in the MRFIT.

Searching the SSA tapes for deaths among the 361,662 screenees yielded data on 6018 males who died within 5 years of their initial screening visit. Death certificates were obtained for 5180 of these deaths (86.1%). Thus, for this preliminary analysis, it is estimated that death certificates are available for 75.6% (0.878) (0.861) (100) of the deaths.

A comparison of the risk variables and other data collected at the initial screening visit of males for whose death a certificate was located and of males for whom the certificate was not located was also performed (not shown). The only difference identified was in the proportion of males who planned to move more than 50 miles away from the clinic at the time of screening. This was expected, since the

September, 1984
American Heart Journal

762 Neaton et al.

Table II. Number of deaths by cause for black and white males in the MRFIT

Cause of death (ICD-9)	Black males			White males		
	No.	Rate/1000	Percent*	No.	Rate/1000	Percent*
Total with death certificates	450	19.2	100.0	4602	14.1	100.0
All cardiovascular diseases	203	8.6	45.1	2226	6.8	48.4
Cerebrovascular diseases (430-438)	30	1.3	6.7	152	0.5	3.3
Myocardial infarction (410)	78	3.3	17.3	1225	3.8	26.6
Other ischemic heart disease (411-414)	29	1.2	6.4	483	1.5	10.5
Hypertensive heart disease (402)	17	0.7	3.8	26	0.1	0.6
Other hypertensive disease (401, 403-405)	1	0.0	0.2	7	0.0	0.1
Other cardiovascular disease (390-459 exclusive of above)	48	2.0	10.7	333	1.0	7.2
All noncardiovascular diseases	247	10.5	54.9	2376	7.3	51.6
Genitourinary diseases (580-629)	0	0.0	0.0	14	0.0	0.3
Diabetes mellitus (250)	5	0.2	1.1	37	0.1	0.8
Neoplastic diseases (140-239)	128	5.4	28.4	1440	4.4	31.3
Gastrointestinal diseases (520-579)	15	0.6	3.3	155	0.5	3.4
Respiratory diseases (460-519)	12	0.5	2.7	124	0.4	2.7
Infectious diseases (001-139)	4	0.2	0.9	16	0.0	0.3
Accidents, suicides, and homicides (800-999)	63	2.7	14.0	455	1.4	9.9
Other disease	20	0.9	4.4	135	0.4	2.9

*Percent of total number of deaths in racial group.

certificates were requested only from the state where the screening was performed. Data in computer-readable form will soon be available from the SSA on location of death; the outstanding death certificates will then be obtained.

To estimate the reliability of the death coding process, the two nosologists independently coded a 5% random sample of death certificates. The cause of death was found to be in agreement for 94.1% of the pairs.

Risk factor levels. The characteristics of black and white males seen at screen 1 are summarized in Table I. Of the 361,662 males seen at the initial screening visit, 23,490 (6.5%) were black and 325,384 (90.0%) were white. The percentage of blacks screened at the clinical centers ranged from less than 1% to approximately 30%. The weighted within-clinical-center difference, given in parentheses in Table I, is similar to the unadjusted difference for each risk factor. The age difference between white and black males is approximately 6 months, the white males being older. The average diastolic blood pressure is 3.3 mm Hg higher for black compared to white males. The average serum cholesterol concentration is 3.9 mg/dl lower for black participants compared to white participants. Among the black males screened, 50% reported smoking cigarettes; 35.9% of white males reported smoking cigarettes. The average number of cigarettes reported to be smoked by cigarette smokers also differed for black and white males. Black cigarette smokers reported smoking 18.5 cigarettes per day on

the average; white cigarette smokers reported smoking 26.9 cigarettes per day.

The difference between white and black males in diastolic blood pressure, serum cholesterol concentration, percentage of cigarette smokers, and number of cigarettes smoked by smokers did not vary by age (not shown).

Mortality results. Among the 23,490 black males, 532 deaths (22.6/1000) were identified through the 5-year follow-up period. For the 325,384 white males, 5340 deaths (16.4/1000) were identified. The ratio (black/white) of the crude 5-year death rates is 1.38. The number of deaths is approximately half that expected with the use of U.S. life tables.[20] Even after adjustment for the incomplete death ascertainment based on the SSA file, the number of deaths is substantially lower than one would expect on the basis of U.S. life tables. The discrepancy is thought to be due to the "healthy worker–volunteer effect."[21, 22] Since a major portion of the screening was done at places of employment, males had to be sufficiently healthy to attend and participate in the screening.

The distribution of the causes of death for black and white males is given in Table II. The number of males dying from each cause is expressed for each racial group as a rate per 1000 and as a percentage of the total number of deaths for which a death certificate was obtained. Within the CVD classification, the CHD mortality rate is lower for black males, and the death rate from cerebrovascular disease is almost three times higher for black males

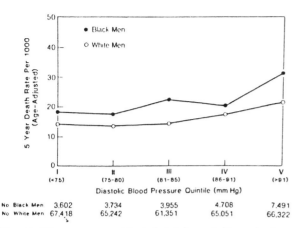

Fig. 1. Five-year age-adjusted total mortality rate (per 1000) by diastolic blood pressure level by race.

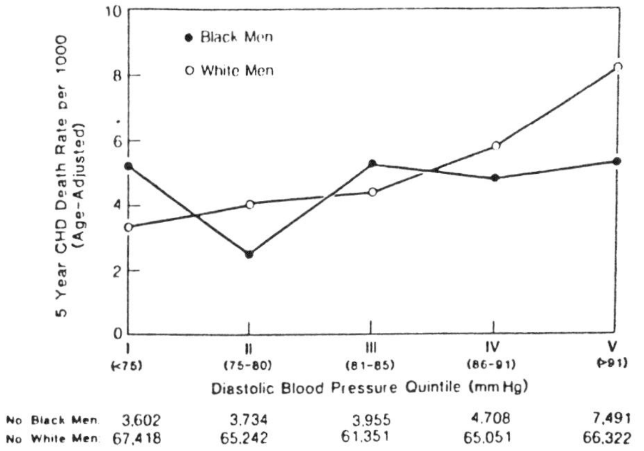

Fig. 2. Five-year age-adjusted CHD mortality rate (per 1000) by diastolic blood pressure level by race.

Table III. Comparison of logistic regression coefficients* for diastolic blood pressure for all-cause and cause-specific mortality for each racial group

		Black		*White*			
	PC	*Coeff*	*SE*	*Coeff*	*SE*	*Difference in coeff*	*SE*
All-cause mortality	1†	0.0195	0.0033	0.0170	0.0013	0.0025	0.0035
	2‡	0.0202	0.0035	0.0171	0.0013	0.0031	0.0037
CVD death	1	0.0261	0.0051	0.0301	0.0019	−0.0040	0.0054
	2	0.0299	0.0055	0.0322	0.0020	−0.0023	0.0058
CHD death	1	0.0188	0.0072	0.0263	0.0021	−0.0075	0.0075
	2	0.0244	0.0078	0.0289	0.0024	−0.0045	0.0082
Death from cerebrovascular disease	1	0.0623	0.0105	0.0372	0.0068	0.0251§	0.0125
	2	0.0624	0.0109	0.0324	0.0072	0.0300§	0.0131

PC = Participant category; Coeff = coefficient; SE = standard error.
*Estimated for fixed age, serum cholesterol, and cigarettes per day.
†Category 1 includes all participants in racial group.
‡Category 2 excludes those participants who reported previous hospitalization for a heart attack or who were taking medication for diabetes.
§$p < 0.05$.

than for white males. Although the proportion of deaths from CVD is similar (48.4% of all deaths for white males and 45.1% for black males), the proportion of deaths classified as CHD (ICD 410-414) is significantly less for black (23.8%) compared to white males (37.1%). With the exception of this difference and differences in the number of strokes (ICD 430-438), hypertensive heart disease (ICD 402), and violent or accidental deaths (ICD 800-999), the distribution of causes of death for black and white males is similar.

Among the black and white males screened, there were 2429 CVD deaths (7.0/1000). The rates for black and white males were 8.6 and 6.8/1000, respectively, yielding a crude risk ratio (black vs white) of 1.26. It can be noted from Table II that this

increased risk of death from CVD among black males arises primarily because of cerebrovascular disease, hypertensive heart disease, and other CVD.

One hundred seven CHD deaths were identified among the black males for whom death certificates were obtained (4.6/1000). The corresponding rate for white males was 5.2/1000. The ratio of the crude 5-year death rates is 0.88, the CHD rate for blacks being 12% lower than that for white males. The distribution of ICD codes that led to the CHD classification is very similar for black and white participants. Approximately 72% of the CHD cases were coded as 410, myocardial infarction, in each racial group.

Thirty deaths (1.3/1000) from cerebrovascular

September, 1984
American Heart Journal

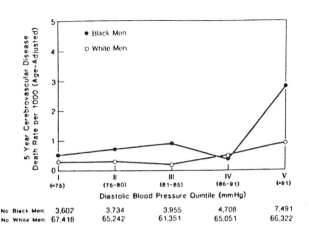

No. Black Men: 3,602   3,734   3,955   4,708   7,491
No. White Men: 67,418   65,242   61,351   65,051   66,322

Fig. 3. Five-year age-adjusted cerebrovascular disease mortality rate (per 1000) by diastolic blood pressure level by race.

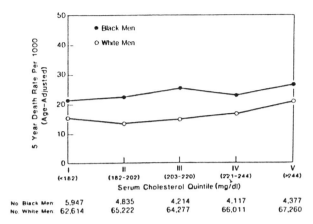

No. Black Men: 5,947   4,835   4,214   4,117   4,377
No. White Men: 62,614   65,222   64,277   66,011   67,260

Fig. 4. Five-year age-adjusted total mortality rate (per 1000) by serum cholesterol level by race.

Table IV. Comparison of logistic regression coefficients* for serum cholesterol concentration for all-cause and cause-specific mortality for each racial group

		Black		White			
	PC	Coeff	SE	Coeff	SE	Difference in coeff	SE
All-cause mortality	1†	0.0016	0.0010	0.0028	0.0003	−0.0012	0.0010
	2‡	0.0013	0.0011	0.0024	0.0004	−0.0011	0.0011
CVD death	1	0.0054	0.0014	0.0072	0.0004	−0.0018	0.0014
	2	0.0059	0.0015	0.0073	0.0005	−0.0014	0.0015
CHD death	1	0.0071	0.0017	0.0079	0.0005	−0.0008	0.0018
	2	0.0079	0.0017	0.0082	0.0005	−0.0003	0.0018
Death from cerebrovascular disease	1	−0.0034	0.0046	0.0023	0.0020	−0.0057	0.0050
	2	−0.0032	0.0047	0.0021	0.0021	−0.0053	0.0051

PC = Participant category; Coeff = coefficient; SE = standard error.
*Estimated for fixed age, diastolic blood pressure, and cigarettes per day
†Category 1 includes all participants in racial group.
‡Category 2 excludes those participants who reported previous hospitalization for a heart attack or who were taking medication for diabetes.

disease for black males were identified; for white males, 152 cerebrovascular deaths (0.5/1000) were identified, yielding a crude risk ratio of 2.6. There was little difference between black and white males in the proportion of cerebrovascular deaths coded as hemorrhage, occlusion, or other cerebrovascular accidents.

Risk factor associations with endpoints

Diastolic blood pressure. Age-adjusted all-cause mortality rates by diastolic blood pressure quintiles are graphed in Fig. 1. Table III summarizes the relationship of diastolic blood pressure to all-cause and cause-specific mortality. The logistic regression coefficients for diastolic blood pressure presented are unstandardized regression coefficients estimated in the presence of (for fixed) age, serum cholesterol

concentration, and number of cigarettes reported smoked per day. For both black and white males, the 5-year mortality rate increases with increasing diastolic blood pressure. The logistic regression coefficients corresponding to diastolic blood pressure estimated for all white and black males are similar and significantly positively associated with all-cause mortality for each racial group (0.0195 vs 0.0170). The findings are similar when males previously hospitalized for a heart attack or taking medication for diabetes are excluded.

The relationship of diastolic blood pressure to CHD death is illustrated in Fig. 2. For both white and black males a significant positive association with CHD death is evident. The regression coefficients in Table III indicate that an increase in

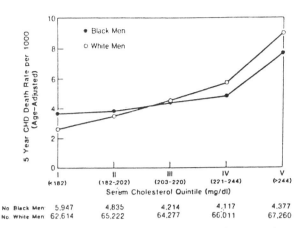

Fig. 5. Five-year age-adjusted CHD mortality rate (per 1000) by serum cholesterol level by race.

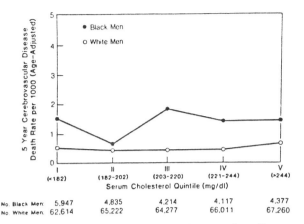

Fig. 6. Five-year age-adjusted cerebrovascular disease mortality rate (per 1000) by serum cholesterol level by race.

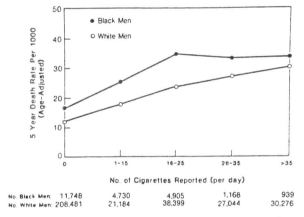

Fig. 7. Five-year age-adjusted total mortality rate (per 1000) by number of cigarettes reported smoked by race.

diastolic blood pressure of 10 mm Hg is associated with a 21% increased risk of CHD death among black males and a 30% increased risk of CHD death among white males. Although the age-adjusted logistic regression coefficients for diastolic blood pressure do not significantly differ for black and white males, it is evident from the plot of 5-year rates by blood pressure quintile that the difference in CHD rates among black and white males is primarily in the upper quintile of diastolic blood pressure, that is, in hypertensive males.

Age-adjusted cerebrovascular disease death rates are plotted in Fig. 3. The association of death from cerebrovascular disease with diastolic blood pressure is significantly positive for both white and black males. With the use of the logistic regression coefficients in Table III for all black and white males, an increase in diastolic blood pressure of 10 mm Hg was estimated to increase the risk of death from cerebrovascular disease by 86% for black males and by 45% for white males. The difference in the regression coefficients for diastolic blood pressure for white and black males is statistically significant ($p = 0.047$). The difference between cerebrovascular disease death rates for black and white males is most marked among those in the upper quintile of diastolic blood pressure; the difference, indicating a higher cerebrovascular disease death rate among black hypertensive males, is in the opposite direction of what was observed for CHD death.

Serum cholesterol concentration. The relationship of serum cholesterol concentration to all-cause mortality is illustrated in Fig. 4. A nonlinear relationship is evident for white participants, whereas for black participants the curve is fairly flat. The logistic regression coefficient (Table IV) for serum cholesterol concentration is small (0.0016 and 0.0028

for black and white participants, respectively) and differs significantly from zero for white males only.

Age-adjusted CHD mortality rates are plotted by quintile of serum cholesterol concentration in Fig. 5. The curves and the logistic regression coefficients are similar for white and black participants: 0.0071 for black males and 0.0079 for white males. These regression coefficients indicate that an increase in serum cholesterol of 20 mg/dl is associated with approximately a 16% increase in the risk of CHD death. The regression coefficients are similar after the exclusion of participants with a previous heart attack or diabetes.

The age-adjusted cerebrovascular disease mortality rates by cholesterol quintile are given in Fig. 6. No consistent relationship is noted for either black or white males.

Cigarette smoking. The relationship between

766   *Neaton et al.*

September, 1984
American Heart Journal

Table V. Comparison of logistic regression coefficients* for number of cigarettes smoked per day for all-cause and cause-specific mortality for each racial group

		Black		White			
	PC	Coeff	SE	Coeff	SE	Difference in coeff	SE
All-cause mortality	1†	0.0244	0.0032	0.0226	0.0008	0.0018	0.0033
	2†	0.0261	0.0034	0.0239	0.0008	0.0022	0.0035
CVD death	1	0.0256	0.0051	0.0223	0.0012	0.0033	0.0052
	2	0.0293	0.0054	0.0248	0.0012	0.0045	0.0055
CHD death	1	0.0309	0.0067	0.0222	0.0013	0.0087	0.0068
	2	0.0324	0.0074	0.0250	0.0014	0.0074	0.0075
Death from cerebrovascular disease	1	0.0103	0.0147	0.0260	0.0042	−0.0157	0.0153
	2	0.0146	0.0147	0.0287	0.0044	−0.0141	0.0153

PC = Participant category; Coeff = coefficient; SE = standard error.
*Estimated for fixed age, diastolic blood pressure, and serum cholesterol.
†Category 1 includes all participants in racial group.
‡Category 2 excludes those participants who reported previous hospitalization for a heart attack or who were taking medication for diabetes.

reported cigarettes per day and all-cause mortality is similar for black and white males (Fig. 7). The regression coefficients (Table V) are 0.0244 and 0.0226, respectively, for black and white males. Both of the regression coefficients differ significantly from zero ($p < 0.001$) and indicate that an increase of 20 cigarettes per day is associated with approximately a 60% increased risk of death.

The age-adjusted 5-year CHD mortality rate by level of cigarette smoking is given in Fig. 8 for black and white participants. The curves are similar except for those smoking 26 to 35 cigarettes per day. Only five CHD deaths occurred among black males in this group. The logistic regression coefficients for all black and white males (0.0309 and 0.0222, respectively) do not differ significantly from each other ($p = 0.20$). Each coefficient reflects a significant positive association between cigarette smoking and CHD mortality. The coefficients are similar to those estimated for the rate of death from any cause. The exclusion of participants with previous heart attack or diabetes does not alter the findings.

The age-adjusted cerebrovascular disease mortality rates, stratified by cigarette smoking levels, are given in Fig. 9. A significant positive association is noted for white males, whereas for black males the association is less clear. An increased mortality rate is observed for black men smoking 16 to 25 and 26 to 35 cigarettes per day, but no cerebrovascular disease deaths were observed among the 939 black men smoking more than 35 cigarettes per day.

Black-white differences in mortality. The effect on the crude relative risk (black vs white) estimates for all-cause and cause-specific mortality is minimal after adjustment for differences in the distribution of diastolic blood pressure, serum cholesterol concentration, and cigarettes smoked per day (column 1 compared to column 2, Table VI). The effect of adjusting for the differential mortality and proportion of blacks among the clinical centers, as well as for these risk factors, is more marked (column 1 compared to column 3, Table VI). These estimates, derived from the use of the Mantel-Haenzel method, correspond to the pooled relative odds over the 352 2 × 2 tables (race vs mortality status) that arise from the subclassification of men (1) into two classes each by age, serum cholesterol concentration, diastolic blood pressure, and cigarettes per day and (2) into 1 of 22 clinics. The adjusted risk estimates are significantly greater than 1.0 for all-cause and CVD mortality. For CHD mortality, each of the relative risk estimates is less than 1.0 but not significantly so. The comparison between the observed and adjusted 5-year risk ratios for cerebrovascular disease mortality was not considered in the same way as those for all-cause, CVD, and CHD mortality because an assumption implicit in using these methods of adjustment is that the association between the risk factors and the endpoint is the same for black and white males. Since the association of cerebrovascular disease death with diastolic blood pressure differs significantly for white and black males, the adjusted relative risk was estimated for a specific blood pressure level. For males in the highest quintile of diastolic blood pressure, the crude relative risk is 2.8; the crude relative risk for men in the lower four quintiles of diastolic blood pressure is 1.8. The corresponding estimates, based on the logistic model and adjusted for age and the three risk factors, are 2.8 and 1.8, respectively.

Volume 108
Number 3, Part 2

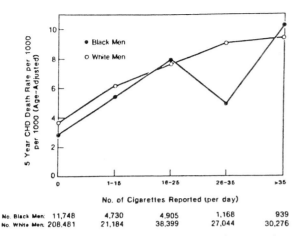

Fig. 8. Five-year age-adjusted CHD mortality rate (per 1000) by number of cigarettes reported smoked by race.

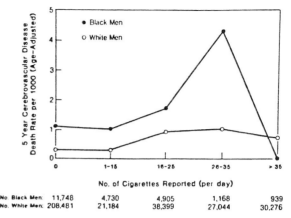

Fig. 9. Five-year age-adjusted cerebrovascular disease mortality rate (per 1000) by number of cigarettes reported smoked by race.

The relative risk (black vs white) of CHD death was examined more closely by classifying black and white males by level of diastolic blood pressure, serum cholesterol concentration, and cigarette smoking and by calculating the relative risk (black vs white) adjusted for age within each of the resulting eight subgroups (Table VII). Among nonhypertensive males, with the exception of those who were nonsmokers with serum cholesterol levels <250 mg/dl, the relative risk (black vs white) estimates are greater than 1.0. Among hypertensive screenees, black males are at a lower risk of CHD death compared to white males in each of the four subgroups. The relative risk of CHD death (black vs white) after adjustment for age, serum cholesterol concentration, and cigarettes per day (by logistic regression) is 1.15 for nonhypertensive (diastolic blood pressure <90 mm Hg) males and 0.69 for hypertensive males. The difference in these relative risk estimates is statistically significant ($p = 0.012$).

DISCUSSION

Risk factor differences. Significant risk factor differences were noted between black and white males. Diastolic blood pressure levels were 3 to 4 mm Hg higher for black males in each age group; the serum cholesterol concentration was 3 to 6 mg/dl lower for black males compared to white males; more blacks reported smoking cigarettes than whites (50.0% vs 35.9%), but black cigarette smokers smoked an average of eight cigarettes per day less than white cigarette smokers.

These results are similar to those of other studies. In the Health and Nutrition Examination Survey of 1971-1974[23] the average diastolic blood pressure for white males 35 to 44 years old and 45 to 54 years old

Table VI. Estimated relative risk (black vs white) of all-cause and cause-specific mortality, observed and adjusted for differences in risk factor levels

	Relative risk (black vs white) estimate		
	Observed	*Using logistic model*	*Using Mantel-Haenzel*
All-cause mortality	1.38*	1.44*	1.24*
CVD death	1.26*	1.28*	1.17*
CHD death	0.88	0.89	0.85

*Significantly different from 1.0 ($p < 0.05$)

was 84.2 and 87.5 mm Hg, respectively. The corresponding estimates for black males were 91.2 and 91.9 mm Hg. The respective differences (black vs white) were 7.0 and 4.4 mm Hg. In the Hypertension Detection and Follow-up Program[24] the average diastolic blood pressure at the initial screening was 4.6 mm Hg higher among black males compared to white males with no reported history of high blood pressure. For males with a reported history of high blood pressure but not currently receiving antihypertensive drugs, the black-white difference was 5.8 mm Hg; for males currently receiving antihypertensive drugs the difference was 3.7 mm Hg.

The 3.9 mg/dl difference in serum cholesterol concentration for black and white males is similar to the 5.4 mg/dl difference found in the Lipid Research Clinics Prevalence Study[25] for total plasma cholesterol for black and white males aged 40 to 59 years.

The difference in smoking habits between black and white males is similar to that found in the National Health Examination Survey,[26] which found that 42.7% of white males aged 45 to 54 years

September, 1984
American Heart Journal

768 *Neaton et al.*

Table VII. Five-year age-adjusted CHD death rates by hypertensive status, cigarette smoking status, and level of serum cholesterol for MRFIT black and white males

Risk factor	No. of men		Age-adjusted rate (5 yr)		
	Black	White	Black	White	Black/white ratio
Diastolic BP <90 mm Hg					
Nonsmoker					
Serum cholesterol <250 mg/dl	6,094	127,864	1.67	2.40	0.70
Serum cholesterol ≥250 mg/dl	1,056	21,182	6.86	6.12	1.12
Smokers					
Serum cholesterol <250 mg/dl	6,215	72,635	6.21	5.62	1.10
Serum cholesterol ≥250 mg/dl	925	14,905	11.08	10.78	1.03
Diastolic BP ≥90 mm Hg					
Nonsmoker					
Serum cholesterol <250 mg/dl	3,669	46,016	2.88	3.86	0.75
Serum cholesterol ≥250 mg/dl	929	13,419	4.92	9.88	0.50
Smokers					
Serum cholesterol <250 mg/dl	3,771	22,010	6.42	11.06	0.58
Serum cholesterol ≥250 mg/dl	831	7,353	9.04	17.49	0.52
Total	23,490	325,384	4.83	5.22	0.93

reported smoking cigarettes, compared to 56.7% of black males in the same age group. The average number of cigarettes reported smoked by smokers in that survey was 22.7 per day for white males and 15.8 per day for black males.

Risk factor associations with all-cause and cause-specific mortality. The relationship of age, diastolic blood pressure, serum cholesterol concentration, and cigarettes per day to all-cause, CVD, and CHD mortality did not differ significantly for white and black males after logistic regression analysis. When the regression analyses were restricted to males who were not taking medication for diabetes and who had not been previously hospitalized for a heart attack, the regression coefficients increased somewhat for each risk factor for both racial groups, but the differences between black and white males were similar. For the endpoint data on death from cerebrovascular disease, a significant difference was found in the regression coefficients for diastolic blood pressure between black and white males. It should be noted that this significant difference was based on only 30 cerebrovascular disease deaths among black males. Additional follow-up will be required to document further the association of these risk factors with cerebrovascular disease death.

Although regression analysis did not reveal significant differences between black and white males in the association of these risk factors with CHD mortality, when black and white males were categorized by hypertensive status at screening (diastolic blood pressure <90 or ≥90 mm Hg), a significant difference between the black/white CHD mortality

risk ratios was observed. Thus this investigation not only confirms the apparent paradoxical situation, observed in other studies,[8,9] that the risk of dying from CHD is lower for black than white males but suggests that the decreased risk is most apparent in hypertensive males.

The all-cause and CVD death rate differences between black and white males after 5 years could not be completely attributed either to risk factor differences between black and white males or to differences in the association of the risk factors with the endpoints. For cerebrovascular disease the difference in the regression coefficients for diastolic blood pressure for the endpoint data on cerebrovascular disease death explains a large part of the difference in the rates between black and white males.

CONCLUSIONS

This follow-up study of males screened as part of the MRFIT presents data on the largest group of blacks ever prospectively studied for the association of diastolic blood pressure, serum cholesterol concentration, and cigarette smoking with CVD mortality. The difference in the relationship of diastolic blood pressure to cerebrovascular disease death for black and white males and the reduced CHD mortality among black hypertensive patients should be studied further. This difference, if real, could reflect a different cause for stroke and CHD mortality in white and black hypertensive males.

REFERENCES

1. The Pooling Project Research Group: Relationship of blood pressure, serum cholesterol, smoking habit, relative weight

Volume 108
Number 3, Part 2

CHD risk factors and mortality in black/white males **769**

and ECG abnormalities to incidence of major coronary events: Final report of the pooling project. J Chronic Dis 31:201, 1978.

2. Keys A: Seven countries: A multivariate analysis of death and coronary heart disease. Cambridge, Mass, 1980, Harvard University Press.

3. Gordon T, Sorlie P, Kannel WB: Coronary heart disease, atherothrombotic brain infarction, intermittent claudication: A multivariate analysis of some factors related to their incidence: Framingham study 16-year follow-up. *In* Kannel WB, Gordon T, editors: The framingham study: An epidemiological investigation of cardiovascular disease, Sect 27. Washington DC, 1971, U.S. Government Printing Office.

4. Brand RJ, Rosenman RH, Sholtz RI, Friedman M: Multivariate prediction of coronary heart disease in the Western Collaborative Group study compared to the findings of the Framingham study. Circulation 53:348, 1976.

5. Tyroler HA, Heyden S, Bartel A, Cassel J, Cornoni JC, Hames CG, Kleinbaum D: Blood pressure and cholesterol as coronary heart disease risk factors. Arch Intern Med **128**:907, 1971.

6. Kleinbaum DG, Kupper LL, Cassel JC, Tyroler HA: Multivariate analysis of risk of coronary heart disease in Evans County, Georgia. Arch Intern Med **128**:943, 1971.

7. Gillum RF, Grant CT: Coronary heart disease in black populations. I. Mortality and morbidity. AM HEART J **104**:852, 1982.

8. Stamler J, Berkson DM, Lindberg HA, Miller W, Hall Y: Racial patterns of coronary heart disease. Geriatrics 16:382, 1961.

9. McDonough JR, Hames CG, Stulb SC, Garrison GE: Coronary heart disease among Negroes and Whites in Evans County, Georgia. J Chronic Dis **18**:443, 1965.

10. MRFIT Group: The Multiple Risk Factor Intervention Trial (MRFIT): A national study of primary prevention of coronary heart disease. JAMA **235**:825, 1976.

11. Sherwin R, Kaelber CT, Kezdi P, Kjelsberg MO, Thomas HE Jr: The Multiple Risk Factor Intervention Trial (MRFIT). II. The development of the protocol. Prev Med **10**:402, 1981.

12. Lipid Research Clinics Program: Manual of operations, vol 1: Lipid and lipoprotein analysis: Washington, DC, 1974, U.S. Department of Health, Education, and Welfare.

13. International Classification of Diseases, 9th revision, Clinical Modification, vol 1. Ann Arbor, Mich, 1981 Edwards Brothers, Inc.

14. Armitage P: Statistical methods in medical research. London, 1973, Blackwell Scientific Publications, Ltd.

15. Fleiss JL: Statistical methods for rates and proportions. New York, 1973, John Wiley & Sons, Inc.

16. Truett J, Cornfield J, Kannel WB: A multivariate analysis of the risk of coronary heart disease in Framingham. J Chronic Dis **20**:511, 1967.

17. Mantel N, Haenzel W: Statistical aspects of the analysis of data from retrospective studies of disease. J Natl Cancer Inst **22**:719, 1959.

18. Wentworth DN, Neaton JD, Rasmussen WL: An evaluation of the Social Security Administration MBR file and the National Death Index in the ascertainment of vital status. Am J Public Health **73**:1270, 1983.

19. Alvey W, Aziz F: Quality of mortality reporting in SSA-linked data: Some preliminary results. Proceedings of the Section on Survey Research Methods, American Statistical Association, Washington, DC, 1979, p 275.

20. National Center for Health Statistics: Mortality, United States, 1977. Washington, DC, 1981, U.S. Government Printing Office.

21. Shindell S, Weisberg RF, Giefer EE: The "healthy worker effect": Fact or artifact. J Occup Med **20**:807, 1978.

22. Fox AJ, Collier PF: Low mortality rates in industrial cohort studies due to selection for work and survival in industry. Br J Prev Social Med **30**:225, 1976.

23. National Center for Health Statistics: Blood pressure levels of persons 6-74 years, United States 1971-1974. Vital and Health Statistics, Series 11, No. 203, 1977.

24. Hypertension Detection and Follow-up Program Cooperative Group: Variability of blood pressure and the results of screening in the Hypertension Detection and Follow-up Program. J Chronic Dis **31**:651, 1978.

25. The Lipid Research Clinics population studies data book, vol I. The Prevalence Study. Washington, DC, 1980, U.S. Department of Health and Human Services.

26. National Center for Health Statistics: Use habits among adults of cigarettes, coffee, asprin, and sleeping pills, United States 1976. Vital and Health Statistics, Series 10, No. 131, 1979.

Consensus Conference

Lowering Blood Cholesterol
to Prevent Heart Disease

● Coronary heart disease is responsible for more than 550,000 deaths in the United States each year. It is responsible for more deaths than all forms of cancer combined. There are more than 5.4 million Americans with symptomatic coronary heart disease and a large number of others with undiagnosed coronary disease, many of them young and highly productive. It has been estimated that coronary heart disease costs the United States more than $60 billion a year in direct and indirect costs.

Coronary heart disease is caused by atherosclerosis, a slowly progressive disease of the large arteries that begins early in life but rarely produces symptoms until middle age. Often the disease goes undetected until the time of the first heart attack, and this first heart attack is often fatal. Modern methods of treatment have improved greatly the outlook for patients having heart attacks, but

---

See also pp 2087, 2091, and 2094.

---

major progress in our battle against this number 1 killer must rest on finding preventive measures.

A number of risk factors have been identified as strongly associated with coronary heart disease. Cigarette smoking, high blood pressure, and high blood cholesterol levels are the most clearly established of these factors. Risk is greater in men, increases with age, and has a strong genetic component. Obesity, diabetes mellitus, physical inactivity, and behavior pattern are also risk factors.

A large body of evidence of many kinds links elevated blood cholesterol levels to coronary heart disease. However, some doubt remains about the strength of the evidence for a cause-and-effect relationship. Questions remain regarding the exact relationship between blood cholesterol and heart attacks and the steps that should be taken to diagnose and treat elevated blood cholesterol levels.

To resolve some of these questions, the National Heart, Lung, and Blood Institute (NHLBI) and the National Institutes of Health Office of Medical Applications of

From the Office of Medical Applications of Research, National Institutes of Health, Bethesda, Md.
Reprint requests to Office of Medical Applications of Research, Bldg 1, Room 216, National Institutes of Health, Bethesda, MD 20205 (Michael J. Bernstein).

Research convened a Consensus Development Conference on Lowering Blood Cholesterol to Prevent Heart Disease from Dec 10 to 12, 1984. After hearing a series of expert presentations and reviewing all of the available data, a consensus panel of lipoprotein experts, cardiologists, primary care physicians, epidemiologists, biomedical scientists, biostatisticians, experts in preventive medicine, and lay representatives considered the evidence and agreed on answers to the following questions:

1. Is the relationship between blood cholesterol levels and coronary heart disease causal?

2. Will reduction of blood cholesterol levels help prevent coronary heart disease?

3. Under what circumstances and at what level of blood cholesterol should dietary or drug treatment be started?

4. Should an attempt be made to reduce the blood cholesterol levels of the general population?

5. What research directions should be pursued regarding the relationship between blood cholesterol and coronary heart disease?

Panel's Conclusions

Elevation of blood cholesterol levels is a major cause of coronary artery disease. It has been established beyond a reasonable doubt that lowering definitely elevated blood cholesterol levels (specifically, blood levels of low-density lipoprotein [LDL] cholesterol) will reduce the risk of heart attacks caused by coronary heart disease. This has been demonstrated most conclusively in men with elevated blood cholesterol levels, but much evidence justifies the conclusion that similar protection will be afforded to women with elevated levels. After careful review of genetic, experimental, epidemiologic, and clinical trial evidence, we recommend treatment of individuals with blood cholesterol levels above the 75th percentile (upper 25% of values). Furthermore, we are persuaded that the blood cholesterol levels of most Americans are undesirably high, in large part because of our high dietary intake of calories, saturated fat, and cholesterol. In countries with diets lower in these constituents, blood cholesterol levels are lower and coronary heart disease is less common. There is no doubt that appropriate changes in our diet will reduce blood cholesterol levels. Epidemiologic data and

---

Editorial Note: The papers referred to as appearing on pp. 2087, 2091 and 2094 have been omitted.

more than a dozen clinical trials allow us to predict with reasonable assurance that such a measure will afford significant protection against coronary heart disease.

For these reasons we recommend the following:

1. Individuals with *high-risk blood cholesterol levels* (values above the 90th percentile) should be treated intensively by dietary means under the guidance of a physician, dietitian, or other health professional; if response to diet is inadequate, appropriate drugs should be added to the treatment regimen. Guidelines for children are somewhat different, as discussed below.

2. Adults with *moderate-risk blood cholesterol levels* (values between the 75th and 90th percentiles) should be treated intensively by dietary means, especially if additional risk factors are present. Only a small proportion should require drug treatment.

3. All Americans (except children younger than 2 years of age) should be advised to adopt a diet that reduces total dietary fat intake from the current level of about 40% of total calories to 30% of total calories, reduces saturated fat intake to less than 10% of total calories, increases polyunsaturated fat intake but to no more than 10% of total calories, and reduces daily cholesterol intake to 250 to 300 mg or less.

4. Intake of total calories should be reduced, if necessary, to correct obesity and adjusted to maintain ideal body weight. A program of regular moderate-level exercise will be helpful in this connection.

5. In individuals with elevated blood cholesterol levels, special attention should be given to the management of other risk factors (hypertension, cigarette smoking, diabetes, and physical inactivity).

These dietary recommendations are similar to those of the American Heart Association and the Inter-Society Commission for Heart Disease Resources.

We further recommend the following:

6. New and expanded programs should be planned and initiated soon to educate physicians, other health professionals, and the public to the significance of elevated blood cholesterol levels and the importance of treating them. We recommend that the NHLBI provide the focus for development of plans for a National Cholesterol Education Program that would enlist participation by and contributions from all interested organizations at national, state, and local levels.

7. The food industry should be encouraged to continue and intensify efforts to develop and market foods that will make it easier for individuals to adhere to the recommended diets, and school food services and restaurants should serve meals consistent with these dietary recommendations.

8. Food labeling should include the specific source or sources of fat, total fat, saturated and polyunsaturated fat, and cholesterol content as well as other nutritional information. The public should be educated on how to use this information to achieve dietary aims.

9. All physicians should be encouraged to include, whenever possible, a blood cholesterol measurement on every adult patient when that patient is first seen; to ensure reliability of data, we recommend steps to improve and standardize methods for cholesterol measurement in clinical laboratories.

10. Further research should be encouraged to compare the effectiveness and safety of currently recommended diets with those of alternative diets; to study human behavior as it relates to food choices and adherence to diets; to develop more effective, better-tolerated, safer, and more economical drugs for lowering blood cholesterol levels; to assess the effectiveness of medical and surgical treatment of high blood cholesterol levels in patients with established clinical coronary artery disease; to develop more precise and sensitive noninvasive artery imaging methods; and to apply basic cell and molecular biology to increase our understanding of lipoprotein metabolism (particularly the role of high-density lipoprotein [HDL] as a protective factor) and artery wall metabolism as they relate to coronary heart disease.

11. Plans should be developed that will permit assessment of the impact of the changes recommended herein as implementation proceeds and provide the basis for changes when and where appropriate.

---

1. Is the Relationship Between Blood Cholesterol Levels and Coronary Heart Disease Causal?—The evidence supporting a causal relationship between blood cholesterol levels and coronary heart disease comes from a wealth of congruent results of genetic, experimental pathologic, epidemiologic, and intervention studies. These data establish beyond any reasonable doubt the close relationship between elevated blood cholesterol levels (as measured in serum or plasma) and coronary heart disease. At the same time, it is equally clear that an elevated blood cholesterol level is not the *only* cause of coronary heart disease. Hypertension, cigarette smoking, diabetes mellitus, obesity, and physical inactivity, along with a number of other risk factors such as age, sex, and family history, are important contributing causes. There probably are other undiscovered contributing causes. However, we shall confine ourselves here primarily to a discussion of elevated blood cholesterol levels.

It is now firmly established that all cholesterol is carried in the bloodstream in several protein-lipid combinations known as lipoproteins and that most of the blood cholesterol in humans is carried by specific LDLs. Some is also present in HDLs and in very low-density lipoproteins. The LDL particles, when present in excess in the blood, are deposited in the tissues and form a major part of a buildup in the artery wall to form atherosclerotic plaque. Atherosclerosis narrows the channels of the coronary arteries, the vessels that furnish the major blood supply to the heart muscle.

Genetic Evidence

Severe coronary heart disease can result from high blood cholesterol levels in the absence of any other contributing risk factors. This is clearly demonstrated by the accelerated and clinically catastrophic coronary heart disease in children with inherited hypercholesterolemia in its most severe form. These children lack the specific receptor that normally removes LDL from the blood, and, as a result, they have very high LDL cholesterol levels from birth. They frequently suffer severe coronary heart disease, and death may occur even in childhood. Careful study of these diseased arteries reveal large quantities of cholesterol in the plaques.

The LDL receptor normally plays a critical role in regulating blood cholesterol levels in all mammals, including humans. It has been purified and fully characterized.

Studies suggest that a number of cases of clinically important coronary heart disease with less severe elevations of blood cholesterol levels may be explained by partial deficiencies of *functioning* LDL receptors, deficiencies induced by dietary and life-style factors. Thus, the basis of high blood cholesterol level in these patients is similar to that in patients with inherited hypercholesterolemia, and, while these levels are less severe, they probably have the same implications.

Experimental Pathology (Animal Model) Evidence

With improved use of the many existing animal models, a number of very important relationships between blood cholesterol, atherosclerosis, and coronary heart disease have been demonstrated:

- Many species (including several nonhuman primates) develop atherosclerosis when fed diets that raise their blood cholesterol levels.
- Studies over time demonstrate that hypercholesterolemic monkeys (and other species) develop intimal lesions that progress from fatty streaks to typical raised plaques to complicated ulcerated plaques resembling those seen in humans suffering from coronary heart disease.
- Hypercholesterolemia augments experimental atherosclerosis when arterial "injury" is present.
- Severe atherosclerosis in rhesus monkeys, usually a progressive process, regresses when the blood cholesterol level is lowered substantially for an extended period by diet or by drugs.

Animal studies thus offer strong and persuasive evidence supporting the causal relationship between blood cholesterol and atherosclerosis.

Epidemiologic Evidence

A large body of epidemiologic evidence supports the direct relationship between blood cholesterol levels and coronary heart disease:

- Comparisons among various populations throughout the world reveal a direct correlation between blood cholesterol levels and the occurrence of coronary heart disease; no population has been reported to have a high rate of coronary heart disease and low blood cholesterol levels.
- People who have migrated to another country with a higher average blood cholesterol level gradually acquire the dietary habits, blood cholesterol concentrations, and coronary heart disease rates of their new country of residence.
- Severity and frequency of raised plaques in the aorta and coronary arteries are strongly correlated with blood cholesterol levels.
- Populations experiencing severe dietary (especially fat) limitations and weight loss have been shown to have less atherosclerosis and coronary heart disease and fewer heart attacks.
- Prospective studies such as the Framingham study have shown that elevated blood cholesterol levels in

healthy people predict the future occurrence of coronary heart disease.

- Evidence emerging from multiple clinical trials, reviewed in the next section, clearly indicates that lowering blood cholesterol levels in patients with hypercholesterolemia decreases the likelihood of fatal and nonfatal coronary heart disease.

Thus, the evidence obtained from genetic, experimental, epidemiologic, and clinical intervention investigations overwhelmingly supports a causal relationship between blood cholesterol levels and coronary heart disease.

2. **Will Reduction of Cholesterol Levels Help Prevent Coronary Heart Disease?**—Our conclusion that reduction of blood cholesterol levels *will* reduce the rate of coronary heart disease is based partly on the evidence for cause-and-effect presented above and partly on the direct evidence from clinical trials noted below.

First, metabolic ward studies establish beyond reasonable doubt three dietary maneuvers that lower blood cholesterol levels: reducing the saturated fat content, increasing the polyunsaturated fat content, and reducing the cholesterol content. Second, a number of drugs have been developed that lower blood cholesterol levels. The issue of whether these interventions also influence coronary heart disease events has been more challenging.

In previous years, more than a dozen randomized trials of the effects of fat-controlled diets or drugs have been reported. Most showed some decrease in coronary heart disease event rates in the treated group, and the dietary trials carried out by Dayton et al and by Leren et al were particularly suggestive, producing 23% and 35% reductions in the incidence of coronary heart disease. However, no study considered individually could be regarded as conclusive: the sample sizes were too small, and there were in some cases unanticipated increases in noncardiovascular deaths, although these were not statistically significant. An aggregate analysis of all unifactor blood cholesterol-lowering trials, while not revealing an effect on total mortality, does indicate that coronary heart disease rates can be reduced by reduction of blood cholesterol levels.

These findings have been extended by two recently reported randomized and blinded clinical trials of the efficacy of the cholesterol-lowering drug cholestyramine resin. One of these studies, the Lipid Research Clinics Coronary Primary Prevention Trial, showed a statistically significant 19% reduction in the combined rate of fatal and nonfatal coronary heart disease in association with a 9% decrease in blood cholesterol level. The other study, the NHLBI Type II Coronary Intervention Study, showed a reduction in the angiographic progression of coronary artery disease. In addition, a third trial (the Coronary Drug Project) has recently presented information extending the earlier published finding that the use of nicotinic acid lowers the rate of recurrent coronary heart disease by demonstrating in long-term follow-up a decrease in overall mortality.

These findings, taken in conjunction with the results of the earlier studies, permit the conclusion that reduction of blood cholesterol levels in people with relatively high initial levels will reduce the rate of coronary heart disease. The clinical trials are too limited to settle the issue of effects on overall mortality. However, the complete evidence, which includes information derived from animal, pathophysiological, metabolic, and epidemiologic studies, makes it reasonable to presume that the reduction in coronary heart disease incidence will be accompanied by a reduction in overall mortality.

The magnitude of the reduction in coronary heart disease risk can be estimated from these clinical trials; they indicate that each 1% reduction in blood cholesterol level yields approximately a 2% reduction in coronary heart disease rates. This is remarkably similar to the magnitude of the beneficial outcome predicted from observational epidemiologic studies. Thus, for example, a 5% reduction in blood cholesterol level resulting from the diets recommended below should reduce coronary heart disease rates by 10%. The absolute magnitude of this benefit should be greater in patients at high risk because of existing coronary heart disease or the presence of other risk factors such as cigarette smoking and hypertension. Reductions in disease rates of as much as 50% may be achievable in patients in the high-risk-cholesterol category who adhere well to a combination of effective drug treatment and a fat-controlled diet.

3. **Under What Circumstances and at What Level of Blood Cholesterol Should Dietary or Drug Treatment Be Started?**

What Is Hypercholesterolemia?

A precise definition of hypercholesterolemia (an abnormally high blood cholesterol level) is difficult to establish. Often, an abnormally high level of a biologic substance is considered to be that level above which is found the upper 5% of the population (the 95th percentile). However, the use of this criterion in defining "normal" values for blood cholesterol levels in the United States is unreasonable; coronary heart disease is our major cause of death because, in part at least, a large fraction of our population probably has too high a blood cholesterol level. A review of available data suggests that levels above 200 to 230 mg/dL are associated with an increased risk of developing premature coronary heart disease. It is staggering to realize that this represents about 50% of the adult population of the United States. The consensus panel has chosen to define two levels of hypercholesterolemia, both of which are associated with an increased coronary heart disease risk, and *both of which should be treated.*

High-Risk Blood Cholesterol Levels (Severe Hypercholesterolemia)

This category is defined as values at approximately the 90th percentile or above as determined by the Lipid Research Clinics Prevalence Study (see the tabulation below for guidelines). It will include individuals with hereditary forms of high blood cholesterol levels, who will require the most aggressive treatment. Withholding treatment subjects these individuals to unnecessary risk.

Moderate-Risk Blood Cholesterol Levels (Moderate Hypercholesterolemia)

This category is defined as values approximately between the 75th to 90th percentiles (see the following tabulation for guidelines). It includes large numbers of people whose elevated blood cholesterol levels are due, in part, to their diet. The intensity of treatment is guided by the clinical and family history and the presence of other risk factors predisposing to coronary heart disease.

Values for Selecting Adults at Moderate and High Risk Requiring Treatment*

Age, yr	Moderate Risk, mg/dL (mM)	High Risk, mg/dL (mM)
20-29	>200 (5.17)	>220 (5.69)
30-39	<220 (5.69)	>240 (6.21)
≥40	>240 (6.21)	>260 (6.72)

*See special guidelines for management of children below.

How Should Adults With Hypercholesterolemia Be Treated

The presence of high-risk and moderate-risk blood cholesterol values should be confirmed by a repeated analysis. Although the initial sample may be obtained without the subject's fasting, the repeated analysis should be obtained after an overnight fast so that a valid triglyceride level also can be determined.

After the secondary causes for hypercholesterolemia (eg, hypothyroidism, nephrotic syndrome, dysproteinemias, diabetes mellitus, and obstructive liver disease) have been excluded, the primary cause should be evaluated. This includes family screening to detect the hereditary forms of elevated blood cholesterol levels and to identify other family members needing treatment. Measurement of HDL cholesterol is often helpful to determine if the elevated blood cholesterol level is due to high levels of HDL (which is associated with a *lower* risk of coronary heart disease). In addition, a low HDL cholesterol level (an independent risk factor) might guide a physician to be more aggressive in treatment of individuals with high or moderately high blood cholesterol levels.

Diet Therapy

The first step in the treatment of persons with high-risk and moderate-risk blood cholesterol levels is diet therapy and caloric restriction for weight normalization in the overweight. Weight loss may reduce blood cholesterol levels, and a moderate level of physical exercise may be helpful in this regard. The dietary approach should be to lower total fat, saturated fat, and cholesterol consumption. The following guidelines are generally consistent with those of the American Heart Association and the Atherosclerosis Study Group of the Inter-Society Commission for Heart Disease Resources. We recommend a diet composed of approximately 30% of the caloric intake from fats and no more than 250 to 300 mg of cholesterol per day. An essential consideration is a reduction of the total saturated fat intake to 10% or less of total calories. It is recommended that polyunsaturated fat intake be increased but to no more than 10% of total calories. These changes can be readily made while intake of protein, vitamins, and minerals is maintained to satisfy the Recommended Dietary Allowances of the Food and Nutrition Board of the National Research Council.

Insufficient response to this diet may necessitate further restrictions of total fat to 20% to 25% of calories, with saturated fat making up 6% to 8% of the calories.

The dietary cholesterol intake should be lowered to 150 to 200 mg/day (equivalent to the American Heart Association Phase II and II diets).

The use of diet as a primary mode of therapy requires a major effort on the part of physicians, nutritionists, dietitians, and other health professionals. Life-style changes are difficult to make without adequate instruction, motivation, and encouragement. Education of physicians, as well as the general public, as to the value of reductions in dietary saturated fat and cholesterol will assist not only in treatment of patients with high- or moderate-risk blood cholesterol levels but also in achieving the goal of reducing the blood cholesterol levels of our entire adult population to less than 200 mg/dL (<180 mg/dL in those younger than 30 years).

Drug Therapy

Drug therapy should be used only after a careful trial of diet modification using the most rigorous diet appropriate for the particular individual. Even when use of drugs seems appropriate, it is important to stress that maximal diet therapy should be continued. Several drugs, used singly or in combination, are now available. These include the bile-acid sequestrants (cholestyramine and colestipol), nicotinic acid, probucol, and the fibric acids (clofibrate and gemfibrozil). Of these, bile-acid sequestrants and nicotinic acid have been shown to reduce the incidence of coronary heart disease. Clofibrate, while effective in treating one rare familial form of lipid abnormality (type III hyperlipoproteinemia), is not recommended because it is not effective in most individuals with a high blood cholesterol level but normal triglyceride level. Moreover, an excess overall mortality was reported in the World Health Organization trial of this drug. We still do not have direct evidence for the safety of any cholesterol-lowering drugs when given over decades; therefore, drug treatment should be undertaken cautiously and its desirability should be periodically reevaluated, particularly in children.

Individuals with high-risk blood cholesterol levels (severe hypercholesterolemia), especially those with the hereditary form, may well require drug therapy in addition to dietary modification. Combined drug treatment (eg, bile-acid sequestrant plus nicotinic acid) may be particularly effective. Several combined treatment regimens are under study. Individuals with moderate-risk blood cholesterol levels will usually respond adequately to diet alone. Judgment on the decision to use drugs in such patients must be made on a case-by-case basis, taking into account family history of coronary heart disease, existing coronary disease in the individual, coexistence of other risk factors, and age of the individual.

Who Should Be Treated?

As described above, individuals with high- and moderate-risk blood cholesterol levels (>75th percentile) should be treated with diet or diet and drugs. Furthermore, it is clearly recognized that it is a goal to encourage reduction of the blood cholesterol level to approximately 180 mg/dL for adults younger than 30 years and to approximately 200 mg/dL for individuals aged 30 years or older. This is recognized as a realistic "target" level that should be

possible to achieve and that would be predicted to have a beneficial effect on coronary heart disease risk. As will be discussed in the following section, it is recommended that all individuals in the population consume a diet composed of approximately 30% of the calories as fat (≤10% saturated fat) and 250 to 300 mg of cholesterol a day in an attempt to shift the blood cholesterol levels in our population toward the lower levels observed in populations having much lower rates of coronary heart disease.

Both men and women at high risk, as defined above, should be treated similarly, even though premenopausal women have an apparent protection and the onset of the disease occurs later than in men. However, as in men, the leading cause of death in women is coronary heart disease, and blood cholesterol is a risk factor. Despite the fact that direct intervention studies have not been conducted in women, there is no reason to propose a separate treatment schedule for women.

Studies are available that indicate a beneficial effect of treating high cholesterol levels in individuals with preexisting clinical disease (secondary intervention) as well as in individuals without preexisting clinical disease (primary intervention). Because of their vulnerability, patients with established disease, including particularly patients with coronary bypass grafts, should be intensively treated. It is encouraging that the progression of established lesions may be retarded by appropriate dietary and drug therapy. The same may apply to the elderly patient. While there is no direct evidence on the benefit to be expected in the elderly, and while blood cholesterol becomes less important as a risk factor in old age, dietary treatment (with due attention to ensure nutritional adequacy) may still be helpful.

Special Guidelines for Management of Children

Identifying and treating children with elevated blood cholesterol levels is a subject for special consideration. It is desirable to begin prevention in childhood because patterns of life-style are developed in childhood. The moderate-fat and moderate-cholesterol diets recommended for the population at large in this report should be suitable for all family members, including healthy children older than 2 years. For children, the diets should provide all nutrients in quantities adequate to ensure growth and development and meet energy requirements. Excessive gain in weight should be avoided. The diet may be inappropriate in children or in the elderly if they are malnourished or have special nutritional requirements. For others, the diet plan is safe and nutritionally adequate.

Children at "high risk" should be identified primarily by carefully obtained family histories rather than routine screening. The history should include parents, grandparents, and all first-degree relatives. A family history of hypercholesterolemia or premature coronary heart disease should alert the physician to obtain at least two blood cholesterol determinations. If the blood cholesterol level in such "high-risk" children is above the 75th percentile (approximately 170 mg/dL for children aged 2 to 19 years), total and HDL cholesterol measurements should be obtained. Those children with blood cholesterol levels between the 75th and 90th percentile (170 to 185 mg/dL) should be counseled regarding diet and other cardiovascular risk factors and then followed up at one-year intervals. Those with levels above the 90th percentile (>185 mg/dL) require special dietary instruction and close supervision with evaluation of other risk factors. A child with a blood cholesterol level above the 95th percentile (>200 mg/dL) on two occasions is in a special category and may have one of the hereditary hypercholesterolemias. Strict dietary intervention is indicated and will be sufficient for many children. Nonresponders should be considered for treatment with a lipid-lowering agent, eg, a bile-acid sequestrant (such as cholestyramine). All family members should be screened.

Dietary management of children with elevated blood cholesterol levels should be part of total management that includes regular exercise programs, maintenance of ideal weight, avoidance of excess salt, and avoidance of cigarette smoking.

What Screening Strategy Should Be Adopted for Finding Subjects With High Blood Cholesterol Levels?

According to data from the National Center for Health Statistics, a high percentage of the American population sees a physician at least once every year. If a cholesterol level were determined in adults at these visits, many of the individuals with cholesterol levels above the 75th percentile would be identified in a relatively short time and should be evaluated and treated as described above. This physician- and clinic-oriented method for screening would be cost-effective. Obviously, some patients may not see a physician for several years, and it would be advisable to educate the public to the importance of knowing one's cholesterol level. In children, only a "family history screening" is recommended, that is, cholesterol levels should be obtained in those at higher risk because of a strong family history, as discussed above. Educational programs developed by voluntary and public health organizations in conjunction with the National Cholesterol Education Program of the NHLBI, as recommended by this consensus panel, should alert all adults to the advisability of learning their cholesterol level.

While we are not at this time recommending mass screening, a feasibility study of various screening methods in adults should be considered. Screening necessitates the availability of laboratories capable of determining precisely and accurately the blood cholesterol and HDL cholesterol levels and of physicians willing and able to manage large numbers of new patients. Thus, preliminary steps are needed before mass screening can be considered.

4. Should an Attempt Be Made to Reduce the Blood Cholesterol Levels of the General Population?

Rationale for Recommendations to the General Population

Many compelling lines of evidence link blood cholesterol to coronary heart disease. There is also strong evidence from epidemiologic studies that the relationship between level of cholesterol and level of risk for coronary heart disease covers virtually the entire cholesterol distribution for the US population. In fact, recent epidemiologic studies suggest that the relationship holds even at the lower end of the spectrum of cholesterol levels found in our population.

The Japanese population, in comparison with the US population, is characterized by a much lower average cholesterol level and a much lower frequency of coronary heart disease. The Finnish, on the other hand, have a much higher average cholesterol level and a much greater risk of coronary heart disease than do US citizens. Furthermore, Japanese who have migrated to Hawaii and to San Francisco have higher cholesterol levels and a higher risk of coronary heart disease than nonmigrants. Compilation of all the available data suggests that it will be beneficial to lower the blood cholesterol of the average American.

In recent years, Americans have been changing their habitual diet in the direction we recommend, that is, by reducing their intake of total fat, saturated fat, and cholesterol and by increasing intake of polyunsaturated fat. This has been accompanied by a substantial reduction in the average blood cholesterol level of the population. In addition, all-cause mortality, cardiovascular mortality, and coronary heart disease mortality have also decreased, but it is difficult to determine with certainty how much, if any, of this decrease is due to changes in diet, blood pressure, and cigarette usage or improved medical care. It is hoped that improved surveillance systems will clarify these issues.

Recommendations

In the general population, the basic intervention should be based on diet rather than drugs. We recommend a shift from the current typical American diet to one that is lower in total fat, saturated fat, and cholesterol. Diets with these characteristics are the usual diets consumed in a number of other countries, eg, Japan and Greece. Life expectancy in these two countries is, at virtually every age, greater than that in the United States. This applies also to the life expectancy in middle age, when mortality from coronary heart disease begins to rise sharply.

The evidence justifies for men, women, and children aged 2 years and older the reduction of calories from fat from the present average level of 40% to 30%, calories from saturated fat to 10% or less, and dietary cholesterol to no more than 250 to 300 mg daily. We recommend that calories from polyunsaturated fat be increased but not exceed 10% of total calories. This diet is generally consistent with the most recent recommendations of the American Heart Association and the Atherosclerosis Study Group of the Inter-Society Commission on Heart Disease Resources. Equally important, individuals, health professionals, and health agencies must recognize the need to control obesity both to aid in controlling blood cholesterol levels and to reduce the other health risks of obesity. Other elements important in the prevention of cardiovascular disease, including avoidance of cigarettes, control of high blood pressure, and maintenance of reasonable levels of physical activity, are recommended.

Means of Implementing Dietary Recommendations in the General Population

• If dietary intervention in the general population is to be effective, the eating habits of the entire family must be changed. Thus, the recommended diet should be available to all family members except those younger than 2 years.

• Educational services that enable adults and children to make informed choices concerning their eating habits should be readily available, including ready availability of data on composition of natural and processed foods.

• Professional educational programs for physicians, dietitians, and other health professionals should be expanded to include adequate material on diet and heart disease.

• Specific food items consistent with the recommended diet should be available, accessible, and affordable.

• The food industry should accelerate its current efforts to develop, produce, and market leaner meats and other foods, including dairy products, with reduced total fat, saturated fat, and cholesterol content.

• Restaurants, including fast-food outlets, should make foods satisfying these diet recommendations available to their customers.

• Government and school food programs should serve meals consistent with these recommendations.

• Food labeling should include total calories, fat source and total fat, saturated fat, polyunsaturated fat, and cholesterol content as well as other essential nutritional information. If necessary, appropriate statutory or other changes to require such labeling should be seriously considered.

• A national cholesterol education program should be implemented for physicians, other health professionals (including those in training), and the public; its effectiveness should be periodically evaluated.

5. What Research Directions Should Be Pursued on the Relationship Between Cholesterol and Heart Disease?—We know that blood cholesterol is causally related to coronary heart disease and that the atherosclerotic process can be influenced by intervention. However, much about lipid metabolism and about the mechanisms of the atherosclerotic process remains unknown.

• *Cellular and Molecular Biology.*—A better understanding of lipoprotein production and removal, lipoprotein receptors, and apolipoproteins is needed. More information is needed with regard to factors controlling the level of HDL and its role in preventing coronary heart disease. To learn whether diets very high in polyunsaturated fatty acids have any adverse effects, more information is needed regarding their biochemical and biologic effects, including those of the highly unsaturated fatty acids found in fish oils. Research is also needed on the biology of vessel wall injury, on the cells that participate in atherosclerosis, and on the events that trigger thrombosis in atherosclerotic vessels.

• *Clinical Investigation.*—Precisely defined diets and pharmacologic interventions to reduce blood cholesterol and other lipids must be studied in individuals under carefully controlled conditions. Research on the effectiveness of regimens to lower blood cholesterol levels and to influence atherosclerosis, including surgical intervention, should also be conducted. Evaluation of these may involve atherosclerotic plaque measurement using safe, precise imaging techniques such as ultrasound, regional radio-scintigraphy, magnetic resonance, and/or computer-enhanced radiography.

• *Pharmacologic Research.*—New compounds that are more effective, economical, and safe for the reduction of blood cholesterol levels are needed. Development of improved, more palatable, and less expensive bile-acid sequestrants also is needed. Similarly, a search for pharmacologic agents that would favorably influence other elements of the atherosclerotic process is highly desirable.

• *Food Product Research.*—The interface of human nutrition and human disease requires collaborative efforts within the agricultural, industrial, and health research communities. More food products that are high in nutritional quality and taste yet low in fat and cholesterol need to be developed.

• *Research in Human Behavior.*—Study of how people choose their diets and how food habits can be improved are necessary. Studies designed to measure and enhance adherence to new nutritional behaviors and treatment programs are needed.

• *Epidemiologic Investigation.*—The search for additional factors that initiate or affect the atherosclerotic process must be continued along with further studies of risk factors in major population subgroups, including blacks. As nutritional practices of the population change and as health professionals improve management of elevated blood cholesterol levels, ongoing monitoring of nutritional patterns, blood cholesterol levels, and disease and death outcomes is essential. An important corollary will be monitoring to assess disease incidence, prevalence, and case fatality rates. Research to assess the effects of blood cholesterol reduction on cardiovascular and all-cause mortality is needed. Overall safety of long-term intervention with diet and drugs should be investigated.

• *Secondary Prevention.*—The effectiveness of lowering blood cholesterol levels by medical or surgical intervention to retard or reverse atherosclerotic lesions in arteries or bypass grafts of patients with established coronary heart disease requires further investigation.

• *Community Applications.*—Community demonstration research to test the effectiveness of nutrition-educational programs that influence food choices and other risk-factor behaviors of the healthy free-living population is needed.

Members of the Consensus Development Panel were Daniel Steinberg, MD, PhD (chairman), La Jolla, Calif; Sidney Blumenthal, MD, New York; Richard A. Carleton, MD, Pawtucket, RI; Nancy H. Chasen, AB, JD, Bethesda, Md; James E. Dalen, MD, MPH, Worcester, Mass; John T. Fitzpatrick, Fairfield, Conn; Stephen B. Hulley, MD, MPH, San Francisco; Robert W. Mahley, MD, PhD, San Francisco; Gregory O'Keefe III, MD, Vinalhaven, Me; Richard D. Remington, PhD, Iowa City; Elijah Saunders, MD, Baltimore; Robert E. Shank, MD, St Louis; Arthur A. Spector, MD, Iowa City; Robert W. Wissler, MD, PhD, Chicago.

Members of the Planning Committee were Basil M. Rifkind, MD, FRCP (chairman), Bethesda, Md; Susan Clark, Bethesda, Md; Charles Gleeck, MD, Cincinnati; William Hazzard, MD, Baltimore; Kenneth Lippel, PhD, Bethesda, Md; Albert Oberman, MD, Birmingham, Ala; Michael J. Bernstein, Bethesda, Md; Larry Blaser, Bethesda, Md.

The conference was sponsored by the National Heart, Lung, and Blood Institute, Claude Lenfant, MD, director; and the Office of Medical Applications of Research, Itzhak Jacoby, PhD, acting director.

JACC Vol. 8, No. 6
December 1986:1245-55

1245

COOPERATIVE STUDIES

Fifteen Year Mortality in Coronary Drug Project Patients: Long-Term Benefit With Niacin

PAUL L. CANNER, PhD,* KENNETH G. BERGE, MD,† NANETTE K. WENGER, MD, FACC,‡
JEREMIAH STAMLER, MD, FACC,§ LAWRENCE FRIEDMAN, MD,‖
RONALD J. PRINEAS, MD, FACC,** WILLIAM FRIEDEWALD, MD,‖ FOR THE CORONARY DRUG
PROJECT RESEARCH GROUP††

The Coronary Drug Project was conducted between 1966 and 1975 to assess the long-term efficacy and safety of five lipid-influencing drugs in 8,341 men aged 30 to 64 years with electrocardiogram-documented previous myocardial infarction. The two estrogen regimens and dextrothyroxine were discontinued early because of adverse effects. No evidence of efficacy was found for the clofibrate treatment. Niacin treatment showed modest benefit in decreasing definite nonfatal recurrent myocardial infarction but did not decrease total mortality.

With a mean follow-up of 15 years, nearly 9 years after termination of the trial, mortality from all causes in each of the drug groups, except for niacin, was similar to that in the placebo group. Mortality in the niacin group was 11% lower than in the placebo group (52.0 versus 58.2%; p = 0.0004). This late benefit of niacin, occurring after discontinuation of the drug, may be a result of a translation into a mortality benefit over subsequent years of the early favorable effect of niacin in decreasing nonfatal reinfarction or a result of the cholesterol-lowering effect of niacin, or both.

(J Am Coll Cardiol 1986;8:1245–55)

The Coronary Drug Project, a long-term study of lipid-influencing drugs in male survivors of myocardial infarction, was concluded as planned in early 1975 (1). Three of the five lipid-influencing regimens studied were discontinued early because of adverse effects. Treatment with the remaining two agents, clofibrate and niacin, did not show convincing evidence of benefit compared with placebo for the primary end point of total mortality during an average period of observation of 6 years. In 1980, the Coronary Drug Project coordinating center systematically began to follow up those patients still alive at the conclusion of the trial. The primary purpose was to determine whether any long-term *adverse* effects were evident in cause-specific mortality several years after the end of the study. This follow-up study was prompted by a possible excess mortality

due to cancer in the Coronary Drug Project low dose estrogen group (2,3) and excess mortality from all causes in the clofibrate regimen of the World Health Organization Clofibrate Trial (4). The findings of this follow-up study are presented in this report.

Methods

Design and methods of the Coronary Drug Project. The background, design and organization of the Coronary Drug Project have been described in detail (1,5,6). The primary objective was to test efficacy and safety of several lipid-influencing drugs in the long-term therapy of coronary heart disease in men with proved previous myocardial infarction. The 53 project clinical centers, located in the United States and Puerto Rico, recruited 8,341 patients who were randomly assigned to six treatment groups: conjugated estrogens at two dosage levels, clofibrate, dextrothyroxine sodium, niacin and a lactose placebo. The allocation schedule was designed to ensure approximately five patients in the placebo group for every two patients in any other group (Fig. 1).

The patients were men aged 30 through 64 years at entry, with verified evidence of one or more myocardial infarctions, categorized in class I or II of the New York Heart Association functional classification (7) and free from a specified list of diseases and conditions (5). All patients

From the *Maryland Medical Research Institute, Baltimore, Maryland; †Mayo Clinic, Rochester, Minnesota; ‡Emory University School of Medicine, Atlanta, Georgia; §Northwestern University Medical School, Chicago, Illinois; ‖National Heart, Lung, and Blood Institute, Bethesda Maryland and **School of Public Health, University of Minnesota, Minneapolis, Minnesota. The Coronary Drug Project was carried out as a collaborative study supported by research grants and other funds from the National Heart, Lung, and Blood Institute, Bethesda, Maryland.

††A list of the key bodies and senior staff members of the Coronary Drug Project Mortality Follow-Up Program is presented in Appendix B.

Manuscript received February 28, 1986; revised manuscript received May 7, 1986, accepted June 6, 1986.

Address for reprints: Paul L. Canner, PhD, Maryland Medical Research Institute, 600 Wyndhurst Avenue, Baltimore, Maryland 21210.

0735-1097/86/$3.50

1246   CANNER ET AL.
LONG-TERM MORTALITY BENEFIT WITH NIACIN

JACC Vol. 8, No. 6
December 1986:1245–55

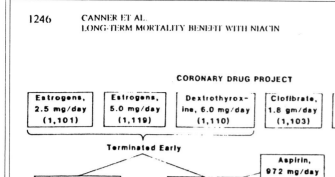

Figure 1. Treatment scheme in the Coronary Drug Project (CDP) and Coronary Drug Project Aspirin Study. Numbers of patients are given in parentheses.

were at least 3 months beyond their most recent myocardial infarction and free of recent worsening of coronary disease or other major illnesses. The study protocol was approved by the human experimentation committees of the coordinating center and all clinical centers' institutions.

The first patient was randomly allocated to treatment in March 1966, and the last in October 1969. Patients were followed up in double-blind fashion with visits every 4 months. Patient follow-up and data collection for the main trial were completed in February 1975. All surviving patients were followed up for at least 4.5 years, and 96% for at least 5 years. The maximal follow-up time was 8.5 years for the participants recruited earliest; the mean follow-up time was 6.2 years. The primary end point was mortality from all causes. Secondary end points included mortality from coronary heart disease, sudden death and incidence of recurrent nonfatal myocardial infarction (5).

The two estrogen regimens and the dextrothyroxine regimen were discontinued before the scheduled end of the trial. High dose estrogen treatment was terminated in 1970 (mean follow-up 1.5 years) because of a significant increase in definite nonfatal myocardial infarction and an unfavorable trend in total mortality (8). Dextrothyroxine was stopped in 1971 (mean follow up 3.0 years) because of increased total mortality, with particularly unfavorable mortality rates in certain patient subgroups (9). Low dose estrogen was terminated in 1973 (mean follow-up 4.7 years) because of an increase in cancer deaths compared with deaths in those receiving placebo and an unfavorable trend in total mortality (2).

Three treatment groups—clofibrate, niacin and placebo—were continued to the scheduled end of the trial (mean follow-up 6.2 years). The clofibrate group showed no benefit with respect to mortality or nonfatal cardiovascular events (1). Niacin had no statistically significant effect on total mortality; however, patients in the niacin group had a significantly lower incidence of definite nonfatal myocardial infarction compared with patients in the placebo group (1).

Coronary Drug Project Aspirin Study. About half the patients in the three groups that were terminated early (1,529 of the 3,330 patients originally assigned to the dextrothyroxine and two estrogen groups) were enrolled between November 1972 and April 1974 in a trial (called the Coro-

nary Drug Project Aspirin Study) comparing aspirin and placebo (Fig. 1). These patients were followed up for a minimum of 10 and a maximum of 28 months (mean 22). Patient follow-up and data collection terminated in February 1975. A difference found in overall mortality between the aspirin and placebo groups was "suggestive of a beneficial effect for aspirin in the treatment of post-myocardial infarction men but not large enough to be conclusive" (10).

Design and methods of the Coronary Drug Project Mortality Follow-up Program. In June 1981, the Coronary Drug Project coordinating center was awarded a contract by the National Heart, Lung, and Blood Institute for mortality follow-up of Coronary Drug Project patients who were alive at the end of the trial. The primary objectives were to determine vital status, at least 5 years after the end of the trial, of all 6,008 Coronary Drug Project patients alive in February 1975, and to relate the findings to previous study treatment group.

*Vital status was ascertained by a variety of means—*information from study investigators; letters (first regular mail and later certified mail) and telephone calls to the patients; telephone calls to the patients' relatives, neighbors, physicians and employers; National Death Index search; Social Security Administration file search; Veterans Administration file search and utilization of the services of a national search agency. (Details concerning these various procedures can be obtained from the senior author.) For all deaths ascertained, attempts were made to obtain death certificates from state offices of vital records so that cause of death could be determined. Other patient information for this post-trial period, such as occurrence of nonfatal cardiovascular events or cardiovascular surgery or use of cholesterol-lowering drugs, was not systematically collected.

Statistical methods. Treatment group comparisons of mortality rates were made by the ordinary test of two proportions (11). This test yields z values defined as the drug-placebo difference in proportions of events divided by the standard error of the difference. A z value exceeding ± 1.96 is generally considered statistically significant at the 5% level of significance; however, adjustment for five drug-placebo comparisons requires a z value on the order of ± 2.58 for statistical significance. Further conservatism is generally considered appropriate in evaluating treatment effects

JACC Vol. 8, No. 6
December 1986:1245-55

Table 1. Vital Status Information by Treatment Group in the Coronary Drug Project and Coronary Drug Project Aspirin Study

Vital Status Information	Coronary Drug Project							Coronary Drug Project Aspirin Study		
	Low Dose Estrogen	High Dose Estrogen	Clofibrate	Dextro-thyroxine	Niacin	Placebo	All	Aspirin	Placebo	All
Number of patients originally enrolled	1,101	1,119	1,103	1,110	1,119	2,789	8,341	758	771	1,529
Deaths reported before end of study in early 1975	317	324	311	308	292	781	2,333	48	71	119
Number of patients in CDP Mortality Follow-up Program	784	795	792	802	827	2,008	6,008	710	700	1,410
Deceased	340	328	326	325	290	842	2,451	255	269	524
	(1)*	(1)	(1)	(0)	(1)	(1)	(5)	(0)	(1)	(1)
Alive	432	461	447	467	523	1,137	3,467	446	423	869
"Assumed alive"†	10	5	13	9	8	21	66	7	8	15
No vital status information	2	1	6	1	6	8	24	2	0	2

*Number of unconfirmed deaths (see text for definition); †as determined from Social Security or Veterans Administration files.

in subgroups. Homogeneity of treatment effects between two categories of a given baseline characteristic was assessed by means of a log odds ratio procedure (11). Adjustment of drug-placebo differences in event rates for baseline covariates was made using multiple linear regression (12). Survival curves were estimated using the Littell method (13), and compared using the log rank test (14).

Results

Ascertainment of vital status (Table 1). Of the 8,341 patients originally enrolled in the Coronary Drug Project, 2,333 were known to have died by the end of the trial in February 1975. Information on vital status as of at least March 1980 was obtained on 5,984 (99.6%) of the other 6,008 patients. For 66 patients, the only information available was "assumed alive" according to either Social Security Administration records as of early 1983 (61 patients) or Veterans Administration records as of early 1985 (5 patients). A total of 3,041 patients were reported by the Social Security Administration as "assumed alive," but 98 (3.2%) of these were found from other sources to be deceased. Thus, it is possible that a small number of the patients for whom the only information is "assumed alive" are actually deceased.

Death certificates have been obtained for 2,227 (97%) of the 2,451 patients identified by one or more of the preceding mechanisms as having died after February 1975. For another 130, death reports were received from two or more independent sources, and for 89 the information concerning the death (including a date of death and often a place of death) was deemed to provide adequate confirmation of the death, even though death certificates could not be obtained. The remaining five identified deaths could not be confirmed

(Table 1). These five patients with unconfirmed death are assumed dead for purposes of this report.

Follow-up period. The mortality findings represent a mean patient follow-up period of about 15 years—6.2 years on the Coronary Drug Project treatment regimen (or less for those in the three treatment groups stopped prematurely) and 8.8 years after termination of the study. The 8.8 years correspond to the interval from August 1974 (midpoint of the period in which the Coronary Drug Project treatment regimen was terminated) to June 1983 (when the Social Security Administration records were searched, identifying the vast majority of the deaths). For patients enrolled in the Coronary Drug Project Aspirin Study, the total follow-up period is 10.2 years—1.8 years on the study regimen and 8.4 years after termination of the study. The mortality findings for patients in the two estrogen and the dextrothyroxine groups—the groups terminated early—include the mortality during the 1.8 years (average) of participation in the Coronary Drug Project Aspirin Study, assigned with equal probability to either aspirin or placebo regimens.

The annual death rates for all six treatment groups combined were 5.1, 4.5 and 4.4%, respectively, for the first 3 years, with a slight but steady increase each year thereafter to 7.1% for the 15th year. The slightly higher rate for the first year may reflect the relative proximity to the qualifying myocardial infarction. The qualifying infarction preceded entry into the study by as little as 3 months and a median of 23 months (5). The rates for the first, second and third 5 year periods were 21.6, 25.0 and 29.5%, respectively, and the cumulative 15 year mortality rate was 58.6%.

Findings in the estrogen, clofibrate and dextrothyroxine groups (Table 2). The mortality follow-up of Coronary Drug Project patients was performed primarily to assess long-term findings in the groups—high and low dose estro-

1248   CANNER ET AL.
LONG-TERM MORTALITY BENEFIT WITH NIACIN

JACC Vol. 8, No. 6
December 1986:1245-55

Table 2. All-Cause Mortality (%) for a Mean Follow-up Period of 15 Years in the Estrogen, Clofibrate, Dextrothyroxine and Placebo Groups

Lipid-Lowering Drug	Drug		Placebo		z Value
	n	%	n	%	
Low dose estrogen	1,101	59.7	2,789	58.2	0.84
High dose estrogen	1,119	58.3	2,789	58.2	0.04
Clofibrate	1,103	57.8	2,789	58.2	-0.25
Dextrothyroxine	1,110	57.0	2,789	58.2	-0.67

gen, dextrothyroxine and clofibrate—found in the Coronary Drug Project or the World Health Organization Clofibrate Trial to have adverse effects. For these four groups, the mortality rate from all causes for a mean follow-up period of 15 years ranged from 57.0% in the dextrothyroxine group to 59.7% in the low dose estrogen group, compared with 58.2% in the placebo group. Mortality in each treatment group was within ± 1.5% of the placebo group mortality, a relative difference of ± 2.6%; none of the drug-placebo differences was statistically significant.

The Coronary Drug Project low dose estrogen group, terminated prematurely because of excess cancer mortality, continues to show a moderate excess of cancer deaths compared with such deaths in the placebo group (5.9 versus 4.4%; z = 1.90, p = 0.057) (Table A2 in Appendix A). However, if cancer deaths before the end of the treatment phase in August 1974 (Table A1) are excluded, the subsequent cancer mortality rate since conclusion of the trial is only slightly higher for the low dose estrogen group (3.9%) than for the placebo group (3.5%). The high dose estrogen group and the clofibrate group both had a somewhat lower cancer mortality rate (3.7 and 3.4%, respectively) than did the placebo group (4.4%) over 15 years (Table A2).

Findings in the aspirin group. The Coronary Drug Project Aspirin Study concluded with a mortality rate from all causes of 5.8% in the aspirin group compared with 8.3% in the placebo group (z = 1.90; p = 0.057), a 30% reduction in mortality (10). An additional 8.4 years after termination of the study, the mortality rate from all causes was 40.0% in the aspirin group and 44.1% in the placebo group (z = -1.63; p = 0.10), a 9% reduction in mortality. Thus, the absolute difference in mortality has subsequently widened somewhat, but the relative difference and degree of statistical significance are diminished.

Findings in the niacin group (Tables 3 to 5). Cumulative mortality from all causes for a mean follow-up period of 15 years was 52.0% in the niacin group compared with 58.2% in the placebo group (Table 3). There were 69 (11%) fewer deaths in the niacin group than expected on the basis of placebo group mortality. The z value for the niacin-placebo difference in mortality from all causes was -3.52, corresponding to a two-sided p value of 0.0004. Survival curves for mortality from all causes are shown for patients

in the niacin and placebo groups in Figure 2; the median survival time from entry into the Coronary Drug Project was 13.03 years for patients in the niacin group compared with 11.40 years for those in the placebo group (p = 0.0012). The survival benefit in the niacin group is primarily evident for death caused by coronary heart disease, with small beneficial trends for each of cerebrovascular, other cardiovascular, cancer, noncardiovascular and noncancer causes of death.

The beneficial effect of niacin on mortality is present in all subgroups of 12 entry characteristics except for probable or definite cardiomegaly, where there is a 0.1% excess mortality in the niacin group (Table 4). There is no statistically significant lack of homogeneity between the niacin treatment effect and the levels of any of these entry characteristics (that is, the niacin-placebo difference in one subgroup is not significantly different from that difference in the complementary subgroup). The largest trend (z = 1.93) toward lack of homogeneity was a greater beneficial effect on mortality in the niacin group compared with placebo in the subgroup with a serum cholesterol level of 250 mg/dl or greater at entry than in those with lower levels.

A multiple linear regression analysis using the niacin treatment variable plus the 12 entry variables given in Table 4 in the model, with total mortality as the dependent variable, yielded an adjusted z value for the niacin effect on total mortality (-3.53), about the same as the unadjusted value reported earlier.

Mortality from all causes in relation to occurrence of

Table 3. Mortality (%) by Cause for a Mean Follow-up Period of 15 Years in the Niacin and Placebo Groups

Cause of Death	Niacin	Placebo	z Value
All causes	52.0	58.2	-3.52
Coronary heart disease	36.5	41.3	-2.80
Cerebrovascular causes	1.4	1.6	-0.34
Other cardiovascular	4.5	4.8	-0.45
Cancer	4.0	4.4	-0.59
Other causes	2.9	3.0	-0.16
Unknown or not coded	2.7	3.0	-0.56
No. of patients	1,119	2,789	

JACC Vol. 8, No. 6
December 1986:1245–55

CANNER ET AL. 1249
LONG-TERM MORTALITY BENEFIT WITH NIACIN

Table 4. All-Cause Mortality by Findings at Entry for Niacin and Placebo Groups

Entry Characteristic	Niacin		Placebo		z Value
	No. Men	% Deaths	No. Men	% Deaths	
Age (yr)					
<55	614	43.2	1,590	49.6	−2.70
≥55	505	62.6	1,199	69.3	−2.71
Cigarette smoker					
No	709	47.2	1,731	53.9	−2.99
Yes	409	59.9	1,056	64.9	−1.77
No. of previous myocardial infarctions					
1	909	48.8	2,231	53.8	−2.54
≥2	209	65.1	555	75.0	−2.72
New York Heart Association class					
I	538	45.2	1,295	49.7	−1.78
II	580	58.1	1,492	65.3	−3.04
Cardiomegaly on chest X-ray film					
No	943	47.9	2,281	54.7	−3.49
Probable or definite	176	73.3	508	73.2	0.02
Diuretic usage					
No	940	48.7	2,321	54.6	−3.04
Yes	179	68.7	468	75.2	−1.67
Serum cholesterol (mg/dl)					
<250	577	53.2	1,481	56.2	−1.22
≥250	541	50.5	1,306	60.2	−3.84
Serum triglycerides (mEq/liter)					
<5	528	51.9	1,375	57.3	−2.13
≥5	590	51.9	1,412	58.8	−2.85
Serum uric acid (mg/dl)					
<7	633	50.2	1,553	55.6	−2.30
≥7	485	54.0	1,234	61.1	−2.69
Plasma fasting glucose (mg/dl)					
<100	630	48.6	1,564	53.5	−2.10
≥100	488	56.1	1,223	63.9	−2.96
Systolic blood pressure (mm Hg)					
<130	526	44.3	1,353	53.4	−3.56
≥130	592	58.6	1,434	52.4	−1.60
Diastolic blood pressure (mm Hg)					
<85	700	49.0	1,763	55.9	−3.11
≥85	418	56.7	1,024	61.7	−1.77

definite nonfatal myocardial infarction during the trial is given for the niacin and placebo groups in Table 5. At the conclusion of the Coronary Drug Project, the incidence of definite nonfatal myocardial infarction was 10.4% for patients in the niacin group and 14.7% for patients in the placebo group. The findings in Table 5 suggest that this beneficial effect of niacin with respect to definite nonfatal myocardial infarction may account for approximately 10 of the 69 fewer deaths in the niacin treatment group. The reasoning for this is as follows: If we assume that the placebo group incidence (14.7%) of definite nonfatal recurrent myocardial infarction had applied to the niacin group of 1,119

men, we would have observed 164 men in the niacin group with such an event, instead of the 116 actually observed. If we then apply the niacin group death rate (81 of 116, or 69.8%) given one or more myocardial infarctions to this group of 164 men, we find that 114 deaths would have been expected. Similar calculations for the noninfarct groups yield a total of 570 deaths expected in the niacin group compared with 560 deaths actually observed.

The percent decrease in mean serum cholesterol from baseline to year 1 was 10.1% in the niacin group (Table 6). Treatment with niacin proved to be the best lipid-lowering regimen among the five Coronary Drug Project treat-

Table 5. All-Cause Mortality by Occurrence of Definite Nonfatal Myocardial Infarction During the Trial in the Niacin and Placebo Groups

No. of Definite Nonfatal Myocardial Infarctions During Trial	Niacin			Placebo		
	No. Men	No. Deaths	% Deaths	No. Men	No. Deaths	% Deaths
None	1,003 (89.6%)*	479	47.8	2,380 (85.3%)	1,285	54.0
One or more	116 (10.4%)	81	69.8	409 (14.7%)	282	68.9
All	1,119	560	50.0	2,789	1,567	56.2
Applying placebo group incidence of definite nonfatal myocardial infarction to niacin group						
None	955 (85.3%)	456	47.8			
One or more	164 (14.7%)	114	69.8			
All	1,119	570†	51.0			

*Percent of men in the particular subgroup given in parentheses; †570 expected deaths minus 560 observed deaths equals 10 niacin deaths saved due to reducing the incidence of definite nonfatal myocardial infarction. Note that deaths that occurred both during the trial (except those before the first Coronary Drug Project follow-up visit, that is, before a nonfatal myocardial infarction could have been reported) and during the period of subsequent follow-up reported in this review are included in this table.

ment regimens. Also, within the niacin group, patients with the largest decrease in serum chlesterol at 1 year experienced a lower subsequent mortality than did those with an increase in serum cholesterol. There was no significant correlation between change in serum triglyceride level and mortality in the niacin group.

As reported earlier by the Coronary Drug Project Research Group (1), niacin therapy was associated with statistically significant increases in serum glutamic oxaloacetic transaminase, serum alkaline phosphatase, plasma fasting and 1 hour glucose and serum uric acid levels, and decreases in plasma urea nitrogen levels and systolic and diastolic blood pressure. Analyses of these response variables in the niacin group failed to demonstrate any correlation between change in values from baseline to 1 year and subsequent mortality.

Discussion

Ascertainment of vital status. The Coronary Drug Project Mortality Follow-up Program has been successful in locating and determining vital status of participants in the Coronary Drug Project 9 years after conclusion of the trial. Definite information concerning vital status was obtained on 98.9% of the 8,341 Coronary Drug Project patients; for 0.8%, death was reported but not confirmed or the patient was "assumed alive"; no information on vital status was obtained for the remaining 0.3% of the patients.

Findings in the estrogen, clofibrate, dextrothyroxine and aspirin groups. The 15 year mortality findings for the two estrogen, the dextrothyroxine, the clofibrate and the aspirin groups compared with the placebo group do not substantially differ qualitatively from those initially reported for each of these treatment groups (1–3, 8–10). There is no evidence of long-term adverse effects in the estrogen- and dextrothyroxine-treated patients beyond those reported at the time these regimens were discontinued. Neither is there evidence of long-term adverse effects of clofibrate. Although the initial findings of the World Health Organization Clofibrate Trial (4) revealed excess mortality from all causes in the patients treated with clofibrate, follow-up data covering a 7.9 year post-trial period showed a moderate attenuation of this excess mortality after the end of treatment (15).

Findings in the niacin group. We are aware of only two randomized placebo-controlled trials of niacin in which

Figure 2. Survival curves for niacin and placebo treatment groups.

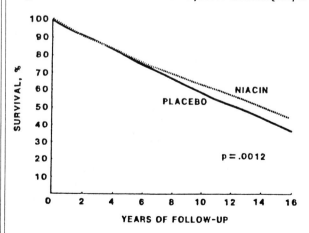

p = .0012

JACC Vol. 8, No. 6
December 1986:1245-55

CANNER ET AL.
LONG-TERM MORTALITY BENEFIT WITH NIACIN

1251

Table 6. Serum Lipid Levels at Baseline and Year 1 for the Treatment and Placebo Groups

Mean Lipid Level	Low Dose Estrogen	High Dose Estrogen	Clofibrate	Dextrothyroxine	Niacin	Placebo
Cholesterol (mg/dl)						
Baseline	250	251	252	250	253	249
Year 1	247	245	239	226	227	254
% change	− 1.3	− 2.3	− 5.1	− 9.7	− 10.1	+ 1.9
Triglycerides (mEq/liter)						
Baseline	6.0	6.1	6.1	5.7	6.4	6.2
Year 1	6.4	7.1	4.3	5.0	4.7	6.3
% change	+ 6.9	+ 17.2	− 23.1	− 12.1	− 26.9	+ 2.1

an attempt was made to assess the efficacy and safety of niacin with respect to mortality. Both studies were of survivors of acute myocardial infarction. The Veterans Administration study (16) of lipid-lowering agents showed, after 3.2 years of follow-up, a slight excess in total mortality in the 77 patients receiving niacin alone compared with the 143 placebo-treated patients. In the Stockholm Ischemic Heart Disease Study (17–19), effects of niacin were confounded with those of clofibrate. The 5 year mortality rate from all causes (21.9%) in 279 patients receiving 2 g/day of clofibrate plus 3 g/day of niacin was 29% lower than that (30.7%) in 267 control group patients (p= 0.036).

In the Coronary Drug Project, the 5 year mortality rate in the niacin group was 21.2%, slightly higher than in the placebo group (20.9%) (1). At the scheduled conclusion of the trial, with a mean follow-up period 6.2 years, mortality in the niacin group was 4% lower than in the placebo group (24.8 versus 25.9%) (Table A1). The published life tables (1) showed that the niacin and placebo mortality rates were almost identical throughout the first 68 months of follow-up, but started to diverge at month 72. Life table curves for definite nonfatal myocardial infarction showed that the niacin group began to diverge in the beneficial direction at about month 28.

The significant benefit in 15 year mortality from all causes in the niacin group in the Coronary Drug Project Mortality Follow-up Program was found even though, during the treatment phase, nearly 30% of the niacin-treated patients adhered poorly to the treatment regimen (that is, took less than 60% of the protocol amount of drug) over the follow up period (1). Thus, therapeutic benefit may have been derived from less than optimal doses of the drug.

Explanations for survival benefits of niacin. The unanticipated finding of a significant long-term survival benefit with niacin may be explained in part by the earlier decrease in definite nonfatal myocardial infarction. However, a more likely explanation stems from the cholesteral-lowering effect of niacin, which was superior to that of the other drugs studied in the Coronary Drug Project. In the niacin group, patients with the largest decrease in serum cholesterol at 1 year had a lower subsequent mortality than did those with

an increase in serum cholesterol. Analyses relating mortality or other outcomes to variables that are themselves affected by the treatment are fraught with hazards and can lead to invalid conclusions (20). Nonetheless, these findings lend support to the suggestion that the cholesterol-lowering effect of niacin may be partly responsible for the reduced mortality. Thus, it is possible that a 10% reduction in serum cholesterol, maintained over 5 to 8 years, may have significantly slowed the progression of coronary atherosclerosis.

Time lag in development of a beneficial trend. While a time lag in development of a beneficial trend in mortality as a consequence of lowering serum cholesterol and slowing coronary atherosclerosis (21) is to be expected, it seems surprising that this lag—for niacin treatment—is of the magnitude of 6 years or more. Both the niacin data during the Coronary Drug Project and the cholestyramine data from the Lipid Research Clinics Coronary Primary Prevention Trial (22) show about a 2 to 3 year delay before the development of a beneficial trend in nonfatal myocardial infarction. Because the atherosclerotic processes underlying nonfatal and fatal myocardial infarction presumably are similar, with the availability of emergency medical services and life support measures often making the difference between a fatal and a nonfatal event, it is puzzling that an additional 3 years of serum lipid-lowering seems to be required for a beneficial trend in *mortality*. However, it is possible that initially, niacin prevents primarily milder, nonlife-threatening infarction. This is suggested by unpublished data from the Coronary Drug Project: among patients with interim nonfatal myocardial infarction, those in the niacin group had greater subsequent mortality during the treatment phase of the trial than did patients in the placebo group. Thus, although patients receiving niacin experienced nonfatal myocardial infarction less frequently than did patients receiving placebo, their nonfatal infarctions were more severe than those of the placebo group, suggesting that milder myocardial infarction may have been prevented by niacin. Then, as the favorable lipid-lowering effect of niacin on the coronary arteries increased over time, more severe life-threatening infarction may have been prevented.

1252   CANNER ET AL.   JACC Vol. 8, No. 6
        LONG-TERM MORTALITY BENEFIT WITH NIACIN   December 1986:1245–55

As an alternative explanation for the 6 year lag, there may have been counterbalancing adverse effects of niacin while patients were taking the drug; the beneficial lipid-lowering effect may be manifest only after the drug is discontinued. The significantly higher incidence of atrial fibrillation and other cardiac arrhythmias in the niacin group (1) may be a possible mechanism for this explanation.

Other explanations for the beneficial effect of niacin. Did patients in the niacin group receive more aggressive medical or surgical treatment of their coronary heart disease after the Coronary Drug Project trial was completed than did patients in the placebo and other treatment groups? No post-trial data are available to answer this question. However, during the Coronary Drug Project trial, patients in the niacin group had a nearly 50% *lower* incidence of cardiovascular surgery than did placebo-treated patients; also, most categories of cardiac medications were prescribed *less* frequently for niacin than for placebo-treated patients during the trial (1). There is no reason to expect these patterns to have changed drastically after the trial was over; thus, such an explanation of the niacin findings seems most improbable.

It is possible that *part* of the observed effect is due to incomplete ascertainment of vital status. However, if the mathematically worst possible scenario occurred (that is, all 6 patients in the niacin group without vital status information and all 8 patients designated as "assumed alive" by Social Security or Veterans Administration information were actually deceased and all 8 and 21 corresponding patients in the placebo group were alive), the z value for the niacin-placebo difference in total mortality would change from −3.52 to −2.81, still a significant difference. Therefore, incomplete ascertainment of vital status does not explain the beneficial effect of niacin.

Conclusion. Follow-up data on patients who participated in the Coronary Drug Project suggest that niacin administered after recovery from myocardial infarction may confer a long-term survival benefit, averaging 1.6 additional years of life. These data are derived from men recovered from myocardial infarction who were prescribed 3 g of niacin daily for an average of 6.2 years, then presumably stopped taking the drug. The maximal difference in survival was attained at about 12 years after initiation of niacin therapy, or an average of about 5.8 years after termination of that regimen. The available data relate only to the use of niacin for 5 to 8 years in survivors or myocardial infarction. There is no information on whether longer-term niacin usage might be helpful or harmful, whether the drug is effective in *women* after myocardial infarction or whether the drug has any value in the *primary* prevention of coronary heart disease. However, in the context of all other information that is available from both epidemiologic and clinical trial sources, the results may indeed be applicable to populations not included in the Coronary Drug Project.

The valuable information obtained from the Coronary Drug Project Mortality Follow-up Program, and especially the totally unexpected findings in the niacin group, suggest the potential usefulness of "reopening the books" on other completed clinical trials to assess long-term treatment effects on mortality.

Appendix A

Detailed Data on Cause-Specific Mortality

Final in-trial cause-specific mortality. The mortality results in the clofibrate, niacin and placebo groups for the treatment phase of the Coronary Drug Project were published in 1975 (1). After that report, a few additional deaths that occurred before August 31, 1974 were brought to the attention of the study investigators. In addition, the cause-specific mortality data reported in 1975 were based on the death reports received from the clinical centers. The coding of all deaths by a Mortality Classification Committee using uniform criteria and without knowledge of treatment assignment was completed subsequently. Table A1 presents this final, committee-coded, detailed cause-specific mortality for the treatment phase of the Coronary Drug Project (that is, all deaths up to the time of the termination of the study treatment in the summer of 1974 or up to August 31, 1974 for patients who dropped out of the study). This table includes patients originally in the two estrogen and dextrothyroxine groups who were subsequently enrolled in the Coronary Drug Project Aspirin Study, as well as patients in those groups not in the Coronary Drug Project Aspirin Study. Thus, the data in Table A1 represent a mean follow-up period of 1.5 years on the high dose estrogen regimen and 4.7 years off this regimen, with 50% of the patients participating in the Coronary Drug Project Aspirin Study for a mean of 1.7 of these years. For dextrothyroxine, there was a mean follow-up on treatment of 3.0 years and 3.2 years off treatment, with 53% of these patients in the Coronary Drug Project Aspirin Study for a mean of 1.7 years. For low dose estrogen, the mean follow-up on treatment was 4.7 years and 1.5 years off treatment, with 35% of these patients participating in the Coronary Drug Project Aspirin Study for a mean of 0.5 years. Finally, the data in Table A1 for the clofibrate, niacin and placebo groups reflect a mean follow-up on study treatment regimen of 6.2 years.

In-trial plus post-trial cause-specific mortality. Table A2 gives cause-specific mortality for the six treatment groups for both the treatment phase covered in Table A1 and the post-trial phase of a mean of 8.8 years. Some difficulties were encountered in attempting to combine cause of death categories used by the Mortality Classification Committee with International Classification of Diseases (ICD) codes used to classify deaths reported during the post-trial follow-up period. The biggest difficulty related to coronary heart disease deaths. The Mortality Classification Committee, using detailed descriptions of the terminal event, carefully classified coronary deaths into those with a recent or acute cardiac event (for example, sudden unexpected death or recent myocardial infarction) and those without a recent or acute cardiac event (for

JACC Vol. 8, No. 6
December 1986:1245–55

CANNER ET AL. 1253
LONG-TERM MORTALITY BENEFIT WITH NIACIN

Table A1. Cause-Specific Mortality During the Coronary Drug Project Treatment Phase

Cause of Death	Low Dose Estrogen (n = 1,101)		High Dose Estrogen (n = 1,119)		Clofibrate (n = 1,103)		Dextrothyroxine (n = 1,110)		Niacin (n = 1,119)		Placebo (n = 2,789)	
	No.	(%)	No.	(%)	No.	(%)	No.	(%)	No.	(%)	No.	(%)
All causes	294	(26.7)	301	(26.9)	288	(26.1)	287	(25.9)	277	(24.8)	723	(25.9)
Cardiovascular	265	(24.1)	279	(24.9)	259	(23.5)	262	(23.6)	250	(22.3)	660	(23.7)
Coronary—acute	230	(20.9)	242	(21.6)	221	(20.0)	225	(20.3)	215	(19.2)	583	(20.9)
Coronary—chronic	20		20		19		26		23		49	
Cerebrovascular	5		10		14		6		6		14	
Pulmonary embolism	1		1		1		1		2		2	
Other cardiovascular	9		6		4		4		4		12	
Cancer	22	(2.0)	13	(1.2)	11	(1.0)	15	(1.4)	14	(1.3)	27	(1.0)
Lung	8		7		3		4		9		12	
Gastrointestinal	5		0		2		3		1		2	
Pancreatic	2		3		1		2		0		2	
Liver, gallbladder	1		0		1		1		0		0	
Genitourinary	2		2		1		1		3		5	
Blood, lymph	0		0		2		0		0		3	
Other cancer	4		1		1		4		1		3	
Other noncardiovascular	6	(0.5)	6	(0.5)	12	(1.1)	9	(0.8)	13	(1.2)	31	(1.1)
Infection	1		0		2		2		1		4	
Lung disease	0		0		1		0		2		5	
Gastrointestinal	1		1		1		2		0		5	
Pancreatitis	1		1		0		0		0		1	
Liver, gallbladder	0		3		2		0		1		0	
Genitourinary	0		0		1		0		1		0	
Blood	0		0		0		0		0		0	
Endocrine, metabolic	0		0		0		0		0		0	
Central nervous system	0		0		0		0		0		0	
Nonmedical*	3		1		5		5		8		15	
Other	0		0		0		0		0		1	
Unknown	1	(0.1)	3	(0.3)	6	(0.5)	1	(0.1)	0	(0.0)	5	(0.2)

*Includes accidents, homicide and suicide.

example, congestive heart failure). It is much more difficult, if not impossible, to make such a distinction using ICD codes. A death certified as "cardiac arrest due to atherosclerotic coronary heart disease," and thus coded 414.0, is more than likely a sudden unexpected cardiac death. However, a death certified as "chronic congestive heart failure due to atherosclerotic coronary heart disease" is also coded 414.0. For purposes of Table A2, all ICD codes 410 to 414 except 414.8 ("chronic myocardial ischemia") plus ICD code 429.2 ("arteriosclerotic cardiovascular disease") were counted as "coronary—acute." Codes 414.8 and 428 were counted as "coronary—chronic."

During the treatment phase (Table A1), 91% of deaths were from cardiovascular causes, while 75% of post-trial deaths were cardiovascular. This highly significant difference ($p = 10^{-48}$) is likely a result of the fact that individuals with serious noncardiovascular disease at the outset were not enrolled in the study.

Appendix B

The key bodies of the Coronary Drug Project Mortality Follow-up Program and the senior staff members are as follows:

Steering and Editorial Review Committee. Jeremiah Stamler, MD (Chairman), Kenneth Berge, MD, Henry Blackburn, MD, William Friedewald, MD, Lawrence Friedman, MD, Adrian Hainline, Jr., PhD, Christian Klimt, MD, DrPH, Charles Laubach, Jr., MD, Ronald Prineas, MB, BS, PhD, Nanette Wenger, MD.

Coordinating Center. Paul Canner, PhD (Principal Investigator), Sandra Forman, MA (Co-Investigator), Joseph Canner, Martha Canner, MS, Rosemary Giro, Elizabeth Heinz, Mary Keiser, Christian Klimt, MD, DrPH, Delores Seldon.

National Heart, Lung, and Blood Institute Staff. William Friedewald, MD, Lawrence Friedman, MD.

Principal Investigators, Clinical Centers. Kenneth Berge, MD, Nicholas Galluzzi, MD, Paul Geller, MD, James Schoenberger, MD, Samuel Baer, MD, Henry Schoch, MD, Ronald Gillilan, MD, Robert Kohn, MD, Bernard Lewis, MD, Richard Jones, MD, Philip Frost, MD, Dean Emanuel, MD, David Morgan, MD, David Berkson, MD, William Bernstein, MD, Ernst Greif, MD, Richard Pyle, MD, Ephraim Donoso, MD, Jacob Haft, MD, Gordon Maurice, MD, Ralph Lazzara, MD, Irving Liebow, MD, Marvin Segal, MD, Charles Moore, MD, John Morledge, MD, Olga Haring, MD, Robert Schlant, MD, Joseph Wagner, MD, Ward Laramore, MD, Donald McCaughan, MD, Robert Ohlath, MD, Peter Gazes, MD, Bernard Tabatznik, MD, Richard Hutchinson, MD, Raphael Sobrino, MD, J. Edward Pickering, MD, Robert Grissom, MD, Ralph Scott, MD, Frank Canosa, MD, Charles Laubach, Jr., MD, Ralph Cole, MD, Thaddeus Prout, MD, Jerome Cooper, MD, Ernest Theilen, MD, C. Basil Williams, MD, Edward Michals, MD, Fred Gilbert, Jr., MD, Sidney Levine, MD, Louis Matthews, Jr., MD, Irving Ershler, MD, Elmer Cooper, MD, Allan Barker, MD, Paul Samuel, MD.

1254   CANNER ET AL.
LONG-TERM MORTALITY BENEFIT WITH NIACIN

JACC Vol. 8, No. 6
December 1986:1245–55

Table A2. Cause-Specific Mortality During and After the Coronary Drug Project Treatment Phase

Cause of Death	Low Dose Estrogen (n = 1,101)		High Dose Estrogen (n = 1,119)		Clofibrate (n = 1,103)		Dextrothyroxine (n = 1,110)		Niacin (n = 1,119)		Placebo (n = 2,789)	
	No.	(%)	No.	(%)	No.	(%)	No.	(%)	No.	(%)	No.	(%)
All causes	657	(59.7)	652	(58.3)	637	(57.8)	633	(57.0)	582	(52.0)	1,623	(58.2)
Cardiovascular	527	(47.9)	540	(48.3)	533	(48.3)	525	(47.3)	474	(42.4)	1,331	(47.7)
Coronary—acute	455	(41.3)	460	(41.1)	466	(42.2)	452	(40.7)	408	(36.5)	1,153	(41.3)
Coronary—chronic	28		32		24		32		26		67	
Cerebrovascular	17		24		24		18		16		44	
Pulmonary embolism	2		2		1		1		3		5	
Other cardiovascular	25		22		18		22		21		62	
Cancer	65	(5.9)	41	(3.7)	37	(3.4)	47	(4.2)	45	(4.0)	124	(4.4)
Lung	23		21		13		16		23		53	
Gastrointestinal	14		6		4		13		6		17	
Pancreatic	8		5		4		2		4		8	
Liver, gallbladder	2		0		1		1		1		2	
Genitourinary	7		5		4		5		5		12	
Blood, lymph	3		0		6		3		0		12	
Other cancer	8		4		5		7		6		20	
Other noncardiovascular	38	(3.5)	34	(3.0)	36	(3.3)	32	(2.9)	33	(2.9)	85	(3.0)
Infection	6		7		7		7		2		10	
Lung disease	7		4		5		5		7		23	
Gastrointestinal	6		5		1		4		1		8	
Pancreatitis	1		1		0		0		1		2	
Liver, gallbladder	2		4		5		1		2		5	
Genitourinary	1		1		1		2		3		4	
Blood	0		1		1		0		0		1	
Endocrine, metabolic	4		3		5		2		3		6	
Central nervous system	2		1		0		3		2		1	
Nonmedical*	8		6		11		8		12		24	
Other	1		1		0		0		0		1	
Unknown	27	(2.5)	37	(3.3)	31	(2.8)	29	(2.6)	30	(2.7)	83	(3.0)

*Includes accidents, homicide and suicide.

We express our gratitude to Joseph Bell, Sandra Carberry, Mary Dorn, Veronica Hartman and Wanda Riggie for their assistance in the preparation of this manuscript.

References

1. Coronary Drug Project Research Group. Clofibrate and niacin in coronary heart disease. JAMA 1975;231:360–81.

2. Coronary Drug Project Research Group. The Coronary Drug Project: findings leading to discontinuation of the 2.5 mg/day estrogen group. JAMA 1973;226:652–7.

3. Coronary Drug Project Research Group. Estrogens and cancer (letter). JAMA 1978;239:2758–9.

4. Committee of Principal Investigators. W.H.O. Cooperative Trial on Primary Prevention of Ischaemic Heart Disease using clofibrate to lower serum cholesterol: mortality follow-up. Lancet 1980;2:379–84.

5. Coronary Drug Project Research Group. The Coronary Drug Project: design, methods, and baseline results. (AHA Monograph No. 38.) Circulation 1973;47(suppl I):I-1–179.

6. Canner PL, Klimt CR. The Coronary Drug Project. Methods and lessons of a multicenter clinical trial. Experimental design features. Controlled Clin Trials 1983;4:313–32.

7. Criteria Committee of New York Heart Association. Diseases of the Heart and Blood Vessels: Nomenclature and Criteria for Diagnosis. 6th ed. Boston: Little, Brown, 1964:112–3.

8. Coronary Drug Project Research Group. The Coronary Drug Project: initial findings leading to modifications of its research protocol. JAMA 1970;214:1303–13.

9. Coronary Drug Project Research Group. The Coronary Drug Project: findings leading to further modifications of its protocol with respect to dextrothyroxine. JAMA 1972;220:996–1008.

10. Coronary Drug Project Research Group. Aspirin in coronary heart disease. J Chronic Dis 1976;29:625–42.

11. Fleiss JL. Statistical Methods for Rates and Proportions. New York: John Wiley, 1973;28:115–7.

12. Draper NR, Smith H. Applied Regression Analysis. New York: John Wiley, 1966:58–67.

13. Littell AS. Estimation of the T-year survival rate from follow-up studies over a limited period of time. Hum Biol 1952;24:87–116.

14. Peto R, Peto J. Asymptotically efficient rank invariant test procedures. J Roy Statist Soc [Series A] 1972;135:185–98.

15. Committee of Principal Investigators. WHO Cooperative Trial on Primary Prevention of Ischaemic Heart Disease with clofibrate to lower serum cholesterol: final mortality follow-up. Lancet 1984;2:600–4.

16. Schoch HK. The U.S. Veterans Administration Cardiology Drug-

JACC Vol. 8, No. 6
December 1986.1245-55

Lipid Study: an interim report. In: Holmes WA, Carlson LA, Paoletti R, eds. Advances in Experimental Medicine and Biology, Vol. 4: Drugs Affecting Lipid Metabolism. New York: Plenum Press, 1969:405-20.

17. Carlson LA, Danielson M, Ekberg I, Klinteman B, Rosenhamer G. Reduction of myocardial infarction by the combined treatment with clofibrate and nicotinic acid. Atherosclerosis 1977;28:81-6.

18. Rosenhamer G, Carlson LA. Effect of combined clofibrate-nicotinic acid treatment in ischemic heart disease. Atherosclerosis 1980; 37:129-38.

19. Rosenhamer G, Carlson LA. Effects of serum lipid-lowering drugs in secondary prevention of coronary heart disease. In: Carlson LA, Olsson AG, eds. Treatment of Hyperlipoproteinemia. New York: Raven Press, 1984.233-6.

20. Coronary Drug Project Research Group. Influence of adherence to treatment and response of cholesterol on mortality in the Coronary Drug Project. N Engl J Med 1980;303:1038-41.

21. Halperin M, Rogot E, Gurian J, Ederer F. Sample sizes for medical trials with special reference to long-term therapy. J Chronic Dis 1968;21:13-24.

22. Lipid Research Clinics Program. The Lipid Research Clinics Coronary Primary Prevention Trial results. 1. Reduction in incidence of coronary heart disease. JAMA 1984;251:351-64.

Original Contributions

Is Relationship Between Serum Cholesterol and Risk of Premature Death From Coronary Heart Disease Continuous and Graded?

Findings in 356 222 Primary Screenees of the Multiple Risk Factor Intervention Trial (MRFIT)

Jeremiah Stamler, MD; Deborah Wentworth, MPH; James D. Neaton, PhD, for the MRFIT Research Group

The 356 222 men aged 35 to 57 years, who were free of a history of hospitalization for myocardial infarction, screened by the Multiple Risk Factor Intervention Trial (MRFIT) in its recruitment effort, constitute the largest cohort with standardized serum cholesterol measurements and long-term mortality follow-up. For each five-year age group, the relationship between serum cholesterol and coronary heart disease (CHD) death rate was continuous, graded, and strong. For the entire group aged 35 to 57 years at entry, the age-adjusted risks of CHD death in cholesterol quintiles 2 through 5 (182 to 202, 203 to 220, 221 to 244, and ≥245 mg/dL [4.71 to 5.22, 5.25 to 5.69, 5.72 to 6.31, and ≥6.34 mmol/L]) relative to the lowest quintile were 1.29, 1.73, 2.21, and 3.42. Of all CHD deaths, 46% were estimated to be excess deaths attributable to serum cholesterol levels 180 mg/dL or greater (≥4.65 mmol/L), with almost half the excess deaths in serum cholesterol quintiles 2 through 4. The pattern of a continuous, graded, strong relationship between serum cholesterol and six-year age-adjusted CHD death rate prevailed for nonhypertensive nonsmokers, nonhypertensive smokers, hypertensive non-smokers, and hypertensive smokers. These data of high precision show that the relationship between serum cholesterol and CHD is *not* a threshold one, with increased risk confined to the two highest quintiles, but rather is a continuously graded one that powerfully affects risk for the great majority of middle-aged American men.

(*JAMA* 1986;256:2823-2828)

AN EXTENSIVE body of scientific knowledge exists demonstrating that serum cholesterol is etiologically related to risk of atherosclerotic disease, particularly coronary heart disease (CHD) in the prime of life. The findings supporting this conclusion come from more than twoscore prospec-

tive epidemiologic studies in many countries throughout the world, from clinical investigations such as angiographic studies, and from postmortem investigations; in addition, powerful concordant evidence is available from animal experimental research in several species, including nonhuman primates.[1-9] However, in recent years, a divergence of opinion has arisen as to whether the association between serum cholesterol and CHD risk is continuous and graded over the whole distribution

of this variable or whether it is a plateaulike relationship with no increase in CHD risk over the lower 10% to 60% of the distribution and with excess risk confined to persons with levels in the upper 40% of the distribution.[10,11]

Recently available data in over 356 000 American men permit evaluation of this issue with a high degree of precision. These data are from the men screened for possible entry into the Multiple Risk Factor Intervention Trial (MRFIT) in a standardized way in 18 cities across the country in the early 1970s. This report presents the findings in this cohort of the relationship between baseline serum cholesterol levels and risk of fatal CHD.

METHODS

The data collection, screening, and follow-up methods used in this research have been published.[12] In brief, from November 1973 to November 1975, 361 662 men aged 35 to 57 years were screened in 18 US cities at 22 MRFIT clinical centers. Several methods of recruitment were used, including screening of employee, civic, and church groups, identification of men by house-to-house canvassing, and screening of respondents to mass media publicity.

Serum cholesterol levels were determined at one of 14 local laboratories using an automated system of chemical analysis (Auto Analyzer II), with standardization by the Lipid Standardiza-

From the MRFIT Coordinating Center, University of Minnesota, Minneapolis.

Reprint requests to MRFIT Coordinating Center, University of Minnesota, 2829 University Ave SE, Suite 508, Minneapolis, MN 55414-3270 (Ms Wentworth).

Table 1.—Quintiles of Serum Cholesterol and Six-Year CHD Mortality for 356 222 Primary Screenees of MRFIT*

Quintile	Serum Cholesterol, mg/dL (mmol/L)	CHD Mortality by Age Group, No. of CHD Deaths (6-y Death Rate per 1000)					
		35-39 y (n=74 077)	40-44 y (n=78 578)	45-49 y (n=84 319)	50-54 y (n=82 544)	55-57 y (n=36 704)	35-57 y (N=356 222)†
1	≤181 (≤4.68)	12 (0.59)	21 (1.28)	43 (2.95)	72 (5.39)	48 (8.31)	196 (3.23)
2	182-202 (4.71-5.22)	11 (0.67)	37 (2.29)	62 (3.72)	108 (6.92)	70 (9.97)	288 (4.18)
3	203-220 (5.25-5.69)	19 (1.37)	52 (3.37)	88 (5.28)	129 (7.73)	107 (14.50)	395 (5.60)
4	221-244 (5.72-6.31)	18 (1.44)	73 (4.72)	123 (6.97)	190 (10.59)	129 (16.05)	533 (7.14)
5	≥245 (≥6.34)	51 (4.57)	112 (7.41)	215 (11.46)	299 (15.78)	169 (19.91)	846 (11.06)
Total		111 (1.50)	295 (3.75)	531 (6.30)	798 (9.67)	523 (14.25)	2258 (6.34)

*CHD indicates coronary heart disease; MRFIT, Multiple Risk Factor Intervention Trial. Analysis is age specific and age standardized.
†Age-standardized six-year death rate per 1000.

Table 2.—Quintiles of Serum Cholesterol and Relative Risk of Six-Year CHD Mortality for 356 222 Primary Screenees of MRFIT*

Quintile	Serum Cholesterol, mg/dL (mmol/L)	Relative Risk of CHD Mortality by Age Group					
		35-39 y	40-44 y	45-49 y	50-54 y	55-57 y	35-57 y
1	≤181 (≤4.68)	1.00	1.00	1.00	1.00	1.00	1.00
2	182-202 (4.71-5.22)	1.14	1.79	1.26	1.28	1.20	1.29
3	203-220 (5.25-5.69)	2.32	2.63	1.79	1.43	1.74	1.73
4	221-244 (5.72-6.31)	2.44	3.69	2.36	1.96	1.93	2.21
5	≥245 (≥6.34)	7.75	5.79	3.88	2.93	2.40	3.42

*CHD indicates coronary heart disease; MRFIT, Multiple Risk Factor Intervention Trial. Analysis is age specific and age standardized.

tion Program, Centers for Disease Control, Public Health Service, Atlanta. Blood pressure was measured according to a standardized protocol by certified technicians, with first and fifth Korotkoff phases recorded as systolic and diastolic pressure, respectively. Three readings were taken with a standard stethoscope and mercury sphygmomanometer. The average of the second and third readings was used in this report. By means of a short questionnaire completed at the time of screening, number of cigarettes currently smoked each day and demographic characteristics were ascertained. Replies were also obtained concerning previous hospitalization of more than two weeks for "heart attack" as well as prescription of medication for diabetes.

Of the 361 662 screenees, 12 866 were eventually enrolled in the randomized clinical trial. The basis of this report, however, is the entire cohort of primary screenees. Vital status of these 361 662 men is being ascertained on an ongoing basis from data provided by the US Social Security System and the National Death Index. For decedents, death certificates are being obtained, abstracted, checked for correct match, and coded by one of two trained nosologists using the ninth revision of the *International Classification of Diseases*

Table 3.—Deciles of Serum Cholesterol and Six-Year CHD Mortality for 356 222 Primary Screenees of MRFIT*

Decile	Serum Cholesterol, mg/dL (mmol/L)	Mean Serum Cholesterol, mg/dL (mmol/L)	CHD Mortality		Relative Risk
			No. of Deaths	Rate per 1000	
1	≤167 (≤4.32)	153.2 (3.962)	95	3.16	1.00
2	168-181 (4.34-4.68)	175.0 (4.526)	101	3.32	1.05
3	182-192 (4.71-4.97)	187.1 (4.838)	139	4.15	1.31
4	193-202 (4.99-5.22)	197.6 (5.110)	149	4.21	1.33
5	203-212 (5.25-5.48)	207.5 (5.366)	203	5.43	1.72
6	213-220 (5.51-5.69)	216.1 (5.588)	192	5.81	1.84
7	221-231 (5.72-5.97)	225.9 (5.842)	261	6.94	2.20
8	232-244 (6.00-6.31)	237.7 (6.147)	272	7.35	2.33
9	245-263 (6.34-6.80)	253.4 (6.553)	352	9.10	2.88
10	≥264 (≥6.83)	289.5 (7.486)	494	13.05	4.13

*CHD indicates coronary heart disease; MRFIT, Multiple Risk Factor Intervention Trial. Analysis is age standardized.

(*ICD 9*). Six-year CHD mortality data (*ICD 9* codes 410-414) are given in this report for men aged 35 to 39, 40 to 44, 45 to 49, 50 to 54, and 55 to 57 years at screening, as well as for the entire cohort aged 35 to 57 years, and were stratified by baseline cigarette use and diastolic blood pressure (DBP) status. For the purposes of this article, which focuses on serum cholesterol, these latter two variables were dichotomized

as follows: cigarette smoking as no or yes and DBP as less than 90 mm Hg or greater than or equal to 90 mm Hg. Other reports deal in greater detail with the relation of these two variables to risk of CHD mortality in this cohort.[13,14] For calculation of CHD death rates for men aged 35 to 57 years, the direct method of standardization was used to adjust for differences in age distribution of subgroups.

Serum Cholesterol—Stamler et al

Table 4.—Quintiles of Serum Cholesterol, DBP, Smoking Status, and Six-Year CHD Death Rate per 1000 for 356 222 Primary Screenees of MRFIT*

Quintile	Serum Cholesterol, mg/dL (mmol/L)	DBP <90 mm Hg			DBP >90 mm Hg			Total		
		No. of Deaths	No. of Men	Rate per 1000	No. of Deaths	No. of Men	Rate per 1000	No. of Deaths	No. of Men	Rate per 1000
				Nonsmokers						
1	≤181 (≤4.68)	47	35 741	1.6	36	9612	3.7	83	45 353	2.1
2	182-202 (4.71-5.22)	82	34 553	2.5	51	11 599	4.0	133	46 152	2.9
3	203-220 (5.25-5.69)	87	31 939	2.7	80	12 839	5.6	167	44 778	3.5
4	221-244 (5.72-6.31)	126	30 431	3.8	94	14 500	5.6	220	44 931	4.4
5	≥245 (≥6.34)	188	26 996	6.4	200	16 930	10.7	388	43 926	8.0
Total		530	159 660	3.3	461	65 480	6.4	991	225 140	4.3
				Smokers						
1	≤181 (≤4.68)	82	20 017	5.2	31	5002	6.3	113	25 019	5.4
2	182-202 (4.71-5.22)	95	19 675	5.5	60	5977	10.0	155	25 652	6.7
3	203-220 (5.25-5.69)	128	18 812	7.3	100	6397	15.5	228	25 209	9.5
4	221-244 (5.72-6.31)	186	19 119	10.2	127	7533	16.6	313	26 652	12.1
5	≥245 (≥6.34)	250	18 907	13.3	208	9643	21.4	458	28 550	16.0
Total		741	96 530	8.4	526	34 552	15.1	1267	131 082	10.3
				All Men						
1	≤181 (≤4.68)	129	55 758	2.8	67	14 614	4.6	196	70 372	3.2
2	182-202 (4.71-5.22)	177	54 228	3.5	111	17 576	6.0	288	71 804	4.2
3	203-220 (5.25-5.69)	215	50 751	4.3	180	19 236	8.8	395	69 987	5.6
4	221-244 (5.72-6.31)	312	49 550	6.2	221	22 033	9.2	533	71 583	7.1
5	≥245 (≥6.34)	438	45 903	9.1	408	26 573	14.4	846	72 476	11.1
Total		1271	256 190	5.2	987	100 032	9.3	2258	356 222	6.3

*DBP indicates diastolic blood pressure; CHD, coronary heart disease; and MRFIT, Multiple Risk Factor Intervention Trial. Analysis is age standardized.

Rates were standardized to the age distribution of the total group of 361 662 screenees.

Mortality rates are presented by quintile and decile of serum cholesterol levels for the 356 222 men free of a history of hospitalization for myocardial infarction. Approximate quintiles and deciles of serum cholesterol levels were determined with use of the entire screened population (361 662 men) and are presented from lowest (quantile 1) to highest (quintile 5 or decile 10). Elevated blood pressure was defined as a mean diastolic reading equal to or greater than 90 mm Hg. Smoking was defined as any use of cigarettes.

RESULTS
Serum Cholesterol Quintiles

Mean serum cholesterol levels for the five serum cholesterol quintiles were 163.7, 192.4, 211.5, 231.7, and 271.2 mg/dL (4.23, 4.98, 5.47, 5.99, and 7.01 mmol/L), respectively. For each of the five age groups (35 to 39 years, 40 to 44 years, 45 to 49 years, 50 to 54 years, and 55 to 57 years), six-year risk of fatal CHD was progressively higher for quintiles 2 through 5 of the serum cholesterol level, compared with quintile 1 (Tables 1 and 2). Range of

relative risk was greater for younger than for older men, eg, 7.75 for men aged 35 to 39 years and 2.40 for men aged 55 to 57 years. However, absolute excess risk, ie, difference in risk between a higher quintile of serum cholesterol level and quintile 1, tended to increase with age. For quintile 5, for example, there was an absolute excess risk at ages 35 to 39 years of 3.98 deaths per 1000 in six years, compared with 11.60 for the age stratum 55 to 57 years.

For the entire cohort of 356 222 men, six-year CHD mortality rates were higher by 29%, 73%, 121%, and 242% for serum cholesterol quintiles 2, 3, 4, and 5, respectively, compared with quintile 1 (Tables 1 and 2). For these five quintiles, the 95% confidence intervals[15] for the age-standardized six-year CHD mortality rates were as follows: quintile 1, 2.8 to 3.7; quintile 2, 3.7 to 4.7; quintile 3, 5.0 to 6.2; quintile 4, 6.5 to 7.7; and quintile 5, 10.3 to 11.9.

Serum Cholesterol Deciles

Age-standardized risk of six-year CHD mortality was also continuous and graded over the range of the deciles of serum cholesterol levels (Ta-

ble 3). The first decile, serum cholesterol level less than or equal to 167 mg/dL (≤4.32 mmol/L), had the lowest death rate (3.16 per 1000); the tenth decile, serum cholesterol equal to or greater than 264 mg/dL (≥6.83 mmol/L), had the highest rate (13.05 per 1000), a rate more than four times higher. Rates were similar for men in the first and second deciles; for men in the third decile (range, 182 to 192 mg/dL [4.71 to 4.97 mmol/L]), the rate was 31% higher than for those in the first decile and was progressively higher for each subsequent decile.

Serum Cholesterol Quintiles Stratified by Cigarette Use and DBP

In each of the nine analyses (Table 4), six-year age-standardized CHD death rates were continuously and progressively higher for men in serum cholesterol quintiles 2 through 5, compared with those in quintile 1. This was the finding for nonsmokers with DBP less than 90 mm Hg and greater than or equal to 90 mm Hg, for smokers with DBP less than 90 mm Hg and greater than or equal to 90 mm Hg, for all nonsmokers and all smokers, and for all men with DBP less than

90 mm Hg and greater than or equal to 90 mm Hg. For the large group of nonsmokers with DBP less than 90 mm Hg (159 660 men, or 45% of the cohort), relative risks for serum cholesterol quintiles 2, 3, 4, and 5 were 1.56, 1.69, 2.38, and 4.00, respectively. These data underscore the key role of serum cholesterol levels above optimal in the causation of premature CHD.

With multiple logistic regression analysis,[16] including age, DBP, cigarette use, and diabetic status, the coefficient for serum cholesterol level and six-year CHD mortality was .0078. This parameter estimate indicates that a higher serum cholesterol level of 20 mg/dL (0.52 mmol/L) is associated with a relative risk of 1.17 (95% confidence interval, 1.15 to 1.19). Since the mean serum cholesterol level for the entire cohort was 214.6 mg/dL (5.55 mmol/L),[12] this translates into an estimate that a 9% higher serum cholesterol level was associated with a 17% greater CHD death rate—that is, a 1% higher serum cholesterol level was associated with an almost 2% higher CHD risk. This is almost certainly an underestimate, since with use of a single serum cholesterol measurement there is bound to be some misclassification due to both intraindividual variability and laboratory error. This estimate is similar to that derived statistically years ago from prospective studies[16] and recently from the intervention experience of the Lipid Research Clinics Coronary Primary Prevention Trial.[17]

The age-specific CHD death rates (Table 1) were used to estimate the number of excess CHD deaths in quintiles 2 through 5, based on the estimated number of CHD deaths that would have occurred if all men of each age group had had the age-specific rate of quintile 1. For all 356 222 men, CHD deaths would have numbered 1143, rather than the observed 2258. Based on their higher rates, estimated numbers of excess CHD deaths for the men aged 35 to 57 years at screening in quintiles 2, 3, 4, and 5 are 66, 167, 290, and 592, totaling 1115 excess CHD deaths in quintiles 2 through 5. Of this total of excess CHD deaths, 6% were in quintile 2, 15% were in quintile 3, 26% were in quintile 4, and 53% were in quintile 5. With a total of 2258 CHD deaths, the estimate is that 49% (1115/2258) are excess deaths attributable to serum cholesterol levels equal to or greater than 182 mg/dL (≥4.71 mmol/L). With control for age, DBP, cigarette use, and diabetes, the estimate of population attributable risk from the multiple logistic analysis is similar—46% of

all CHD deaths in this cohort were excess deaths attributable to serum cholesterol levels equal to or greater than 180 mg/dL (≥4.65 mmol/L).

For men in each of the five quintiles of serum cholesterol levels, CHD mortality was higher for cigarette smokers than for nonsmokers, without or with high blood pressure. Most risk ratios for smokers compared with nonsmokers were greater than 2.0—overall, 2.4 (Table 4, last column, 10.3/4.3). Similarly, for men in each of the five quintiles of serum cholesterol levels, whether nonsmokers or smokers, CHD mortality was higher for those with DBP greater than or equal to 90 mm Hg compared with those with DBP less than 90 mm Hg, with risk ratios in the range of 1.2 to 2.3 or 1.8 overall (Table 4, last row, 9.3/5.2). The extremes of risk based on the three factors, as stratified in Table 4, ranged from 21.4 per 1000 to 1.6, the former being 13.4 times greater than the latter. Only 35 741 men (10%) of the entire cohort of 356 222 were in the lowest risk group, ie, had a serum cholesterol level equal to or less than 181 mg/dL (≤4.68 mmol/L), had a DBP less than 90 mm Hg, and were not cigarette smokers. If their six-year age-standardized CHD mortality rate of only 1.6 per 1000 had prevailed for the whole cohort, the estimate is that CHD deaths would have numbered 560 instead of the total 2258. The estimated number of excess deaths attributable to serum cholesterol levels equal to or greater than 182 mg/dL (≥4.71 mmol/L), cigarette smoking, and elevated blood pressure in various combinations is 1698, which is 75% of all CHD deaths.

An additional estimate of excess CHD mortality in this cohort was made based on the following five criteria for optimal risk: serum cholesterol level equal to or less than 181 mg/dL (≤4.68 mmol/L), systolic pressure less than 120 mm Hg, DBP less than 76 mm Hg, no cigarette smoking, and no history of diabetes. A DBP of less than 76 mm Hg was used since this was the cut point for the lowest quintile of DBP; for the men in this quintile, six-year age-adjusted CHD death rate was lower than that for men in the four other DBP quintiles. Of the entire cohort of 356 222 men, only 7948 (2.2%) met all five of these criteria. Among these 7948 men, CHD deaths numbered only six, and the six-year age-adjusted CHD mortality rate was only 0.8 per 1000. If the entire cohort of 356 222 men had had a rate of 0.8 per 1000, there would have been only 285 CHD deaths, rather than the 2258 observed. Thus, based on this estimate, 1973 CHD deaths (87%

of the total) were excess deaths attributable to above optimal levels of the five established major CHD risk factors, prevalent in various combinations among 98% of the cohort.

COMMENT

The data of this large prospective study clearly demonstrate that for American men aged 35 to 57 years in 1973 to 1975, the relationship between serum cholesterol and six-year risk of CHD death was continuous, graded (dose-related), and strong over the entire range of the distribution of this variable. In age-specific analyses for men aged 35 to 39, 40 to 44, 45 to 49, 50 to 54, and 55 to 57 years at screening and in age-standardized analyses with stratification based on cigarette use and DBP, risk of CHD rose steadily for men in the second, third, fourth, and fifth quintiles, compared with the first quintile; this was the consistent finding without exception. Overall, based on the data for the entire cohort of 356 222 men, for men in quintile 2 with serum cholesterol levels of 182 to 202 mg/dL (4.71 to 5.22 mmol/L) and for men in quintile 3 with serum cholesterol levels of 203 to 220 mg/dL (5.25 to 5.69 mmol/L), six-year age-standardized death rates were 29% and 73% higher, respectively, than for men in quintile 1. With CHD deaths numbering 288 and 395 for quintiles 2 and 3, respectively, and 196 for quintile 1, these estimates of relative risk have a high degree of precision. Thus, they lend powerful support—along with the data from the other quintile analyses and the decile analysis and data from other studies[1-9,11]—to the conclusion that the relationship of serum cholesterol to CHD in the US population is a *graded one* and *not* a threshold (plateaulike) one. That is, the great majority of adults in the United States are at increased CHD risk because of their status in regard to this trait, and not only those in the highest or the two highest quintiles of the distribution. Specifically, serum cholesterol levels of about 180 mg/dL (4.65 mmol/L) and above are associated with increased risk for middle-aged American men, and not only levels equal to or greater than 220 or 240 mg/dL (5.69 or 6.21 mmol/L).

Quantitative estimates, based on these data, of the distribution of excess CHD risk across serum cholesterol quintiles 2 through 5 lend further weight to the importance of the foregoing conclusion. Thus, while 53% of the estimated excess CHD deaths attributable to serum cholesterol levels above optimal were derived from quintile 5, about 21% were distributed across quintiles 2 and 3 and another 26% were in quintile 4. Therefore, a high-risk-only strategy—based on the idea of a threshold relationship, hence dealing only with severe hypercholesterolemia—has only a limited potential to have an impact on the totality of excess risk. This is the case, for example, when hypercholesterolemia requiring treatment is defined solely as 2 SD above the mean (2.5% of the population), or the cut point used is the 95th or 90th percentile (5% or 10% of the population) or a level equal to or greater than 265 mg/dL ($\geq$6.85 mmol/L) (approximately the tenth decile cut point for the MRFIT cohort) or a level equal to or greater than 240 or 245 mg/dL (6.21 or 6.34 mmol/L) (approximately the fifth quintile cut point here). Even with this last cut point, 47% of the estimated excess risk, distributed across quintiles 2 through 4, would be neglected.

Since the first American Heart Association statement on diet and CHD in 1961,[7,18] the emphasis of recommendations by expert groups for coronary prevention in the United States has been on a two-pronged strategy, involving advice for improved eating habits for the whole population, to shift the serum cholesterol distribution of the whole population downward, plus special approaches for individuals and families at higher risk.[1-7,9] This is also the strategy set down in the Report of the World Health Organization Expert Committee on the Prevention of Coronary Heart Disease[8] and in the several reports on public policy emanating from other industrialized countries concerned with the epidemic of premature CHD.[8,19-23]

It is a reasonable inference that the steady and marked decline in CHD mortality in the United States since the late 1960s—greater than for any other country in the world (many countries have been steady in their rates, and others have registered rising rates)—is related to the improvements in nutrition and serum cholesterol distribution, as well as in other major risk factors (eg, cigarette use, blood pressure).[3,5,10,23-28]

The US Department of Health and Human Services, in a recent report, *Health United States 1983—and Prevention Profile*, set the goal for 1990 of a further nutrition-related decline in mean serum cholesterol levels for American adults, to less than 200 mg/dL (<5.17 mmol/L).[27] Correspondingly, the National Heart, Lung, and Blood Institute, in accordance with the recommendations of two recent major reports,[3,9,27,29] has launched a National Cholesterol Education Program. The massive data set reported herein is yet another scientific underpinning for these goals and endeavors.

This research was carried out in the MRFIT Centers as a collaborative research undertaking with contract support from the National Heart, Lung, and Blood Institute (NHLBI), Bethesda, Md.

The principal investigators and senior staff of the clinical, coordinating, and support centers, the NHLBI, and members of the MRFIT Policy Advisory Board and Mortality Review Committee are as follows.

American Health Foundation, New York
C. B. Arnold, MD, MPH (principal investigator), R. Mandriota, MS, MEd, R. P. Ames, MD, J. Ruff Eisenbach, RN.
Boston University, Boston
H. E. Thomas, Jr, MD (principal investigator), W. B. Kannel, MD (co-principal investigator), R. Rotondo, MA, J. Connors, RD.
Cox Heart Institute, Kettering, Ohio
P. Kezdi, MD (principal investigator), E. L. Stanley, MD (co-principal investigator), W. L. Black, MD, F. A. Ernst, PhD.
Dade County Department of Public Health, Miami
G. Christakis, MD, MPH (principal investigator); J. M. Burr, MD, T. A. Gerace, PhD (co-principal investigators); M. E. Wilcox, RD, MEd.
Dalhousie University, Halifax, Nova Scotia (MRFIT Electrocardiography Center)
P. M. Rautaharju, MD, PhD (principal investigator), H. Wolf, PhD.
Harvard University, Boston
R. C. Benfari, PhD (principal investigator); K. M. McIntyre, MD, JD, O. Paul, MD (co-principal investigators); E. Danielson, MA, J. Ockene, PhD.
Kaiser Foundation Research Institute, Portland, Ore
J. B. Wild, MD (principal investigator); M. Greenlick, PhD, J. Grover, MD (co-principal investigators); S. Lamb.
Lankenau Hospital, Philadelphia
W. Holmes, PhD (principal investigator), J. E. Pickering, MD (co-principal investigator), E. L. Duffy, RD, G. B. Rubel, RD.
National Centers for Disease Control, Atlanta
G. R. Cooper, PhD, MD (principal investigator), D. T. Miller, PhD.
New Jersey Medical School, Newark
N. L. Lasser, MD, PhD (principal investigator),

N. Hymowitz, PhD (co-principal investigator), K. C. Mezey, MD, B. Munves, PhD, RD.
Northwestern University, Chicago
J. Stamler, MD (principal investigator), D. Moss, MS, RD, V. Persky, MD, E. Robinson, MS, RD, L. Van Horn, PhD, RD.
University of Chicago
L. Cohen, MD (principal investigator), J. Morgan, PhD (co-principal investigator), G. Grundmann, MS, RD, T. D. Vestal, PA.
St Joseph's Hospital, Chicago
D. M. Berkson, MD (principal investigator), G. Lauger, MS, S. Grujic, MD, D. Obradovic, MD.
Institutes of Medical Sciences, University of California, San Francisco, and Berkeley
J. Billings, PhD, MPH (principal investigator); S. B. Hulley, MD, MPH, W. M. Smith, MD, MPH, S. L. Syme, PhD (co-principal investigators).
Institutes of Medical Sciences, San Francisco Central Laboratory
G. M. Widdowson, PhD, G. Z. Williams, MD, S. B. Hulley, MD, MPH (co-principal investigators); M. L. Kuehneman (laboratory manager).
Rush-Presbyterian–St Luke's Medical Center, Chicago
J. A. Schoenberger, MD (principal investigator), J. C. Schoenenberger, PhD, R. B. Shekelle, PhD, G. S. Neri, MD, T. A. Dolecek, MS, RD.
Rutgers Medical School, Piscataway, NJ
N. H. Wright, MD, MPH (principal investigator), S. A. Kopel, PhD (co-principal investigator), K. R. Suckerman, PhD, M. Schorin, MPH, RD.
St Louis Heart Association
N. Simon, MD (principal investigator), J. D. Cohen, MD (co-principal investigator), E. Bunkers, RD, B. Ronchetto, RN.
University of Alabama in Birmingham
H. W. Schnaper, MD (principal investigator), G. H. Hughes, PhD (co-principal investigator), A. Oberman, MD, C. C. Hill, PhD.
University of California, Davis
N. O. Borhani, MD (principal investigator), C. Sugars, RD, K. Kirkpatrick, M. Lee, MD.
University of Maryland, Baltimore
R. W. Sherwin, MB, BChir (principal investiga-

tor), M. S. Sexton, PhD, MPH (co-principal investigator), P. C. Dischinger, PhD.
University of Minnesota, Minneapolis
R. H. Grimm, Jr, MD, MPH (principal investigator); M. Mittelmark, PhD, R. S. Crow, MD, H. Blackburn, MD (co-principal investigators); D. Jacobs, PhD (co-investigator).
University of Minnesota Electrocardiography Coding Center
R. J. Prineas, MB, PhD (director), R. C. Crow, MD (associate director).
University of Minnesota Nutrition Coding Center
I. M. Buzzard, PhD (director), P. V. Grambsch (former director).
University of Minnesota Coordinating Center
M. O. Kjelsberg, PhD (principal investigator); G. E. Bartsch, ScD, J. D. Neaton, PhD (co-principal investigators); D. N. Wentworth, MPH.
University of Pittsburgh
L. H. Kuller, MD, DPH (principal investigator); R. McDonald, MD, A. Caggiula, PhD, RD, L. Falvo-Gerard, MN, MPH (co-principal investigators).
University of South Carolina, Columbia
W. K. Giese, PhD (principal investigator); J. F. Martin, MD, J. A. Keith, PhD (co-principal investigators); H. H. Harrison, RN.
University of Southern California, Los Angeles
E. Fishman, MD (principal investigator), L. Wampler, PhD, G. Newmark, MA, RD, E. Rosenfield, MPH.
Policy Advisory Board
W. Insull, Jr, MD (chairperson), J. W. Farquhar, MD, C. D. Jenkins, PhD, E. Rapaport, MD, D. J. Thompson, PhD, H. A. Tyroler, MD, P. W. Willis III, MD, W. T. Friedewald, MD, W. Zukel, MD.
Mortality Review Committee
J. T. Doyle, MD (chairman), H. B. Burchell, MD, P. N. Yu, MD, P. W. Willis III, MD (former member).
NHLBI Staff
W. T. Friedewald, MD (program director); C. D. Furberg, MD (project office director); J. A. Cutler, MD (scientific project officer); E. R. Passamani, MD, C. T. Kaelber, MD (former scientific project officers).

References

1. Stamler J: *Lectures on Preventive Cardiology.* New York, Grune & Stratton, 1967.
2. Gotto AM, Witterls EH: Diet, serum cholesterol, lipoproteins, and coronary heart disease, in Kaplan NM, Stamler J (eds): *Prevention of Coronary Heart Disease: Practical Management of the Risk Factors.* Philadelphia, WB Saunders Co, 1983, pp 33-50.
3. Working Group on Arteriosclerosis of the National Heart, Lung, and Blood Institute: *Report of the Working Group on Arteriosclerosis of the National Heart, Lung, and Blood Institute,* US Dept of Health and Human Services publication (NIH) 81-2035. Bethesda, Md, US Public Health Service, 1981, vol 2.
4. Inter-Society Commission for Heart Disease Resources, Atherosclerosis Study Group and Epidemiology Study Group: Primary prevention of the atherosclerotic diseases. *Circulation* 1970; 42:55A-95A.
5. Inter-Society Commission for Heart Disease Resources, Atherosclerosis Study Group: Optimal resources for primary prevention of atherosclerotic diseases. *Circulation* 1984;70:153A-205A.
6. American Heart Association Steering Committee for Medical and Community Program: Risk factors and coronary disease: A statement for physicians. *Circulation* 1980;62:449A-455A.
7. Grundy SM, Bilheimer D, Blackburn H, et al: Rationale of the Diet-Heart Statement of the American Heart Association: Report of the Nutrition Committee. *Circulation* 1982;65:839A-854A.
8. WHO Expert Committee on the Prevention of Coronary Heart Disease: *Prevention of Coronary Heart Disease,* World Health Organization Technical Report Series 678. Geneva, Switzerland, World Health Organization, 1982.
9. NIH Consensus Development Conference: Lowering blood cholesterol to prevent heart disease. *JAMA* 1985;253:2080-2086.
10. Oliver MF: Serum cholesterol: The knave of hearts and the joker. *Lancet* 1981;2:1090-1095.
11. Castelli WP: Epidemiology of coronary heart disease: The Framingham study. *Am J Med* 1984;76:4-12.
12. Benfari RC, Sherwin R: The Multiple Risk Factor Intervention Trial (MRFIT): The methods and impact of intervention over four years. *Prev Med* 1981;10:387-553.
13. Multiple Risk Factor Intervention Trial Research Group (Neaton JD, Kuller LH, Wentworth D, et al): Total and cardiovascular mortality in relation to cigarette smoking, serum cholesterol concentration, and diastolic blood pressure among black and white males followed for five years. *Am Heart J* 1984;108:759-769.
14. Stamler J: Epidemiology; established major risk factors and the primary prevention of coronary heart disease, in Parmley WW, Chatterjee K, Cheitlin M, et al (eds): *Cardiology.* New York, JB Lippincott, in press.
15. Armitage P: *Statistical Methods in Medical Research.* Boston, Blackwell Scientific Publications Inc, 1973, p 387.
16. Cornfield J: Joint dependence of risk of coronary heart disease on serum cholesterol and systolic blood pressure: A discriminant function analysis. *Fed Proc* 1962;21(suppl 2):58-61.
17. Lipid Research Clinics Program: The Lipid Research Clinics Coronary Prevention Trial results: II. The relationship of reduction in incidence of coronary heart disease to cholesterol lowering. *JAMA* 1984;251:365-374.
18. American Heart Association Central Committee for Medical and Community Program: *Dietary Fat and Its Relation to Heart Attacks and Strokes.* New York, American Heart Association, EM 180, 1961.
19. Stamler J: Primary prevention of coronary heart disease: The last 20 years: Keynote address, 11th Bethesda Conference. *Am J Cardiol* 1981; 47:722-735.
20. Rose G, Ball K, Catford J, et al: *Coronary Heart Disease Prevention: Plans for Action (The Canterbury Report).* London, Pitman Books, 1984.
21. Committee on Medical Aspects of Food Policy: *Report of the Panel on Diet in Relation to Cardiovascular Disease: Diet and Cardiovascular Disease,* Department of Health and Social Security Report on Health and Social Subjects 28. London, Her Majesty's Stationery Office, 1984.
22. *European Conference on Primary Prevention of Coronary Heart Disease, Anacapri, Oct 15-19, 1984.* Geneva, Switzerland, World Health Organization, ICP/NCD 001/15, October 1984.
23. Pyörälä K, Epstein FH, Kornitzer M: Changing trends in coronary heart disease mortality: Possible explanations. *Cardiology* 1985;72:4-104.
24. Stamler J, Liu K: The benefits of prevention, in Kaplan NM, Stamler J (eds): *Prevention of Coronary Heart Disease: Practical Management of the Risk Factors.* Philadelphia, WB Saunders, 1983, pp 188-207.
25. Stamler J: The marked decline in coronary heart disease mortality rates in the United States, 1968-1981: Summary of findings and possible explanations. *Cardiology* 1985;72:11-22.
26. Stamler J: Coronary heart disease: Doing the 'right things.' *N Engl J Med* 1985;312:1053-1055.
27. *Health United States 1983—and Prevention Profile, 1983,* US Dept of Health and Human Services publication (PHS) 84-1232. Hyattsville, Md, US Public Health Service, National Center for Health Statistics, 1983.
28. Working Group on Arteriosclerosis of the National Heart, Lung, and Blood Institute: *Report of the Working Group on Arteriosclerosis of the National Heart, Lung, and Blood Institute: Summary, Conclusions, and Recommendations,* US Dept of Health and Human Services, publication (NIH) 81-2034. Bethesda, Md, US Public Health Service, 1981.
29. Lenfant C: A new challenge for America: The National Cholesterol Education Program. *Circulation* 1986;73:855-856.

Original Contributions

Beneficial Effects of Combined Colestipol-Niacin Therapy on Coronary Atherosclerosis and Coronary Venous Bypass Grafts

David H. Blankenhorn, MD; Sharon A. Nessim, DrPH; Ruth L. Johnson, RD, MA; Miguel E. Sanmarco, MD; Stanley P. Azen, PhD; Linda Çashin-Hemphill, MD

The Cholesterol-Lowering Atherosclerosis Study (CLAS) was a randomized, placebo-controlled, angiographic trial testing combined colestipol hydrochloride and niacin therapy in 162 nonsmoking men aged 40 to 59 years with previous coronary bypass surgery. During two years of treatment there was a 26% reduction in total plasma cholesterol, a 43% reduction in low-density lipoprotein cholesterol, plus a simultaneous 37% elevation of high-density lipoprotein cholesterol. This resulted in a significant reduction in the average number of lesions per subject that progressed ($P<.03$) and the percentage of subjects with new atheroma formation ($P<.03$) in native coronary arteries. Also, the percentage of subjects with new lesions ($P<.04$) or any adverse change in bypass grafts ($P<.03$) was significantly reduced. Deterioration in overall coronary status was significantly less in drug-treated subjects than placebo-treated subjects ($P<.001$). Atherosclerosis regression, as indicated by perceptible improvement in overall coronary status, occurred in 16.2% of colestipol-niacin treated vs 2.4% placebo treated ($P=.002$).

(*JAMA* 1987;257:3233-3240)

THE Cholesterol-Lowering Atherosclerosis Study (CLAS) was a randomized placebo-controlled, selectively blinded, angiographic trial designed to test the lipid hypothesis; namely, that aggressive lowering of low-density lipoprotein (LDL) cholesterol with concomitant increase in high-density lipoprotein (HDL) cholesterol will reverse or retard the growth of atherosclerotic lesions. The study was designed to determine whether combined therapy with colestipol hydrochloride plus niacin will produce clinically significant change in coronary, carotid, and femoral artery atherosclerosis and coronary bypass graft lesions. Additional objectives were to determine possible correlations between lesion change and plasma lipid and lipoprotein cholesterol levels and to explore interrelationships of atherosclerosis change in femoral, coronary, and carotid arteries.

The rationale for CLAS was lack of convincing evidence that blood cholesterol lowering has directly beneficial effects on human atherosclerotic lesions. Blood cholesterol levels influence the prevalence of atherosclerotic heart disease in human populations,[1] and two large clinical trials have indicated that morbidity and mortality from ischemic heart disease are reduced by blood cholesterol-lowering therapy.[2,3] Blood cholesterol reduction ameliorates experimental atherosclerosis in animal models,[4] but the two largest human studies with angiographic observation of arterial lesion change have not demonstrated significant treatment effects.[5,6] Favorable but inconclusive treatment trends were observed in four angiographic trials not controlled by randomization[7-10] and one too small for evaluation of randomized groups.[11]

In CLAS, combined coronary, femoral, and carotid angiograms were obtained before and after two years of blood cholesterol-lowering therapy. In this study we report the effect of treatment on our primary, per-subject, cardiac end point, the global coronary change score. In a subsequent report we will evaluate per-lesion treatment effects in native coronary arteries and bypass grafts. Additional, later reports will describe interrelationships of lipoprotein and apolipoprotein levels to change in atherosclerosis in femoral and carotid arteries.

From the Atherosclerosis Research Institute, the Department of Medicine (Drs Blankenhorn, Sanmarco, and Cashin-Hemphill), and the Department of Preventive Medicine (Drs Nessim and Azen), University of Southern California School of Medicine, Los Angeles.
Reprint requests to the Department of Medicine, Atherosclerosis Research, University of Southern California, 2025 Zonal Ave, Los Angeles, CA 90033 (Dr Blankenhorn).

MATERIALS AND METHODS
Study Population

The population under study consisted of nonsmoking men, 40 to 59 years of age, with progressive atherosclerosis (confirmed through angiographic review), who had coronary bypass surgery not involving valve replacement (performed at least three months prior to the study admission date) and who had entry fasting blood cholesterol levels in the range of 185 to 350 mg/dL (4.81 to 9.10 mmol/L). Eligibility criteria were chosen to produce (1) a relatively homogeneous group with respect to the outcome measures, (2) a group expected to have a good response to blood cholesterol–lowering medication, and (3) a group with proved atherosclerosis expected to have low two-year mortality. Exclusion criteria included bilateral femoral artery surgery, diabetes mellitus, hypertension (diastolic blood pressure>115 mm Hg), thyroid disease, renal insufficiency, fasting blood triglyceride levels of 500 mg/dL (5.50 mmol/L) or greater, congestive heart failure, major arrhythmia, QRS width exceeding 0.12 s, and weight exceeding 1.5 times ideal weight as determined by Multiple Risk Factor Intervention Trial criteria.[12]

The number of subjects recruited was based on power calculations derived from computerized measures of femoral atherosclerosis.[13,14] These required 188 subjects (94 per treatment group) to be randomized to the study in expectation that 80 per group would complete two years of therapy and two angiograms. The power of the trial was 81% for detecting a 40% treatment effect employing a one-sided test with a significance level set at .05. Power calculations were not performed for coronary or carotid end points because the necessary data were not available. A more detailed presentation of the subject population, entry criteria, and trial design will be reported elsewhere.[15]

Screening and Prerandomization Trial

The screening period consisted of five clinic visits, which included a prerandomization trial of study drugs. At the first three visits, CLAS was explained, informed consent was obtained, a complete medical evaluation (including a resting electrocardiogram) was conducted, and measurements of fasting blood lipid levels, weight, and blood pressure were made. Diet composition was evaluated and diet intervention started at screening visit 2.

At the third screening visit, subjects began a six-week trial-period regimen of colestipol and niacin. To be randomized, subjects must have demonstrated sufficient response (at least a 15% reduction in total blood cholesterol level) to the study drugs. The prerandomization drug trial also evaluated subject ability and willingness to adhere to the drug regimen, as well as subject tolerance to the medications. One disadvantage of this procedure was that subjects were exposed to the gamut of symptomatic side effects of colestipol and niacin during the prerandomization drug trial and therefore were better able to distinguish between placebo and active treatment later. An advantage of the prerandomization trial was selection of compliant and responsive subjects.

Randomization and Treatment Groups

Prior to randomization, subjects were scheduled for angiography to obtain baseline data on the atherosclerotic disease of the carotid, femoral, and coronary arteries, as well as of the coronary bypass grafts. Selective coronary angiography was performed by the percutaneous femoral technique. Simultaneous biplane views obtained with a 17.8-cm cesium-iodide intensifier were recorded at 60 frames per second on 35-mm cine film. The contrast medium was 76% meglumine diatrizoate (Renografin 76). Standardized 30° right anterior oblique and 60° lateral anterior oblique views were obtained in the same sequence in all subjects in each of the coronary arteries and bypass grafts. Additional views were obtained when standard views did not suffice. On repeated angiography, identical views were repeated in the original sequence by the same angiographer using the same roentgenographic equipment. Subjects were not premedicated. If a subject developed angina during a procedure, sublingual nitroglycerin (usually 0.4 mg) was administered and the time and dose recorded. This dose of nitroglycerin was administered during the same stage of any later procedure. All angiographic procedures will be described in more detail elsewhere.[15]

Eligible candidates (n=188) were randomized to either the drug group (30 g of colestipol hydrochloride plus 3 to 12 g of niacin daily, titrated individually on the basis of blood cholesterol response) or to the placebo group (methyl cellulose images of colestipol and niacin). Niacin was to be taken three times a day in the middle of a meal. Five grains of aspirin before breakfast was prescribed for the first 14 days to reduce the severity of flushes. Regular doses of aspirin were stopped after 14 days and for the duration of the trial. Colestipol was prescribed in two 15-g doses 30 to 60 minutes after morning and evening meals. One teaspoon of mineral oil nightly was prescribed for the first 14 days as a precaution against constipation. The dosage of mineral oil was adjusted as necessary and stopped as soon as bowel habits became normal. No lipid-lowering agents except study medications were allowed; anticoagulants and platelet-active drugs also were not allowed.

Both groups received diet intervention. The target diet for the drug group included less than 125 mg of cholesterol per day and provided 22% of energy as fat, 10% as polyunsaturated fat, and 4% as saturated fat. The target diet for the placebo group included less than 250 mg of cholesterol per day and provided 26% of energy as fat, 10% as polyunsaturated, and 5% as saturated fat. Different diet composition was prescribed for drug and placebo groups to enhance the differential in blood cholesterol responses between the two groups. Cholesterol responses to the diets were projected using the Keys and Hegsted[16] formulas. Total fasting blood cholesterol level reduction goals were 30% to 40% for the drug group and 7% to 8% for the placebo group. The randomization process included balancing on drug and placebo within blocks of age groups (40 to 44, 45 to 49, 50 to 54, and 55 to 59 years) and the three hospitals where study angiograms were performed.

Blinding

Both study subjects and clinic staff were blinded to the prerandomization study drug trial lipid responses. Study subjects were blinded to treatment assignment. Subjects and clinic staff were not blinded to on-trial lipid values because fasting blood cholesterol response was used as a compliance measure. The effectiveness of blinding was reduced by symptoms secondary to niacin therapy and knowledge of on-trial fasting blood lipid levels. Evaluation of the study end points was carried out by staff and consultants who were blinded to treatment group assignment, as well as the temporal ordering of angiographic data.

Treatment and Follow-up

Subjects were seen monthly for the first six months and then at two-month intervals. Clinic visits consisted of nutritional counseling and measurement of weight, blood pressure, and levels of fasting blood lipids and lipoproteins. All health-related events were recorded at each visit and all nonstudy medications at six-month intervals. Physical examinations, including urinalysis and

Table 1.—Distribution of Entry Characteristics by Treatment Group (All Randomized Subjects)

Entry Characteristic	Drug (n = 94)	Placebo (n = 94)	P
Age, y	53.9 ± 0.5*	54.5 ± 0.5	.42
Age at bypass, y	50.2 ± 0.5	50.9 ± 0.5	.33
Weight, kg	83.1 ± 1.2	80.7 ± 1.1	.13
Relative weight	1.20 ± 0.02	1.18 ± 0.01	.32
Quetelet Index	26.9 ± 0.3	26.4 ± 0.3	.24
Systolic BP, mm Hg	123.7 ± 1.5	125.1 ± 1.5	.50
Diastolic BP, mm Hg	81.1 ± 1.0	80.1 ± 1.0	.80
Pulse, beats per min	65.9 ± 1.0	66.3 ± 1.2	.82
No. of drinks per week	10.0 ± 1.2	8.1 ± 1.0	.22
Race (% white)	93	95	.54†
Marital status (% married)	87	90	.48
Educational level (% completed college)	48	40	.28
Employment status (% employed)	88	87	.84
Never smoked, %	28	30	.74
Receiving antihypertensive medications, %	41	37	.54
Vasectomy, %	38	42	.60

*Mean ± SEM, group differences tested using the independent Student's t test against a two-sided alternative.
†Differences in percentages tested using the χ² test with continuity correction against a two-sided alternative.

Table 2.—Mean [SEM] Baseline and On-Trial Fasting Lipid Levels by Treatment Group*

Lipid or Lipoprotein	Treatment Group	Lipid Level, mg/dL (mmol/L)		Change†	
		Baseline	On-Trial	Difference	%
Total cholesterol	D	246 [4] (6.35 [0.09])	180 [3] (4.65 [0.09])	− 66 [3]‡(− 1.70 [0.08])	− 26 [1]
	P	243 [4] (6.28 [0.10])	232 [4] (6.00 [0.10])	− 11 [2]‡(− 0.28 [0.06])	− 4 [1]
Triglycerides	D	151 [9] (1.71 [0.10])	110 [5] (1.25 [0.06])	− 41 [6]‡(− 0.46 [0.07])	− 22 [2]
	P	154 [10] (1.74 [0.11])	141 [9] (1.59 [0.10])	− 13 [4]‡(− 0.15 [0.04])	− 5 [2]
LDL cholesterol	D	171 [3] (4.42 [0.09])	97 [3] (2.51 [0.07])	− 74 [3]‡(− 1.91 [0.08])	− 43 [1]
	P	169 [3] (4.36 [0.09])	160 [3] (4.13 [0.08])	− 9 [2]‡(− 0.23 [0.06])	− 5 [1]
HDL cholesterol	D	44.6 [1.0] (1.15 [0.03])	60.8 [1.4] (1.57 [0.04])	16.2 [0.9]‡(0.42 [0.02])	37 [2]
	P	43.7 [1.0] (1.13 [0.03])	44.4 [0.9] (1.15 [0.02])	0.7 [0.6] (0.02 [0.01])	2 [1]
LDL/HDL ratio	D	4.0 [0.1]	1.7 [0.1]	− 2.3 [0.1]‡	− 57 [1]
	P	4.0 [0.1]	3.7 [0.1]	− 0.3 [0.1]‡	− 6 [2]

*Eighty subjects were receiving drug (D); 82, placebo (P).
†Group differences were significant at P<.001 using the independent Student's t test against a two-sided alternative.
‡Significant at P<.001 using a paired Student's t test against a two-sided alternative.

Table 3.—Percent Distribution of Global Change Score by Treatment*

Group	Global Score†							Mean	Median
	−3	−2	−1	0	1	2	3		
Drug	0.0	0.0	16.2	45.0	30.0	8.8	0.0	0.3	0
Placebo	0.0	0.0	2.4	36.6	36.6	23.2	1.2	0.8	1

*Eighty subjects were receiving drug; 82, placebo.
†Positive numbers denote a worsening of disease.

Table 4.—Evaluation of Global Change Score Category With Measures of Change in Native Vessels and Grafts

Parameter	Global Change Category			P
	Better or No Change (−3 to 0)	Mild Worsening (1)	Moderate Worsening (2, 3)	
No. of subjects	82	54	26	...
Native vessels				
No. of lesions/subject	10.5	11.6	11.8	.19*
% Subjects with new lesions	4	24	38	<.001
% Subjects with new closures	6	20	31	.001
No. of lesions with increased stenosis/subject	0.3	1.7	3.0	<.001*
Grafts				
No. of grafts/subject	2.7	2.6	2.8	.78*
% Subjects with new lesions	5	33	65	<.001
% Subjects with new closures	1	7	27	<.001
% Subjects with any adverse change	7	44	81	<.001

*Differences among global change categories tested using the Kruskal-Wallis analysis of variance test procedure. All other differences among global change categories were tested using the χ² test for association.

blood safety monitoring studies, were performed annually.

Lipid assay procedures were total cholesterol, triglycerides, and cholesterol from the HDL, isolated by precipitation of the low-density species[17] and analyzed by Lipid Research Clinic's methodology.[18] These were standardized throughout the trial against reference materials supplied by the Standardization Program of the National Centers for Disease Control. Low-density lipoprotein was calculated as follows: LDL = cholesterol − HDL − triglyceride/5.[19]

The major on-treatment compliance measure used was the change in fasting blood cholesterol level from baseline. Additional compliance measures included number of missed clinic visits, subjective response to treatment tabulated with a behavioral checklist adapted from the Multiple Risk Factor Intervention Trial dietary compliance checklist,[20] and measurement of the niacin metabolite, n-methyl-2-pyridone, in 24-hour urine specimens. To monitor and improve dietary compliance, a computerized pictorial diet record system[21] was used (Nutrition Scientific, 1510 Oxley St, Suite F, South Pasadena, Calif). Nicotine and cotinine levels were measured in 24-hour urine collections every six months to test for smoking recidivism.

A repeated angiogram was performed at two years by the same angiographer, who was blinded to treatment assignment. Complications following the 356 study angiograms were one arteriovenous fistula that was repaired surgically and three hematomas that subsided during outpatient observation.

Coronary Evaluation—the Global Change Score

Film pairs, showing identical coronary artery views with temporal order masked, were evaluated to determine a global measure of change, the *global change score*. This was done by a panel of expert angiographers who viewed films without knowledge of a subject's demographic or clinical characteristics, his treatment assignment, or the temporal order of the angiograms. They did not review ventriculograms or other angiograms. Two angiographers and a moderator viewed pairs of films using two 35-mm cine angiographic projectors (Vanguard Instruments Inc, Melville, NY) that magnified the image sixfold.

First or second angiograms from drug- or placebo-treated subjects were assigned at random to the left-hand projector. Panelists began with the left-hand film and worked independently, recording their findings on individualized, predrawn diagrams of the native coronary arteries and grafts. Each reader identified lesions in the native arteries and recorded the maximal percent stenosis (percent reduction of lumen diameter at the narrowest point compared with an adjacent normal diameter, ranging from 0% to 100%). Each bypass graft was divided into proximal, middle, and distal thirds, excluding a short proximal and distal anastomotic point. Percent stenosis and the length of each segment involved were estimated for each third of each graft. Percent stenosis of proximal and distal anastomotic points was also recorded. After each reader evaluated the left-hand film independently, panelists discussed this film to arrive at a consensus regarding the degree and location of all stenotic lesions. This consensus was recorded by the moderator on a consensus diagram.

For the right-hand film, panelists used the consensus diagram and worked independently to evaluate all diagrammed lesions for change. If there was change, the new degree of stenosis was estimated. Any lesion not previously noted (on the left-hand film) was recorded with an estimate of percent stenosis. Each reader recorded a global evaluation of the films on a four-point scale that combined changes in both grafts and native coronary arteries. A score of 0 indicated no demonstrable change; a score of 1, definitely discernible change; a score of 2, intermediate change; and a score of 3, extreme change. Working independently, panelists also recorded which film exhibited the greater extent and severity of obstructive atherosclerosis in native coronary arteries and/or abnormality of grafts. Later, when the code for film order was broken, this information was used to attach a sign to global change scores (− was assigned to pairs showing regression, + to pairs showing progression). It will be shown later (Table 5) that, on average, 11.1 lesions in native coronary arteries and 2.7 grafts were evaluated in each angiogram. Twenty-eight film pairs, selected at random, were evaluated as unknowns by duplicate panel reading. An in-depth analysis of the performance of the panelists in evaluating change in native coronary arteries and bypass grafts will be the subject of a separate report.

As a last step, panelists reviewed and discussed both films together. A consensus as to change in each lesion, percent stenosis for each new lesion, a consensus coronary global change score, and agreement as to which film showed the greatest extent of lesions in native coronary arteries and/or grafts was recorded by the moderator. Consensus global change score, the overall judgment of both panelists integrating all changes seen in the film pair, is the primary, per-subject end point measure reported in this study. As in the case of individual panelists' change scores, a direction for change (− for regression, + for progression) was assigned after the code for film sequence was broken. The 28 random duplicate consensus global change scores showed complete agreement in 20 pairs, a difference of one grade in seven pairs, and a difference of two grades in one pair. The eight differences in duplicate global change score did not result in a change in classification from "regression" to "progression."

Statistical Methods

All analyses were done based on treatment assigned at randomization without regard to compliance. All testing of hypotheses utilized parametric or nonparametric methods available in a standard statistical programming package.[32] Significance was established at the .05 level. Drug vs placebo comparison of baseline characteristics was made using the independent Student's t test or a χ^2 test with continuity correction.

On trial, averages for each fasting blood lipid or lipoprotein were obtained from values weighted according to the scheduled interval (either one or two months) between treatment visits. Baseline values were the unweighted averages obtained at the first three screening visits. Change in fasting blood lipid values was expressed both as a difference from baseline and as a percent difference from baseline. Within a group, the average change in blood lipid levels was tested using the paired Student's t test; between groups, the difference in average change in blood lipid levels was tested using the independent Student's t test. Tests of treatment effects on lipids were two-sided. Comparisons of drug and placebo event rates for major medical events, symptoms, and abnormal blood chemistries were made using a Fisher's exact test.

The primary end point, coronary global change score, was tested for treatment effect using the normal approximation (with continuity correction) to the Wilcoxon rank sum test.[33] Tests for treatment effects on other measures of coronary change (eg, new

Table 5.—Evaluation of Treatment Effect on Measures of Change in Native Vessels and Grafts

Parameter	Treatment		
	Drug (n = 80)	Placebo (n = 82)	P
Global score	0.3	0.8	.001*
Native vessels			
No. of lesions/subject	10.9	11.2	.30*
% Subjects with new lesions	10	22	.03
% Subjects with new closures	13	16	.35
No. of lesions with increased stenosis/subject	1.0	1.4	.03*
Grafts			
No. of grafts/subject	2.7	2.7	.21*
% Subjects with new lesions	18	30	.04
% Subjects with new closures	5	10	.20
% Subjects with any adverse change	24	39	.03

*Group differences tested using the normal approximation (with continuity correction) to the Wilcoxon rank sum test against a one-sided alternative. All other group differences were tested using the χ^2 test with correction for continuity.

lesions, new closures, and increase in stenosis) were made using either the χ^2 test with continuity correction or the Wilcoxon rank sum test. Tests of treatment effects on coronary measures were all one sided. The associations of global change categories with measures of coronary change were tested using either a χ^2 test or a Kruskal-Wallis nonparametric analysis of variance.[33]

The choice of one- or two-sided testing was made during the design phase of the study prior to unblinding treatment results. One-sided testing was selected for treatment effects on atherosclerosis end points because the study was designed to learn if treatment can ameliorate this disease. Two-sided testing was selected for entry characteristics, blood lipid and lipoprotein change, event rates of major medical events, event rates of reported symptoms, and rate of new abnormal blood chemistries because we were interested in detecting relative increase or decrease in either group.

RESULTS

Subjects were recruited through various mechanisms. At the time that CLAS began, a log of coronary bypass patients in Los Angeles was available to the research team. These patients were contacted and interviewed for possible participation in CLAS. Additionally, advertisements were placed in Los Angeles–area newspapers. Several public service radio and television announcements advertised the study. The most consistent recruitment method was found to be a 4 × 3.25-in advertisement placed in the news section of the *Los Angeles Times*, each of which, on the average, resulted in 76.1 telephone inquiries about the program, 19.4 first screening visits, and randomization of 5.0 subjects.

Table 6.—Global Change Score by Treatment and Baseline Cholesterol

Treatment Group	No.	Mean (SEM)	Median	P
Cholesterol level 185-240 mg/dL (4.81-6.24 mmol/L) (mean = 216 mg/dL [5.62 mmol/L])				
Drug	31	0.3 (0.1)	0	.03
Placebo	47	0.7 (0.1)	0	...
Cholesterol level 241-350 mg/dL (6.26-9.10 mmol/L) (mean = 270 mg/dL [7.02 mmol/L])				
Drug	49	0.3 (0.1)	0	.001
Placebo	35	0.9 (0.2)	1	...

Table 7.—Event Rates (%) of Major Medical Events by Treatment Group (All Randomized Subjects)

Medical Event*	Drug (n = 94)	Placebo (n = 94)
Cardiovascular		
Cardiac death	0	1
Myocardial infarction	1	4
New or increased angina	13	13
All other cardiac events	7	4
All other vascular events	4	3
Cancer	2	1
Gastrointestinal	4	2
Gouty arthritis	5	0
Urologic	2	3
Hepatic	3	0
Ophthalmologic	2	1

*Group comparisons were nonsignificant except for gouty arthritis (P<.03).

Table 8.—Event Rates (%) of Reporting of Symptoms by Treatment Group (All Randomized Subjects)*

Symptom	Drug Ever†	Drug Recurrent‡	Placebo Ever	Placebo Recurrent
Skin				
Flushing	91	63	6	0
Skin feels warm	69	31	1	0
Itching	60	24	10	1
Rash	37	11	14	1
Skin tingles	26	2	4	0
Dry skin	15	1	1	0
Gastrointestinal				
Constipation	31	7	11	2
Nausea	23	9	4	0
Stomach discomfort	23	3	8	0
Heartburn	20	3	6	0
Diffuse abdominal pain	15	2	3	0
Sore throat	14	2	2	0
Vomiting	6	0	0	0

*Ninety-four subjects were receiving drug; 94, placebo.
†P values for ever reported were all significant with P<.01.
‡Recurrent symptoms are defined as those reported on three or more occasions.

Demographic and prerandomization clinical characteristics for the 188 subjects recruited for the study are summarized in Table 1. There were no significant differences between the treatment groups. On the average, subjects were 54 years old, white, married, employed, and well educated. As a group they were approximately 20% overweight, and although blood pressures were normal, 39% of the subjects were taking antihypertension medication. Seventy-one percent were ex-smokers. Smoking recidivism (as judged by urinalysis for nicotine and cotinine) occurred in three drug and two placebo subjects during the study; one drug and one placebo subject had positive results from nicotine/cotinine urinalysis on two occasions; two drug subjects and one placebo subject had positive results on one occasion. Forty percent of the subjects had vasectomy at an average interval (estimated from the clinical records of 52 subjects) of 18.5 years before study entry. The prevalence of vasectomy among men of our study subjects' age has been reported to approximate 30% in a four-city survey that included Los Angeles.[24] There was no significant difference in the interval between vasectomy and study entry in treatment and control groups.

Of the 188 randomized subjects, 162 (86%) completed the study (80 in the drug group and 82 in the placebo group). Twenty-six subjects dropped out of the study (14 from the drug group and 12 from the placebo group). Causes were refusal to have a second angiogram (four drug subjects and four placebo subjects), dislike of medication (five drug subjects and two placebo subjects), health-related reasons (one drug subject with congestive heart failure and one placebo subject with sudden cardiac death), administrative disagreement over hospital charges (one drug subject and one placebo subject), moved out of state (one drug subject and one placebo subject), missed study visits (two drug subjects), work related (one placebo subject), lost angiogram (one placebo subject), and attitude after discovery of smoking recidivism (one placebo sub-

ject). There were no significant differences between the subjects who completed the study and those who did not complete the study when all attributes listed in Table 1 and study entry lipid and lipoprotein levels were compared.

Table 2 summarizes entry and on-trial fasting blood lipid and lipoprotein values for the subjects who completed the study. There were no significant differences in baseline fasting blood lipid levels between the study groups. After treatment by drug, there were large, statistically significant decreases in total cholesterol level (26%), levels of triglycerides (22%) and LDL cholesterol (43%), and LDL/HDL ratio (57%) and a large, statistically significant increase in HDL cholesterol level (37%). In the diet group, modest yet statistically significant decreases were found for total cholesterol level (4%), levels of triglycerides (5%) and LDL cholesterol (5%), and LDL/HDL ratio (6%). High-density lipoprotein cholesterol did not change significantly after placebo treatment (2%). When comparing the changes in lipids between the two treatment groups, large significant differences were found for all lipids (P<.001). These differences reflect an average on-trial colestipol hydrochloride dose of 29.5 ± 6.0 g SD per day and a niacin dose of 4.3 ± 1.9 g SD per day. These differences may also reflect a change in body weight in both drug- and placebo-treated subjects. Body weight at entry was 117% ± 3% SEM of ideal in the 82 drug subjects completing the trial. This was reduced by the end of the trial to 113% ± 2% SEM of ideal. Body weight at entry was 119% ± 1% SEM of ideal in the 82 placebo subjects completing the trial. This was reduced to 118% ± 1% SEM of ideal. The difference between average weight losses in the two groups was significant (P<.001).

Table 3 summarizes the percent distribution of the global change score obtained after two years for each of the treatment groups. The distribution for the drug group was shifted toward lower scores (less disease progression) as compared with that for the placebo group. Sixty-one percent of the drug

subjects (as compared with 39% of the placebo subjects) improved or remained the same (global change score, −1 to 0). Also, 16.2% of the drug subjects vs 2.4% of the placebo subjects showed regression (global change score, −1). A Fisher's exact test performed after inspection of Table 3 showed a significant difference in percentage of subjects with regression (P = .002).

To determine which factors contributed to the coronary panel global change score, coronary measures in the native vessels and grafts (eg, new lesions, new closures, increase in stenosis, and any other adverse change) were related to a global change category (better or no change, mild worsening, and moderate worsening). As shown in Table 4, there is a strong significant relationship between the global change category and all coronary change measures. Larger global scores (worsening disease) were significantly related to increased change rates in new lesions and new closures in both the native arteries and grafts, increased stenosis per subject in the native arteries, and increased incidence of adverse change in the grafts. These data strongly support the rationale of the global scoring method.

Table 5 summarizes treatment effect on coronary change measures. There was a significant benefit due to use of the drug. The average global change score was significantly smaller (less disease progression) for the drug group than for the placebo group ($P<.001$). In the native vessels, the drug group had a significant reduction in the average number of lesions that progressed per subject ($P<.03$) and in the percentage of subjects with new lesions ($P<.03$). No significant difference in the rates of new closure was found, however. In the bypass grafts, the drug group had a significant reduction in the percentage of subjects with any adverse change ($P<.03$) and the percentage of subjects with new lesions ($P<.04$). Again, there was no significant group difference in the rates of new closure. The mean baseline stenosis in the native arteries that progressed to complete occlusion was 79%; in the bypass grafts it was 45%.

The treatment effect on coronary disease was also seen after stratification of the treatment groups by baseline total cholesterol levels into a "low" entry subgroup (range = 185 to 240 mg/dL [4.81 to 6.24 mmol/L]) with a mean baseline of 216 mg/dL (5.62 mmol/L) and a "high" entry total cholesterol subgroup (range = 241 to 350 mg/dL [6.26 to 9.10 mmol/L]) with a mean baseline of 270 mg/dL (7.02 mmol/L) (Table 6). In the drug group, mean total cholesterol values were reduced from 214 mg/dL to 165 mg/dL (5.56 to 4.29 mmol/L) in the "low" subgroup and from 266 mg/dL to 189 mg/dL (6.91 to 4.91 mmol/L) in the "high" subgroup. Tests for treatment effect are significant in each total cholesterol subgroup.

Table 7 summarizes the major events for all randomized subjects. There were no group differences in potential treatment-related adverse clinic event rates except for gouty arthritis, where there was a significantly higher occurrence in the drug group ($P<.03$). Events classified as "all other cardiac events" in the drug group were four cases of transient arrhythmia and one case each of recurrent atrial fibrillation, repeated coronary bypass surgery, and coronary angioplasty; in the placebo group, one case each of pacemaker replacement, recurrent atrial fibrillation, congestive heart failure, and coronary angioplasty. Events classified as "all other vascular events" in the drug group were two cases with abdominal aneurysm repair and one case each of carotid endarterectomy and ileofemoral bypass grafting; in the placebo group, two cases of carotid endarterectomy and one case of retinal vein thrombosis. Cancer in the drug group consisted of one recurrent cancer of the bladder and one basal cell carcinoma of the skin; in the placebo group there was one subject with chronic lymphatic leukemia. The drug group had two cases of an undiagnosed moderately severe, single episode of abdominal pain and one case each of bleeding gastric ulcer, new duodenal ulcer, renal calculus requiring surgery, chronic glomerulonephritis, cystoid macular edema, and iridocyclitis. The cystoid macular edema resolved when niacin therapy was withdrawn; the subject continued to receive colestipol alone. The placebo group had one case each of an undiagnosed moderately severe, single episode of abdominal pain, rectal discomfort leading to hemorrhoidectomy, renal calculus treated medically, urinary tract infection, transurethral resection of the prostate, and cataract. Hepatic events in the drug group were extreme elevations of levels of liver enzymes that subsided when niacin therapy was discontinued.

Symptoms that were significantly more common in the treatment group cluster into skin related or gastrointestinal (Table 8). Except for flushing, skin warmth, itching, rash, nausea, and constipation in drug-treated subjects, all symptoms were preponderantly transient, being reported no more than twice in two years. Table 8 demonstrates the large difference in recurrent symptoms between the two groups.

In the drug group there was a significantly higher prevalence of subjects with new abnormal levels (increased) of alkaline phosphatase, aspartate aminotransferase, and uric acid and (decreased) thyroxin and carotene. The prevalence of new abnormal values of total bilirubin, creatine phosphokinase, glucose, urea nitrogen, potassium, sodium, red blood cell count, white blood cell count, hemoglobin, hematocrit, and urinary albumin did not differ significantly between the two treatment groups.

COMMENT

The Cholesterol-Lowering Atherosclerosis Study has demonstrated that aggressive lowering of LDL cholesterol levels with concomitant increase in HDL cholesterol levels produced significant benefit to both native coronary arteries and venous bypass grafts. Deterioration of average global coronary change scores was significantly reduced in drug-treated subjects as compared with placebo-treated, and atherosclerosis regression, as indicated by perceptible improvement in overall coronary status, occurred in 16.2% of colestipol-niacin–treated subjects vs 2.4% of placebo-treated subjects (Table 3). In contrast to previous trials, CLAS tested blood lipid–lowering therapy in a setting that minimized the effects of other major nonlipid risk factors. All subjects in this trial were nonsmokers during the experimental period, and average blood pressure levels were within the range of normal. Also, drug-treated CLAS subjects had greater changes in blood lipid levels for longer periods than in any previous trial.

The global coronary change score, our primary per-subject measure of treatment effect, represented the consensus of expert coronary angiographer panelists who are broadly experienced and nationally known. Panelists reviewed pairs of angiograms from the same subject without knowledge of the order of angiograms or treatment and identified all lesions and all lesion change. A global score (scaled from -3 to $+3$) was obtained after panelists had recorded all changes in a film pair and were asked to assess overall coronary status, using clinical judgment to designate which film of the pair exhibited the greater extent of obstructive stenosis in native coronary arteries and/or abnormality of bypass grafts. Global change scores were uniformly consistent with changes observed in native coronary arteries and grafts (Table 4).

When all study angiograms had been evaluated and the code of examination sequence and treatment assignment was broken, a strong and consistent trend toward benefit from therapy was apparent. Average global coronary change score among drug-treated subjects was 0.3 as compared with 0.8 in placebo-treated subjects ($P<.001$). Treatment produced significant reduction in progression of atherosclerosis in native coronary arteries, both in average number of lesions that progressed per subject ($P<.03$) and in the percentage of subjects with new atheroma formation ($P<.03$). Treatment also significantly reduced the percentage of subjects with any adverse change ($P<.03$) or new lesions ($P<.04$) in venous bypass grafts (Table 5).

The clinical implications of CLAS coronary results are that therapy after coronary bypass surgery should routinely include measures to lower blood cholesterol levels. Follow-up of large numbers of postbypass patients indicates that with current medical therapy 44% of patients with venous bypass grafts will need a repeated operation in ten years,[25] but patients whose lesions do not show progression have improved chances of survival and lower rates of myocardial infarction.[26] The CLAS results indicate that it is possible to reduce long-term adverse change in both native coronary arteries and grafts. Thirty-nine percent of nonsmoking men with normal blood pressures and fasting blood cholesterol levels between 185 mg/dL and 350 mg/dL (4.81 to 9.10 mmol/L) who were treated by diet plus placebo had stable or improved coronary status while following a moderate-fat and cholesterol-restricted diet similar to the American Heart Association phase 2 diet (Table 3). Sixty-one percent of randomly selected men with identical risk factors at entry who were aggressively treated with a more rigorous diet plus combined colestipol-niacin therapy had stable or improved coronary status. The more aggressive regimen was acceptable for two years to 90% of those assigned to it, although they had a significant increase in skin and abdominal complaints (Table 8). Other less likely, but more serious, side effects were cystoid macular edema, gouty arthritis, gastric ulcer with bleeding, and duodenal ulcer. There was no difference in the prevalence of malignancy in the two CLAS study groups.

The CLAS results significantly extend what is known from previous studies testing blood cholesterol lowering as therapy for atherosclerosis. The largest previous body of evidence indicating benefit from reduction of blood cholesterol levels was obtained in the Lipid Research Clinics Primary Prevention Trial, where hyperlipoproteinemic men with no previous evidence of ischemic heart disease were treated for five years with cholestyramine resin, a bile acid-binding resin.[2] Cholestyramine resin treatment produced an average 8.5% differential total cholesterol level reduction (as compared with placebo treatment) and a significant reduction in mortality from ischemic heart disease and/or nonfatal myocardial infarction (P<.05). Supporting trends indicating therapeutic benefit were significantly reduced incidence of angina pectoris (P<.01) or positive results from treadmill exercise tests (P<.001).[27] However, the Lipid Research Clinics Trial did not include observations on the subjects' coronary arterial status, and so the mechanism underlying these benefits remains unknown.

Additional evidence for benefit from blood cholesterol-lowering therapy in humans was obtained by long-term follow-up of subjects in the Coronary Drug Project who were randomized to niacin treatment.[3] In this trial, 1119 male survivors of myocardial infarction were randomized to 3 g/d of niacin (which produced a 10% reduction in blood cholesterol levels) and 2789 men were randomized to placebo. After six years, niacin therapy reduced nonfatal recurrences of myocardial infarction but not total mortality. Nine years after termination of the trial, follow-up data indicated an 11% reduction in the 15-year mortality rate as compared with placebo (P = .0004).[28] Again, vessel status was not evaluated, and, as in the case of the Lipid Research Clinics Primary Prevention Trial, the mechanism of benefit remains unknown. The CLAS study, which demonstrates a direct effect of lipid-lowering therapy on the process of atherogenesis at the level of the arterial wall, offers a logical, mechanical explanation for benefits from blood cholesterol-lowering therapy.

The Cholesterol-Lowering Atherosclerosis Study is the first angiographic study providing clear evidence of a treatment effect on human atherosclerotic lesions. Cohn and coworkers,[6] who randomized 24 subjects to clofibrate therapy (2.0 g/d, which produced a 13.7% reduction in blood triglyceride level) and 16 to placebo, concluded that there was no significant reduction in the progression of atherosclerosis. Brensike and coworkers[5] found that 25% of 116 subjects with type II hyperlipoproteinemia treated with 24 g/d of cholestyramine resin (which produced a 26% reduction in LDL cholesterol levels) showed definite evidence of lesion progression after five years as compared with 35% of placebo-treated; this result did not achieve statistical significance. A favorable effect at the 5% significance level was found when comparison was confined to subjects with progression of lesions greater than 50% stenosis or definite manifestations of progression were pooled with equivocal manifestations of progression.[29] The Leiden Intervention Trial, a nonrandomized study, tested dietary effects in 39 subjects with angina pectoris and demonstrated stability of lesions after 39 months. There was significant correlation of lesion growth with total cholesterol/HDL cholesterol ratio (r = .50, P = .001).[7]

The CLAS results indicate a clear therapeutic effect (P<.001) when the outcome is analyzed on a per-subject basis according to treatment assignment without regard to degree of treatment adherence. The power of the CLAS study to detect a therapeutic effect was greater than that of previous angiographic trials, because more subjects completed two angiograms than in any previous study. In addition, we produced and maintained larger changes in LDL and HDL levels than any previous study through use of a prerandomization drug trial to select compliant and responsive subjects, plus unblinded prospective monitoring of each subject's on-trial fasting blood cholesterol level. The overriding consideration in adopting these procedures was to obtain large on-trial treatment changes in cholesterol level. The rationale supporting these procedures is that they simulate conditions of careful clinical practice and do not reduce the strength of a randomized trial when the end-point measurement is derived from observers blinded as to therapy assignment. Although the largest change we produced was in the ratio LDL/HDL, there were significant changes in levels of all other plasma lipids and lipoproteins; the differential reduction in total cholesterol level between drug and placebo groups was 26%; in triglyceride level, 22%. Weight loss, which occurred in both drug and placebo groups and was more pronounced in the drug group, was of minor degree and unlikely to have contributed to change in atherosclerosis, except as it contributed to change in blood lipid and lipoprotein levels.

The CLAS study findings indicate that global coronary change score and all contributing angiographic changes (except progression to complete occlusion) can be significantly reduced in subjects with pretreatment cholesterol levels ranging from 185 to 350 mg/dL (4.81 to 9.10 mmol/L). Evidence for benefit retained strong statistical significance after our results were divided to compare treatment effects separately when entry cholesterol levels were above or below 240 mg/dL. This evidence implicates the entire range of cholesterol levels between 185 and 350 mg/dL (4.81 and 9.10 mmol/L) as coronary risk factors that should be reduced through appropriate medical treatment. The data also support and extend treatment goals cited in December 1984 at the National Institutes of Health Consensus Conference, "Lowering Blood Cholesterol Level to Prevent Heart Disease."[30]

In the CLAS study, large changes in fasting blood cholesterol levels were produced in an attempt to achieve arterial changes that could be clearly recognized within two or four years. Within two years, evidence of atherosclerosis regression, as measured by a perceptible improvement in global coronary status, occurred in 16.2% of colestipol plus niacin-treated subjects vs 2.4%

of placebo-treated subjects (Table 3). At this time, we advocate measures to lower blood cholesterol levels in all post-coronary bypass patients. We have shown that combined therapy with colestipol plus niacin provides significant benefits in nonsmoking men selected on the basis of response to a six-week trial of this therapy. However, we caution that the aggressive regimen that we used requires close supervision because of recognized side effects due to the use of colestipol plus niacin.

CLAS II—AN OPTIONAL TWO-YEAR EXTENSION OF THE TRIAL

Following the second angiogram in CLAS, subjects were offered the option of continuing to take their assigned medication (either colestipol-niacin or placebo) for two additional years and having a third angiogram. Seventy-four colestipol-niacin–treated subjects and 62 placebo-treated subjects elected to do this. The coronary results we describe in this report dictate that we offer an alternative for placebo to subjects in CLAS II. This step, which effectively terminated angiographic observations in CLAS II, has been taken following consultation with our extramural advisory committee and with advisors at the National Heart, Lung, and Blood Institute. Results from subjects who completed CLAS II and had repeated angiography before the trial was terminated will be reported later.

This study was supported by National Heart, Lung, and Blood Institute Program Project Grant HL23619 and by The Upjohn Company.

We wish to acknowledge the commitment of volunteer participants in this clinical trial. Key CLAS personnel involved in the results reported here are as follows: Program Director: David H. Blankenhorn, MD. Clinical Staff: Ruth L. Johnson, RD; Linda Cashin-Hemphill, MD; Laura I. Vailas, RD; Barbara J. Stokes, RN; Donald W. Crawford, MD; Christine J. Gesselman; Donna J. Conover, RN; Chao-ran Liu, MD; and Rosalinda Baca. Biostatistics Laboratory: Sharon A. Nessim, DrPH; Emily Wickham, MA; Stanely P. Azen, PhD; and Lydia A. Gonzalez. Coronary Film Panelists: Miguel E. Sanmarco, MD; George G. Rowe, MD; Peter R. Mahrer, MD; Ivan L. Bunnell, MD; William J. French, MD; C. Richard Conti, MD; J. Michael Criley, MD; Harold T. Dodge, MD; David G. Greene, MD; W. David Johnston, MD; and K. Ramaswamy, MD. Angiographers: Miguel E. Sanmarco, MD, and Robert B. Chesne, MD. Lipid Laboratory: H. P. Chin, PhD; Dalila Q. Pirott; and Valentina Karamanoikian. Administration: C. Joan Darnall. The CLAS Advisory Committee: William Insull, Jr, MD; Chairman; Elmer C. Hall, PhD; and J. Ward Kennedy, MD.

References

1. Keys A (ed): Coronary heart disease in seven countries. *Circulation* 1970;41(suppl 1):I-1–I-211.
2. Lipid Research Clinics Program: The Lipid Research Clinics Coronary Primary Prevention Trial results: I. Reduction in incidence of coronary heart disease. *JAMA* 1984;251:351-364.
3. The Coronary Drug Project Research Group: Clofibrate and niacin in coronary heart disease. *JAMA* 1975;231:360-381.
4. Malinow MR, Blaton V: Regression of atherosclerotic lesions. *Arteriosclerosis* 1984;4:292-295.
5. Brensike JF, Levy RI, Kelsey SF, et al: Effects of therapy with cholestyramine on progression of coronary arteriosclerosis: Results of the NHLBI Type II Coronary Intervention Study. *Circulation* 1984;69:313-324.
6. Cohn K, Sakai FJ, Langston MF Jr: Effect of clofibrate on progression of coronary disease: A prospective angiographic study in man. *Am Heart J* 1975;89:591-598.
7. Arntzenius AC, Kromhout D, Barth JD, et al: Diet, lipoproteins, and the progression of coronary atherosclerosis: The Leiden Intervention Trial. *N Engl J Med* 1985;312:805-811.
8. Nikkila EA, Viikinkoski P, Valle M, et al: Prevention of progression of coronary atherosclerosis by treatment of hyperlipidaemia: A seven year prospective angiographic study. *Br Med J* 1984;289:220-223.
9. Nash DT, Gensini G, Esente P: Effect of lipid-lowering therapy on the progression of coronary atherosclerosis assessed by scheduled repetitive coronary arteriography. *Int J Cardiol* 1982;2:43-55.
10. Kuo PT, Hayase K, Kostis JB, et al: Use of combined diet and colestipol in long-term (7-7½ years) treatment of patients with type II hyperlipoproteinemia. *Circulation* 1979;59:199-211.
11. Duffield RG, Lewis B, Miller NE, et al: Treatment of hyperlipidaemia retards progression of symptomatic femoral atherosclerosis: A randomised controlled trial. *Lancet* 1983;2:639-642.
12. Sherwin R, Kaelber CT, Kezdi P, et al: The Multiple Risk Factor Intervention Trial (MRFIT) II: The development of the protocol. *Prev Med* 1981;10:402-425.
13. Brooks SH, Blankenhorn DH, Chin HP, et al: Design of human atherosclerosis studies by serial angiography. *J Chronic Dis* 1980;33:347-357.
14. Blankenhorn DH, Brooks SH: Angiographic trials of lipid-lowering therapy. *Arteriosclerosis* 1981;1:242-249.
15. Blankenhorn DH, Johnson RL, Nessim SA, et al: The Cholesterol Lowering Atherosclerosis Study (CLAS): Design, methods, and baseline results. *Controlled Clin Trials*, in press.
16. Keys A, Anderson JT, Grande F: Serum cholesterol response to changes in the diet: I. Iodine value of dietary fat versus 2S-P. *Metabolism* 1965;14:747-758.
17. Burstein M, Samaille J: Sur un dosage rapide du cholesterol lie aux a et au b-lipoproteines du serum. *Clin Chim Acta* 1960;5:609.
18. Lipid Research Clinics Program: *The Manual of Laboratory Operations: Lipid and Lipoprotein Analysis*, publication NIH 75-628. Bethesda, Md, National Institutes of Health, 1974.
19. Friedewald WT, Levy RI, Fredrickson DS: Estimation of the concentration of low-density lipoprotein cholesterol in plasma, without use of the preparative ultracentrifuge. *Clin Chem* 1972;18:499-502.
20. Multiple Risk Factor Intervention Trial Research Group: Multiple Risk Factor Intervention Trial: Risk factor changes and mortality results. *JAMA* 1982;248:1465-1477.
21. Johnson RL, Selzer R, Blankenhorn DH, et al: Nutrient Analysis System—a computerized seven-day food record system. *J Am Diet Assoc* 1983;83:667-671.
22. *SAS User's Guide: Statistics*, ed 5. Cray, NC, SAS Institute Inc, 1985.
23. Siegel S: *Nonparametric Statistics for the Behavioral Sciences*. New York, McGraw-Hill International Book Co, 1956.
24. Massey FJ Jr, Bernstein GS, O'Fallon WM, et al: Vasectomy and health: Results from a large cohort study. *JAMA* 1984;252:1023-1029.
25. Loop FD, Cosgrove DM: Repeat coronary bypass surgery: Selection of cases, surgical risks, and long-term outlook. *Mod Concepts Cardiovasc Dis* 1986;55:31-36.
26. Moise A, Bourassa MG, Theroux P, et al: Prognostic significance of progression of coronary artery disease. *Am J Cardiol* 1985;55:941-946.
27. Lipid Research Clinics Program: The Lipid Research Clinics Coronary Primary Prevention Trial results: II. The relationship of reduction in incidence of coronary heart disease to cholesterol lowering. *JAMA* 1984;251:365-374.
28. Canner PL, Berg KG, Wegner NK, et al: Fifteen year mortality in Coronary Drug Project patients: Long-term benefit with niacin. *J Am Coll Cardiol* 1986;8:1245-1255.
29. Detre KM, Levy RI, Kelsey SF, et al: Secondary prevention and lipid lowering: Results and implications. *Am Heart J* 1985;110:1123-1127.
30. Lowering blood cholesterol to prevent heart disease, CONSENSUS CONFERENCE. *JAMA* 1985;253:2080-2086.

The New England
Journal of Medicine

Volume 317   NOVEMBER 12, 1987   Number 20

HELSINKI HEART STUDY: PRIMARY-PREVENTION TRIAL WITH GEMFIBROZIL IN MIDDLE-AGED MEN WITH DYSLIPIDEMIA

Safety of Treatment, Changes in Risk Factors, and Incidence of Coronary Heart Disease

M. Heikki Frick, M.D., Olli Elo, M.D., Kauko Haapa, M.D., Olli P. Heinonen, M.D., D.Sc.,
Pertti Heinsalmi, M.D., Pekka Helo, M.D., Jussi K. Huttunen, M.D., Pertti Kaitaniemi, M.D.,
Pekka Koskinen, M.D., Vesa Manninen, M.D., Hanna Mäenpää, M.D., Marjatta Mälkönen, M.Sc.,
Matti Mänttäri, M.D., Seppo Norola, M.D., Amos Pasternack, M.D., Jarmo Pikkarainen, M.D.,
Matti Romo, M.D., Tom Sjöblom, M.D., and Esko A. Nikkilä, M.D.*

Abstract In a randomized, double-blind five-year trial, we tested the efficacy of simultaneously elevating serum levels of high-density lipoprotein (HDL) cholesterol and lowering levels of non-HDL cholesterol with gemfibrozil in reducing the risk of coronary heart disease in 4081 asymptomatic middle-aged men (40 to 55 years of age) with primary dyslipidemia (non-HDL cholesterol $\geq$200 mg per deciliter [5.2 mmol per liter] in two consecutive pretreatment measurements). One group (2051 men) received 600 mg of gemfibrozil twice daily, and the other (2030 men) received placebo.

Gemfibrozil caused a marked increase in HDL cholesterol and persistent reductions in serum levels of total, low-density lipoprotein (LDL), and non-HDL cholesterol and triglycerides. There were minimal changes in serum lipid levels in the placebo group. The cumulative rate of cardiac end points at five years was 27.3 per 1000 in the gemfibrozil group and 41.4 per 1000 in the placebo group — a reduction of 34.0 percent in the incidence of coronary heart disease (95 percent confidence interval, 8.2 to 52.6; P<0.02; two-tailed test). The decline in incidence in the gemfibrozil group became evident in the second year and continued throughout the study. There was no difference between the groups in the total death rate, nor did the treatment influence the cancer rates.

The results are in accord with two previous trials with different pharmacologic agents and indicate that modification of lipoprotein levels with gemfibrozil reduces the incidence of coronary heart disease in men with dyslipidemia. (N Engl J Med 1987; 317:1237-45.)

AN elevated serum level of low-density lipoprotein (LDL) cholesterol is a factor etiologically related to atherosclerotic vascular disease, and in particular to coronary heart disease.[1-5] A protective effect against coronary heart disease of elevated serum high-density lipoprotein (HDL) has been observed in several epidemiologic and clinical studies.[6-11] A low serum level of HDL cholesterol appears to be an important risk factor, particularly in populations whose serum level of total cholesterol is high.

Clinical trials aimed at reducing elevated serum total cholesterol (and hence LDL cholesterol) have demonstrated that whether the reduction is achieved by dietary or pharmacologic means, the incidence of coronary heart disease is reduced.[12-15] There is a positive correlation between the extent to which LDL choles-

terol is lowered and the incidence of coronary heart disease.[16] No such conclusive data are so far available on the effect of induced changes in the serum level of HDL cholesterol on the incidence of coronary heart disease.

Gemfibrozil belongs to the group of fibric acid derivatives, but is structurally different and possesses biologic actions distinct from those of clofibrate.[17,18] Gemfibrozil reduces levels of total and LDL cholesterol and triglycerides, but also raises HDL cholesterol levels both in normal subjects and in patients with various forms of hyperlipoproteinemia.[19-28] The short-term toxicity of gemfibrozil is low, and no adverse effects due to long-term use have been reported.[20]

The Helsinki Heart Study was launched to investigate the effect of this agent on the incidence of coronary heart disease in a randomized, double-blind, five-year trial in middle-aged men who were free of coronary symptoms on entry and were at high risk because of abnormal concentrations of blood lipids.[29] The present report documents the changes in risk factors and the reduction in the incidence of coronary

From the First and Third Departments of Medicine, University of Helsinki; National Public Health Institute, Helsinki; Department of Medicine, University of Tampere, Finland; Finnish Railways, Posts and Telecommunications, and the following industrial companies: A. Ahlström, Enso-Gutzeit, Kaukas (Kymmene), Neste, and Veitsiluoto. Address reprint requests to Prof. Frick at the First Department of Medicine, University of Helsinki, SF-00290 Helsinki, Finland.

*Deceased, September 21, 1986.

1238 THE NEW ENGLAND JOURNAL OF MEDICINE Nov. 12, 1987

heart disease, and provides an analysis of the major safety aspects of the trial.

METHODS

General Design

The design of the Helsinki Heart Study has been described in detail elsewhere.[30] The study was a randomized, double-blind, placebo-controlled trial of gemfibrozil (600 mg twice daily) against placebo, lasting for five years. In addition to drug treatment, a cholesterol-lowering diet was recommended to all participants. An increase in physical activity as well as a reduction in smoking and body weight was also encouraged.

The study protocol was approved by the Ethics Committee of the Faculty of Medicine, University of Helsinki; the National Board of Health in Finland; the U.S. Food and Drug Administration; and the trade unions and management of the public-sector and private-sector industries by whom the participants were employed. The study had a central office in Helsinki for its day-to-day management. There were 37 clinics, all of which followed the same protocol.

Screening and Follow-up Procedures

On the basis of a pilot study,[30] non-HDL cholesterol, which is defined as total cholesterol minus HDL cholesterol (i.e., the sum of LDL and very-low-density lipoprotein [VLDL] cholesterol) was selected as the lipid whose level would determine acceptance into the study. Non-HDL cholesterol was considered to represent the atherogenic fractions in both the low-density and very-low-density regions of the lipoprotein distribution. The acceptance level was set at ≥200 mg per deciliter (5.2 mmol per liter). To ascertain that the lipid disorder was stable, the participant had to meet the acceptance criterion in two successive measurements.

The purpose of the screening was to identify at least 4000 healthy middle-aged men who satisfied the lipid acceptance criterion and were willing to participate in a five-year trial.[30] The participants were selected from 23,531 men 40 to 55 years of age who were employed by the Finnish Posts and Telecommunications agency, the Finnish State Railways, and five industrial companies in Finland. Complete screening of the civil service group was carried out during the first half of 1981, and the screening of the industrial employees one year later. A total of 18,966 men (80.6 percent) agreed to participate in the first screening. Subjects were excluded if they had any clinical manifestations of coronary heart disease or electrocardiographic abnormalities (713 men), congestive heart failure, or any other disease that could have had an influence on the study outcome. Subjects with hypertension and mild non-insulin-dependent diabetes were accepted.

The screening procedure was conducted in three steps and was completed in three to five months. During the first screening visit, blood pressure was measured and a blood sample with the subject not fasting was taken for the determination of serum levels of total and HDL cholesterol. Subjects fulfilling the lipid acceptance criterion and without reasons for exclusion (6903 men) were invited to the second screening visit, during which a medical examination was carried out and electrocardiography performed. A complete lipid profile in the fasting state and a multichannel laboratory analysis were obtained. At the third (base-line) visit, 4081 men who met the acceptance criterion twice and were willing to participate were randomly assigned to receive either gemfibrozil or placebo.

The subjects visited the clinics at three-month intervals. Data on compliance with the study regimen, adverse events, smoking, adherence to dietary recommendations, hospitalization, major illness, other medication, and any symptoms suggesting myocardial infarction were recorded, as were body weight and blood pressure. In any cases of suspected myocardial infarction, 12-lead electrocardiography was performed with the subject resting. In addition, routine electrocardiography was performed each year in conjunction with the annual medical examination.

Smoking habits were recorded in terms of the daily consumption of tobacco. Occupational and leisure-time physical activities were assessed with use of a four-point scale adapted from the Gothenburg study.[41] A modification of the Finnish version of the original Bortner rating scale for Type A behavior[42] was applied. Alcohol consumption was recorded according to the Scandinavian drinking survey.[43]

Medication and Maintenance of Study Blinding

Subjects were randomly assigned to receive either gemfibrozil or placebo capsules in blocks distributed to each of the 37 clinics. The capsules were supplied by Parke–Davis Pharmaceutical Research Division, Pontypool, United Kingdom. Unused capsules were returned and counted. Gemfibrozil was measured in urine to check compliance, and the results were kept blinded for later analysis. A microdose of digoxin (2.2 μg per capsule) was used as a marker in both active and placebo capsules.[34] Urinary digoxin levels were measured in all participants during the last quarter of the third[35] and fifth study years.

Every effort was made to maintain the double-blindness of the study. A four-member safety committee had access to safety data. The committee reviewed the end points of the study according to treatment group only once during the trial. The end points, along with the codes, were sealed and kept in a safe until all patients had completed the trial.

Laboratory Methods

A venous blood sample was drawn into a vacuum tube at every visit. A sample in the fasting state was required during the semiannual visits only, when the serum concentration of triglycerides was determined. Serum samples were sent to the central laboratory (at the National Public Health Institute in Helsinki) daily by mail. The interval from sampling to analysis ranged from one to five days. The total cholesterol was measured directly in the serum, and HDL cholesterol was measured after precipitation of VLDL and LDL with dextran sulfate–magnesium chloride by an enzymatic method.[30] The concentration of triglycerides in serum was determined by measuring glycerol after an enzymatic hydrolysis with lipase-esterase.[30] The LDL cholesterol concentration was calculated according to the formula LDL cholesterol = total cholesterol minus HDL cholesterol minus triglycerides divided by 5.[36]

The mean coefficients of variation from day to day for total cholesterol and HDL cholesterol were 0.9 percent and 2.0 percent, respectively. External quality assessments were made in collaboration with the World Health Organization Lipid Research Center in Prague. The mean deviation from reference values was ±0.5 percent, and the range was −1.5 to 1.0 percent for the total cholesterol level. The accuracy of the cholesterol method was further tested against quality-control serum samples analyzed by mass spectrometry. The deviation from the reference cholesterol value was ±0.4 percent.

Because the triglyceride concentration was not measured at the base-line visit (the last before treatment), the base-line values for LDL cholesterol were calculated on the basis of total cholesterol and HDL cholesterol values at the base-line visit and triglyceride values determined at the second screening visit. Triglyceride values of 700 mg per deciliter or higher were excluded from the LDL calculations.[36] LDL cholesterol values under 100 mg per deciliter (e.g., negative values) were deemed outliers and were excluded.

In addition to hemoglobin measurements, white-cell counts, and strip tests for urinary sugar and protein performed in local laboratories twice a year, a package analysis was carried out once in the central laboratory to measure the following: alkaline phosphatase, aspartate aminotransferase, bilirubin, calcium, creatinine, iron, latent iron-binding capacity, and uric acid.

Cardiovascular End Points

Fatal and nonfatal myocardial infarction and cardiac death were the principal end points. All end-point assessments were made without knowledge of the subject's treatment. Classifications could not be altered once the treatment codes were broken. "Fatal myocardial infarction" was diagnosed when a death certificate or hospital record described the cause of death and there was either preterminal hospitalization with definite myocardial infarction or an autopsy finding of acute myocardial infarction. "Sudden cardiac death" was diagnosed when a death certificate described coronary heart disease and death occurred within one hour after the onset of symptoms.

Vol. 317　No. 20　　THE NEW ENGLAND JOURNAL OF MEDICINE　　1239

"Unwitnessed cardiac death" was diagnosed when a death certificate described coronary heart disease and there was no evidence to justify a classification of sudden cardiac death.

"Definite nonfatal myocardial infarction" was diagnosed in hospitalized patients when there was a diagnostic electrocardiogram at the time of the event (Minnesota codes[17] 1-1, or 1-2 plus 5-1 or 5-2, and excluding 1-2.6 and 1-2.8) or ischemic cardiac pain and diagnostic enzyme levels (levels of aspartate aminotransferase, creatine kinase, creatine kinase MB, or lactate dehydrogenase exceeding at least twice the upper limit of the reference values) or ischemic cardiac pain and equivocal enzyme levels (elevated but not fulfilling the diagnostic criteria) and an equivocal electrocardiogram (Minnesota codes 1-2 or 1-3, 4-1-1 to 4-1-3, 5-1 to 5-2, or 7-1). In patients not hospitalized, the diagnosis was confirmed when a patient reporting chest pain, breathlessness, or syncope had a diagnostic electrocardiogram at the time of the event or when annual routine electrocardiography indicated new changes consistent with myocardial infarction.

Hospitalized patients with ischemic cardiac pain and equivocal enzyme levels or an equivocal electrocardiogram were classified as having a "possible myocardial infarction," whereas among patients not hospitalized, ischemic cardiac pain and an electrocardiogram that was equivocal for reasons other than S-T-segment or T-wave changes were sufficient criteria. Possible myocardial infarction was not considered a cardiovascular end point. The classification of definite and possible cases was made by a senior board-certified cardiologist. A more detailed description of the end-point definitions has been published.[30]

The Minnesota coding of the electrocardiograms was performed by two specially trained technicians. All positive findings were checked by an independent board-certified cardiologist, who also had no clinical information about the participants. To check the reliability of negative findings, a review committee, consisting of two independent cardiologists with experience in cardiovascular epidemiology and clinical cardiology, reviewed a random sample of Minnesota codings. A board-certified cardiologist who was a member of the research group made the end-point assessment, using the Minnesota coding and all relevant clinical information, including data on enzymes.

The review committee evaluated the classification of all end points. In the few cases in which there was a difference of opinion between the designated cardiologist and the review committee, the final assessment of an end point was made by the four-member safety committee, consisting of experts in clinical cardiology and cardiovascular epidemiology.

Statistical Methods

The log-rank (Mantel–Haenszel) statistic[38] was used to compare the survival (or failure) curves in the treatment groups. The nominal P value derived by this procedure is reported, as well as the corresponding two-tailed 5 percent critical chi-square value derived by the sequential procedure of Lan and DeMets.[39] This procedure has been recommended for the analysis of survival-type data in long-term clinical trials.[40] In determining the Lan–DeMets critical value, time in the study was approximated by calendar time. Thus, the one interim analysis occurred in 71.4 percent of the way through the study. The 5 percent alpha-error rate was "spent" with use of the function $a * (t)$, to approximate the O'Brien–Fleming boundaries.[41] The Kaplan–Meier method was used to construct life-table plots.[42]

RESULTS

Success of Random Assignment

A total of 18,966 subjects were screened, and 4081 were included in the trial (Table 1). They were randomly assigned to receive either gemfibrozil (2051 men) or placebo (2030 men). With the exception of serum lipids, the levels of other cardiovascular risk factors were almost identical in the screened population and in the two treatment groups. Because the first screening was not carried out in the fasting state, tri-

Table 1. Characteristics of the Screened Population and the Treatment Groups at the First Screening in the Helsinki Heart Study.*

CHARACTERISTIC	SCREENED POPULATION	TREATMENT GROUP	
		GEMFIBROZIL	PLACEBO
No. of subjects	18,966	2051	2030
		mean ±SD	
Age (yr)	47.3±4.7	47.2±4.6	47.4±4.6
Body-mass index (kg/m²)	26.3±3.2	26.6±3.2	26.6±3.2
Blood pressure (mm Hg)			
Systolic	141.0±17.1	142.1±16.6	141.3±16.4
Diastolic	90.3±10.5	91.5±10.2	91.0±10.2
Cholesterol (mg/dl)†			
Total	244.7±45.1	289.1±32.9	288.7±31.3
HDL	49.4±11.9	47.1±10.5	47.1±11.0
Non-HDL‡	195.4±45.9	242.1±32.2	241.7±30.8
Triglycerides (mg/dl)§	ND	175.3±117.8	176.6±120.5
		percent of total	
Hypertension¶	12.9	14.5	13.4
Diabetes	2.6	2.4	2.9
Nonsmokers	40.2	37.2	35.7
Ex-smokers	27.5	26.4	28.5
Smokers	32.3	36.5	35.8
Fredrickson type			
IIa	ND	63.3	63.7
IIb	ND	27.9	27.5
IV	ND	8.8	8.5

*HDL denotes high-density lipoprotein, and ND not determined in the first screening.

†To convert values to millimoles per liter, multiply by 0.02586.

‡Total cholesterol minus HDL cholesterol.

§To convert values to millimoles per liter, multiply by 0.01129.

¶Hypertension was defined as one screening blood pressure of ≥170/≥100 mm Hg, or a diastolic pressure >105 mm Hg; it was also considered present if the patient was taking antihypertensive medication.

glyceride values were available for only 6903 subjects who participated in the second screening — i.e., whose non-HDL cholesterol level was ≥200 mg per deciliter (5.2 mmol per liter) at the first screening. Their mean serum triglyceride level was 171.7 mg per deciliter (1.94 mmol per liter) — slightly below the value in the two treatment groups.

The mean blood pressure, the rate of smoking, and the prevalence of hypertension, diabetes, and the customary Fredrickson lipoprotein types IIa, IIb, and IV were similar in the two treatment groups (Table 1). The gemfibrozil and placebo groups were also similar with regard to their scores on the Bortner behavior-rating scale, alcohol consumption, and family history of myocardial infarction and angina pectoris.[30] The leisure-time physical-activity score was significantly higher in the placebo than in the gemfibrozil group. Finally, the predicted five-year incidences of coronary heart disease according to the multiple logistic risk functions were similar in both treatment groups, as they were when analyzed in subgroups of occupational affiliation and geographic area.[30]

Study Participation and Compliance with Medication Regimen

Of the total 4081 subjects initially randomized, 2859 (70.1 percent) continued in the trial until its completion. In the gemfibrozil group, the annual dropout rates among subjects remaining in the study from the previous year were 14.7, 6.6, 5.3, 4.7, and 4.5 percent, respectively. In the placebo group, the rates were 12.6, 6.4, 4.5, 4.3, and 4.4 percent. All the subjects initially randomized were followed for five years and included in the analysis; none were lost to follow-up.

According to the three-month capsule counts, the proportions of prescribed capsules taken annually in the gemfibrozil group were 85, 85, 84, 84, and 82 percent. The respective figures for the placebo group were 85, 86, 86, 86, and 83 percent. The digoxin-marker study also indicated that the compliance with the regimen was good.[35]

Blood Lipids

The last of the three pretreatment lipid values, measured when the drug or placebo was dispensed, was chosen to represent the base-line value for the subsequent follow-up, since there was a declining trend during the screening period, except for HDL, which did not change. Before the intervention, triglycerides were measured only during the second screening.

During treatment, the placebo group had only minimal and random changes from the base-line values and particularly clear seasonal variations. Gemfibrozil rapidly increased the HDL cholesterol level by more than 10 percent; this was followed by a small decline with time. The total cholesterol level was initially reduced by 11 percent, the level of LDL cholesterol by 10 percent, that of non-HDL cholesterol by 14 percent, and that of triglycerides by 43 percent; these changes were followed by a consistent level of total and of LDL cholesterol and a small increase in the triglyceride level during the last years of the trial (Fig. 1; Table 2). These changes resulted in significant and sustained elevations in the ratios of HDL cholesterol to LDL cholesterol and of HDL cholesterol to total cholesterol.

Selected Cardiovascular Risk Factors

Systolic and diastolic blood pressure, body mass, and smoking habits remained similar in both treatment groups throughout the study. Changes in blood pressure were within 1 mm Hg, changes in body-mass index were within 0.2 kg per square meter, and smoking decreased 3 to 4 percent in both treatment groups.

Cardiac End Points

The mean follow-up period was 60.4 months, and the total follow-up period was 20,541 person-years. The total dropout rate was 29.9 percent. If the dropouts are taken into account, the total exposure to gemfibrozil was 8194 person-years, as opposed to 8372 person-years for the placebo.

The total number of cardiac end points in the gemfibrozil group was 56 (27.3 per 1000), as compared with 84 in the placebo group (41.4 per 1000) (Table

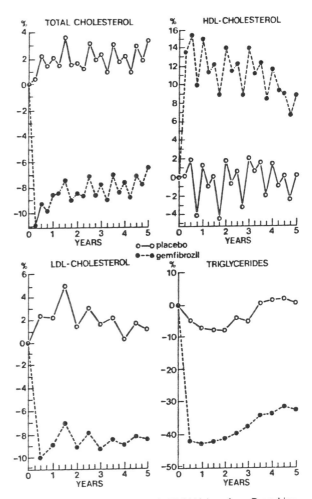

Figure 1. Percentage Changes in Lipid Values from Base Line, According to Treatment Group and Time.

3), yielding a log-rank chi-square of 6.0, with a nominal $P < 0.02$ (two-tailed). The significance was also tested according to the Lan–DeMets procedure, taking into account the interim evaluation of the data at three years. With this conservative procedure, the difference between the two groups was also statistically significant (critical value = 4.02; $P < 0.05$; two-tailed). The overall reduction in the frequency of cardiac end points in the gemfibrozil group was 34.0 percent (95 percent confidence interval, 8.2 to 52.6).

The greatest reduction in end-point rates (37 percent; $P < 0.05$) was noted in the group with nonfatal myocardial infarction (21.9 per 1000 vs. 35.0 per 1000; $P < 0.02$). The results were essentially similar when the analysis excluded the patients who dropped out. The end-point rates in the civil service group were 25.2 per 1000 for gemfibrozil and 44.3 per 1000 for placebo. The respective values in the industrial group were 31.3 per 1000 and 35.9 per 1000. The distribution of end points from clinic to clinic favored gemfibrozil in 29 of the 37 centers in the study; most of the remaining centers showed equal distributions of the end points.

The Kaplan–Meier life-table values for the cumula-

Vol. 317   No. 20   THE NEW ENGLAND JOURNAL OF MEDICINE   1241

Table 2. Lipid Values According to Treatment Group and Time.*

| SERUM LIPID | | GEMFIBROZIL | | | PLACEBO | | |
	Interval (mo) ⟶	BASE LINE	0–24	≥25	BASE LINE	0–24	≥25
Cholesterol (mg/dl)							
Total	Mean	269.9	244.7	246.9	269.6	272.5	272.6
	SE	0.78	0.76	0.85	0.78	0.71	0.78
	No.	2051	1973	1611	2030	1958	1638
HDL	Mean	47.1	52.1	51.2	47.6	46.8	47.0
	SE	0.24	0.26	0.29	0.25	0.23	0.26
	No.	2051	1973	1611	2030	1958	1638
Non-HDL†	Mean	222.9	192.6	195.7	222.1	225.7	225.5
	SE	0.78	0.80	0.89	0.78	0.72	0.78
	No.	2051	1973	1611	2030	1958	1638
LDL	Mean	189.2	172.8	173.5	188.2	193.6	191.4
	SE	0.76	0.72	0.77	0.76	0.70	0.76
	No.	2004	1885	1590	1991	1887	1616
Cholesterol ratio							
HDL to total	Mean	0.18	0.22	0.21	0.18	0.17	0.17
	SE	0.00	0.00	0.00	0.00	0.00	0.00
	No.	2051	1973	1611	2030	1958	1638
HDL to LDL	Mean	0.26	0.32	0.31	0.26	0.25	0.26
	SE	0.00	0.00	0.00	0.00	0.00	0.00
	No.	2004	1885	1590	1991	1887	1616
Triglycerides (mg/dl)‡	Mean	175.3	102.7	114.8	176.7	166.6	177.7
	SE	2.60	1.38	1.68	2.67	2.10	2.34
	No.	2050	1885	1590	2030	1891	1618

*Values are means of readings made during the indicated intervals. HDL denotes high-density lipoprotein, and LDL low-density lipoprotein. To convert cholesterol values to millimoles per liter, multiply by 0.02586. To convert triglyceride values to millimoles per liter, multiply by 0.01129.

†Total cholesterol minus HDL cholesterol.

‡Not determined at base line. Values shown were obtained at the second screening.

tive incidence of definite cardiac end points, as well as the actual annual number of definite end points, are shown in Figure 2. No meaningful difference was observed during the first two years. Thereafter, the curves began to separate, with a progressive decrease in the gemfibrozil group, whereas the annual endpoint rate in the placebo group remained virtually unaltered throughout the study. From the third to fifth years of the trial, the number of end points in the gemfibrozil group was about one-third to one-half their number in the placebo group. In the fifth year, there were 6 end points in the gemfibrozil group and 18 in the placebo group when analysis was performed on an intention-to-treat basis. If the dropouts were excluded, the corresponding numbers of end points were 4 and 16, respectively.

There were 31 cases of possible myocardial infarction (15 in the gemfibrozil group and 16 in the placebo group). When these cases were included in the analyses, the difference in end-point rates between treatment groups was still statistically significant.

Mortality

There were 45 deaths (rate, 21.9 per 1000) in the gemfibrozil group and 42 deaths (rate, 20.7 per 1000) in the placebo group (Table 4). This difference was not statistically significant. Neither were there significant differences between the treatment groups in any of the specific causes of death. There were fewer deaths due to ischemic heart disease and more deaths due to violence, accidents, and intracranial hemorrhage in the gemfibrozil group, but the dif-

ferences were not statistically significant.

Cancers

There was no significant difference in the total number of cancers (31 vs. 26) between the two treatment groups (Table 5). In the subgroup analysis, there were five basal-cell carcinomas of the skin in the gemfibrozil group and none in the placebo group. This difference was of borderline statistical significance according to Fisher's exact test (P = 0.062). The expected numbers of basal-cell carcinomas calculated from the national cancer statistics of Finland[43] were 4.8 cases in the gemfibrozil group and 4.7 in the placebo group. No statistically significant differences were found in any of the analyses of other specific cancer types.

Surgical Operations and Hospital Admissions

In the subgroup analyses according to type of operation, there were no significant differences between the treatment groups in the numbers of any major surgical operations. In particular, gemfibrozil did not significantly increase the number of gallstone operations (18 in the gemfibrozil group vs. 12 in the placebo group). However, when all gastrointestinal operations, including hemorrhoidectomies, were combined, there was a statistically significant difference (81 in the gemfibrozil group vs. 53 in the placebo group, P<0.02). Eye operations were somewhat more common in the gemfibrozil group (17 vs. 12), mainly because of cataract operations (7 vs. 3), but the differences were not statistically significant. The same applied to coronary-bypass surgery (7 vs. 6).

When hospital admissions for the treatment of acute myocardial infarction were excluded, there were no statistically significant differences between the two treatment groups in the total numbers of hospitalizations or in the numbers of hospitalizations for gastrointestinal diseases or symptoms.

Adverse Events

During the first year, 11.3 percent of the subjects in the gemfibrozil group reported various moderate to severe upper gastrointestinal symptoms, whereas the corresponding rate for the placebo group was 7.0 percent (P<0.001). During subsequent years, these rates decreased to 2.4 and 1.2 percent (P<0.05), respectively. No significant differences between treatment groups were observed in the occurrence of constipation, diarrhea, or nausea and vomiting.

Similarly, no differences between the two treatment

1242   THE NEW ENGLAND JOURNAL OF MEDICINE   Nov. 12, 1987

Table 3. Cardiac End Points and Cases of Possible Myocardial Infarction According to Treatment Group and Participation Status.

CORONARY EVENT	SUBJECTS RECEIVING TREATMENT		SUBJECTS WITHDRAWN FROM TREATMENT		TOTAL	
	GEMFIBROZIL	PLACEBO	GEMFIBROZIL	PLACEBO	GEMFIBROZIL	PLACEBO
					no. (rate/1000)	
Definite						
Nonfatal myocardial infarction	40	61	5	10	45 (21.9)	71 (35.0)
Fatal myocardial infarction	3	7	3	1	6 (2.9)	8 (3.9)
Sudden cardiac death	3	3	2	1	5 (2.4)	4 (2.0)
Unwitnessed death	0	1	0	0	0 (0.0)	1 (0.5)
Total	46	72	10	12	56 (27.3)	84 (41.4)*
Possible	14	12	1	4	15 (7.3)	16 (7.9)

*Log-rank chi-square = 6.0, nominal P value <0.02 (two-tailed). Lan-DeMets sequential-procedure critical value = 4.02; overall P value <0.05 (two-tailed).

groups were observed in levels of hemoglobin, urinary protein, or urinary sugar or in laboratory multichannel analyses.

DISCUSSION

The total rate of cardiac end points during the five-year study was 27.3 per 1000 in the gemfibrozil group and 41.4 per 1000 in the placebo group (log-rank P<0.02, two-tailed). The number of definite cardiac end points was 56 in the gemfibrozil group and 84 in the placebo group. Despite a 26 percent lower mortality from coronary heart disease (19 vs. 14), there were slightly more deaths overall in the gemfibrozil

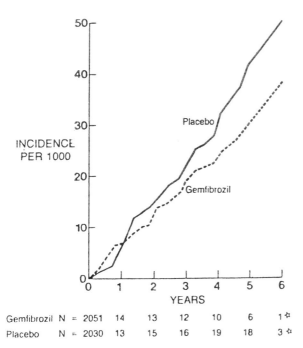

Gemfibrozil N = 2051   14   13   12   10   6   1 ☆
Placebo   N = 2030   13   15   16   19   18   3 ☆

Figure 2. Kaplan–Meier Cumulative Incidence (per 1000) and Annual Number of Cardiac End Points, According to Treatment Group and Time.

Data for the sixth year (stars) were derived from 305 person-years of observation for gemfibrozil and from 316 person-years of observation for placebo.

than in the placebo group (45 vs. 42). The size of the study population and the length of observation were not, however, sufficient to allow conclusions about the possible effects of changes in cardiac mortality on total mortality. The higher number of deaths in the gemfibrozil group was mainly due to accidents or violence and intracranial hemorrhage. An excess number of violent deaths in subjects treated with lipid-lowering regimens has also been observed in other studies[44] but has been interpreted to be a chance finding. No significant difference was observed between the groups in the occurrence of neoplasms.

A 30 percent reduction in the incidence of coronary heart disease was considered during the planning stage of the study to be the minimal change necessary to justify the use of long-term medication in subjects without symptoms. The observed reduction was 34 percent over the entire study period and more than 50 percent during years three to five. The difference during the latter half of the study may represent the long-term effect of the drug, since earlier studies[14,44] also suggest a lag of one to three years between the start of lipid-lowering treatment and effects on morbidity from coronary heart disease. A latent period between the changes in lipid values and changes in morbidity has also been predicted on the basis of epidemiologic studies[45] and may in fact be expected, because of the slow progress of the underlying atherosclerotic process.[46,47]

The incidence of events related to coronary heart disease in the placebo group was lower than expected — 41 per 1000 as compared with a predicted rate of 75 per 1000 in five years. Estimates of the incidence of coronary heart disease in men with similar dyslipidemia were based on coronary-register data collected in the 1970s.[30] This lower-than-predicted rate has also been observed in several previous clinical trials and may be due to a number of factors, including stringent selection processes, better health monitoring, and the concurrent decline in mortality and morbidity from coronary heart disease in the general population.

Previous dietary and pharmacologic trials have attempted to show that modification of lipid levels results in decreased morbidity and mortality from coronary heart disease. A statistically significant reduction was observed in patients on a fat-modified diet in the Finnish mental hospital study[12] and in conjunction with an antismoking program in the Oslo study.[13] Earlier pharmacologic trials, such as the World Health Organization's study of clofibrate[14] and the Lipid Research Clinic's (LRC) Coronary Primary Prevention Trial of cholestyramine[44] have both demonstrated that lowering cholesterol levels with drugs

Vol. 317   No. 20   THE NEW ENGLAND JOURNAL OF MEDICINE   1243

Table 4. Deaths According to Treatment Group and Cause.*

CAUSE OF DEATH	GEMFIBROZIL		PLACEBO	
	NO.	RATE/1000	NO.	RATE/1000
Ischemic heart disease	14†	6.8	19‡	9.4
Ischemic cerebral infarction	1	0.5	3	1.5
Intracranial hemorrhage	5§	2.4	1	0.5
Other vascular cause	2	1.0	0	0.0
Malignant neoplasm	11	5.4	11	5.4
Other medical cause	2	1.0	4	2.0
Accident/violence	10	4.9	4	2.0
Total	45	21.9	42	20.7

*The differences in rates between the treatment groups were not statistically significant.

†Three subjects died later in the study after surviving initial myocardial infarction.

‡Six subjects died later in the study after surviving initial myocardial infarction.

§One subject had pulmonary embolism and hemorrhage after streptokinase treatment.

significantly decreases the incidence of major coronary events. In the World Health Organization study there was, however, an increase in mortality due to a variety of causes, with no particular disease predominating. This excess of deaths diverted attention from the principal study finding — i.e., that reduction of plasma cholesterol lowered the incidence of coronary heart disease.

The LRC cholestyramine study was a multicenter, randomized, double-blind investigation to test the efficacy of cholesterol lowering in reducing the risk of coronary heart disease in 3806 asymptomatic men with hypercholesterolemia that had not responded to simple dietary management.[15,44] In many respects, the LRC trial and the Helsinki heart study are similar. In both studies, the participants (in the LRC study, men 35 to 59 years of age; in the Helsinki study, men 40 to 55) were initially free of overt coronary heart disease and other major disabilities. The LRC study had as its initial entry criteria a total cholesterol level over 265 mg per deciliter (6.85 mmol per liter) and an LDL cholesterol level over 175 mg per deciliter (4.53 mmol per liter) after a period of dietary intervention. Subjects were excluded if they had serum triglyceride levels over 300 mg per deciliter (3.4 mmol per liter), hypertension, or some other diseases.

Table 5. Cancers According to Treatment Group.*

CANCER	GEMFIBROZIL		PLACEBO	
	NO.	RATE/1000	NO.	RATE/1000
Lung	5	2.4	5	2.5
Colon/rectum	3	1.5	4	2.0
Stomach	1	0.5	4	2.0
Leukemia	2	1.0	1	0.5
Skin: basal-cell carcinoma	5	2.4	0	0.0
Other	15†	—	12‡	—
Total	31	15.1	26	12.8

*The differences in rates between treatment groups were not statistically significant, except for the differences in basal-cell carcinoma (P = 0.032 by Fisher's exact test).

†Cancers of the brain, bladder, bile duct, esophagus, gall bladder, liver, nasopharynx, prostate, kidney, and thyroid, and femoral fibrosarcoma, glioblastoma, lymphoma, melanoma, and myeloma.

‡Anaplastic cancer, carcinoid tumor of the small intestine, fibrosarcoma, intestinal mesothelioma, myeloma (two cases), pancreatic cancer (two), peritoneal fibrosarcoma, renal cancer (two), and type not specified (one).

Thus, all the patients in the LRC trial had Type II hyperlipoproteinemia.

Both the initial and final criterion of the Helsinki heart study was a level of non-HDL cholesterol equal to or greater than 200 mg per deciliter (5.2 mmol per liter). This criterion yielded 9 percent patients with Type IV hyperlipoproteinemia, 28 percent with Type IIb, and 63 percent with Type IIa. In spite of these differences, the initial mean lipid values were almost identical in the two studies. On the other hand, the two drugs used have distinctly different effects and mechanisms of action. Cholestyramine, a nonabsorbable sequestrant of bile acid, effectively lowers LDL cholesterol but has only minimal effects on VLDL and HDL cholesterol. In contrast, gemfibrozil elevates HDL cholesterol and reduces LDL and VLDL cholesterol.[17-28]

The cholestyramine-treated subjects in the seven-year LRC study had average reductions in plasma levels of total and LDL cholesterol of 13 and 20 percent, respectively, and an average increase in HDL cholesterol of 3 percent. A 21 percent reduction (38 vs. 30) in definite coronary deaths and a 17 percent reduction (187 vs. 155) in all definite end points for coronary heart disease were observed. Treatment with gemfibrozil in the Helsinki heart study over the five-year period induced mean reductions in serum total cholesterol, LDL cholesterol, non-HDL cholesterol, and triglycerides, respectively, of 8, 8, 12, and 35 percent, and an increase of more than 10 percent in HDL cholesterol. All lipid responses in the Helsinki heart study were obvious three to six months after the start of drug treatment. The differences between the gemfibrozil and placebo groups were maintained throughout the five-year study. These changes were accompanied by a 26 percent reduction in definite coronary deaths (19 vs. 14) and a 34 percent reduction in all definite end points for coronary heart disease (84 vs. 56).

It is generally agreed that ideal total cholesterol values should be below 200 mg per deciliter (5.2 mmol per liter)[48,49] and that active treatment should certainly be instituted in subjects with values in excess of 250 mg per deciliter (6.5 mmol per liter). On the other hand, no such definite guidelines have been generated for levels of HDL cholesterol. The study group of the European Atherosclerosis Society provisionally set a cutoff point of 35 mg per deciliter for the lower limit of plasma HDL cholesterol.[48] Several sources indicate that levels of HDL cholesterol should be at least 20 percent of total cholesterol in populations with high levels of non-HDL cholesterol.[7,10,11] In view of the growing evidence of the protective role of HDL in atherogenesis,[6-11] it is logical to raise the level of this lipoprotein either by nonpharmacologic means (exercise and weight reduction) or by pharmacologic means, at least in persons with high levels of non-HDL cholesterol. The present results are in agreement with such an approach. A simultaneous increase in HDL cholesterol and reduction in non-HDL choles-

1244 THE NEW ENGLAND JOURNAL OF MEDICINE Nov. 12, 1987

terol with gemfibrozil significantly reduced the incidence of coronary heart disease in middle-aged men.

The greatest relative change in serum lipid levels (approximately 35 percent) that was observed in this study was that in serum triglycerides. The role of triglycerides as a coronary risk factor is still controversial. The existing information suggests that in the presence of normal cholesterol levels, small elevations of plasma triglyceride levels do not necessarily increase the risk of cardiovascular disease. However, triglyceride levels exceeding 250 mg per deciliter (2.8 mmol per liter) may be associated with an increased risk of coronary heart disease, particularly in young subjects.[50-52] Whether the association is causal and the treatment of hypertriglyceridemia, either by dietary or pharmacologic means, is justified remains to be established.

The cancer mortality was identical in the two treatment groups. The small excess in the incidence of basal-cell carcinomas in the gemfibrozil group will require further evaluation, since the rate in the placebo group was exceptionally low.[43] The incidence of other neoplasms did not differ between the study groups.

The use of gemfibrozil resulted in several gastrointestinal side effects, although these were also common in the placebo group. Although according to one study gemfibrozil is less lithogenic than clofibrate,[18] it increases biliary cholesterol saturation in healthy persons,[53] and this may cause more gallstones and necessitate more cholecystectomies. There were slightly more cases of eye surgery, mainly involving cataracts, in the gemfibrozil than in the placebo group. None of the differences between the two study groups in the numbers of surgical operations for specific causes were statistically significant.

In conclusion, specifically modifying the lipoprotein profile with gemfibrozil resulted in a marked reduction in the incidence of coronary heart disease without evoking any critical adverse events. These findings are in accord with those of two previous primary-prevention trials using lipid-modulating agents with different pharmacologic effects,[14,15,44] and furnish additional and conclusive evidence of the role of lipid modification in preventing coronary heart disease.

We are indebted to the participants in the study for their understanding and trust; to the nurses for their excellent care; to Stephen Preston, M.D., John Gorringe, M.D., Robert Hodges, M.D., and Mr. Joseph Dresner for overseeing the initial phases of the study and for subsequent help; to David Evans, M.D., and Mr. Roy Couch for extremely valuable contributions; to Terry Goodburn, Ph.D., and his department in Pontypool, United Kingdom, who supplied the drugs; to Ms. Kaija Javela and her staff for excellent work at the Central Laboratory of the Public Health Institute; to Sven Punsar, M.D., Ritva Halonen, R.N., and Outi Marila, R.N., for the excellent quality of the electrocardiogram reading and the Minnesota coding; to Pentti Ristola, M.D., and Olli Suhonen, M.D., who liberally gave their time and expertise for the independent end-point revision; to Mr. Joe Dresner (director), Mr. Harry Haber, Ms. Janet Ward, and the whole staff of the data-processing section in Ann Arbor, Michigan, for excellent service in managing well over half a million case reports and other information collected during the study; and to the Warner–Lambert Company and all the Finnish participating institutions for their generous support.

Tables concerning selected risk factors and their changes during the study, as well as surgical operations and gastrointestinal side effects, can be obtained on request from the authors.

REFERENCES

1. Keys A. Seven countries: a multivariate analysis of death and coronary heart disease. Cambridge, Mass.: Harvard University Press, 1980.
2. Dawber TR. The Framingham Study: the epidemiology of atherosclerotic disease. Cambridge, Mass.: Harvard University Press, 1980.
3. American Heart Association Steering Committee for Medical and Community Program. Risk factors and coronary disease: a statement for physicians. Circulation 1980; 62:449A-455A.
4. Ross R. The pathology of atherosclerosis — an update. N Engl J Med 1986; 314:488-500.
5. Martin MJ, Hulley SB, Browner WS, Kuller LH, Wentworth D. Serum cholesterol, blood pressure, and mortality: implications from a cohort of 361 662 men. Lancet 1986; 2:933-6.
6. Barr DP, Russ EM, Eder HA. Protein-lipid relationships in human plasma. II. In atherosclerosis and related conditions. Am J Med 1951; 11:480-93.
7. Nikkilä E. Studies on the lipid-protein relationships in normal and pathological sera and the effect of heparin on serum lipoproteins. Scand J Clin Lab Invest [Suppl] 1953; 5:Suppl 8:1-101.
8. Miller GJ, Miller NE. Plasma-high-density-lipoprotein concentration and development of ischaemic heart-disease. Lancet 1975; 1:16-9.
9. Miller NE, Førde OH, Thelle DS, Mjøs OD. The Tromsø Heart-Study: high-density lipoprotein and coronary heart-disease: a prospective case-control study. Lancet 1977; 1:965-7.
10. Gordon T, Castelli WP, Hjortland MC, Kannel WB, Dawber TR. High density lipoprotein as a protective factor against coronary heart disease. Am J Med 1977; 62:707-14.
11. Castelli WP, Garrison RJ, Wilson PWF, Abbott RD, Kalousdian S, Kannel WB. Incidence of coronary heart disease and lipoprotein cholesterol levels: the Framingham Study. JAMA 1986; 256:2835-8.
12. Turpeinen O, Karvonen MJ, Pekkarinen M, Miettinen M, Elosuo R, Paavilainen E. Dietary prevention of coronary heart disease: the Finnish Mental Hospital Study. Int J Epidemiol 1979; 8:99-118.
13. Hjermann I, Velve Byre K, Holme I, Leren P. Effect of diet and smoking intervention on the incidence of coronary heart disease: report from the Oslo Study Group of a randomized trial in healthy men. Lancet 1981; 2:1303-10.
14. Oliver MF, Heady JA, Morris JN, et al. A co-operative trial in the primary prevention of ischaemic heart disease using clofibrate: a report from the Committee of Principal Investigators. Br Heart J 1978; 40:1069-118.
15. Lipid Research Clinics Program. The Lipid Research Clinics Coronary Primary Prevention Trial results. II. The relationship of reduction in incidence of coronary heart disease to cholesterol lowering. JAMA 1984; 251:365-74.
16. Peto R, Yusuf S, Collins R. Cholesterol-lowering trial results in their epidemiologic context. Circulation 1985; 72:III-451. abstract.
17. Gemfibrozil: a new lipid lowering agent: proceedings of an International Symposium held by Parke, Davis & Company at The Royal Society of Medicine on 15–16 June 1976. Proc R Soc Med 1976; 69:Suppl 2:1-120.
18. Newton RS, Krause BR. Mechanisms of action of gemfibrozil: comparison of studies in the rat to clinical efficacy: In: Fears R, ed. Pharmacological control of hyperlipidaemia. Barcelona, Spain: J.R. Prous, 1986: 171-86.
19. Nikkilä EA, Ylikahri R, Huttunen JK. Gemfibrozil: effect on serum lipids, lipoproteins, postheparin plasma lipase activities, and glucose tolerance in primary hypertriglyceridaemia. Proc R Soc Med 1976; 69:Suppl 2:58-63.
20. Olsson AG, Rössner S, Walldius G, Carlson LA. Effect of gemfibrozil on lipoprotein concentrations in different types of hyperlipoproteinaemia. Proc R Soc Med 1976; 69:Suppl 2:28-31.
21. Manninen V, Mälkönen M, Eisalo A, Virtamo J, Tuomilehto J, Kuusisto P. Gemfibrozil in the treatment of dyslipidaemia: a 5-year follow-up study. Acta Med Scand [Suppl] 1982; 668:82-7.
22. Glueck C. Influence of gemfibrozil on high-density lipoproteins. Am J Cardiol 1983; 52:31B-34B.
23. Kesäniemi YA, Grundy SM. Influence of gemfibrozil and clofibrate on metabolism of cholesterol and plasma triglycerides in man. JAMA 1984; 251:2241-6.
24. Turner PR, Cortese C, Wootton R, Marenah C, Miller NE, Lewis B. Plasma apolipoprotein B metabolism in familial type III dysbetalipoproteinaemia. Eur J Clin Invest 1985; 15:100-12.
25. Saku K, Gartside PS, Hynd BA, Kashyap ML. Mechanism of action of gemfibrozil on lipoprotein metabolism. J Clin Invest 1985; 75:1702-12.
26. Meinertz H. Effects of gemfibrozil on plasma lipoproteins in patients with type II hyperlipoproteinaemia and familial hypercholesterolaemia. R Soc Med Int Congr Symp Ser 1986; 87:15-21.

Vol. 317   No. 20   THE NEW ENGLAND JOURNAL OF MEDICINE   1245

27. Weintraub MS, Eisenberg S, Breslow JL. Different patterns of postprandial lipoprotein metabolism in normal, type IIa, type III, and type IV hyperlipoproteinemic individuals: effects of treatment with cholestyramine and gemfibrozil. J Clin Invest 1987; 79:1110-9.

28. Pasternack A, Vänttinen T, Solakivi T, Kuusi T, Korte T. Normalization of lipoprotein lipase and hepatic lipase by gemfibrozil results in correction of lipoprotein abnormalities in chronic renal failure. Clin Nephrol 1987; 27:163-8.

29. Manninen V. Clinical results with gemfibrozil and background for the Helsinki Heart Study. Am J Cardiol 1983; 52:35B-38B.

30. Mänttäri M, Elo O, Frick MH, et al. The Helsinki Heart Study: Basic design and randomization procedure. Eur Heart J 1987; 8:Suppl 1:1-29.

31. Wilhelmsen L, Tibblin G, Fodor J, Werkö L. A multifactorial primary prevention trial in Gothenburg, Sweden. In: Larsen OA, Malmborg RO, eds. Coronary heart disease and physical fitness. Copenhagen: Munksgaard, 1971:266-70.

32. Bortner RW. A short rating scale as a potential measure of pattern A behavior. J Chronic Dis 1969; 22:87-91.

33. Simpura J. Scandinavian drinking survey: construction of indices of alcohol intake. Report 46. Oslo: National Institute for Alcohol Research, 1981.

34. Mäenpää H, Pikkarainen J, Javela K, Mälkönen M, Heinonen OP, Manninen V. Minimal doses of digoxin: a new marker for compliance to medication. Eur Heart J 1987; 8:Suppl 1:31-7.

35. Mäenpää H, Manninen V, Heinonen OP. Comparison of the digoxin marker and compliance questionnaire methods in a clinical trial. Eur Heart J 1987; 8:Suppl 1:39-43.

36. Friedewald WT, Levy RI, Fredrickson DS. Estimation of the concentration of low-density lipoprotein cholesterol in plasma, without use of the preparative ultracentrifuge. Clin Chem 1972; 18:499-502.

37. Blackburn H, Keys A, Simonson E, Rautaharju P, Punsar S. The electrocardiogram in population studies: a classification system. Circulation 1960; 21:1160-75.

38. Kalbfleisch JD, Prentice RL. The statistical analysis of failure time data. New York: John Wiley, 1980.

39. Lan KKG, DeMets DL. Discrete sequential boundaries for clinical trials. Biometrika 1983; 70:659-63.

40. Lan KKG, DeMets DL, Halperin M. More flexible sequential and nonsequential designs in long-term clinical trials. Commun Stat Theory Methods 1984; 13:2339-53.

41. O'Brien PC, Fleming TR. A multiple testing procedure for clinical trials. Biometrics 1979; 35:549-56.

42. Kaplan EL, Meier P. Nonparametric estimation from incomplete observations. J Am Stat Assoc 1958; 53:457-81.

43. Cancer incidence in Finland 1982. Helsinki, Finland: Cancer Society of Finland, 1986. (Publication no. 34.)

44. Lipid Research Clinics Program. The Lipid Research Clinics Coronary Primary Prevention Trial results. I. Reduction in incidence of coronary heart disease. JAMA 1984; 251:351-64.

45. Rose G. Incubation period of coronary heart disease. Br Med J 1982; 284:1600-1.

46. Frick MH, Valle M, Harjola P-T. Progression of coronary artery disease in randomized medical and surgical patients over a 5-year angiographic follow-up. Am J Cardiol 1983; 52:681-5.

47. Canner PL, Berge KG, Wenger NK, et al. Fifteen year mortality in Coronary Drug Project patients: long-term benefit with niacin. J Am Coll Cardiol 1986; 8:1245-55.

48. Strategies for the prevention of coronary heart disease: a policy statement for the European Atherosclerosis Society. Eur Heart J 1987; 8:77-88.

49. Steinberg D, NIH Consensus Development Panel. Lowering blood cholesterol to prevent heart disease. JAMA 1985; 253:2080-6.

50. Åberg H, Lithell H, Selinius I, Hedstrand H. Serum triglycerides are a risk factor for myocardial infarction but not for angina pectoris: results from a 10-year follow-up of Uppsala Primary Prevention Study. Atherosclerosis 1985; 54:89-97.

51. Carlson LA, Böttiger LE. Risk factors for ischaemic heart disease in men and women: results of the 19-year follow-up of the Stockholm Prospective Study. Acta Med Scand 1985; 218:207-11.

52. Hamsten A, Wiman B, de Faire U, Blombäck M. Increased plasma levels of a rapid inhibitor of tissue plasminogen activator in young survivors of myocardial infarction. N Engl J Med 1985; 313:1557-63.

53. Leiss O, von Bergmann K, Gnasso A, Augustin J. Effect of gemfibrozil on biliary lipid metabolism in normolipemic subjects. Metabolism 1985; 34:74-82.

European Heart Journal (1988) **9**, 571–600

The recognition and management of hyperlipidaemia in adults: A policy statement of the European Atherosclerosis Society

STUDY GROUP, EUROPEAN ATHEROSCLEROSIS SOCIETY*

Contents

KEY WORDS: Action limits, case finding, coronary heart disease, hyperlipidaemia, hypolipidaemic drugs, lipid-lowering diets, prevention, risk factors.

The control of coronary heart disease (CHD) depends primarily on its prevention at an early stage. It is generally agreed that this depends upon the elimination or treatment of the known risk factors for CHD. Among these, hyperlipidaemia occupies a central position. The diagnosis and treatment of this condition is the subject of this statement.

Before initiating therapy for primary hyperlipidaemia the common causes of secondary hyperlipidaemia are sought and dealt with, including diabetes, hypothyroidism, over-use of alcohol, renal and liver diseases and certain drugs. Next, an assessment of all risk factors for CHD is carried out, i.e. family history of CHD, smoking, hypertension, high density lipoprotein (HDL) cholesterol measurement, diabetes mellitus and overweight. More intensive therapy is called for in patients with multiple risk factors than in those with lone hyperlipidaemia, and also after successful bypass operation or after coronary angioplasty. Evaluation of hyperlipidaemia in the patient's family is often appropriate. The diagnosis and follow-up of the hyperlipidaemic patient depend on reliable and well-controlled laboratory support.

The primary hyperlipidaemias include several distinct diseases that are characterized by elevated serum levels of cholesterol and/or triglyceride with or without abnormally low levels of HDL cholesterol. From these

---

*The members of the study group are listed in Appendix 5.

Requests for reprints should be addressed to: Professor Barry Lewis, Division of Chemical Pathology and Metabolic Disorders, St Thomas's Hospital, Medical School, London SE1 7EH, U.K.

0195-668X/88/050571 + 30 $02.00/0

measurements, low-density lipoprotein (LDL) cholesterol levels are calculated [except when triglyceride levels are > 500 mg dl^{-1} (5·6 mmol l^{-1})]. Elevated LDL levels are causally important in atherosclerosis, and occur in three disorders: familial hypercholesterolaemia, familial combined hyperlipidaemia and common hypercholesterolaemia. The finding of elevated serum triglyceride without marked hypercholesterolaemia may occur in familial hypertriglyceridaemia and sometimes in familial combined hyperlipidaemia.

Elevation of serum cholesterol and triglyceride can have several genetic bases, including remnant (type III) hyperlipidaemia and familial combined hyperlipidaemia. The characteristic feature of remnant (type III) hyperlipidaemia (demonstrated by ultracentrifugation in a specialized laboratory) is the presence of cholesterol and triglyceride-rich very low density lipoproteins (VLDL), whereas combined (mixed) hyperlipidaemia is diagnosed when both VLDL (of normal composition) and LDL levels are elevated. Investigation of other family members is necessary to make the diagnosis of familial combined hyperlipidaemia. It depends on the identification of different lipoprotein profiles in affected members of the same family.

In two rare disorders, the chylomicronaemia syndrome and severe primary familial hypertriglyceridaemia, gross elevation of triglyceride is found to levels above 1000 mg dl^{-1} (11 mmol l^{-1}). Such patients are at risk of pancreatitis and should be promptly and effectively treated.

Therapy of hyperlipidaemia always starts with dietary counselling. The general principles of the lipid-lowering diet are: (1) weight reduction in overweight subjects [body mass index (weight/height^2) > 27]; (2) a lipid-lowering diet providing 55% of calories from carbohydrates, 10–15% from protein and up to 30% from fat comprising 10% each of saturated, monounsaturated and polyunsaturated fatty acids, cholesterol < 300 mg day^{-1} and 35 g day^{-1} of fibre derived largely from legumes and other vegetables, and fruit. Further reduction of fat consumption to 20–25% of total energy and of cholesterol to < 150 mg day^{-1} may be attempted when patients respond inadequately to the standard diet.

The goal of treatment is to minimize the risk of CHD and of pancreatitis. Where possible, a level of LDL cholesterol of 135 mg dl^{-1} (3·5 mmol l^{-1}) is the aim in hypercholesterolaemic patients with multiple or severe risk factors and of 155 mg dl^{-1} (4 mmol l^{-1}) in the absence of other risk factors. Some patients with hyperlipidaemia do not respond adequately to diet and correction of underlying causes; drug treatment is then additionally required, but careful attention to diet is continued.

Five treatment groups are defined:

Group A consists of subjects with mild hypercholesterolaemia [serum cholesterol 200–250 mg dl^{-1} (5·2–6·5 mmol l^{-1}), serum triglyceride < 200 mg dl^{-1} (2·3 mmol l^{-1})]. Diet alone is effective and drug therapy is rarely necessary.

Group B subjects have serum cholesterol levels in the range 250–300 mg dl^{-1} (6·5–7·8 mmol l^{-1}). If the response to a thorough trial of diet is not satisfactory, drug therapy should be considered, e.g. bile acid sequestrants at low dosage.

Group C comprises subjects with hypertriglyceridaemia [serum cholesterol < 200 mg dl^{-1} (5·2 mmol l^{-1}), plasma triglyceride 200–500 mg dl^{-1} (2·3–5·6 mmol l^{-1})]. Many of these patients also have low HDL-cholesterol levels. Management is primarily by control of underlying causes, particularly overweight and excessive intake of alcohol. A lipid-lowering diet is prescribed. Drug therapy is usually withheld, but may be considered when persisting high triglyceride levels are due to familial combined hyperlipidaemia or other high-risk subgroups.

Group D consists of patients with elevated serum levels of both cholesterol and triglyceride [serum cholesterol 200–300 mg dl^{-1} (5·2–7·8 mmol l^{-1}) and serum triglyceride 200–500 mg dl^{-1} (2·3–5·6 mmol l^{-1})]. Such patients may have familial combined hyperlipidaemia, the diagnosis of which depends on a family study (see text). Although the lipid elevation is often mild, this disorder is associated with increased risk of CHD. Management is by control of underlying causes, weight reduction, if necessary, and a lipid-lowering diet. Drug treatment together with controlled diet is necessary in a minority of patients. A drug combination is sometimes necessary.

Group E includes patients with severe hyperlipidaemia [serum cholesterol above 300 mg dl^{-1} (7·8 mmol l^{-1}) and/or serum triglyceride greater than 500 mg dl^{-1} (5·6 mmol l^{-1})]. Patients with serum cholesterol levels > 300 mg dl^{-1} (7·8 mmol l^{-1}) and with normal triglyceride commonly have familial hypercholesterolaemia and are at especially high risk of CHD. Therapy usually comprises diet and one or two drugs, e.g. bile acid sequestrants often together with a fibrate, or cholesterol synthesis inhibitor, or nicotinic acid. For the chylomicronaemia syndrome there is no satisfactory drug therapy, and it is managed by a low fat diet.

Remnant (type III) hyperlipidaemia usually manifests with marked increase in cholesterol and triglyceride. It is associated with coronary and peripheral atherosclerosis and most patients require treatment with diet and a drug, usually a fibrate. Familial hypertriglyceridaemia, like the chylomicronaemia syndrome, may lead to acute pancreatitis. It is treated by weight control, diet and, when severe, a fibrate or nicotinic acid. It is often accompanied by diabetes mellitus.

Introduction

This account of the diagnosis and management of the hyperlipidaemic patient is intended for all medical practitioners. Those involved in primary care, and hospital doctors in selected specialities may find it of particular use.

Recently, the European Atherosclerosis Society (EAS) published a statement of policy on 'Strategies for the prevention of coronary heart disease (CHD)'[1], describing two complementary approaches directed to the population as a whole and to individuals at particular risk; these are the 'population strategy' and the 'individual' or 'high-risk strategy'. Both aim to reduce the well-established risk factors for CHD, but by different means. While the population strategy seeks to improve the health-oriented behaviour of the entire population, individual strategy is based on identifying persons at high risk with a view to effective individual therapy; the latter is a major responsibility for clinicians in meeting the goals of preventive medicine.

The risk of CHD increases steeply when more than one risk factor is present. Prevention of CHD in individuals at high risk involves management of all modifiable risk factors. In the EAS policy statement on the prevention of CHD, particular attention was given to lipids and lipoproteins as important causes of coronary atherosclerosis. In this report, the diagnosis of hyperlipidaemia is based on clinical findings and measurements of cholesterol, triglyceride and high-density lipoprotein (HDL) cholesterol. Management, primarily by diet and correction of underlying causes, is dependent on diagnosis of the lipid disorders and is influenced by overall risk of CHD; the medications for additional treatment by lipid-lowering drugs are discussed.

The plasma lipoproteins

Plasma lipoproteins are water-soluble complexes of high molecular weight composed of lipids (cholesterol, triglyceride, phospholipids), and one or more specific proteins called apolipoproteins. Five major classes of lipoproteins are defined and subclasses exist within these. All lipoproteins have their origin in the liver or intestine, or both.

The largest of the lipoproteins, *chylomicrons*, can be defined in various ways, but the term is best applied to both large and small triglyceride-rich lipoproteins produced by the intestinal mucosa. After entering the general circulation via the thoracic duct, chylomicrons have a half-life of only a few minutes, being degraded to remnant particles by the enzyme lipoprotein lipase, especially found in muscle and adipose tissue. The remnants of chylomicrons are taken up by the liver. In health, chylomicrons are present in plasma after a fat-containing meal and not in the fasted state.

The liver secretes triglyceride into the circulation in *very low-density lipoproteins (VLDL)*. These particles undergo degradation in the circulation by lipoprotein lipase, to *intermediate-density lipoproteins (IDL)*. In turn, these are in part converted to *low-density lipoproteins (LDL)* in the liver. Control of the synthesis of VLDL and regulation of the conversion progress are complex and not fully understood. In certain metabolic conditions, remnants of VLDL and IDL accumulate in plasma and this is associated with increased risk of atherosclerosis.

Approximately 60–70% of the total serum cholesterol is transported in LDL. Apolipoprotein B is the principal protein component of LDL. Increased concentration of LDL cholesterol in serum, due to oversynthesis or diminished catabolism, is causally related to atherosclerosis. LDL receptors at the surface of numerous cells are important in regulating cholesterol content of cells and of plasma. Control of hepatic LDL receptors by diet, hormones, and drugs importantly influences LDL cholesterol concentrations in plasma, thereby affecting risk of atherosclerosis.

High-density lipoproteins (HDL) usually transport 20–30% of the total cholesterol. The precise mechanisms of their synthesis and catabolism are not yet understood in detail. In several epidemiological studies, serum levels of HDL cholesterol were inversely correlated with risk of coronary heart disease.

Action limits for lipids and lipoproteins, and the assessment of risk of coronary heart disease

The European Atherosclerosis Society has established simplified action limits for plasma lipids and lipoproteins in adults as guidelines for choosing suitable levels of therapy. The choice of therapy depends on the patient's overall risk of CHD (or of acute pancreatitis). CHD risk is influenced by a number of characteristics and these need to be taken into account, as well as the lipid profile, in deciding on the need for and the level of therapy for hyperlipidaemia. While lipid levels are a guide to therapy, clinical judgement must be exercised and it is the patient, not the hyperlipidaemia, that should be treated. Individual care of the hyperlipidaemic patient is provided against a background of health education in diet, smoking avoidance and suitable exercise, directed to the entire population. According to the type and the severity of the hyperlipidaemia, five Treatment Groups (A–E) may be distinguished[11].

The action limits shown in Table 1 for cholesterol are based on longitudinal epidemiological studies, particularly a study of 361 000 men screened for entry into the MRFIT study (Fig. 1). While the relation of mild hypertriglyceridaemia to CHD is less well established, triglyceride appears to be an independent CHD risk factor in men and women who have low levels of HDL cholesterol (Fig. 2).

The preferred treatment appropriate for patients with lipid levels in the ranges shown in Table 1 is modified by the several risk-related characteristics shown in Table 2.

The modifiable risk factors shown in Table 2 interact with hypercholesterolaemia and with each other by increasing the risk of CHD. They require correction in their own right. In addition, hyperlipidaemia requires more vigorous treatment when it co-exists with one or more of the characteristics shown in Table 2. The presence of other risk determinants in Table 2, including male sex, also influences the level of therapy. At all times the physician's judgement of the balance between the risk of CHD and the untoward effects of treatment is central to such therapeutic decisions.

The presence, number and severity of these risk-related characteristics are all taken into account in choosing a suitable level of therapy. Many of these characteristics vary in degree (e.g. a family history of CHD in several relatives, and/or onset at a particularly young age, severe current hypertension, or a long history of diabetes also justify particular attention).

Table 1   Action limits

Treatment group	Cholesterol		Triglyceride (fasted)	
	(mmol l⁻¹)	(mg dl⁻¹)*	(mmol l⁻¹)	(mg dl⁻¹)*
A	5·2–6·5	200–250	<2·3	<200
B	6·5–7·8	250–300	<2·3	<200
C	<5·2	<200	2·3–5·6	200–500
D	5·2–7·8	200–300	2·3–5·6	200–500
E	>7·8	>300 and/or	>5·6	>500

*Approximate equivalents.

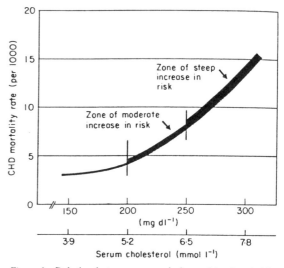

Figure 1   Relation between serum cholesterol level and risk of fatal coronary heart disease in a longitudinal study of over 361 000 men screened for entry into the Multiple Risk Factor Intervention Trial (based on data of Martin *et al.*[2]).

In the presence of two or more of these characteristics, or of any one in severe degree, the therapy of hyperlipidaemia in Treatment Groups B and D, and on occasion even in Treatment Groups A and C, should be more stringent (pp. 578–9). This implies progression to a more restrictive diet and/or use of lipid-active drugs, if necessary, to achieve or approach target levels of plasma lipids.

At all ages, CHD incidence is higher in men than in women, and this may influence the choice of therapy. In younger women, on the other hand, it must be borne in mind that CHD relative risk is increased by use of oral contraceptives, particularly in cigarette smokers. Furthermore, women affected

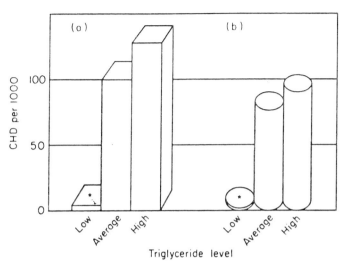

Figure 2 Relation between serum triglyceride level and incidence of coronary heart disease in men and women with low levels of HDL cholesterol in the Framingham Study (based on data of Castelli[3]). (a) Men, HDL cholesterol < 40 mg dl^{-1} ($< 1\cdot04$ mmol l^{-1}): low triglyceride < 94 mg dl^{-1} ($< 1\cdot1$ mmol l^{-1}); average triglyceride 94–144 mg dl^{-1} ($1\cdot1$–$1\cdot6$ mmol l^{-1}); high triglyceride $\geqslant 145$ mg dl^{-1} ($> 1\cdot6$ mmol l^{-1}). (b) Women, HDL cholesterol < 50 mg dl^{-1} ($< 1\cdot30$ mmol l^{-1}): low triglyceride < 88 mg dl^{-1} ($< 1\cdot0$ mmol l^{-1}); average triglyceride 88–135 mg dl^{-1} ($1\cdot0$–$1\cdot5$ mmol l^{-1}); high triglyceride $\geqslant 136$ mg dl^{-1} ($> 1\cdot5$ mmol l^{-1}).* < 85 individuals per group.

Table 2 Factors affecting therapy of hyperlipidaemia

Modifiable risk factors	Other factors
Hypertension	Family history of CHD or peripheral
Cigarette smoking	vascular disease
Diabetes mellitus	Personal history of early onset CHD
Obesity	Revascularization procedures
Low HDL cholesterol	Male sex
	Younger age

by hypertriglyceridaemia *and* diabetes mellitus are at increased risk of CHD. The presence of early onset CHD, and of CHD or other atherosclerotic disease treated by a revascularization procedure, justify more vigorous correction of hyperlipidaemia. Detection and effective treatment of hyperlipidaemia at an early age affords the best chance of preventing atherosclerosis progression; though there is no basis for witholding treatment of hyperlipidaemia in older patients, it is generally agreed that less vigorous therapy is appropriate (e.g. reduction of overweight, moderate dietary change). The overall state of health ('biological age') should take precedence over the chronological age.

Therapeutic groups

TREATMENT GROUP A

The risk of CHD is increased about two-fold in persons with cholesterol levels of 250 mg dl^{-1} ($6\cdot5$ mmol l^{-1}), compared with those with levels of 200 mg dl^{-1} ($5\cdot2$ mmol l^{-1}) or less. Dietary counselling is provided, to achieve an estimated LDL cholesterol value of about 135–155 mg dl^{-1} ($3\cdot5$–4 mmol l^{-1}). Typically, the corresponding target serum cholesterol will be around 200 mg dl^{-1} ($5\cdot2$ mmol l^{-1}). Any other modifiable risk factors also require attention. As levels in this range are common, a substantial proportion of all CHD arises in this group. Drug therapy is rarely appropriate and would be considered only in the presence of other marked risk-related characteristics. In individuals at high risk of CHD, it is particularly important to achieve serum cholesterol levels in the vicinity of 200 mg dl^{-1} ($5\cdot2$ mmol l^{-1}) or LDL cholesterol levels close to 135 mg dl^{-1} ($3\cdot5$ mmol l^{-1}) (see Tables 3 and 4).

TREATMENT GROUP B

The risk of CHD is high and increases steeply in the range 250–300 mg dl^{-1} ($6\cdot5$–$7\cdot8$ mmol l^{-1})

Table 3   A therapeutic classification

Treatment Group	Diagnostic levels	Investigation	Management
A	Cholesterol 200–250 mg dl⁻¹ (5·2–6·5 mmol l⁻¹) Triglyceride < 200 mg dl⁻¹ (< 2·3 mmol l⁻¹)	Assess overall risk of CHD, taking into account family history of CHD, hypertension, diabetes, male sex, younger age, smoking, low HDL cholesterol e.g. < 35 mg dl⁻¹ (< 0·9 mmol l⁻¹)	Restrict food energy if overweight; give nutritional advice (lipid lowering diet) and correct other risk factors if present; if LDL response inadequate, consider additional therapy in individuals at very high risk; therapeutic goal: see Table 4; unless at high overall risk, no follow-up; if at high risk, manage as Group B
B	Cholesterol 250–300 mg dl⁻¹ (6·5–7·8 mmol l⁻¹) Triglyceride < 200 mg dl⁻¹ (< 2·3 mmol l⁻¹)	Assess overall risk of CHD as under A	Restrict food energy if overweight; prescribe lipid-lowering diet and monitor response and compliance; if cholesterol remains high, reinforce lipid-lowering diet; if this fails, consider drugs; correct other risk factors if present; therapeutic goal: see Table 4
C	Cholesterol < 200 mg dl⁻¹ (< 5·2 mmol l⁻¹) Triglyceride 200–500 mg dl⁻¹ (2·3–5·6 mmol l⁻¹)	Seek underlying causes of hypertriglyceridaemia, e.g. obesity, excessive alcohol intake, diuretics, beta blockers, exogenous oestrogens, diabetes	Restrict dietary energy if overweight; deal with underlying causes if present; prescribe and monitor lipid-lowering diet; monitor cholesterol and triglyceride levels; correct other risk factors, if present; therapeutic goal: see Table 4
D	Cholesterol 200–300 mg dl⁻¹ (5·2–7·8 mmol l⁻¹) Triglyceride 200–500 mg dl⁻¹ (2·3–5·6 mmol l⁻¹)	Assess overall risk of CHD as in A. Seek underlying causes of hypertriglyceridaemia as in C	Restrict dietary energy if overweight; deal with underlying causes of hypertriglyceridaemia if present and proceed according to A or C; prescribe and monitor lipid-lowering diet; correct other risk factors, if present; if serum lipid response is inadequate and overall CHD risk is high, consider use of lipid-lowering drug; therapeutic goal: see Table 4
E	Cholesterol > 300 mg dl⁻¹ (> 7·8 mmol l⁻¹) and/or Triglyceride > 500 mg dl⁻¹ (> 5·6 mmol l⁻¹)	Make full diagnosis on clinical and laboratory data	Dietary treatment and, commonly, drug therapy needed with ongoing supervision to maximize response; referral to specialist for diagnosis and initiation of therapy may be considered; particular attention is required to correction of other risk factors; guidelines for treatment appear in pp. 585–93 and Tables 4 and 5

cholesterol. Treatment is initiated by diet, with ongoing dietary reinforcement and plasma lipid monitoring. Drug therapy is additionally required in a minority, if severe risk-related characteristics are present and if thorough trial of diet over several months has failed to achieve target values (Tables 5–7). Rapid advances are being made in the drug therapy of lipid disorders. The guidelines in Table 5 are those currently recommended.

It is possible to estimate LDL cholesterol concentration in most patients by measuring serum cholesterol, HDL cholesterol and fasting serum triglyceride (see p. 579). Since this is the main atherogenic fraction of cholesterol it is appropriate to design therapy on LDL cholesterol levels rather than serum cholesterol.

TREATMENT GROUP C

Aggressive treatment of triglyceride levels of 200–500 mg dl⁻¹ (2·3–5·6 mmol l⁻¹) is unjustified by current evidence. However, in many individuals, such levels are associated with obesity, alcohol overindulgence or diabetes, conditions justifying treatment in their own right. A lipid-lowering diet is

Table 4   Goals of treatment: these target values are associated with low risk of CHD; they can be attained in many patients using the management suggested; however, they are not always achievable, and clinical judgement must be exercised in balancing expected benefit against untoward effects

	No other marked risk factor		Other marked or multiple risk factors present*	
	(mg dl⁻¹)	(mmol l⁻¹)	(mg dl⁻¹)	(mmol l⁻¹)
LDL cholesterol	155	4	135	3·5
Serum cholesterol	200–215	5·2–5·6	200	5·2
Serum triglyceride†	200	2·3	200	2·3

*See Table 2.
†The relation between triglyceride levels and CHD is incompletely defined, and the value shown here is necessarily arbitrary at the present time. In the chylomicronaemia syndrome and in severe familial hypertriglyceridaemia, the goal of treatment is to minimize the risk of acute pancreatitis, which requires that triglyceride levels be reduced to <1000 mg dl⁻¹ (<11 mmol l⁻¹), and preferably to <500 mg dl⁻¹ (<5·6 mmol l⁻¹).

prescribed. Drug therapy is seldom indicated, but may be required in selected patients at high risk of CHD if dietary treatment is unsuccessful (see pp. 593–4).

TREATMENT GROUP D

The risk of CHD is high. Management is essentially similar to that of Treatment Group B, with additional attention to underlying causes of hypertriglyceridaemia as specified for Group C.

TREATMENT GROUP E

Many patients in this category have major genetic diseases of lipid metabolism (see pp. 581–4). Some of these confer very high risk of CHD; others (causing marked hypertriglyceridaemia) can lead to recurrent acute pancreatitis. Full diagnosis is necessary to define the natural history and to select optimal therapy. Primary hyperlipidaemia of this severity requires dietary treatment and, in many patients, medication.

Technical procedures

BASIC INVESTIGATION OF THE HYPERLIPIDAEMIC PATIENT

The usual repertoire of tests for characterizing the nature of the lipid disorder is measurement of cholesterol, triglyceride and HDL cholesterol. This also has the advantage of permitting calculation of the LDL cholesterol; this is of particular value in

assessing CHD risk and in judging the effectiveness of therapy.

BLOOD SAMPLING

As plasma lipid levels show considerable biological variation from day to day, the diagnosis of elevated lipid levels should be based on two consistent lipid analyses; particularly in Groups B–E, the finding of a cholesterol level >250 mg dl⁻¹ (6·5 mmol l⁻¹) is confirmed by obtaining a second blood sample in the fasted state 1–3 weeks later, in which cholesterol, triglyceride and HDL cholesterol are measured. Similarly, major changes in therapy should be based on trends in lipid levels rather than on single measurements.

For cholesterol and HDL-cholesterol measurements it is unnecessary for the patient to fast. Triglyceride is, by convention, measured in samples obtained after overnight (12–14 h) fasting; water or other fat-free fluids are permitted. The patient should have followed his/her habitual weight-maintaining diet for at least three weeks. Measurements should be deferred for three weeks after intercurrent minor illness, and for three months after major illness, e.g. myocardial infarction or surgery. Cholesterol may be measured within 24 h of onset of chest pain in myocardial infarction. Pregnancy is associated with physiological hyperlipidaemia.

Venous samples should be drawn without prolonged stasis; a cuff may be applied briefly for

Table 5   Precis of guidelines to therapy of hyperlipidaemia (see text for details)

Management	No other marked risk factor	Other marked or multiple risk factors present*
Group A		
Step 1	Lipid-lowering diet, with weight control if necessary. Regular follow-up not essential.	Lipid-lowering diet, with weight control if necessary. Control of associated risk factors.
Step 2		Reassess in 6 months: (a) if treatment goal achieved, reassess in 2–5 years; (b) if treatment goal not achieved, review and encourage diet compliance.
Step 3		Reassess in 6–12 months; as in Step 2.
Step 4		Reassess in 12 months: (a) if treatment goal achieved, reassess in 2–5 years; (b) if LDL cholesterol 135–155 mg dl^{-1} (3·5–4 mmol l^{-1}), encourage diet compliance; (c) if LDL cholesterol > 155 mg dl^{-1} (4 mmol l^{-1}) despite good dietary compliance, additional use of drug therapy occasionally appropriate.
Long term	Consider reassessment after 5 years.	Reassess at 2–5-year intervals if on diet therapy alone. If on diet and drug therapy, reassess at 3-month intervals increasing to 1-year intervals. Continue medication only if justified by response.
Group B		
Step 1	Lipid-lowering diet with weight control if necessary. Correct underlying causes.	Lipid-lowering diet with weight control if necessary. Correct underlying causes. Control associated risk factors.
Step 2	Reassess at 2–4 months: (a) if treatment goal achieved, reassess at 1 year; (b) if treatment goal not achieved, review diet and encourage compliance.	Reassess at 2–4 months: (a) if treatment goal achieved, reassess at 1 year; (b) if treatment goal not achieved, review diet and encourage compliance.
Step 3	Reassess at 3–6 months. As Step 2.	Reassess at 3–6 months: (a) if treatment goal achieved, reassess at 1 year; (b) if treatment goal not achieved, consider addition of drug therapy.
Step 4	Reassess at 3-6 months: (a) if treatment goal achieved, reassess at 1 year; (b) if treatment goal not achieved despite good dietary compliance, consider addition of drug therapy.	Reassess at 2–4 months. If treatment goal not achieved, consider increase of drug dosage if appropriate. Encourage dietary compliance.
Long term	Reassess at 1–3-year intervals if on dietary treatment alone, and at 3-month increasing to one-year intervals if on diet and drug therapy.	
Group C		
Step 1	Correct underlying causes. Correct overweight. Prescribe lipid-lowering diet. Control associated risk factors.	
Step 2	Reassess in 6-12 months: (a) if goal of treatment achieved, follow-up in 3–5 years; (b) if goal of treatment not achieved, encourage compliance to all measures listed in Step 1.	
Step 3	As Step 2.	
Step 4	If treatment goal achieved, follow-up in 3-5 years. If goal of treatment not achieved despite dietary compliance, consider referral to specialized centre or investigate lipid levels in parents, siblings and adult children. If evidence is obtained of familial combined hyperlipidaemia, or if other marked or multiple risk factors (Table 2), consider use of drugs in addition to diet. Drug treatment for moderate hypertriglyceridaemia is a subject of controversy.	
Long term	Reassess at 1–5-year intervals if treatment by diet alone and at 3 months, increasing to 1-year intervals if treated by drug and diet. Continue drug therapy only if justified by response.	

Table 5 (Continued)

Management	No other marked risk factor	Other marked or multiple risk factors present*
Group D		
Step 1	Lipid-lowering diet with weight control if necessary. Correct underlying causes.	Lipid-lowering diet with weight control if necessary. Correct underlying causes. Control associated risk factors.
Step 2	Reassess at 2–4 months: (a) if treatment goal achieved reassess at 6-12 months; (b) if treatment goal not achieved, review and encourage weight control and dietary compliance and check control of underlying causes, reassess at 3-6 months.	Reassess at 2–4 months: (a) if treatment goal achieved reassess at 6-12 months; (b) if treatment goal not achieved, review and encourage weight control and dietary compliance and check control of underlying causes, reassess at 3-6 months.
Step 3	As Step 2.	(a) If treatment goal achieved reassess at 1 year. (b) If treatment goal not achieved, consider drug therapy in addition to existing measures. Reassess at 3 months if drug therapy instituted.
Step 4	(a) If treatment goal achieved reassess at 1 year. (b) If treatment goal not achieved, consider drug therapy in addition to existing measures.	(a) If treatment goal achieved reassess at 1 year. (b) If treatment goal not achieved, consider drug therapy in addition to existing measures. Reassess at 3 months if drug treatment instituted.
Long term	Reassess at 1–5-year intervals if treatment by diet alone, and at 3-month intervals increasing to 1-year if treatment by diet and drug. Continue drug therapy only if justified by response.	Reassess at 1–5-year intervals if treated by diet alone, and at 3-month intervals increasing to 1-year if treated by diet and drug. Continue drug therapy only if justified by response.
Group E		
Investigations	Investigate for and correct underlying causes. Make precise diagnosis of primary lipid disorder wherever possible. Consider referral to specialized centre for diagnosis and initiation of treatment.	
Step 1	Lipid-lowering diet, with weight control if necessary (except for chylomicronaemia syndrome for which prescribe low-fat diet). Control associated risk factors.	
Step 2	Reassess at 1–3 months. Encourage compliance to weight control and lipid-lowering diet. (a) If treatment goal achieved, reassess at 4–6 months. (b) If treatment goal not achieved, drug therapy probably required in addition to existing measures. Choice of drug largely dependent on diagnosis of primary lipid disorder (see Table C and text). Check that any associated risk factors are controlled.	
Step 3	Reassess lipid response and assess side effects at 1–2 months. (a) If treatment goal achieved, reassess at 4–6 months. (b) If treatment goal not achieved, adjust dosage if appropriate and maximize diet compliance. Check that underlying causes corrected. Check that any associated risk factors are controlled.	
Step 4	As Step 3.	
Step 5	Reassess at 2–4 months. (a) If treatment goal achieved, reassess at 1 year. (b) If treatment goal not achieved, adjust dose and/or consider introduction of second drug.	
Long term	Reassess at 3 months, increasing to 1 year. Continue drug only if justified by response. Assess cardiovascular status at 1–5-year intervals.	

*See Table 2.

insertion of the needle and released before the sample is withdrawn. Posture should be standardized. It is most convenient to take the blood sample after the patient has been seated for 5–10 min. Plasma lipid levels are about 4% lower than serum levels, therefore, the choice of sample must be consistent.

Despite improvements in quality control, variation between laboratories remains a problem. A further sample should be analyzed if an apparently aberrant result is obtained.

Lipid analyses are possible using dry chemistry techniques on capillary blood samples. These are rapid, cheap and convenient. In the future, these procedures may greatly facilitate management of lipid disorders.

CALCULATION OF LDL CHOLESTEROL

Today, most laboratories calculate LDL cholesterol from total plasma cholesterol, plasma triglyceride and HDL cholesterol. This calculation

580   *The European Atherosclerosis Society*

Table 6   The choice of lipid-lowering drugs

Treatment Group	Treatment
Group A	Drug treatment rarely indicated; if required for patients at extremely high CHD risk, selection as in Group B.
Group B	Single-drug treatment considered for persistent LDL cholesterol elevation despite prolonged effort at dietary control: bile acid sequestrants, usually at low dosage *or either* nicotinic acid *or* fibrate group *or* HMGCoA reductase inhibitors (when approved).
Group C	Drug treatment controversial (see text): *either* nicotinic acid, *or* fibrate group.
Group D	Drug treatment considered if LDL cholesterol and/or triglyceride elevation persist despite prolonged effort at dietary control: (a) cholesterol remains elevated, triglyceride within limits — nicotinic acid, *or* fibrid group, *or* bile acid sequestrants, *or* HMGCoA reductase inhibitors (when approved); (b) triglyceride elevated, cholesterol within limits —nicotinic acid, *or* fibrate; (c) cholesterol and triglyceride elevated — nicotinic acid, *or* fibrate, *or* fibrate plus bile acid sequestrants, *or* HMGCoA reductase inhibitors (when approved).
Group E	Choice of drug treatment depends on diagnosis of primary lipid disorder: (a) familial hypercholesterolaemia — bile acid sequestrants, *or* HMGCoA reductase inhibitors (when approved), *or* nicotinic acid; for non-responders use combination therapy — bile acid sequestrants with *either* nicotinic acid, *or* with fibrate, *or* with probucol, *or* HMGCoA reductase inhibitors with bile acid sequestrants; (b) remnant hyperlipidaemia — fibrate, *or* nicotinic acid; (c) familial hypertriglyceridaemia — nicotinic acid *or* fibrate; (d) familial combined hyperlipidaemia — drug treatment as under Group D; (e) primary chylomicronaemia — drug treatment rarely indicated.

Table 7   Summary of Tables 4 and 5: goal of treatment

Treatment Group	No other marked risk factors	Other marked or multiple risk factors
	Cholesterol <200–215 mg dl^{-1} ($<5 \cdot 2$–$5 \cdot 6$ mmol l^{-1}) LDL cholesterol <155 mg dl^{-1} (4 mmol l^{-1}) Triglyceride <200 mg dl^{-1} ($5 \cdot 2$ mmol l^{-1})	Cholesterol <200 mg dl^{-1} ($5 \cdot 2$ mmol l^{-1}) LDL cholesterol <135 mg dl^{-1} ($3 \cdot 5$ mmol l^{-1}) Triglyceride <200 mg dl^{-1} ($5 \cdot 2$ mmol l^{-1})
Group A	Lipid-lowering diet, weight control if needed, drugs rarely indicated; follow-up optional.	Lipid-lowering diet, weight control if needed; re-assess in 6 months; if treatment goal not achieved reinforce dietary advice, consider use of drugs in individuals at highest risk.
Group B	Lipid-lowering diet, weight control; reassess in 2–4 months, if treatment goal not achieved reinforce dietary advice; consider use of drugs if diet response persistently inadequate.	Lipid-lowering diet, weight control; reassess in 2–4 months; if treatment goal not achieved reinforce dietary advice; drug therapy if diet response persistently inadequate.
Group C	Correct underlying causes, lipid-lowering diet, weight control if needed; reassess in 12 months; if treatment goal achieved, reassess in 1–5 years; if treatment goal not achieved reinforce diet.	Correct underlying causes, lipid-lowering diet, weight control if needed; reassess in 6 months; if treatment goal achieved reassess in 1 year, if treatment goal not achieved reinforce diet; consider drug if response to diet therapy persistently inadequate.
Group D	Correct underlying causes, lipid-lowering diet, weight control if needed; reassess in 2–4 months; if treatment goal not achieved despite dietary compliance consider use of drugs.	Correct underlying causes, lipid-lowering diet, weight control if needed, reassess in 2–4 months, if treatment goal not achieved implement drug therapy.
Group E	Correct underlying causes, make precise diagnosis of primary lipid disorder; lipid-lowering diet (low-fat diet for chylomicronaemia), weight control if needed, control associated risk factors; reassess in 1–3 months; if treatment goal not achieved despite dietary compliance implement drug therapy or consider referral to specialized centre.	

is commonly performed using the Friedewald formula (for nomogram see Appendix 3):

LDL cholesterol (mg dl^{-1}) =
cholesterol − triglyceride/5 − HDL cholesterol
LDL cholesterol (mmol l^{-1}) =
cholesterol − triglyceride/2·2 − HDL cholesterol.

This is valid for LDL cholesterol determination, when triglyceride is measured in the fasted state, and does not exceed 500 mg dl^{-1} (5·6 mmol l^{-1}). In specialized centres, LDL cholesterol can be measured directly using ultracentrifugation. As LDL is particularly important in the development of atherosclerosis, its measurement permits a more reliable assessment of CHD risk than does measurement of total serum cholesterol. However, where cost is a consideration, serum cholesterol is usually adequate for monitoring the dietary treatment of raised cholesterol levels, except in Groups D and E.

Classification of hyperlipidaemias

A large number of genetic and acquired diseases can result in hyperlipidaemia. This account focusses on the most important of these. Their initial classification is into primary and secondary hyperlipidaemic states. Primary disorders are listed in Table 8, roughly in decreasing order of prevalence, together with their major clinical and laboratory characteristics. In a minority of hyperlipidaemic patients the disorder is secondary to other diseases, and, not infrequently, primary and secondary hyperlipidaemias coexist (e.g. familial and alcohol-related hypertriglyceridaemia).

RECOGNITION OF THE PRIMARY HYPERLIPIDAEMIAS, AND THEIR NATURAL HISTORY

The disorders listed in Table 8 differ in the risk of major complications, in their optimal therapy, and in their prevalence. Though it is not always possible to make a rigorous diagnosis, this should be the goal in order to provide optimal treatment and to facilitate prognosis. Family screening provides a genetic diagnosis and may detect relatives requiring treatment. Newer techniques in genetics are likely to enable more precise diagnosis within the next few years.

The diagnostic features are usually elicited from the family history, physical examination, lipid and lipoprotein measurements and, where appropriate, family screening. Specific diagnostic tests based on ultracentrifugation, apolipoprotein analysis, enzyme measurements and receptor studies are available in specialized centres; most patients can be managed satisfactorily, without recourse to such procedures.

Among the several disorders listed some are exceedingly common and others rare. As a rule of thumb, most patients with mild hyperlipidaemia will prove to have common ('polygenic') hypercholesterolaemia, familial combined hyperlipidaemia or hypertriglyceridaemia associated with obesity or alcohol overuse. Familial hypercholesterolaemia and remnant hyperlipidaemia are relatively commonly encountered causes of severe hyperlipidaemia.

Common ('polygenic') hypercholesterolaemia

This is by far the most frequent cause of cholesterol levels exceeding the cut-off values defined on p. 574. It reflects an interaction between multiple genes (including those coding for apo E and apo B) and dietary and other environmental factors, and has more than one metabolic basis. Variation in its prevalence is the main reason for differences between countries in plasma cholesterol distribution and in CHD prevalence.

At present common hypercholesterolaemia can only be diagnosed by exclusion of other causes of hypercholesterolaemia (Tables 8 and 9). It is usually mild to moderate in degree. Xanthomas do not occur. Persons with a positive family history of CHD, corneal arcus or xanthomas, and obese persons, are more likely to have elevated plasma cholesterol levels than persons without these characteristics.

Familial hypercholesterolaemia (FH)

This is a serious disease, in which affected men have an 8–10-fold greater risk of CHD than unaffected men. Heart disease may present in the fourth or even the third decade of life. The condition is present in one of 20 patients presenting with myocardial infarction before age 60. It is among the commonest of major genetic diseases, affecting one person in 500. The hypercholesterolaemia is due to increased levels of LDL resulting from impaired function of LDL receptors.

Hypercholesterolaemia is usually severe (350–460 mg dl^{-1}, 9–12 mmol l^{-1}), but values > 300 mg dl^{-1} (7·8 mmol l^{-1}) in adults or > 260 mg dl^{-1} (6·7 mmol l^{-1}) up to age 16 are compatible with the diagnosis. The presence of LDL cholesterol > 190 mg dl^{-1} (4·9 mmol l^{-1}) is similarly compatible. The diagnosis can be made at birth on umbilical-cord blood. Triglyceride is normal or

Table 8   *Primary hyperlipidaemias*

	CHD risk	Risk of pancreatitis	Plasma cholesterol	Plasma triglyceride	Lipoprotein phenotype	Physical signs (if present)
Common ('polygenic') hypercholesterolaemia	+	−	↑	N	IIa	Corneal arcus, xanthelasma
Familial combined hyperlipidaemia	++	−	↑ or N	↑ or N	IIa, IIb or IV	Corneal arcus, xanthelasma
Familial hypercholesterolaemia	+++	−	↑↑↑	N or ↑	IIa or IIb	Tendon xanthomas (finger extensors, Achilles tendons), corneal arcus, xanthelasmas, aortic stenosis
Remnant hyperlipidaemia	+++	±	↑↑↑	↑↑	III	Tuberous xanthomas (elbows), striate xanthomas (palm creases), tendon xanthomas
Chylomicronaemia syndrome	−	+++	↑	↑↑↑	I or V	Eruptive xanthomas (buttocks, elbows), retinal lipaemia, hepatosplenomegaly
Familial hypertriglyceridaemia	?	++	↑	↑↑	IV or V	Eruptive xanthomas (buttocks, elbows), retinal lipaemia, hepatosplenomegaly
HDL hypercholesterolaemia	−	−	↑	N	(Increased HDL cholesterol)	—

Table 9 Some causes of secondary hyperlipidaemia

	Main lipid abnormality	Lipoprotein changes			
		Chylomicrons	VLDL	LDL	HDL
Diabetes mellitus	↑ triglyceride	↑	↑		↓
Alcohol abuse	↑ triglyceride	↑	↑		
Drugs	↑ triglyceride and/or ↑ cholesterol				
Hypothyroidism	↑ cholesterol			↑	
Chronic renal failure	↑ triglyceride		↑	↑ or N	
Nephrotic syndrome	↑ cholesterol and ↑ triglyceride		↑	↑	
Cholestasis	↑ cholesterol			↑	↓
Bulimia	↑ triglyceride	↑	↑		

slightly elevated. These findings, coupled with the presence of tendon xanthomas in the patient or in a relative, provide a definite diagnosis. These lesions can be quite small, and need to sought specifically as part of routine examination. Tendon xanthomas are not always present, and a probable diagnosis can be made on the lipid findings listed, coupled with appropriate observations in the family: a definite history of myocardial infarction occurring before age 60 in a first-degree relative (patient, sibling or offspring), or before age 50 in a second-degree relative; an alternative criterion is a cholesterol level of >300 mg dl^{-1} (7·8 mmol l^{-1}) in a first-degree relative. The disease is transmitted by autosomal dominant inheritance.

These are the features of the heterozygous form of the disease. Homozygous FH, affecting about one person per million in most countries, leads to cholesterol levels of 600–1000 mg dl^{-1} (15–25 mmol l^{-1}) and, untreated, to CHD and aortic stenosis in childhood or adolescence. It requires management in specialized centres.

Remnant hyperlipidaemia

This disorder, also known as type III hyperlipidaemia, is a less common but also serious cause of early onset CHD and peripheral vascular disease. Typically, there is marked elevation of both cholesterol and triglyceride levels (combined hyperlipidaemia); the severity varies, however, and in young, lean patients moderate hypertriglyceridaemia may be the only manifestation. Cardiovascular manifestations often present in the fourth or fifth decades.

The disorder has been diagnosed in childhood but is usually expressed in adult life. When marked increase in cholesterol and triglyceride is associated with typical skin xanthomas, particularly in the palmar creases and over the elbows, a presumptive diagnosis may be made. Chronic cholestasis and myelomatosis in which similar skin lesions may occur, should be excluded. Xanthomas are not invariably present. Laboratory confirmation (at a specialized centre) requires either demonstration of the E2/2 pattern of apo E or of cholesterol enrichment of VLDL by preparative ultracentrifugation (showing a molar ratio of cholesterol to triglyceride exceeding 0·6). Electrophoresis of lipoproteins may be misleading. An abnormal phenotype of apo E is found quite commonly but hyperlipidaemia usually develops in such persons only when an associated abnormality such as obesity, hypothyroidism, diabetes or a co-existent genetic lipid disorder is present.

Familial combined hyperlipidaemia (FCH)

Families are commonly encountered in which many members develop CHD and in which often-mild inherited hyperlipidaemia is present. It may be the commonest genetic disorder of lipoprotein metabolism associated with CHD. Xanthomas do not occur. Production of apo B, the structural protein of VLDL and LDL, is increased, and levels of both these lipoproteins, or either alone, are elevated. The condition may, therefore, manifest in various ways, either as a moderate increase in cholesterol and triglyceride, or as hypercholesterolaemia alone, or as hypertriglyceridaemia alone. In an affected individual, the pattern of hyperlipidaemia may vary. Thus the condition should be suspected when moderate hyperlipidaemia is accompanied by a personal or family history of CHD.

Diagnosis depends, at present, on a family study. A strong family history of CHD is usually present. The disorder is strongly inherited and each generation is affected; diversity of the pattern of hyperlipidaemia within a family is characteristic, and at least one family member manifests combined (mixed) hyperlipidaemia. The majority of patients have elevated plasma levels of apo B.

In patients with high cholesterol and triglyceride concentrations, the differential diagnosis includes FCH, remnant hyperlipidaemia, FH (in which moderate elevation of triglyceride, often associated with an underlying cause, is not unusual) and a secondary hyperlipidaemia.

The chylomicronaemia syndrome

This is an uncommon cause of severe hypertriglyceridaemia presenting in childhood or adult life. It is caused by deficiency of the enzyme lipoprotein lipase or of apolipoprotein C-II. The natural history is of recurrent episodes of acute pancreatitis and/or crops of eruptive xanthomas, and in adults there is often a history of attacks of undiagnosed abdominal pain dating from childhood or infancy. Occasionally the disorder is clinically silent.

Despite gross hypertriglyceridaemia and very low levels of HDL cholesterol there is no excess risk of CHD. Transmission is by autosomal recessive inheritance; hyperlipidaemia and pancreatitis in family members are unusual except in offspring of a consanguineous marriage. Characteristic physical signs are eruptive xanthomas on extensor surfaces, retinal lipaemia and hepatosplenomegaly; these run a fluctuating course.

Gross hypertriglyceridaemia and relatively mild hypercholesterolaemia can usually be shown by the stored plasma test to be due to chylomicronaemia; in adults there is also often a modest increase in VLDL. The simplest investigation in hospital is the fat-deprivation test. A positive test is an 80% reduction in plasma triglyceride, and virtual disappearance of chylomicronaemia, within three days of instituting an isocaloric diet containing <5 g fat day^{-1}. The two usual causes, namely gross deficiency of lipoprotein lipase (measured in plasma obtained 10 min after heparin 40 µ kg^{-1} by i.v.i.) or

absence of normal apo C-II, may be tested for in specialized centres. Plasma amylase measurements may give falsely low results in lipaemic plasma, and abdominal pain should be investigated by the urinary amylase/creatinine ratio.

Familial hypertriglyceridaemia

This is a clinically similar disorder to the chylomicronaemia syndrome. Primary endogenous hypertriglyceridaemia may be pronounced or relatively mild. Lesser degrees of triglyceride elevation reflect increased VLDL levels; in more severe form there is usually also chylomicronaemia. The metabolic defect is unknown. There is probably no excess risk of CHD, but recurrent pancreatitis is a common manifestation of the disorder in its florid form. There is an association with venous thrombosis. In some patients, diabetes mellitus may be present, representing co-existence of two diseases or, possibly, recurrent pancreatic damage. A family study will reveal a similar pattern of hyperlipidaemia, distributed by autosomal dominant transmission. The disorder seldom manifests until adult life. Unlike the chylomicronaemia syndrome, familial hypertriglyceridaemia is not ameliorated by, and may be exaggerated during, the fat deprivation test. Lipoprotein lipase activity may be normal or slightly subnormal.

Elevated HDL cholesterol

Not uncommonly, mild hypercholesterolaemia proves to be due to unusually high levels of HDL cholesterol. This is evidently a benign abnormality, not requiring treatment, and has been termed the 'longevity syndrome'. Levels of other lipoproteins are normal. It may be seen in postmenopausal women receiving oestrogen replacement, but can also be familial, and can be due to microsomal enzyme-inducing drugs, e.g. phenytoin, phenobarbitone.

Elevated apolipoprotein B

In case-control studies, elevated levels of apo B are well recognized to be present in many patients with CHD. Our knowledge of this entity is not yet sufficient to justify treatment in the absence of hyperlipidaemia.

RECOGNITION OF SECONDARY HYPERLIPIDAEMIAS

The most common causes of the secondary hyperlipidaemias are listed in Table 9. The recognition of these causes can lead to the diagnosis of a serious and treatable underlying disease; conversely, management of the causal condition will, in most cases, correct or ameliorate the hyperlipidaemia. The risk of CHD may be less marked in secondary disorders than in primary ones, because the duration is shorter. However, there is no reason to doubt that the increased risk of CHD and peripheral vascular disease in diabetes mellitus is mediated in part by lipoprotein abnormalities; acute pancreatitis is a common manifestation of severe secondary hypertriglyceridaemia.

Underlying causes can most often be detected from the history and clinical findings. Hypothyroidism may be evident from a history of cold intolerance, constipation, lack of sweating, deafness and amnesia and a slow relaxation phase of tendon reflexes, but appropriate laboratory investigation (e.g. TSH) is necessary. A family history of thyroid disease is common. Alcohol use is often under-reported but is usually revealed by skilled history taking. Hypertriglyceridaemia of fluctuating severity is characteristic. The syndrome of bulimia, gross hypertriglyceridaemia and pancreatitis, only recently defined, is probably underdiagnosed; it is a serious illness requiring clinical acumen for its prompt recognition. Commonly used drugs that can cause moderate hyperlipidaemia include thiazide and other diuretics, combined oral contraceptives, retinoids and corticosteroids. Anabolic steroids and progestogens may lead to elevated LDL-cholesterol levels. Elevated HDL cholesterol may be due to oestrogen use, phenytoin, phenobarbitone, cimetidine, rifampicin and alcohol, and is also seen in lean, highly trained athletes. Cardiovascular disease is a frequent complication in patients with chronic renal failure treated with maintenance dialysis or after renal transplantation. This increased risk is probably related, at least in part, to the high incidence of hyperlipidaemia. Overproduction of VLDL, and consequently LDL, seems to account for hyperlipidaemia in the nephrotic syndrome.

Many causes of secondary hyperlipidaemia will be recognized if a biochemical profile is requested when the patient is first seen. Rarer causes of secondary hyperlipidaemia include severe liver dysfunction and anorexia nervosa (elevated cholesterol), myelomatosis (elevated cholesterol and triglyceride) and glycogen storage disease (elevated triglyceride).

When hyperlipidaemia is secondary, the underlying disease should be treated, where possible, and lipid values should be evaluated several weeks later.

Similarly, drugs causing hyperlipidaemia should be replaced if a suitable alternative is available.

Dietary and drug treatment of hyperlipidaemia

Comprehensive management of hyperlipidaemia has several components. The following summary serves as a check-list that may be considered for every patient:

(a) accompanying modifiable risk factors (Table 2, left-hand column) should be sought and treated;

(b) underlying treatable causes of hyperlipidaemia (Table 9) should be identified and corrected;

(c) the goal of treatment (e.g. reduction in CHD risk, avoidance of pancreatitis) should be clearly explained to the patient and the risks conferred by untreated hyperlipidaemia should be clarified. The patient should understand the strength of the evidence for these statements (see Fig. 1 and pp. 596–7);

(d) the essential component in the treatment of all primary hyperlipidaemias is the institution of and supervision of an appropriate lipid-lowering diet, with ongoing efforts by doctor and dietitian to encourage maximum compliance and offer support;

(e) for a minority of patients it is necessary to combine dietary and drug therapy, in order to achieve or approach target levels of plasma lipids; the decision to introduce drug treatment should not be taken lightly; such therapy is likely to be lifelong. The decision will be influenced by clinical judgement, taking into account the patient's overall risk of CHD (Table 2), age and cardiovascular status;

(f) when there is increased risk of CHD, particular attention should be paid to history-taking for symptoms suggesting cardiovascular disease and, if necessary, appropriate investigations performed;

(g) although it has not been shown in clinical trials that CHD risk can be reduced by increasing HDL-cholesterol levels, several measures that are desirable in their own right are known to elevate HDL cholesterol, i.e. correction of obesity, ceasing to smoke, adequate appropriate physical exercise and control of diabetes. Similarly, raised triglyceride levels are often lowered by these measures and especially by avoiding overuse of alcohol.

DIETARY MANAGEMENT

Weight reduction

Correction or reduction of obesity are effective in reducing elevated levels of triglyceride and, to a lesser extent, cholesterol. Reduction of overweight also enhances the responsiveness of elevated plasma lipids to other therapy. Doctor and patient should jointly agree on a target weight; the preferred goal is a weight conforming with a body-mass index in the range 20–25 (see Appendix 2). The patient should understand that the appropriate rate of weight loss is 0·5–1 kg week⁻¹, and the duration of dieting to achieve the goal may be estimated. Most physicians encourage patients to accompany dieting by a programme of exercise suitable to age, cardiorespiratory and musculoskeletal health and fitness level.

Positive support and encouragement are of real value in facilitating diet compliance, and the patient should be seen as frequently as possible.

A typical energy intake during weight reduction is 1000 kcal day⁻¹, but more is appropriate if the patient's work or recreation entail very heavy energy expenditure; and an intake of 800 kcal day⁻¹ may be appropriate for the very sedentary patient, or if the rate of weight loss is inadequate. The intention is to achieve a calorie deficit of about 1000 kcal day⁻¹. The composition of the diet is similar to the lipid-lowering diet. Little or no alcohol should be taken until weight loss has been completed. During prolonged reducing diets many physicians prescribe vitamin and potassium supplements.

General lipid-lowering diet

The seven principles of this diet and the necessary nutrient composition are given in Table 10. A sample diet sheet is given in Appendix 1.

In a patient consuming a typical western diet who adopts the lipid-lowering diet with complete compliance, the average fall in plasma cholesterol may be calculated to be about 20–25%; however, there is considerable individual variation in responsiveness. Additional plasma cholesterol reduction may be expected in overweight patients who successfully lose weight. Although the effect of the lipid-lowering diet on plasma lipid levels becomes complete within about three weeks, it takes considerably longer to achieve a maximum response in clinical

practice. This is because learning the diet is an extended process, involving the entire family and comprising changes in food preference and portion size, cooking techniques, shopping and ordering habits in restaurants, etc.

To obtain maximal reduction of plasma lipids an extended period of several months may be required. The trend in lipid levels is measured; optimally the analysis is performed shortly before the patient is seen, e.g. by a dry chemistry procedure on a fingerprick blood sample. In the light of the observed trend, supplementary dieting counselling is provided at each visit by the dietitian and/or doctor. It may be helpful to inquire briefly about recent intake of the major food groups if the response is inadequate: how often in the past day/week did the patient consume red meat/low-fat meats (chicken, turkey, veal, game) and fish, high-fat/low fat dairy products, fruit, vegetables, saturated fats (butter, hard margarine)/unsaturated fats (olive oil, seed oils and their products), manufactured and convenience food (tinned meats, pizzas, sausages, hamburgers, cakes, biscuits, pastries), and alcohol? The diet should be tailored as far as possible to meet individual food preferences.

The professional dietitian is best able to instruct patients in the details of food selection. Particularly when the therapeutic goal is not at first achieved, counselling by a dietitian is advantageous. However, in many countries it is necessary for the doctor to be able to provide dietary counselling and to issue written dietary guidelines (see Appendix 1). At all times the doctor's role is essential in informing the patient about the purpose and principles of treatment, e.g. in explaining that dietary cholesterol and saturated fats are not essential to healthy nutrition. Above all the doctor provides ongoing motivation and support to the patient with hyperlipidaemia. For patients who travel extensively or use restaurants frequently the dietitian should provide guidance on appropriate menu items. Suitable items are clear soups, grilled or poached fish, veal, chicken, turkey or game, vegetables and salads, fruit salads and sorbets. The patient needs to order such foods without dressings, sauces, butter or cream, and should specify grilled or poached entrees wherever possible. Boiled rice is preferable to fried rice, and boiled or jacket potatoes are suitable while roast or fried potatoes are not.

In the management of hypercholesterolaemia a further reduction of total fat, saturated fatty acids and cholesterol in the diet as well as an increase in fibre may be needed if target values of serum choles-

Table 10 The general lipid-lowering diet: principles, nutrient composition and sources

Principle	Sources
Decreased total fat intake and reduction of saturated fats	Butter, hard margarine, whole milk, cream, ice cream, hard cheese, cream cheese, visible meat fat, usual cuts of red meat and pork, duck, goose, usual sausage, pastry, usual coffee whiteners, coconut, coconut oil and palm oil-containing foods
Increased use of high protein, low saturated fat foods	Fish, chicken, turkey, game, veal
Increased complex carbohydrate and fruit, vegetable and cereal fibre, with some emphasis on legumes	All fresh and frozen vegetables, all fresh fruit, all unrefined cereal foods, lentils, dried beans, rice
Moderately increased use of polyunsaturated and monounsaturated fats	Sunflower oil, corn oil, soybean oil and products unless hardened (hydrogenated), olive oil
Decreased dietary cholesterol	Brain, sweetbreads, kidneys, tongue; eggs (limit to 1–2 yolks per week); liver (limit to twice per month)
Moderately decreased sodium intake	Salt, sodium glutamate, cheese, tinned vegetables and meats, salt-preserved foods (ham, bacon, kippers), high-salt mineral waters, many convenience foods

Nutrient composition (%)	
Carbohydrates	50–60*
Protein	10–20
Fat	⩽ 30
Saturated fatty acids	⩽ 10
Monounsaturated fatty acids	⩽ 10
n-6 and n-3 polyunsaturated fatty acids†	⩽ 10
Fibre‡	ca. 35 g day⁻¹
Cholesterol	< 300 mg day⁻¹

*Percentage of total dietary energy (excluding alcohol) contributed by each nutrient.
†These nutrients should be obtained from natural foods.
‡At least half derived from fruit, pulses and other vegetables, and oats.

terol are not at first achieved. It is most likely to benefit those patients who, for incompletely understood reasons, show a less-than-average response of plasma lipid metabolism to dietary change. This diet is more stringent (semi-vegetarian) and not every patient will tolerate the restrictions.

Low-fat diet for chylomicronaemia

Entirely distinct from the fat-modified lipid-lowering diet, the low-fat diet is indicated for the rare chylomicronaemia syndrome. Its content of fats comprising all long-chain fatty acids is far lower than that of lipid-lowering diets for hyperlipidaemic states, ranging from 10–20% dietary energy. The contents of carbohydrate and protein are high, and the diet is usually supplemented with medium-chain triglyceride. The use of low-fat diets is described in the section on treatment of the chylomicronaemia syndrome.

DRUG TREATMENT

When lipid-lowering drugs are used, this is always in conjunction with on-going careful attention to diet therapy. Indications for their use appear on pp. 591–4. Here their individual characteristics are described. Combination therapy is not infrequently needed and is discussed on p. 590. The balance between benefit and risks of therapy should be borne in mind. In managing severe hypertriglyceridaemia, the goal is determined largely by the risk of pancreatitis; this risk becomes very low if levels can be maintained below 1000 mg dl⁻¹ (11 mmol l⁻¹). The following is a brief description of the more important drugs. The use and common side effects are reviewed. On pp. 596–7 the large-scale clinical trials of these agents are described. For patients at very high risk, particularly those in Group E, introduction of drug therapy often proves necessary at a relatively early stage. For the majority of patients, however, early drug therapy is not appropriate, and an extended attempt should be made (e.g. for 9–12 months) to maximize the effect of dietary measures and control of underlying causes. The following should be read in conjunction with the manufacturer's recommendations on dosage and precautions.

Bile acid sequestrant resins

These are well-tried drugs, widely used in the treatment of heterozygous familial hypercholesterolaemia in adults and children, and of patients with common hypercholesterolaemia who have proved refractory to a thorough trial of dietary therapy during several months. They are not absorbed and function by reducing intestinal reabsorption of bile acids. Increased production of bile acids ensues, depleting liver cells of cholesterol and, thereby, inducing increased LDL receptor activity on these cells. As a result, LDL catabolism is increased and plasma cholesterol levels fall by 20–30%. Triglyceride and HDL cholesterol levels may increase moderately.

The major side effects are constipation (which is common in adults but can usually be offset by increased intake of wheat fibre) and gastrointestinal discomfort. The drugs interfere with absorption of folic acid, of several other drugs including thyroxin, digoxin, warfarin, probucol and fibrates, and of fat-soluble vitamins. Folate supplements (5 mg day^{-1}) are given throughout growth, and to adults with increased requirements (e.g. during pregnancy and lactation) 1–2 h before the next dose of the resin. Other than folic acid, clinically significant vitamin deficiencies are unlikely to occur in patients with normal intestinal and hepatic function. Other drugs too must be so scheduled that they are taken 1–4 h before or 4 h after resins. Rarer side effects are diarrhoea, steatorrhoea, intestinal obstruction and severe abdominal pain.

Two resins are currently in use, cholestyramine which is presented in sachets containing 4 g and colestipol, presented in 5-g sachets. Newer, more convenient presentations are likely to be forthcoming. Resins are, at present, supplied in granular form and are taken in doses of 1–3 sachets, dispersed in fluid. Many patients find their preparation and consumption troublesome, and successful therapy requires careful instruction of the patients in their use to minimize inconvenience and side effects. It is usual to commence with a low dosage, e.g. one sachet twice daily and to increase progressively to effective or maximum-tolerated dosage over 1–3

months. Initial dyspepsia and nausea may prove transient. In common hypercholesterolaemia the daily dosage is 2–4 sachets per day. Resins are taken in at least two divided doses per day; it is recommended that they be taken with meals to avoid dyspepsia (preferably the largest meals of the day). Most patients prefer to take them at or near commencement of the meal.

In powder form, resins are taken dispersed in fruit juice or water. The drug is conveniently prepared as a day's batch, by sprinkling it onto the requisite amount of fruit juice in a wide-necked jar, shaking thoroughly, storing it in the refrigerator and consuming it the following day in two or three doses. Use of a blender is preferred by some patients. A dosage of 4–6 sachets a day usually results in 20–30% lowering of LDL cholesterol.

Fibrate drugs (phenoxyisobutyrates)

Different members of this group (which includes beclobrate, bezafibrate, ciprofibrate, clofibrate, fenofibrate and gemfibrozil, listed alphabetically) are licensed for use in various countries. Clofibrate and gemfibrozil have been subjected to large-scale clinical trials of CHD prevention (see pp. 596–7). Biochemically, the fibrates vary in potency and, therefore, in dosage. They increase the activity of lipoprotein lipase, enhancing catabolism of VLDL triglyceride and promoting transfer of cholesterol to HDL. VLDL production appear to be decreased. Some, including clofibrate, increase biliary excretion of cholesterol. In consequence, plasma triglyceride is effectively decreased (due to lowering of VLDL and IDL levels) and HDL cholesterol variably increases. LDL cholesterol is decreased by 5–25% (except in hypertriglyceridaemic patients in whom initially low levels tend to increase). Plasma cholesterol reduction by fibrates is due to decreased VLDL and IDL, and, to a variable extent, lower LDL lipids.

The drugs are usually well tolerated. Untoward effects include gastrointestinal discomfort, potentiation of warfarin, an increase in creatine kinase sometimes accompanied by a reversible myopathy with pain and stiffness in large muscle groups, impotence and increased hepatocellular enzymes. Clofibrate increases the incidence of cholesterol gallstones; this lithogenic effect appears to be less marked with other fibrates. In one of two large-scale clofibrate trial, non-cardiovascular deaths from a variety of causes increased. Impaired renal function is a relative contraindication for fibrate drugs; if used at all, to treat renal hyperlipidaemias, a reduced dose should be used and creatinine clearance closely monitored.

Nicotinic acid

Nicotinic acid, a B vitamin, is a potent lipid-lowering agent when used in pharmacological dosage, decreasing VLDL and LDL production.

Triglyceride and, to a smaller but still substantial extent, cholesterol levels decrease. VLDL levels fall and HDL cholesterol increases; LDL cholesterol decreases except in some hypertriglyceridaemic patients in whom the response is variable. The dose of nicotinic acid can be adjusted according to response.

Nicotinic acid is thus a useful drug, but requires experience in its use because of numerous acute and chronic side effects. In the first 7–14 days of therapy severe flushing and itching follow each dose; these wane with continued use and cease in most patients. To minimize side effects, treatment is started with a low dose, e.g. 0·25 g or even 0·1 g four times a day with meals for 3–7 days; the dose is slowly increased up to 1 g four times daily as a maintenance dose at a rate dependent on side effects. To minimize flush, the drug should be taken without fluid at the end of the meal. The flushing is mediated by prostaglandins and can be reduced by premedication with even a low dose of aspirin. Other side effects are gastro-intestinal discomfort, hyperuricaemia and precipitation of acute gout, a macular rash, urticaria, and acanthosis nigricans, increased liver enzymes, cholestasis, and impairment of glucose tolerance (the last is seldom of clinically significant extent).

In addition to nicotinic acid, derivatives and sustained-release preparations are available that may cause less flushing and gastrointestinal discomfort, but may be less potent in lipid reduction.

Cholesterol synthesis inhibitors

Cholesterol synthesis inhibitors, which act by inhibition of the enzyme HMGCoA reductase, are the most promising of the current generation of cholesterol-lowering drugs, now at an advanced stage of evaluation. Their potency is remarkable. Among them, lovastatin, pravastatin and simvastatin have been most extensively studied; simvastatin is the most potent in inhibiting HMGCoA reductase *in vitro*, and appears fully effective by once-daily dosage after the evening meal. A large-scale, long-term evaluation is awaited before their place in therapy is defined.

Serum cholesterol is reduced by 30–40%, and LDL cholesterol by 35–45%; triglyceride is moderately reduced and HDL slightly elevated.

The drugs are usually well tolerated. Dyspepsia is infrequent and mild. Until the possibility of an increased incidence of lens opacities has been fully excluded, ophthalmological monitoring (including slit-lamp examination) at baseline and at six-month intervals is indicated. No loss of visual acuity has been reported. Hepatocellular enzymes, particularly alanine transaminase (ALT), may increase, usually to a mild extent, with some drugs in this class. This is uncommon but should also be monitored at intervals of, for example, 4–6 weeks for 15 months, and at the present state of knowledge the drug should be withdrawn if ALT exceeds three times the upper limit. Symptomatic liver disease has not occurred. A mild and usually transient increase in creatine kinase is not uncommon with some synthesis inhibitors; symptomatic myopathy is rare and requires withdrawal of the drug.

Lovastatin is given at a dosage of 20–80 mg daily in single or divided dose, pravastatin at 20 mg twice daily and simvastatin at 20–40 mg daily.

Probucol

Probucol is, on average, a cholesterol-lowering agent of moderate effectiveness, but there is a wide variation in responsiveness. The dosage is 0·5 g twice daily. Reduction of cholesterol results from a decrease in both LDL (5–15%) and HDL (up to 25%). It accumulates in the core of lipoprotein particles, presumably altering their structure in a way that enhances their uptake by cells. This enhanced uptake is not dependent on LDL receptors, hence the drug is effective in some patients with homozygous familial hypercholesterolaemia who lack LDL receptors.

Side effects include diarrhoea and dyspepsia or nausea. Prolongation of the corrected QT interval occurs uncommonly, but the drug should not be used in patients with a ventricular arrhythmia, or with a prolonged QT prior to therapy; the ECG should be monitored in the first year or two of therapy.

As the desired lipoprotein effect is reduction of LDL, levels of LDL cholesterol must be monitored and shown to decrease substantially if treatment is to be continued. The fall in HDL cholesterol is not desired, but there is no evidence to indicate whether or not it increases progression of atherosclerosis. Xanthomas in tendons and skin regress during probucol treatment, providing possible reassurance concerning HDL changes.

Probucol is also a potent antioxidant. As peroxidation of LDL may be an important step in its atherogenic role, the theoretical possibility exists that the drug may protect against atherosclerosis progression through this mechanism, but as yet this is unsupported by persuasive evidence.

Omega-3 fatty acids

Omega-3 fatty acids present in marine oils are effective, in large doses, in treating hypertriglyceridaemia due to elevated VLDL levels; they act by decreasing VLDL production. They may also lessen the risk of thrombosis, partly by modifying prostaglandin metabolism. Epidemiologically there is an inverse relation between fish consumption and CHD mortality but it is by no means established that this is a result of differences in intake of omega-3 fatty acids.

Marine oil preparations (based on carcass extracts; not of liver origin) are well tolerated. There is, as yet, a paucity of large-scale, long-term studies. Protection against CHD and long-term safety have not been established in man, and animal studies have been somewhat inconsistent. At very high dosage (20–30 g day^{-1}) marine oils can reduce LDL as well as VLDL levels. At usually recommended doses of 5–10 g twice daily, however, the beneficial effect is confined to marked reduction of VLDL lipids; LDL cholesterol and LDL apo B tend to increase as VLDL levels fall in familial hypertriglyceridaemia and familial combined hyperlipidaemia. As a rise in LDL is undesirable, LDL cholesterol should be monitored regularly. Highly unsaturated fatty acids are prone to lipid peroxidation, the products being toxic. It is essential to prevent this by addition of antioxidant to marine oil preparations. More extensive long-term evaluation is desirable before widespread use of marine oil preparations.

COMBINED LIPID-LOWERING DRUG THERAPY

Single lipid-lowering drug therapy in combination with diet not infrequently fails to achieve an adequate reduction in plasma cholesterol or triglyceride and, indeed, may produce undesirable changes in addition to the required response in the lipoprotein profile. In these situations combined lipid-lowering drug therapy may be warranted.

The bile acid sequestrant drugs are often used in combination therapy. In combination with nicotinic acid further reductions can be obtained in serum cholesterol, triglyceride and LDL cholesterol, while HDL cholesterol rises. Similar effects are seen during combined therapy with resins and the fibrates. In some patients the combined use of a bile acid sequestrant with probucol leads to marked serum cholesterol reduction. Combination therapy with sequestrant resins and cholesterol synthesis inhibitors results in striking reductions in serum LDL cholesterol of up to 50%. Their combined effects are often a powerful therapeutic approach to the treatment of severe hypercholesterolaemia.

While two-drug therapy may prove essential to achieve full control of existent hyperlipidaemia, it must be remembered that side effects are more likely and that costs can become very substantial. Before adding a second drug, increasing the dose (of a resin or nicotinic acid) may be considered, or substitution of an alternative drug may prove more effective.

Management of the patient with primary hyperlipidaemia

COMMON HYPERCHOLESTEROLAEMIA

In most patients nutrition plays a central role in the pathogenesis, hence the mainstay of treatment is diet. Aggravating factors include obesity and diuretic therapy. Most patients in this category fall into Groups A or B. Mild hypercholesterolaemia due to elevated HDL cholesterol levels must be excluded. If possible the patient should be managed with the assistance of a dietitian.

Accompanying reversible risk factors (Table 2) should be dealt with. Management of associated hypertension, if drugs are needed, should emphasize agents that lack potentially adverse lipoprotein effects. Suitable drugs include ACE inhibitors, calcium channel blockers, prazosin, and beta-blockers possessing intrinsic sympathomimetic activity.

If the patient is overweight (body mass index > 25, see Appendix 2) an energy-restricted lipid-lowering diet is prescribed.

Long-term management is by a lipid-lowering diet providing energy sufficient to maintain desirable weight. The general lipid lowering diet (see Appendix 1) is similar to that recommended for general use in countries with high CHD incidence; its use must be particularly emphasized for patients with documented hypercholesterolaemia. A diet sheet should be provided. When cholesterol levels are in the range 200–250 mg dl^{-1} (5·2–6·5 mmol l^{-1}), the management amounts to a strong reinforcement of advice given to the population as a whole.

In teaching the diet to the patient with cholesterol levels > 250 mg dl^{-1} (6·5 mmol l^{-1}), the doctor (and dietitian) will take into account food preferences and relevant aspects of life style (frequent travelling, use of restaurants). The patient should know suitable menu items. Although the diet is not radically altered, re-education of the patient and spouse in eating habits, shopping, menu selection and cooking methods may take up to 6–9 months; at 2–4 follow-up visits, therefore, cholesterol is measured and, as necessary, food intake is assessed and aspects of the diet reemphasized. Dietary compliance is progressively enhanced by these means and by a positive encouraging approach.

Patients achieving a plasma cholesterol level close to 200 mg dl^{-1} (5·2 mmol l^{-1}) may be discharged if pre-treatment levels were in the range 200–250 mg dl^{-1} (5·2–6·5 mmol l^{-1}), but those with baseline values of 250–300 mg dl^{-1} (6·5–7·8 mmol l^{-1}) (whose risk was greater) should be followed-up at intervals of six months to three years to verify ongoing good control.

Two options are available for treatment of hypercholesterolaemia persisting after 6–9 months of use of the diet. One is to restrict intake of saturated fats and cholesterol further by eliminating from the diet, or severely curtailing, those discretionary foods listed in column 2 of the diet sheet (Appendix 1). For those patients who find this diet acceptable, this is the preferred option.

The alternative approach that may require consideration is most appropriate for younger patients, and for those whose overall risk of CHD is judged to be high (on the basis of lipid levels and other risk-related characteristics) (Table 2). This option is to introduce drug therapy. For example, one may use a low dose of a non-absorbable drug. Colestipol 5 g or cholestryamine 4 g, given one to three times daily with meals, is combined with ongoing attempts to maximize the response to diet. This approach should rarely be necessary in Treatment Group A, and only where patients are deemed to be at particularly high risk. However, a substantial minority of patients in Treatment Group B will benefit from this approach. The response should be monitored, and the drug continued only if it is seen to be effective. Alternative drugs are shown in Table 6 and may be preferred in subjects with borderline high triglyceride and low HDL cholesterol.

FAMILIAL HYPERCHOLESTEROLAEMIA

Heterozygous familial hypercholesterolaemia is the commonest cause of severe hypercholesterolaemia, and confers a serious increase in the risk of premature CHD. The great majority of these patients fall into Group E. As the hypercholestero-

laemia is often gross, dietary treatment alone is rarely adequate; but most patients can be well controlled by a combination of careful dietary control and one or two lipid-lowering drugs.

Management of accompanying risk factors is especially important in FH in view of the particularly high risk of CHD caused by their interaction: most FH heterozygotes who develop CHD before age 30 also smoke cigarettes or are hypertensive.

Careful history taking all too frequently reveals the presence of symptomatic CHD when the condition is first diagnosed in early middle age. As a result of the high prevalence of CHD in familial hypercholesterolaemia, exercise electrocardiography of asymptomatic patients is recommended, and often detailed cardiologic evaluation is required.

The baseline should first be established. Initial therapy should at present be the lipid-lowering diet. Failure to respond within two months should result in institution of drug therapy without further delay while diet is continued.

The measures described under 'Common hypercholesterolaemia' to maximize dietary compliance are particularly important to the FH patient. Follow-up measurements are, of course, mandatory. The use of drug therapy should never allow lessened attention to diet.

Currently, the preferred initial drug is a bile acid sequestrant resin because this group is the most effective of the currently available agents in FH and large-scale trials have established no serious side effects. When they are approved, HMGCoA reductase inhibitor drugs may become the first choice.

Resin therapy in relatively high dosage is effective, though problems of compliance tend to limit the average reduction of plasma cholesterol to about 25%. The appropriate dosage of cholestyramine is 16–24 g day^{-1}, and that of colestipol 20–30 g day^{-1}, in divided doses, always taken with food; if tolerated, higher dosage may improve the response where necessary. The patient should receive a careful explanation of the use of the drug. Most experts start treatment at low dosage, e.g. one sachet twice daily, increasing over 1–2 months to an effective dose. With experience, the physician will be able to achieve successful resin therapy in a majority of patients, but patience and attention to detail are necessary. Newer formulations of resins are likely to facilitate their use considerably.

In the more severely hypercholesterolaemic FH patient, achieving target lipid levels will require of the order of 50% reduction in plasma cholesterol. If it is necessary to introduce higher dosage resin therapy, the plasma cholesterol response to each measure should be monitored; stringent dieting and high-dosage resins should be continued only if an incremental reduction in cholesterol level justifies such treatment.

Although cholestyramine and colestipol have similar modes of action the patient will often have a strong preference for one resin. The physician should readily offer the alternative drug if tolerance problems arise.

There are two indications for introduction of a second drug in the treatment of heterozygous FH. The more common is failure to approach target cholesterol levels in an adequate trial of diet and a single drug. The other is marked and persistent hypertriglyceridaemia occurring during resin therapy, despite attention to diet and to underlying causes of elevated triglyceride levels.

Several drug combinations have been reported in FH. The effects of a resin and a fibrate on hypercholesterolaemia are strongly additive and also provide control of elevated triglyceride levels. Resins may be combined very effectively with nicotinic acid. The combination of an HMGCoA reductase inhibitor with a resin is probably the most potent means of reducing hypercholesterolaemia. In some patients therapy with a resin and probucol is of value.

In specialized centres, homozygous familial hypercholesterolaemia and (experimentally) heterozygous familial hypercholesterolaemia are treated, for example, by serial LDL apheresis in which plasma is passed through LDL-adsorbing columns or other special procedures.

REMNANT (TYPE III) HYPERLIPIDAEMIA

This is, in most patients, readily treated. As it is associated with premature atherosclerosis affecting the heart and peripheral arteries, its early diagnosis is important to permit effective therapy before the appearance of cardiovascular complications. Most patients fall into Group E, though some appear in Group D or even C.

The condition is relatively responsive to dietary treatment, but only in a minority of patients is the elevated VLDL cholesterol level adequately corrected by diet alone. Most patients are effectively treated by diet together with either a drug of the fibrate family or nicotinic acid; a preliminary report suggests that HMGCoA reductase inhibitors may also be suitable.

The disorder requires for its expression both a genetic predisposition together with an additional cause, often acquired; successful management requires that such causes be identified and treated. In particular, obesity, hypothyroidism, or diabetes need appropriate management, and their continued presence explains most therapeutic failures.

Dietary treatment includes the correction of overweight and institution of the lipid-lowering diet. Particularly in patients with relatively mild hyperlipidaemia the lipid response to this regime should be followed before introducing medication.

The response to introduction of drug therapy is often remarkable, with 60–70% reduction of plasma triglyceride and cholesterol. The most widely used drugs are those of the fibrate group, including gemfibrozil and bezafibrate.

FAMILIAL HYPERTRIGLYCERIDAEMIA

Endogenous hypertriglyceridaemia of mild degree (Treatment Group C) may be secondary to underlying causes (Table 2), or may be primary and familial, or may reflect the interacton of genetic with environmental causes.

When triglyceride levels are elevated, an important task for the clinician is to identify and deal with reversible underlying causes. Prominent among these are obesity and over-use of alcohol, the latter being commonly under-reported. A lipid-lowering diet is prescribed; to provide supplementary omega-3 fatty acids, use of fish including salmon, mackerel, sardines, tuna and herring is emphasized.

In hypertriglyceridaemia of greater severity (triglyceride > 500 mg dl^{-1}, > 5·6 mmol l^{-1}) there is often an accumulation of both endogenous and dietary triglyceride. This is a difficult, but fortunately uncommon, therapeutic problem. The majority of such patients may best be investigated and initially treated in a specialized centre. Triglyceride levels are notoriously labile, and fluctuations in food intake, or alcohol use, can lead to large day-to-day changes in plasma triglyceride, so that a level of 500 mg dl^{-1} (5·6 mmol l^{-1}) can increase to one capable of precipitating acute pancreatitis (> 1000 mg dl^{-1}, > 11 mmol l^{-1}) within a short period of time.

The initial approach to treatment is the same as that for milder hypertriglyceridaemia; obesity and other underlying causes are dealt with. Gradual reduction of overweight lessens hypertriglyceridaemia. It should be emphasized to the patient that triglyceride levels can rise steeply and potentially dangerously if weight is regained, hence steady but progressive correction of obesity is the necessary strategy. The fat-modified lipid-lowering diet is prescribed with some emphasis on the use of fish. If the lipoprotein analysis indicates that a large proportion of the excess circulating triglyceride is carried in the chylomicron fraction, stepwise further reduction in dietary fat intake (to 25% or 20% of dietary energy) may prove effective. However, this must be carried out under close supervision because the attendant rise in dietary carbohydrate can lead to an increase in the endogenous component of the hypertriglyceridaemia. As hypertriglyceridaemia is frequently associated with hyperinsulinaemia, regular aerobic physical exercise may be of use.

Medication is introduced if serial measurements do not indicate adequate reduction in plasma triglyceride levels, while assiduous attention to diet is continued. There is controversy as to the use of drug treatment for moderate degrees of hypertriglyceridaemia. Wherever possible treatment should be based on correction of obesity, removal of underlying causes, and maximizing compliance to the lipid-lowering diet. Drug treatment of resistant hypertriglyceridaemia is appropriate when the abnormality is a manifestation of remnant hyperlipidaemia or familial combined hyperlipidaemia (discussed elsewhere in this section).

The treatment options in hypertriglyceridaemia include a fibrate drug, nicotinic acid or one of its derivatives. It is difficult to predict which drug will be most effective in an individual patient. Occasionally it proves necessary to use a combination of two of these drugs.

Many patients present with the combination of familial hypertriglyceridaemia and diabetes mellitus, the two disorders resulting in gross hypertriglyceridaemia. It is helpful to assess pancreatic islet cell reserve by an intravenous glucagon test, a flat plasma insulin response indicating the need for insulin therapy (see also the section on diabetic hyperlipidaemia).

CHYLOMICRONAEMIA SYNDROME

These patients, always in Group E, are best investigated and initially treated in a specialized centre. Before making the diagnosis of this rare genetic disorder, several underlying causes of chylomicronaemia must be excluded, such as uncontrolled diabetes mellitus, hypothyroidism and glycogen storage disease.

Initiation of treatment usually takes place in hospital. If the patient has presented with acute pancreatitis he or she will have received intravenous fluids, followed by fat-free oral feeding. If seen in an interval, the diagnostic work-up will probably include a three-day fat deprivation test (<5 g fat day^{-1}). In either case initial dietary therapy will then comprise isocaloric feeding with a low fat content such as 10% of dietary energy. Plasma triglyceride is measured daily after a 12–14 h overnight fast, and it is convenient also to identify chylomicronaemia in each sample by the stored plasma test.

At intervals of about one week, small stepwise increases in fat intake are allowed, while plasma triglyceride monitoring continues. Patients may tolerate 15–25% of energy intake as dietary fat without increasing triglyceride levels. Optimally, plasma triglyceride is maintained at <500 mg dl^{-1} (<5.6 mmol l^{-1}). An undesirable increase in VLDL triglyceride can be induced by the high carbohydrate content of very low fat diets. A substantial protein intake (15–18% of energy) permits a somewhat lower intake of carbohydrate. For most patients the diet must remain a restricted one, with a relatively limited range of permitted foods. When an optimal fat intake has been identified, intake of normal dietary long-chain fatty acids may be supplemented by medium-chain triglyceride for use in cooking or as salad dressing.

Drug treatment seldom has a place in the chylomicronaemia syndrome. An occasional indication arises if the tolerance of fat is very low and marked carbohydrate-induced elevation of VLDL triglyceride becomes a problem; nicotinic acid or a fibrate drug may then be tried, under close observation.

Potentially deleterious medication such as oestrogen preparations, propranolol or thiazides should be avoided. The endogenous hypertriglyceridaemia that may result competes with dietary triglyceride for compromised removal mechanisms, and may lead to rapid build-up of dangerous plasma triglyceride levels. The disorder may be gravely exacerbated during pregnancy.

FAMILIAL COMBINED HYPERLIPIDAEMIA

Although the elevation of plasma cholesterol and/or triglyceride levels is usually only moderate, this disorder can present a therapeutic problem. Most patients fall into Treatment Group D. Underlying causes are identified and dealt with. Initial treatment is by diet, which provides adequate response in the majority of patients; management is then similar to that of common hypercholesterolaemia. Weight control is particularly relevant because correction of obesity lessens the underlying metabolic defect, i.e. the overproduction of VLDL and LDL. Dietary management should be persevered with, using all efforts to reinforce good compliance.

In some patients serial lipid measurements nevertheless show persisting hyperlipidaemia, and consideration should then be given to additional drug therapy. The selection of a suitable drug regime may, however, impose some difficulty. If the persisting hyperlipidaemia takes the form of hypercholesterolaemia with low triglyceride levels, a bile acid-binding resin should be used at minimum effective dosage; as an example, colestipol may be tried at a dosage of 5 g twice or three times daily. Unfortunately some patients show a good cholesterol response but develop a reciprocal increase in plasma triglyceride. If marked this may require additional treatment with a fibrate drug or nicotinic acid.

Conversely, treatment of patients with diet-resistant hypertriglyceridaemia by a fibrate may normalize triglyceride levels but in some will result in increased plasma cholesterol and LDL cholesterol; again it may prove necessary to resort to two-drug therapy, including a bile acid binding resin in the regime.

For monotherapy, the most effective currently available drug appears to be nicotinic acid, which can substantially decrease both triglyceride and cholesterol levels (see Part 8). Unfortunately the drug is relatively difficult to use, having a number of side effects.

Limited available evidence suggests that HMGCoA inhibitors may be very effective against familial combined hyperlipidaemia. Omega-3 fatty acids have been reported to be effective at very high dosage (20–30 g marine oil per day); at more usual dosage, however, triglyceride and VLDL levels are reduced but cholesterol and LDL levels may increase.

DIABETIC HYPERLIPIDAEMIA

Diabetics have a 1·5–3-fold increased CHD risk, and it is likely that this is mediated, at least in part, by lipoprotein abnormalities. In the untreated diabetic, hypertriglyceridaemia is the major abnormality and may be gross enough to lead to eruptive xanthomas, enlargement of liver and spleen, and retinal lipaemia. In such patients the hyperlipidaemia is chiefly due to accumulation of chylomicrons and VLDL and the most serious complication is acute pancreatitis; if this occurs the short-term management is with intravenous clear fluids followed by a virtually fat-free diet, and insulin may be required.

In more mildly affected patients, serum triglyceride is moderately elevated due to increased level of VLDL. HDL cholesterol tends to be low; IDL levels may be elevated.

In non-insulin-dependent diabetes (NIDDM) LDL cholesterol has been found to be normal in some studies and elevated in others; increased triglyceride levels are the rule. In addition, the composition of LDL may be modified, partly due to the addition of glucose to its apolipoprotein B, thereby altering its metabolism. All these lipoprotein abnormalities could contribute to the enhanced risk of CHD and of peripheral vascular disease. The recent European Consensus on NIDDM stated: 'In view of the importance of cholesterol *and* triglyceride as risk factors for macrovascular disease in NIDDM it is strongly recommended that total cholesterol, HDL-cholesterol and triglyceride are checked annually. If results are abnormal and intervention is appropriate, values should be checked 3 monthly'. Their goals of treatment are similar to those expressed in this report.

The lipoprotein changes revert towards normal with effective treatment of hyperglycaemia. The insulin-treated diabetic often attains a fully satisfactory lipoprotein pattern. Treatment of NIDDM, however, does not always correct the lipoprotein disorder. Often this is explained by persisting obesity; in other patients it reflects co-existence of primary familial hypertriglyceridaemia with diabetes.

The management of diabetic hyperlipidaemia depends initially on effective control of hyperglycaemia. In NIDDM, every effort should be made to deal with overweight, aiming at steady, gradual weight reduction. The diabetic diet now includes a high content of vegetable-derived fibre and a relatively low content of saturated fat; both features are common to the lipid-lowering diet and, therefore, deserve particular emphasis.

When hyperlipidaemia persists despite satisfactory compliance with these measures, a co-existing primary hyperlipidaemia may be suspected and may be confirmed by a family study. In practice, in view of the high risk of CHD, it is appropriate to introduce a lipid-lowering drug. Fibrates are the first choice and among them bezafibrate mildly improves carbohydrate tolerance.

Hyperlipidaemia may also be secondary to renal failure or nephrotic syndrome complicating the diabetes.

Monitoring therapy

Patients in Treatment Groups B, D and E, and all patients receiving hypolipidaemic drug therapy require indefinite follow-up. The purposes are to ensure good dietary and drug compliance, and hence maximize the response of elevated lipid levels to therapy, to monitor for untoward effects of drugs, to achieve and maintain control of associated risk factors and, especially, to ensure an on-going lipid response.

The initial frequency of follow-up attendance varies with the severity of the lipid abnormality and the vigour with which treatment is pursued; the patient may be seen 3–6 times in the first year. When a stable, satisfactory response is achieved, patients receiving drug treatment are usually seen twice a year or at least annually; after 2–3 years of medication, drug therapy may be discontinued for a short period to validate its further usefulness. Patients treated by diet alone are seen annually, or at least every 2–3 years after stability of control is established.

Follow-up of patients in Treatment Groups A and C, with pretreatment cholesterol levels of 200–250 mg dl^{-1} (5·2–6·5 mmol l^{-1}) or triglyceride levels of 200–500 mg dl^{-1} (2·3–5·6 mmol l^{-1}) depends, in part, on the resources available. Such lipid levels are very common in many populations. In an ideal world regular follow-up would be carried out and it is certainly preferable to see such patients at least once or twice after the initial visit. As a compromise, where restricted time prevents long-term follow-up of all patients, those in Groups A and C who are considered at high overall risk of CHD deserve regular monitoring at intervals of 1–2 years, increasing to 5 years. If resources are limited, there is justification for providing follow-up at least to younger patients in Groups A and C.

Family screening

In most patients in Groups D and E, examination of the patient should be accompanied by lipid measurements on accessible first-degree relatives (children, brothers, sisters, parents). This serves two purposes: (1) it permits early detection of affected relatives and their treatment; and (2) by identifying the pattern of inheritance it often characterizes the genetic disorder in the family. As primary hyperlipidaemia, dependent on its precise origin, may be associated with high risk of atherosclerotic diseases and as it may require life-long treatment, all efforts

should be made to establish or exclude the familial nature of the disease.

In most primary hyperlipidaemias, abnormal lipid values become manifest in adult life. An important exception is familial hypercholesterolaemia where high LDL cholesterol values (>95 percentile) are already detectable in cord blood. The demonstration of a high LDL cholesterol concentration in children should always raise the suspicion of familial hypercholesterolaemia.

In remnant (type III) hyperlipoproteinaemia, correct diagnosis of primary hyperlipidaemia requires more specialized diagnostic procedures. The determination of apolipoprotein E polymorphism is needed to establish that mixed hyperlipidaemia (Groups D or E) as observed in these patients is a consequence of an abnormal apolipoprotein E isoform (apolipoprotein E-2 homozygosity). Another isoform, apolipoprotein E-4, is frequently observed in hypercholesterolaemia (Group B). Apo E-4 heterozygosity occurs with a frequency of 20% in the West German population and of 30% in the Finnish population. It is a major genetic factor accounting for differences in serum cholesterol distribution between populations.

The lipid abnormality in first-degree relatives does not necessarily resemble that of the proband. Familial combined hyperlipidaemia in a single affected family member may fall into any of Groups A–E. In the absence of a genetic or biochemical marker, the diagnosis of familial combined hyperlipidaemia depends upon demonstration of hypercholesterolaemia, hypertriglyceridaemia, or both, in several first-degree relatives. Hyperlipidaemia is not apparent in affected relatives until adult life.

Early detection of high-risk persons is of key importance in primary prevention. In the specialized laboratory, investigation of genes, apolipoproteins, lipoprotein receptors and lipolytic enzymes has become an invaluable tool to diagnose familial lipoprotein disorders correctly. This is a justification for patients in Group E always, and patients in the other groups occasionally, being referred to the specialized physician for correct diagnosis and initiation of treatment.

Clinical trials of reduction of serum lipids

This section summarizes the major clinical trials carried out to establish whether it is possible to achieve a reduction in morbidity and mortality from CHD or to demonstrate regression or non-progression of atherosclerosis, by lowering cholesterol over a relatively short period of time.

TRIALS OF DIET TO CONTROL HYPERCHOLESTEROLAEMIA

There have been at least 10 trials in which dietary modification has been used as the method of intervention to lower cholesterol levels in the hope of reducing CHD. The majority were carried out in patients with established CHD with entry into the trials at variable times after myocardial infarction. Dietary advice differed in the various studies. Individual trials have suffered problems of statistical power; but when the results of all dietary studies that employed a randomized design are aggregated, a clear and highly significant trend emerges: a 10% reduction in cholesterol is associated with a reduction of $13 \pm 6\%$ of all coronary heart disease despite the relatively short duration of the trials. The moderate extent of CHD reduction almost certainly reflects this short period of intervention.

In three more recent studies an attempt was made to modify diet together with other risk factors (multi-factor intervention trials). In the European Collaborative Trial, health education was introduced into factories randomly selected from pairs, the non-selected of the pair serving as a control. Overall reduction in coronary heart disease mortality in the 'experimental' factories as compared with controls was only 7·4%, but results from individual centres showed that change in mortality was strongly related to the extent of risk-factor modification. Where intervention was most successful, CHD incidence showed a more pronounced fall.

In Oslo, men at high risk of CHD [as a result of smoking and/or having a cholesterol level in the range 290–380 mg dl^{-1} (7·5–9·8 mmol l^{-1})] were divided into two groups; half received intensive dietary education and advice to stop smoking, the other half served as a control group. An impressive reduction (31 *vs* 57 per 1000 over a five-year period) in the total number of coronary events was observed in association with a 13% fall in cholesterol and a reduction in tobacco consumption. The beneficial effect of intervention was reflected in improved total mortality.

The potentially important American Multiple Risk Factor Intervention Trial (MRFIT) which also included men at high risk of CHD unfortunately produced unhelpful results. The 'control' group showed cholesterol changes in the same direction as the intervention group to the extent that the difference in cholesterol between the two groups became only 3%.

TRIALS OF LIPID-LOWERING DRUGS

Of the many drugs shown to lower blood lipids, only clofibrate, niacin, cholestyramine, colestipol and gemfibrozil have been investigated in appropriate randomized clinical trials. The Coronary Drug Project (CDP) included 8000 patients with previous myocardial infarction who received oestrogen, clofibrate, dextrothyroxine, niacin or placebo. Oestrogen and dextrothyroxine were discontinued. Clofibrate led to a non-significant reduction in coronary heart disease. Niacin was associated with a significant reduction in non-fatal myocardial infarction that has persisted during a 15-year follow-up.

The World Health Organization trial of clofibrate showed a significant reduction in major coronary heart disease in those taking the drug as compared with the control group in association with a 9% reduction of cholesterol. However, clofibrate was associated with an increased risk of gallstones, and a significant increase in all-cause mortality due to a wide variety of causes, with no relation between excess mortality and cholesterol lowering. In the Coronary Drug Project, there was no excess of cancer death in the clofibrate group.

The Lipid Research Clinics Coronary Primary Prevention Trial of cholestyramine in 3806 asymptomatic men with primary hypercholesterolaemia not responding to dietary management is particularly relevant to clinical practice. The cholestyramine group showed average plasma total and LDL-cholesterol reductions of 13% and 20%, respectively. There was a 24% reduction in fatal CHD and a 19% reduction in non-fatal myocardial infarction, and in those who complied fully with medication a 39% reduction in all CHD events. The reduction of CHD incidence in the cholestryamine group appeared to be mediated by reduction in total and LDL cholesterol. Deaths from accidents and violence occurred more frequently (though not significantly so) in the cholestryamine group. All other causes of death were similar in the two groups.

The results of the double-blind Helsinki Heart Study have recently become available. In this study 4081 asymptomatic men with LDL plus VLDL cholesterol > 200 mg dl^{-1} (5·2 mmol l^{-1}) received a lipid-lowering diet and were randomized to gemfibrozil or placebo groups. The majority had raised LDL (type IIa). The mean serum triglyceride level fell by 38%, cholesterol by 9% and LDL cholesterol by 9%, while HDL cholesterol increased by 9%. Nonfatal myocardial infarction was decreased by 37% overall ($P < 0.02$) with a 1–2 year latency; thus reduction in years 3–5 was more than 50%. There were six fatal myocardial infarctions in the drug group and eight in the controls. Upper gastrointestinal symptoms were the only side effects which were significantly over-represented in the drug group, but due to usually modest and non-significant increases in various non-cardiac diseases, the total mortality did not decrease. There was a non-significant increased frequency of gall-bladder surgery in the drug group. This study of gemfibrozil showed a greater reduction in CHD incidence then and the cholestyramine trial referred to; the latter drug chiefly affected LDL cholesterol. There is evidence that decreasing LDL cholesterol and increasing HDL cholesterol by gemfibrozil are associated with reduction of CHD.

Interestingly, when the results of all the drug trials were aggregated, the beneficial effect of cholesterol, lowering with regard to CHD was similar to that observed as a consequence of dietary change; *viz.* a 10% reduction was accompanied by a highly significant reduction, $16 \pm 3\%$, in CHD incidence.

NON-CARDIAC MORTALITY AND
CHOLESTEROL-LOWERING

Some studies have shown an increase in non-cardiac causes of mortality. However, the increase in mortality from 'other causes' has been trivial in extent, when compared with the reduction in incidence and mortality from CHD. This benefit is specific, highly statistically significant, pro-portional to the cholesterol lowering achieved and in keeping with the epidemiological evidence. On the other hand, the small excess in deaths from other causes was non-specific (no single cause of death has been predominant or consistent), not related to the degree of cholesterol lowering and not in keeping with the epidemiological evidence. In no instance were the trials formally designed to contain sufficient numbers to look at non-cardiovascular end-points as well as total mortality.

EFFECT OF CHOLESTEROL REDUCTION ON
ATHEROSCLEROSIS

Regression of atherosclerosis in association with cholesterol lowering has been well demonstrated in animal experiments. Several studies in man have shown that reduction of blood lipids can retard the progression of both femoral and coronary atherosclerosis, and one study has shown regression of coronary lesions.

References

[1] Assmann G, Lewis B, Mancini M, Paoletti R, Schettler G. (co-chairmen). Strategies for the prevention of coronary heart disease. A policy statement of the European Atherosclerosis Society. Eur Heart J 1987; 8: 77–88.
[2] Martin MJ, Hulley SB, Browner WS, Kuller LH, Wentworth D. Serum cholesterol, blood pressure and mortality: implications from a cohort of 361 662 men. Lancet 1986; ii: 933–6.
[3] Castelli WP. The triglyceride issue: a view from Framingham. Am Heart J 1986; 112: 432–7.
[4] Bray GA (ed.). Obesity in America. Proceedings of the Second Fogarty International Center Conference on Obesity, No. 79. Washington: USDHEW, 1979.
[5] Royal College of Physicians of London. Report on Obesity. J R Coll Physicians Lond 1983; 17: 3–58.

Appendix 1

Below is an example of a lipid-lowering diet sheet.

(1) *'Advisable'* foods are generally low in fat and/or high in fibre. These should be used regularly as part of your diet. (2) Foods listed under *'in moderation'* contain polyunsaturated fats or smaller quantities of saturated fats. As your diet should be low in fat, these foods are allowed only in moderation. For example: (a) red meat not more than 3 times week^{-1}; (b) medium fat cheeses and meat and fish pastes once a week; (c) homemade cake, biscuits and pastries made with suitable polyunsaturated margarine or oil twice a week; and (d) chips or roast potatoes cooked in suitable oil once a fortnight. (3) Foods *'not advised'* contain large proportions of saturated fats and, therefore, should be avoided wherever possible.

	Advisable	In moderation	Not advised
Fats	All fats should be limited.	Oils or margarine labelled 'high in polyunsaturates'. Sunflower oil, corn oil, soya oil, safflower oil, olive oil, cottonseed oil. Low fat spreads.	Butter, dripping, lard, suet, palm oil, coconut oil, margarines not 'high in polyunsaturates' cooking or vegetable oil of unknown origin. Hydrogenated fats and oils.

598 *The European Atherosclerosis Society*

Appendix 1 — (*Continued*)

	Advisable	In moderation	Not advised
Meat	Chicken, turkey, veal, rabbit, game.	Lean beef, bacon, ham, pork, lamb, lean mince, good quality burgers, liver and kidney.	Visible fat on meat (including crackling), breast of lamb, belly pork, streaky bacon, sausages, salami, pate, luncheon meat, scotch egg, duck, goose, pork pies, meat pasties. Skin on poultry.
Dairy products	Skimmed milk, low-fat cheeses: e.g. cottage cheese, quark (skimmed milk soft cheese), curd cheese. Egg white. Low-fat yoghurt.	Semi-skimmed milk. Medium-fat cheeses: e.g. Edam, Camembert, Gouda, Brie, cheese spreads, processed cheese, Parmesan in small quantities. Half-fat cheeses, 1–3 whole eggs a week.	Full cream milk, evaporated or condensed milk, cream, imitation cream. Full-fat cheeses: e.g. Stilton, Cheddar, Cheshire, cream cheeses. Full-fat yoghurt.
Fish	All white fish: e.g. cod, haddock, plaice. Oily fish: e.g. herring, mackerel, sardines, tuna, salmon.	Fish fried in suitable oil. Shellfish.	Fish roe.
Fruit/ vegetables	All fresh and frozen vegetables. Peas, beans, sweetcorn, dried beans of all kinds: e.g. haricot, red kidney, butter beans, lentils, chick peas, are particularly high in 'soluble fibre'. Jacket or boiled potatoes, eat skins wherever possible. Fresh fruit, unsweetened tinned fruit, dried fruit.	Chips and roast potatoes if cooked in suitable polyunsaturated fat. Avocado pears, fruit in syrup, crystallized fruit.	Chips or roast potatoes cooked in unsuitable oil or fat. Oven chips. Potato crisps.
	Walnuts, chestnuts.	Almonds, brazil nuts, hazelnuts.	Coconut.
Cereal foods	Wholemeal flour, wholemeal bread, wholegrain cereals, oatmeal, cornmeal, porridge oats, sweetcorn, wholegrain rice & pasta, crispbreads, oatcakes, matzos.	White flour, white bread, sugary breakfast cereals, muesli, white rice & pasta, plain semi-sweet biscuits, water biscuits.	Fancy breads: e.g. croissants, brioche, savoury cheese biscuits, bought pastry.
Prepared foods	Low-fat puddings: e.g. jelly, sorbet, skimmed milk pudding, low-fat yoghurt, low-fat sauces.	Cakes, pastry, puddings, biscuits & sauces made with suitable margarine or oil. Home made snacks made with polyunsaturated fat.	Cakes and pastry puddings and biscuits made with saturated fats. Suet dumplings and puddings, butter and cream sauces. All proprietary puddings and sauces. Deep-fried snacks. Dairy ice-cream.
Beverages	Tea, coffee, mineral water, slimline or sugar-free soft drinks, unsweetened fruit juice. Clear soups, homemade vegetable soup. Low alcohol beer.	Sweet soft drinks, low-fat malted drinks or low-fat drinking chocolate, occasionally. Packet soups, meat soups, alcohol.	Irish coffee. Full-fat malted drinks, drinking chocolate. Cream soups.
Preserves, spreads, sweets	Clear pickles. Sugar-free sweeteners: e.g. saccharin tablets or liquid aspartame sweetener.	Sweet pickles & chutney, jam, marmalade, honey, syrup, marzipan, peanut butter & lemon curd. Boiled sweets, pastilles, peppermints, sugar, sorbitol, glucose, fructose.	Chocolate spreads, mincemeat containing suet. Toffees, fudge, butterscotch, chocolate, coconut bars.
Miscellaneous	Herbs, spices, mustard, pepper, vinegar. Low-fat dressings: e.g. lemon or low-fat yoghurt.	Meat & fish pastes. Low-calorie salad cream or low-calorie mayonnaise, bottled sauces. French dressing, sparingly. Soy sauce.	Ordinary salad cream, mayonnaise, cream or cream cheese dressings.

Modified from, and with acknowledgement to, the Nutrition and Dietetic Department, The John Radcliffe Hospital, Oxford, U.K.

Appendix 2

Guidelines for body weight (based on Bray[4], and Royal College of Physicians of London[5]. The minimum level for diagnosing obesity is taken as 20% above the upper limit of the acceptable weight range.

Height without shoes (m)	Men Weight without clothes (kg)			Women Weight without clothes (kg)		
	Acceptable average	Acceptable weight range	Obese	Acceptable average	Acceptable weight range	Obese
1·45				46·0	42–53	64
1·48				46·5	42–54	65
1·50				47·0	43–55	66
1·52				48·5	44–57	68
1·54				49·5	44–58	70
1·56				50·4	45–58	70
1·58	55·8	51–64	77	51·3	46–59	71
1·60	57·6	52–65	78	52·6	48–61	73
1·62	58·6	53–66	79	54·0	49–62	74
1·64	59·6	54–67	80	55·4	50–64	77
1·66	60·6	55–69	83	56·8	51–63	78
1·68	61·7	56–71	85	58·1	52–66	79
1·70	63·5	58–73	88	60·0	53–67	80
1·72	65·0	59–74	89	61·3	55–69	83
1·74	66·5	60–75	90	62·6	56–70	84
1·76	68·0	62–77	92	64·0	58–72	86
1·78	69·4	64–79	95	65·3	59–74	89
1·80	71·0	65–80	96			
1·82	72·6	66–82	98			
1·84	74·2	67–84	101			
1·86	75·8	69–86	103			
1·88	77·6	71–88	106			
1·90	79·3	73–90	108			
1·92	81·0	75–93	112			
BMI	22·0	20·1–25·0	30·0	20·8	18·7–23·8	28·6

Appendix 3

Nomogram for the determination of LDL-C (in mg dl^{-1}).

To convert cholesterol mg dl^{-1} to mmol l^{-1}, divide by 38·6.

Appendix 4

Dosage range and untoward effects of lipid-lowering drugs.

Drug	Daily dosage	Contraindications	Adverse effects	Drug interactions
Cholestyramine	2–6 × 4 g	A 9, 10, 15	B 1	C 1, 3, 4, 5, 6, 7, 8, 9, 10
Colestipol	2–6 × 5 g	A 9, 10, 15	B 1	C 1, 3, 4, 5, 6, 7, 8, 9, 10
Lovastatin	20–80 mg	A 1, 3, 4, 14	B 1, 2, 4, 8, 11	
Simvastatin	20–40 mg	A 1, 3, 4, 14	B 1, 2, 4, 8, 11	
Nicotinic acid	3 × 1–2 g	A 1, 6, 7, 8, 16	B 1, 2, 7, 8, 12, 13, 14	C 2
Probucol	2 × 500 mg	A 1, 3, 4, 12, 17	B 1, 5, 8, 11, 16	
Bezafibrate	3 × 200 mg or 1 × 400 mg	A 1, 2, 3, 4, 5, 14	B 1, 2, 3, 4, 5, 6	C 1
Ciprofibrate	100–200 mg	A 1, 2, 3, 4, ? 5, 14	B 1, 2, 3, 4, 5, 8	C 1
Clofibrate	3–4 × 500 mg	A 1, 2, 3, 4, 5, 14	B 1, 2, 3, 4, 5, 6, 8	C 1
Fenofibrate	3 × 100 mg or 1 × 250 mg	A 1, 2, 3, 4, 5, 14	B 1, 2, 3, 4, 5, 6	C 1
Gemfibrozil	2 × 600 mg	A 1, 2, 3, 4, 5, 14	B 1, 2, 3, 4, 5, 6	C 1, 2

Based upon Physician's Desk Report, Rote Liste, and other sources.

(A) Contraindications: 1, hepatic dysfunction, hepatitis; 2, severe renal dysfunction; 3, pregnancy; 4, lactation; 5, gallbladder disease; 6, congestive heart failure; 7, recent myocardial infarction; 8, acute haemorrhage; 9, nephrolithiasis; 10, hyperparathyroidism; 11, hypothyroidism; 12, cholestasis; 13, inflammatory bowel disease; 14, hypersensitivity; 15, acute peptic ulcer; 16, gout; 17, arrhythmia.

(B) Adverse reactions: 1, gastrointestinal disorders; 2, hepatic dysfunction, increased liver enzymes; 3, cholelithiasis or increased lithogenicity; 4, myositis or increased creatine phosphokinase; 5, disturbance of potency; 6, hair loss; 7, severe flushing; 8, pruritus, urticaria or rash; 9, feeling of anxiety; 10, tachycardia; 11, transient headache; 12, hyperacidity; 13, hypotension; 14, impaired glucose tolerance; 15, cardiac arrhythmias; 16, QT prolongation in the ECG.

(C) Drug interactions: 1, coumarin anticoagulants; 2, oral hypoglycaemics; 3, digitalis glycosides; 4, thyroid hormones; 5, tetracyclines; 6, phenylbutazone; 7, propranolol; 8, chlorothiazide; 9, phenobarbitone; 10, penicillin G.

Appendix 5

MEMBERS OF THE STUDY GROUP

Co-chairmen: G. Assmann (F.R.G.), B. Lewis (U.K.), M. Mancini (Italy), Y. Stein (Israel).

Members of Panel: R. Carmena (Spain), G. Crepaldi (Italy), G. De Backer (Belgium), J. L. de Gennes (France), S. Eisenberg (Israel), D. Galton (U.K.), A. M. Gotto (U.S.A.) (adviser), J. F. Goodwin (U.K.), H. Greten (F.R.G.), M. Hanefeld (G.D.R.), J. K. Huttunen (Finland), B. Jacotot (France), M. B. Katan (The Netherlands), J. I. Mann (U.K.), T. A. Miettinen (Finland), K. R. Norum (Norway), R. G. Oganov (U.S.S.R.), A. G. Olsson (Sweden), R. Paoletti (Italy), D. Pometta (Switzerland), K. Pyorala (Finland), G. Schettler (F.R.G.), J. Shepherd (U.K.), P. Schwandt (F.R.G.), M. J. Tikkanen (Finland).

Special Article

Report of the National Cholesterol Education Program Expert Panel on Detection, Evaluation, and Treatment of High Blood Cholesterol in Adults

The Expert Panel

• This report of an expert panel of the National Cholesterol Education Program provides new guidelines for the treatment of high blood cholesterol in adults 20 years of age and over. Total cholesterol levels are classified as follows: <200 mg/dL —"desirable blood cholesterol"; 200 to 239 mg/dL—borderline–high blood cholesterol; ≥240 mg/dL—high blood cholesterol. The guidelines detail which patients should go on to have lipoprotein analysis, and which should receive cholesterol-lowering treatment on the basis of their low density lipoprotein (LDL)–cholesterol levels and status with respect to other coronary heart disease risk factors. Dietary therapy is the primary cholesterol-lowering treatment. The report specifies the LDL-cholesterol levels at which dietary therapy should be started and the goals of therapy, and provides detailed guidance on the nature of the recommended dietary changes. If, after six months of intensive dietary therapy, LDL-cholesterol exceeds specified levels, drug treatment should be considered.

(*Arch Intern Med* 1988;148:36-69)

OVERVIEW AND SUMMARY

Increased blood cholesterol levels, or, more specifically, increased levels of low density lipoprotein (LDL)–cholesterol, are causally related to an increased risk of coronary heart disease (CHD). Coronary risk rises progressively with an increase in cholesterol level, particularly when cholesterol levels rise above 200 mg/dL (for Système International [SI] conversions throughout text, refer to Appendix I, Table 1). There is also substantial evidence that lowering total and LDL-cholesterol levels will reduce the incidence of CHD.

Two approaches can be used to lower blood cholesterol levels. The first is the subject of this report: a patient-based approach that seeks to identify individuals at high risk who will benefit from intensive intervention efforts. The goal here is to establish criteria that define the candidates for medical intervention and to provide guidelines on how to detect, set goals for, treat, and monitor

Accepted for publication Sept 28, 1987.
From the National Cholesterol Education Program, National Heart, Lung, and Blood Institute, Bethesda, Md.
Reprint requests to Coordinator, National Cholesterol Education Program, National Heart, Lung, and Blood Institute, Bldg 31, Room 4A 05, Bethesda, MD 20892 (Dr Cleeman).

these patients over time. The second approach, the population (public health) strategy, aims to shift the distribution of cholesterol levels in the entire population to a lower range. These two approaches are complementary and, together, represent a coordinated strategy aimed at reducing cholesterol levels and coronary risk.

Case finding: Initial Classification by Total Blood Cholesterol (Table 1)

Serum total cholesterol should be measured in all adults 20 years of age and over at least once every five years; this measurement may be made in the nonfasting state. Levels below 200 mg/dL are classified as "desirable blood cholesterol," those 200 to 239 mg/dL as "borderline–high blood cholesterol," and those 240 mg/dL and above as "high blood cholesterol." The cutpoint that defines high blood cholesterol (240 mg/dL) is a value above which risk of CHD rises steeply, and corresponds approximately to the 75th percentile for the adult US population. The cutpoints recommended in this report are uniform for adult men and women of all ages.

MEMBERS OF THE NATIONAL CHOLESTEROL EDUCATION PROGRAM EXPERT PANEL ON DETECTION, EVALUATION, AND TREATMENT OF HIGH BLOOD CHOLESTEROL IN ADULTS

Panel Chairman.—DeWitt S. Goodman, MD
Prevalence, Detection, Diagnosis, and Evaluation Subcommittee.—*Chairman*: Stephen B. Hulley, MD, MPH; Luther T. Clark, MD; C. E. Davis, PhD; Valentin Fuster, MD; John C. LaRosa, MD; Albert Oberman, MD; Ernst J. Schaefer, MD; Daniel Steinberg, MD, PhD.
Diet Treatment Subcommittee.—*Co-Chairmen*: W. Virgil Brown, MD, and Scott M. Grundy, MD, PhD; Diane Becker, RN, MPH, ScD; Edwin Bierman, MD; Jacqueline Sooter-Bochenek, RD, MS; Rebecca Mullis, RD, PhD; Neil Stone, MD.
Drug Treatment Subcommittee.—*Chairman*: Donald B. Hunninghake, MD; Jacqueline M. Dunbar, RN, PhD; Henry N. Ginsberg, MD; D. Roger Illingworth, MD, PhD; Harold C. Sadin, MD; Gustav Schonfeld, MD.
Executive Director of the Panel.—James I. Cleeman, MD.
Ex-Officio Members.—H. Bryan Brewer, Jr, MD; Nancy Ernst, MS, RD; William Friedewald, MD; Jeffrey M. Hoeg, MD; Basil Rifkind, MD.
Consultant.—David Gordon, MD, PhD.

Table 1.—Initial Classification and Recommended Followup Based on Total Cholesterol*	
Classification, mg/dL	
<200	Desirable blood cholesterol
200 to 239	Borderline–high blood cholesterol
≥240	High blood cholesterol
Recommended followup	
Total cholesterol, <200 mg/dL	Repeat within five years
Total cholesterol, 200-239 mg/dL	
Without definite CHD or two other CHD risk factors (one of which can be male sex)	Dietary information and recheck annually
With definite CHD or two other CHD risk factors (one of which can be male sex)	Lipoprotein analysis; further action based on LDL-cholesterol level
Total cholesterol ≥240 mg/dL	

*CHD indicates coronary heart disease; LDL, low density lipoprotein.

Table 2.—Classification and Treatment Decisions Based on LDL-Cholesterol*		
Classification, mg/dL		
<130	Desirable LDL-cholesterol	
130 to 159	Borderline-high-risk LDL-cholesterol	
≥160	High-risk LDL-cholesterol	
	Initiation Level, mg/dL	Minimal Goal, mg/dL
Dietary treatment		
Without CHD or two other risk factors†	≥160	<160‡
With CHD or two other risk factors†	≥130	<130§
Drug treatment		
Without CHD or two other risk factors†	≥190	<160
With CHD or two other risk factors†	≥160	<130

*LDL indicates low density lipoprotein; CHD, coronary heart disease.

†Patients have a lower initiation level and goal if they are at high risk because they already have definite CHD, or because they have any two of the following risk factors: male sex, family history of premature CHD, cigarette smoking, hypertension, low high density lipoprotein (HDL)–cholesterol, diabetes mellitus, definite cerebrovascular or peripheral vascular disease, or severe obesity.

‡Roughly equivalent to total cholesterol level of <240 mg/dL‡ or <200 mg/dL.

§As goals for monitoring dietary treatment.

Along with cholesterol testing, all adults should also be evaluated for the presence of other CHD risk factors, including hypertension, cigarette smoking, diabetes mellitus, severe obesity, and a history of CHD in the patient or of premature CHD in family members. Patients with other risk factors should be given other forms of preventive care as appropriate.

Patients with desirable blood cholesterol levels (<200 mg/dL) should be given general dietary and risk reduction educational materials, and advised to have another serum cholesterol test within five years. Patients with cholesterol levels 200 mg/dL or greater should have the value confirmed by repeating the test; the average of the two test results is then used to guide subsequent decisions. Patients with high blood cholesterol (≥240 mg/dL) should undergo lipoprotein analysis, as should those with a borderline–high blood cholesterol (200 to 239 mg/dL) who are at high risk because they have definite CHD or two other CHD risk factors; in this report male sex is considered a risk factor for the purpose of estimating risk status. Patients with confirmed borderline–high blood cholesterol levels who do not have CHD or two other risk factors do not need further evaluation and active medical therapy; they should be given the dietary information designed for the general population and reevaluated at one year.

Some experts believe that patients in the borderline–high blood cholesterol group who have one other risk factor (eg, hypertension), or who are of younger age (20 to 39 years), should also undergo lipoprotein analysis. Although this is not recommended here as a general approach for the borderline–high blood cholesterol group, it is clear that individualized clinical judgment and patient management is appropriate for this group.

Deciding to Treat: Classification by LDL-Cholesterol (Table 2)

Once someone is identified as requiring lipoprotein analysis, the focus of attention should shift from total cholesterol to LDL-cholesterol. The ultimate objective of case finding and screening is to identify individuals with elevated LDL-cholesterol levels. Similarly, the specific goal of treatment is to lower LDL-cholesterol levels. Hence, the level of LDL-cholesterol will serve as the key index for clinical decision making about cholesterol-lowering therapy.

Lipoprotein analysis involves measurement of the fasting levels of total cholesterol, total triglyceride, and high density lipoprotein (HDL)–cholesterol. From these values, LDL-cholesterol is calculated as follows: LDL-Cholesterol = Total Cholesterol − HDL-Cholesterol − (Triglyceride/5).

Levels of LDL-cholesterol of 160 mg/dL or greater are classified as "high-risk LDL-cholesterol," and those 130 to 159 mg/dL as "borderline–high-risk LDL-cholesterol." Patients with high-risk LDL-cholesterol levels, and those with borderline-high-risk LDL-cholesterol levels who have definite CHD or two other risk factors (one of which can be male sex), should have a complete clinical evaluation and then begin cholesterol-lowering treatment. A basic principle adopted in this report is that the presence of other risk factors or definite CHD warrants initiating treatment at lower LDL-cholesterol levels and the setting of lower LDL-cholesterol treatment goals. In this scheme, a low level of HDL-cholesterol (below 35 mg/dL) is considered another risk factor (like hypertension) that will affect the assessment of overall coronary risk, and, in this way, influence clinical decisions about treatment.

The clinical evaluation should include a complete history, physical examination, and basic laboratory tests. This workup will aim to determine whether the high LDL-cholesterol level is secondary to another disease or a drug, and whether or not a familial lipid disorder is present. The patient's total coronary risk and clinical status, as well as age and sex, should be considered in developing a cholesterol-lowering treatment program.

Dietary Treatment

Treatment begins with dietary therapy. The minimal goals of therapy are to lower LDL-cholesterol to levels below the cutpoints for initiating therapy, ie, to below 160 mg/dL, or to below 130 mg/dL if definite CHD or two other CHD risk factors are present. Ideally, even lower levels of LDL-cholesterol should be attained, if possible, to achieve a further reduction in risk.

Although the goal of therapy is to lower the LDL-cholesterol level, most patients can be managed during dietary therapy on the basis of their total cholesterol levels. This has the advantage of avoiding the additional costs and the need for a fasting blood specimen involved in the measurement of LDL-cholesterol levels. Serum total cholesterol levels of 240 and 200 mg/dL correspond roughly to LDL-cholesterol levels of 160 and 130 mg/dL, respectively. Thus, the monitoring goals during dietary therapy are to lower the serum total cholesterol level to below 240 mg/dL for patients with an LDL-cholesterol goal of <160 mg/dL, or to below 200 mg/dL for patients with an LDL-cholesterol goal of <130 mg/dL.

The general aim of dietary therapy is to reduce elevated cholesterol levels while maintaining a nutritionally adequate eating pattern. Dietary therapy should occur in two steps, the Step-One and Step-Two Diets, that are designed to progressively reduce intakes of saturated fatty acids and cholesterol, and to promote weight loss in patients who are overweight by eliminating excess total calories. The Step-One Diet should be prescribed and explained by the physician and his or her staff. This diet involves an intake of total fat less than 30% of calories, saturated fatty acids less than 10% of calories, and cholesterol less than 300 mg/d. The Step-Two Diet, used if the response to the Step-One Diet is insufficient, calls for a further reduction in saturated fatty acid intake to less than 7% of calories and in cholesterol to less than 200 mg/d. The Step-One Diet calls for the reduction of the major and obvious sources of saturated fatty acids and cholesterol in the diet; for many patients this can be achieved without a radical alteration in dietary habits. The Step-Two Diet requires careful attention to the whole diet so as to reduce intake of saturated fatty acids and cholesterol to a minimal level compatible with an acceptable and nutritious diet. Involvement of a registered dietitian is very useful, particularly for intensive dietary therapy such as the Step-Two Diet.

After starting the Step-One Diet, the serum total cholesterol level should be measured and adherence to the diet assessed at four to six weeks and at three months. If the total cholesterol monitoring goal is met, then the LDL-cholesterol level should be measured to confirm that the LDL goal has been achieved. If this is the case, the patient enters a long-term monitoring program, and is seen quarterly for the first year and twice yearly thereafter. At these visits total cholesterol levels should be measured, and dietary and behavior modifications reinforced.

If the cholesterol goal has not been achieved with the Step-One Diet, the patient should generally be referred to a registered dietitian. With the aid of the dietitian, the patient should progress to the Step-Two Diet, or to another trial on the Step-One Diet (with progression to the Step-Two Diet if the response is still not satisfactory). On the Step-Two Diet, total cholesterol levels should again be measured and adherence to the diet assessed after four to six weeks and at three months of therapy. If the desired goal for total cholesterol (and for LDL-cholesterol) lowering has been attained, long-term monitoring can begin. If not, drug therapy should be considered. A minimum of six months of intensive dietary therapy and counseling should usually be carried out before initiating drug therapy; shorter periods can be considered in patients with severe elevations of LDL-cholesterol (>225 mg/dL) or with definite CHD. Drug therapy should be added to dietary therapy, and not substituted for it.

Drug Treatment

Drug therapy should be considered for an adult patient who, despite dietary therapy, has an LDL-cholesterol level of 190 mg/dL or higher if the patient does not have definite CHD or two other risk factors (one of which can be male sex). If the patient does have definite CHD or two other risk factors, then drug therapy should be considered at LDL-cholesterol levels of 160 mg/dL or higher. The goals of drug therapy are the same as those of dietary therapy: to lower LDL-cholesterol to below 160 mg/dL, or to below 130 mg/dL if definite CHD or two other risk factors are present. These are minimal goals; if possible, considerably lower levels of LDL-cholesterol should be attained.

Individualized clinical judgment is needed for patients who do not meet these criteria for drug therapy, but have not attained their minimal goals on dietary therapy. These patients include those without definite CHD or two other risk factors whose LDL-cholesterol levels remain in the range of 160 to 190 mg/dL, and patients with CHD or two other risk factors whose LDL-cholesterol levels remain in the range of 130 to 160 mg/dL, on adequate dietary therapy. In general, maximal efforts should be made in this group to achieve lower cholesterol levels and lower CHD risk by means of nonpharmacologic approaches. Consideration should also be given to the use of low doses of bile acid sequestrants in these patients, especially in males. Moreover, many experts feel that patients with definite CHD should receive drug therapy if their minimal LDL-cholesterol goal (<130 mg/dL) has not been reached.

The drugs of first choice are the bile acid sequestrants (cholestyramine, colestipol) and nicotinic acid. Both cholestyramine and nicotinic acid have been shown to lower CHD risk in clinical trials, and their long-term safety has been established. However, these drugs require considerable patient education to achieve effective adherence. Nicotinic acid is the preferred drug in patients with concurrent hypertriglyceridemia (triglyceride levels ≥250 mg/dL), because bile acid sequestrants tend to increase triglyceride levels.

A new class of drugs, to be considered after the bile acid sequestrants and nicotinic acid, is the 3-hydroxy-3-methyl glutaryl coenzyme-A (HMG CoA) reductase inhibitors (eg, lovastatin). These drugs are very effective in lowering LDL-cholesterol levels, but their effects on CHD incidence and their long-term safety have not yet been established.

Other available drugs include gemfibrozil, probucol, and clofibrate. Gemfibrozil and clofibrate are fibric acid derivatives; they are primarily effective for lowering elevated triglyceride levels, but are not approved by the Food and Drug Administration for routine use in lowering cholesterol levels.

After starting drug therapy, the LDL-cholesterol level should be measured at four to six weeks, and then again at three months. If the response to drug therapy is adequate (ie, the LDL-cholesterol goal has been achieved), then the patient should be seen every four months, or more frequently when drugs requiring closer followup are used, in order to monitor the cholesterol response and possible side effects of therapy. For long-term monitoring, serum total cholesterol alone can be measured at most follow-up visits, with lipoprotein analysis (and LDL-cholesterol estimation) carried out once a year.

If the response to initial drug therapy is not adequate, the patient should be switched to another drug, or to a combination of two drugs. The combination of a bile acid sequestrant with either nicotinic acid or an HMG CoA reductase inhibitor has the potential of lowering LDL-cholesterol levels by 40% to 50% or more. The combination of colestipol and nicotinic acid has been shown to beneficially influence coronary atherosclerotic lesions. For most patients, the judicious use of one or two drugs should be able to provide an adequate LDL-cholesterol–lowering effect.

Drug therapy is likely to continue for many years, or for a lifetime. Hence, the decision to add drug therapy to the regimen should be made only after vigorous efforts at dietary treatment have not proven sufficient. The patient must be well informed about the goals and side effects of medication and the need for long-term commitment. In the ideal treatment setting, the management of high-risk cholesterol levels would call on the expertise of a variety of professionals. The office nurse or physician's assistant can help greatly in promoting adherence to dietary and drug therapy. A registered dietitian can be of great value in dietary therapy. The pharmacist can help to provide counseling and promote adherence with drug therapy. Consultation with a lipid specialist is useful for patients with unusually severe, complex, or refractory lipid disorders.

CLASSIFICATION, PREVALENCE, DETECTION, AND EVALUATION
Background and Introduction

This report provides practical guidelines for clinicians to use in measuring and reducing blood cholesterol in adult patients. (This report addresses patients 20 years of age and above; a separate panel will provide guidelines for children and adolescents.) The report adds a more specific set of recommendations to basic policies set forth by previous bodies, notably the National Institutes of Health (NIH) Consensus Development Conference on Lowering Blood Cholesterol to Prevent Heart Disease.[1] While it is recognized that approaches for modifying the cholesterol levels in whole population groups are important, this report focuses on caring for individual patients.

Basic Description of Lipids and Lipoproteins.—Cholesterol is a fatlike substance (lipid) that is a key component of cell membranes and a precursor of bile acids and steroid hormones. Cholesterol travels in the circulation in spherical particles containing both lipids and proteins called lipoproteins. The cholesterol level in blood plasma is determined partly by inheritance and partly by the fat and cholesterol content of the diet. Other factors such as obesity and physical inactivity may also play a role.

Three major classes of lipoproteins can be measured in the serum of a fasting individual: very low density lipoproteins (VLDL), LDL, and HDL. The LDL are the major atherogenic class, and, typically, contain 60% to 70% of the total serum cholesterol. The HDL usually contain 20% to 30% of the total cholesterol, and their levels are inversely correlated with risk for CHD. The VLDL, which are largely composed of triglycerides, contain 10% to 15% of the total serum cholesterol.

Because most of the cholesterol in the serum is found in the LDL, the concentration of total cholesterol is closely correlated with the concentration of LDL-cholesterol. Thus, while LDL-cholesterol is the actual target of cholesterol-lowering efforts, total cholesterol can be used in its place in the initial stages of evaluating a patient's serum lipids. Testing for serum total cholesterol is more available and less expensive and does not require that the patient be fasting. On the other hand, LDL-cholesterol offers more precision as a risk factor and is therefore preferred for clinical decisions about interventions to lower blood cholesterol, especially in patients who may be candidates for cholesterol-lowering drugs.

Rationale for Intervention.—*The Evidence That LDL-Cholesterol Is a Cause of CHD.*—The conclusion that high levels of LDL-cholesterol are a cause of coronary athero-

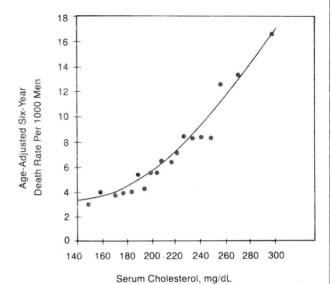

Fig 1.—Relationship of serum cholesterol to coronary heart disease (CHD) death in 361 662 men 35 to 57 years of age during an average followup of six years. Each point represents median value for 5% of the population.[5] Key points are as follows: (1) risk increases steadily, particularly above levels of 200 mg/dL; and (2) the magnitude of the increased risk is large, fourfold in the top 10% as compared with the bottom 10%.

sclerosis and produce an increased risk of CHD comes from the congruent results of many studies.

EPIDEMIOLOGIC EVIDENCE.—A large body of epidemiologic evidence supports a direct relationship between the level of serum total and LDL-cholesterol and the rate of CHD.[2-4] Comparisons among various populations throughout the world reveal a direct correlation between serum cholesterol levels and CHD rates. People who have migrated to a country that has a higher average serum cholesterol level gradually acquire the dietary habits, serum cholesterol level, and CHD rates of their new country. Prospective studies of the individuals within a population have uniformly shown that serum cholesterol levels predict the future occurrence of CHD morbidity and mortality. This association is continuous throughout the range of cholesterol levels in the population (Fig 1).[5,6] At higher levels of serum cholesterol, the relationship becomes particularly strong. For persons with cholesterol values in the top 10% of the population distribution, the risk of CHD mortality is four times as high as the risk in the bottom 10% of the population.

GENETIC AND PHYSIOLOGIC EVIDENCE.—Premature CHD can result from high LDL-cholesterol levels even in the absence of any other risk factors.[7] This is most clearly demonstrated in children who have the rare homozygous familial hypercholesterolemia, a disorder characterized by the absence of the specific cell-surface receptors that normally remove LDL from the circulation.[8] The LDL-cholesterol levels can be as high as 1000 mg/dL, and severe atherosclerosis and CHD can develop during the first two decades of life. Patients with the more common heterozygous form of familial hypercholesterolemia and partial deficiencies of LDL-receptor function commonly develop premature CHD in the middle decades of life.

ANIMAL MODEL EVIDENCE.—Animal models have demonstrated important relationships between LDL-cholesterol and atherosclerosis.[9] Many animal species (including monkeys and baboons) develop atherosclerosis when fed diets that raise their serum cholesterol levels. These hypercholesterolemic animals develop intimal lesions that progress from fatty streaks to complicated ulcerated plaques resembling those of human atherosclerosis. Severe atherosclerosis in monkeys regresses when the blood cholesterol is lowered substantially for an extended period by diet or drugs. These studies thus support a causal relationship between LDL-cholesterol and atherosclerosis, and suggest that this process may be reversible under some circumstances.

The Evidence That Reducing LDL-Cholesterol Levels Will Prevent CHD.—The evidence noted above from epidemiologic, genetic, and animal investigations strongly supports a causal link between elevated serum cholesterol levels and CHD. In addition, clinical trials have shown that this risk can be altered—that lowering LDL-cholesterol in men with high levels decreases the incidence of CHD.

The issue of whether lowering LDL-cholesterol levels by dietary and drug interventions can reduce the incidence of CHD has been addressed in more than a dozen randomized clinical trials. One of the largest, the Coronary Primary Prevention Trial, which compared the cholesterol-lowering drug cholestyramine with a placebo, produced statistically significant reductions in LDL-cholesterol levels and in the incidence of CHD.[10] An aggregate analysis that pools the results of serum cholesterol-lowering trials confirms an effect on CHD incidence. Moreover, the Coronary Drug Project has shown a significant decrease in overall mortality (compared with the placebo group) in a long-term followup of men treated with nicotinic acid after myocardial infarction.[11] In addition, a recent angiographic study showed that cholesterol-lowering dietary and drug therapy slowed the progression and produced regression of coronary atherosclerosis in men with bypass grafts.[12]

In summary, these findings support the conclusion that lowering total and LDL-cholesterol levels will reduce the subsequent incidence of CHD events. Moreover, the pooled analysis of clinical trial findings suggests that intervention is as effective in secondary prevention (preventing recurrent myocardial infarction and death in patients who have had a heart attack) as it is in primary prevention. The direct evidence from clinical trials is strongest in middle-aged men with high initial cholesterol levels. However, the complete set of evidence, including the epidemiologic observations and animal experiments, strongly supports the generalization that reducing total and LDL-cholesterol levels is also likely to reduce CHD incidence in younger and older men, in women, and in individuals with more moderate elevations of cholesterol.

The Magnitude of the Reduction in CHD.—Epidemiologic studies and clinical trials are remarkably consistent in supporting the projection that for individuals with serum cholesterol levels initially in the 250 to 300 mg/dL range, each 1% reduction in serum cholesterol level yields approximately a 2% reduction in CHD rates.[13] Thus, for example, it is reasonable to estimate that a 10% to 15% reduction in serum cholesterol level resulting from the diets recommended in this report should reduce CHD risk by 20% to 30%.

The *absolute magnitude* of these benefits will probably be greatest in patients who are at high risk because of the presence of other risk factors, such as cigarette smoking and hypertension. This concept is illustrated in Table 3 using data from the Multiple Risk Factor Intervention Trial (MRFIT). Among nonsmokers with normal blood pressure, the risk of CHD death per 1000 men in the six years of observation was 6.4 in the top quintile of serum cholesterol and 1.6 in the bottom quintile, a difference of

Table 3.—Coronary Heart Disease Deaths per 1000 in Men 35 to 57 Years of Age With an Average Followup of Six Years According to Serum Cholesterol Quintile and Presence or Absence of Other Risk Factors.[14] The Difference in Absolute Risk in the Highest vs the Lowest Quintile of Serum Cholesterol Is Greater in Patients Who Are at High Risk for Other Reasons

Serum Cholesterol Quintile, mg/dL	Normotensive Nonsmoker	Hypertensive Smoker
<182	1.6	6.3
182 to 202	2.5	10.0
203 to 220	2.7	15.5
221 to 244	3.8	16.6
≥245	6.4	21.4

4.8. Among smokers with hypertension, the comparable figures were 21.4 and 6.3, a difference of 15.1. Thus, an intervention that lowered cholesterol levels from the highest to the lowest quintile should have three times the benefit (15 vs five deaths prevented per thousand persons) when applied to men who have the other two risk factors (assuming no change in those other risk factors). These risk relationships are the basis for recommending lower cholesterol cutpoints and goals for treating patients who, for other reasons (in addition to cholesterol), are at high risk for developing CHD.

Classification of Patients by Total and LDL-Cholesterol Levels.—Population distributions for serum total cholesterol and LDL-cholesterol levels in the United States are provided in Appendix I, Tables. To convert serum values to plasma, multiply by 0.97. To convert cholesterol values in milligrams per deciliter to millimoles per liter, multiply by 0.02586. To convert triglyceride values in milligrams per deciliter to millimoles per liter, multiply by 0.01129.

The classification system (Fig 2) begins with measurement of the total cholesterol level. Serum is most frequently used for this measurement, and cholesterol levels in this report are stated as serum values. (Cholesterol levels can also be measured on plasma. If, as is customary, ethylenediaminetetraacetic acid [EDTA] is used as an anticoagulant, the results should be multiplied by 1.03 to arrive at the serum equivalent.) Levels below 200 mg/dL are classified as "desirable blood cholesterol," those 200 to 239 mg/dL as "borderline-high blood cholesterol," and those 240 mg/dL and above (corresponding to approximately the top 25% of the entire adult population 20 years of age and above) as "high blood cholesterol."

Patients with high blood cholesterol need additional evaluation and are further classified for the purposes of clinical decisions about possible dietary and drug treatment by performing lipoprotein analysis and estimating the more specific determinant of CHD risk, the LDL-cholesterol level. Levels of LDL-cholesterol that are 160 mg/dL and above are classified as "high-risk LDL-cholesterol."

Because the relationship between serum cholesterol level and CHD is a continuous and steadily increasing one (Fig 1), these cutpoints are necessarily somewhat arbitrary. However, this is also true of other risk factors, such as blood pressure, and the success of basing clinical decisions on whether or not a patient is classified as hypertensive indicates the value of establishing cutpoints for clinical decisions. The 240 mg/dL cutpoint for total serum cholesterol is a level at which CHD risk is almost double that at 200 mg/dL, and is rising steeply. Patients with cholesterol levels at or above this cutpoint have sufficiently high risk

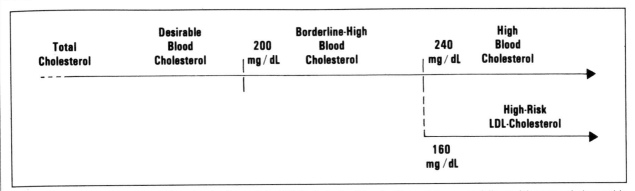

Fig 2.—Classification by total and low density lipoprotein (LDL)–cholesterol levels. Key points are as follows: (1) serum cholesterol is used for initial classification; (2) low density lipoprotein–cholesterol is used for those with high levels.

to warrant more detailed evaluation and possible treatment.

Other Risk Factors for CHD.—Coronary heart disease is a disease of multifactorial etiology, and other risk factors should also be considered in preventive medical efforts. These include modifiable factors like hypertension and cigarette smoking, which are appropriate targets for intervention efforts. (Assistance in intervention efforts aimed at hypertension and cigarette smoking may be obtained from two National Heart, Lung, and Blood Institute publications: "The 1984 Report of the Joint National Committee on Detection, Evaluation, and Treatment of High Blood Pressure" [to be updated in 1988]; and "Clinical Opportunities for Smoking Intervention—A Guide for the Busy Physician.") Everyone tested for blood cholesterol should also be examined for other risk factors (Table 4), and intervention should be undertaken as appropriate. All patients should receive educational materials that describe general dietary and life-style approaches to reducing the risk of CHD. (These materials may be obtained from a variety of sources—see the list in the National Cholesterol Education Program publication "Cholesterol Resources for the Physician.") Advice to quit smoking is particularly important because it has the potential not only to reduce CHD risk by 50%, but also to prevent cancer and chronic lung disease.

In addition to being candidates for intervention, these modifiable factors increase the absolute level of CHD risk and thereby enhance the potential value of reducing cholesterol levels. This is also true for the fixed risk factors like older age, male sex, family history of premature CHD, and CHD in the patient. Two other lipid and lipoprotein factors that have a bearing on CHD, HDL-cholesterol and triglyceride, are not dealt with in this report as direct targets for intervention but enter into clinical decisions in ways that are discussed in the sections that follow and in Appendix II.

The Patient-Based Approach and the Population-Based Approach.—The 1984 Consensus Conference and other groups have recommended two major strategies for preventing CHD by lowering blood cholesterol levels.[1,13-15] One is the subject of this report: a patient-based approach that seeks to identify individuals at high risk who will benefit from intensive intervention efforts. The goal here is to establish total and LDL-cholesterol cutpoints that define the candidates for medical intervention, and to provide guidelines on how to detect, set goals for, treat, and monitor these patients over time.

The other strategy is the population-based approach that

Table 4.—Risk Status Based on Presence of CHD Risk Factors Other Than LDL–Cholesterol
The patient is considered to have a high risk status if he or she has one of the following:
Definite CHD: the characteristic clinical picture and objective laboratory findings of either:
Definite prior myocardial infarction, or
Definite myocardial ischemia, such as angina pectoris
Two other CHD risk factors:
Male sex*
Family history of premature CHD (definite myocardial infarction or sudden death before 55 years of age in a parent or sibling)
Cigarette smoking (currently smokes more than ten cigarettes per day)
Hypertension
Low HDL–cholesterol concentration (below 35 mg/dL confirmed by repeated measurement)
Diabetes mellitus
History of definite cerebrovascular or occlusive peripheral vascular disease
Severe obesity (≥30% overweight)

*Male sex is considered a risk factor in this scheme because the rates of CHD are three to four times higher in men than in women in the middle decades of life and roughly two times higher in the elderly. Hence, a man with one other CHD risk factor is considered to have a high-risk status, whereas a woman is not so considered unless she has two other CHD risk factors.

seeks to lower the mean serum cholesterol level by modifying the dietary habits of the entire population. This strategy has the general goal of lowering the serum cholesterol levels of the population at large.

These two strategies are complementary, not competitive, and the National Cholesterol Education Program is considering both in the development of its activities. This report is the product of an expert panel focused on the patient-based approach. Another panel is charged with examining the scientific evidence and making recommendations for the population-based approach.

The Importance of a Multidisciplinary Team Approach.—This report presents guidelines for interventions that are partly the responsibility of the physicians, dietitians, nurses, pharmacists, and other health professionals who must work together as a team to decide on the best approach for testing and treating each patient, and for implementing and following up these recommendations. The interventions are also the responsibility of the patient, for whom the challenge is to make the dietary and other life-style changes that are needed for successful reduction of CHD risk.

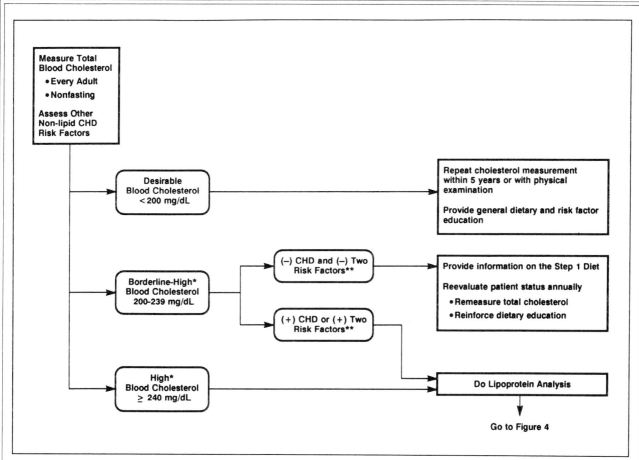

Fig 3.—Initial classification based on total cholesterol. CHD indicates coronary heart disease; asterisk, must be confirmed by obtaining repeated measurements and then using the average value; double asterisks, one of which can be male sex (Table 4).

Detection and Evaluation

Who Should Be Tested.—The total cholesterol level should be measured in all adults 20 years of age and over at least once every five years. Although screening programs that have the specific purpose of inviting the public to receive this test can be used (provided that care is taken to assure that the screening determination is accurate and that there is appropriate followup for further tests and treatment), the usual approach is through case finding. Case finding is defined as testing the cholesterol level as part of any medical examination.

Classification of Patients.—*Initial Classification Based on Total Cholesterol Level.*—The schedule for evaluation and followup of serum cholesterol concentration is shown in Fig 3. The schedule begins with measurement of the nonfasting serum total cholesterol level and an assessment of other nonlipid risk factors including blood pressure, smoking, and history of CHD in the patient or of premature CHD in family members. The presence of a high cholesterol level is confirmed with a second test and then the fasting LDL-cholesterol level is measured in order to provide a more precise estimate of risk on which to base treatment. Patients should be asked not to change their eating habits during this series of baseline tests.

Patients with a *desirable blood cholesterol* level at this initial test (<200 mg/dL) should be given advice and educational materials on the diet recommended for the general population and advised to have another serum cholesterol test within five years. As with all patients,

these individuals should also have been evaluated for hypertension, cigarette smoking, and other risk factors, and should be given other forms of preventive medical care as appropriate.

Patients with a serum cholesterol level of 200 mg/dL or greater should have the measurement repeated in one to eight weeks. If the level is within 30 mg/dL of the first result, the average of the two values can be used to guide subsequent decisions; otherwise, a third test should be obtained within another one to eight weeks, and the average of the three values used. Getting more than one cholesterol measurement at the outset of treatment is extremely important to assess the patient's serum cholesterol status accurately, because cholesterol levels can fluctuate considerably from day to day in a given individual. (The standard deviation of repeated measurements in an individual over time has been reported as 18 mg/dL for total cholesterol[16] and 15 mg/dL for LDL-cholesterol.[17])

Most patients with *borderline–high blood cholesterol* levels (200 to 239 mg/dL) confirmed by two or more readings are given dietary education designed to lower their serum cholesterol level and are followed up annually. However, those individuals in the 200-239 mg/dL range who have definite CHD or two other nonlipid CHD risk factors (as defined in Table 4) should have lipoprotein analysis and their LDL-cholesterol level determined.

All patients with *high blood cholesterol* levels (240 mg/dL or greater), as well as those with levels from 200 to 239 mg/dL who have definite CHD or two other

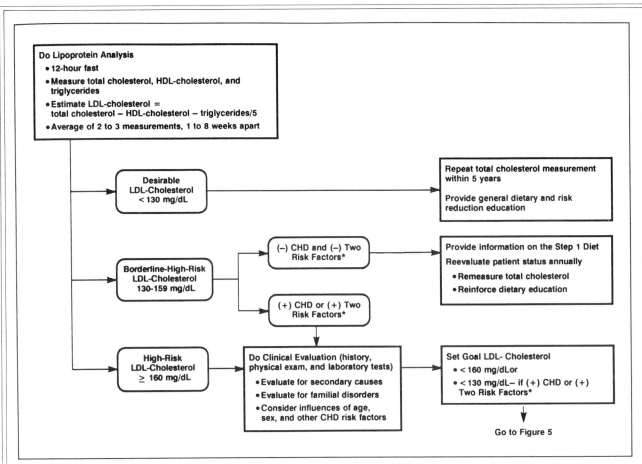

Fig 4.—Classification based on low density lipoprotein (LDL)—cholesterol. Asterisk indicates one of which can be male sex (Table 4); CHD, coronary heart disease; HDL, high density lipoprotein.

CHD risk factors (Table 4), should be tested for the serum level of LDL-cholesterol.

Subsequent Classification Based on LDL-Cholesterol Level.—The action scheme based on LDL-cholesterol level is shown in Fig 4. Two measurements of LDL-cholesterol after an overnight fast are made one to eight weeks apart, and the average is used for clinical decisions unless the two values differ by more than 30 mg/dL (in which case a third test is carried out, and the average of all three is used). The repeated testing of LDL-cholesterol is important for the same reasons given earlier for total cholesterol—the variability of the level from day to day, and the importance of establishing an accurate baseline on which to design the best treatment program. It is possible, however, to save time and effort by making the first LDL-cholesterol measurement on the same specimen that is used for the second test of total cholesterol; this is an especially attractive option for patients with very high levels of total cholesterol (above 260 mg/dL) on the first test.

The LDL-cholesterol levels are classified on the basis of average values as *desirable* (below 130 mg/dL), *borderline-high-risk* (130 to 159 mg/dL), or *high-risk* (160 mg/dL or greater). Patients with desirable LDL-cholesterol fall into the same class as those with desirable total cholesterol levels (<200 mg/dL), and are given general educational materials and tested again within five years. Those with borderline-high-risk LDL-cholesterol (130 to 159 mg/dL) are given information about and advised to follow a fat-modified diet; they are reevaluated annually unless they

have definite CHD or two other risk factors (one of which can be male sex [Table 4]). Such patients (with borderline-high-risk LDL-cholesterol who do have CHD or two other risk factors), together with all patients in the high-risk LDL-cholesterol group (≥160 mg/dL), are clinically evaluated as described below, and then enter a cholesterol-lowering treatment program.

Methods of Detection.—Serum *total cholesterol* levels can be measured at any time of day in the nonfasting state, since total cholesterol concentrations do not change appreciably after a fat-containing meal. Patients should be following their ordinary eating habits and be in their usual state of health. Patients who are acutely ill, are losing weight, are pregnant, or have had a myocardial infarction within the past three months should be rescheduled; the cholesterol levels obtained in such patients may not be representative of their usual levels. To prevent an effect of posture or stasis on the cholesterol determination, venipuncture should be carried out on patients who have been in the sitting position for at least five minutes, and the tourniquet should be used for as brief a period as possible. The blood may be collected either as serum (no anticoagulant) or as plasma (in EDTA). If blood is obtained without anticoagulant, it should be allowed to clot for 30 minutes at room temperature, and the clot should be detached from the wall of the tube prior to centrifuging. Rapid capillary blood (fingerstick) methodology for cholesterol measurement is currently under development and evaluation. Should this methodology prove reliable, it could be suitable for initial cholesterol determinations.

Low density lipoprotein–cholesterol determinations can also be carried out on either serum or plasma, provided that, as with total cholesterol measurements, plasma values are multiplied by 1.03 to correct them to the serum cutpoints specified in this report. However, because the LDL-cholesterol value is estimated from measurements of other lipids, including triglyceride, blood samples should be collected from patients who have fasted for at least 12 hours (except for water or black coffee).

The LDL-cholesterol level is estimated from measurements of the levels of total cholesterol, total triglycerides, and HDL-cholesterol. If the triglyceride value is below 400 mg/dL, then this value can be divided by five to estimate the VLDL-cholesterol level. Since total cholesterol is the sum of LDL-cholesterol, HDL-cholesterol, and VLDL-cholesterol, LDL-cholesterol can be calculated as follows (all quantities are in milligrams per deciliter): LDL-Cholesterol = Total Cholesterol − HDL-Cholesterol − (Triglyceride/5).[18] (A recent report suggests that, in this formula, dividing the triglyceride value by 6, rather than 5, may provide a more accurate estimation of the LDL-cholesterol level.[19] Further studies may validate the use of triglyceride/6 as the preferred way of estimating LDL-cholesterol.) If the triglyceride value is above 400 mg/dL, LDL-cholesterol estimation by the above formula becomes less accurate. For such patients, ultracentrifugation in a specialized laboratory can be used to give a more accurate LDL-cholesterol level; it may be appropriate to refer such patients to a lipid specialist.

The choice of laboratory is an important issue because there is considerable variability in the accuracy with which laboratories measure cholesterol. This measurement variability is another reason for recommending that more than one cholesterol measurement be obtained and average values be used at key decision points in this report. All recommendations about cholesterol levels in this report presuppose accurate and reliable measurements. The physician should seek a laboratory that participates in a suitable standardization program. The issue of laboratory methods and their standardization is being addressed by the Laboratory Standardization Panel of the National Cholesterol Education Program.

Clinical Evaluation.—All patients with an LDL-cholesterol level ≥160 mg/dL, and those with a level of 130 to 159 mg/dL and high risk status, as defined in Table 4, should be evaluated clinically. They should then be assigned a goal LDL-cholesterol level and enter the program for cholesterol-lowering treatment.

The clinical evaluation, which includes a history, physical examination, and basic laboratory tests, has three aims. The first is to determine whether the high LDL-cholesterol level is caused by another disease or by a drug. The second is to determine whether a genetic disorder may underlie the elevated LDL-cholesterol. The third aim is to ensure that the patient is fully characterized with regard to age, sex, and the presence or absence of definite CHD and of other CHD risk factors, in order to use this information in decisions about treatment directed at LDL-cholesterol.

Secondary High Blood Cholesterol.—The clinical evaluation for secondary (and possibly reversible) forms of high-risk LDL-cholesterol includes consideration of, and, where appropriate, ruling out, the following conditions: hypothyroidism; nephrotic syndrome; diabetes mellitus; obstructive liver disease; and drugs that may raise LDL-cholesterol levels, particularly progestins and anabolic steroids. High blood cholesterol secondary to other diseases or drugs can be detected by clinical evaluation and, when indicated, by the following laboratory tests: urinalysis, complete blood cell count, and serum thyroid-stimulating hormone (TSH), glucose, alkaline phosphatase, and albumin. When one of the causes of secondary high cholesterol is present, the usual approach is to treat the disease or discontinue the drug (if possible) and then to reevaluate the LDL-cholesterol level.

Familial Disorders.—In most cases, high blood cholesterol is not secondary to some other condition, and the patient has a primary form of LDL-cholesterol elevation. This can be either genetic (familial) or sporadic (often diet induced), and the next step is to consider which of these possibilities is more likely. Diagnosing genetic disorders helps clarify the etiology and management of LDL-cholesterol elevations in affected patients, and emphasizes the desirability of measuring cholesterol in first-degree relatives (parents, siblings, children) in order to identify those who may need cholesterol-lowering treatment.

The genetic hyperlipidemias are described in Appendix II; two important ones are summarized here. One of these is familial hypercholesterolemia (FH), an autosomal dominant disorder of the LDL receptor. Heterozygotes with this disorder have a population frequency of about one in 500 and often have serum cholesterol levels greater than 300 mg/dL, tendon xanthomas, and premature CHD. Another important genetic cause of high-risk LDL-cholesterol levels is familial combined hyperlipidemia (FCHL). Affected family members may have high serum levels of LDL-cholesterol, or of triglyceride, or both. Such patients generally do not have tendon xanthomas, but premature CHD is common. The prevalence of these two familial disorders among survivors of myocardial infarction under 60 years of age is 5% for FH and 15% for FCHL.[20]

Other Lipid Risk Factors.—The level of plasma HDL-cholesterol is inversely related to CHD rates in most epidemiologic studies even after adjustment for the influence of other risk factors (see Appendix II). Although there is no direct experimental evidence that raising HDL-cholesterol levels reduces the risk of CHD, the life-style interventions that raise the level of this lipoprotein—quitting smoking, reducing obesity, and exercising—are good advice for other reasons and should be recommended to all patients regardless of their HDL-cholesterol levels. One other life-style approach to increasing the level of HDL-cholesterol—increasing the intake of alcohol—is not recommended because of the possibility of encouraging excessive intake. The issue of low HDL-cholesterol and its management is discussed further in Appendix II.

Reliance on a ratio of either total or LDL-cholesterol to HDL-cholesterol as a key factor in decisions regarding treatment is not a practice recommended in this report. Blood pressure and smoking are not combined into a single number because the clinician needs to know both facts separately in order to recommend an intervention. Similarly, HDL-cholesterol and LDL-cholesterol are independent risk factors with different determinants, and combining them into a single number conceals information that may be useful to the clinician. The HDL-cholesterol level does, however, contribute to decisions about treatment for LDL-cholesterol, because a low level increases the CHD risk of the patient (Table 4).

The level of plasma triglyceride is also a risk factor for CHD in most epidemiologic studies. In general, however, it is not an independent risk factor, ie, the association usually disappears when statistically adjusted for plasma total cholesterol and HDL-cholesterol levels. In the Framingham Study, however, the plasma triglyceride level was found to be an independent predictor of CHD risk in women.[21] The recommended approach to the problem of hypertriglyceridemia is described in the report of the National Institutes of Health Consensus Development Conference on Treatment of Hypertriglyceridemia,[22] and is summarized in Appendix II. In the absence of pathophysiologic or animal evidence that triglyceride is atherogenic or that lowering the plasma level lowers the risk of CHD, intervention specifically directed at this lipid (except in the rare patient with a very high level that may cause pancreatitis) is not generally recommended at this time. On the other hand, many individuals with elevated triglyceride levels have associated low levels of HDL-cholesterol and/or high levels of LDL-cholesterol, which do influence decisions about intervention to reduce the risk of CHD in ways described in this report. Moreover, hypertriglyceridemia alone may be a marker for familial combined hyperlipidemia, which warrants therapy to prevent CHD.

Other Major (Nonlipid) Risk Factors.—Information on whether CHD or its other risk factors are present is used to assess whether the patient has reasons unrelated to LDL-cholesterol for being at high risk of a CHD event or death. The search is important because modifiable risk factors such as hypertension and cigarette smoking are themselves important targets for intervention. In addition, the presence of any risk factor, whether modifiable or not, influences clinical decisions about LDL-cholesterol because the increased absolute level of risk may increase the potential benefit from lowering the level of LDL-cholesterol (Table 3).

This principle can be used in a general way by the clinician, and also as a specific rule in the decision schemes set out in Figs 3 and 4. In Fig 4 the presence of high risk status due to factors other than LDL-cholesterol establishes a lower cutpoint for triggering intervention and a lower therapeutic goal for LDL-cholesterol. The definitions of high-risk status are given in Table 4. Because the presence of CHD is by far the strongest factor that influences the risk of recurrent CHD events or death, it is particularly important in clinical decisions for treating LDL-cholesterol. Thus, this report emphasizes the importance of both primary and secondary prevention.

Race, Sex, and Age.—The percentage of adults with high blood cholesterol by age, race, and sex is given in Table 5. The prevalence rises with age to plateau at about 50 years of age, and does not vary appreciably by race or sex except for the higher prevalence in older women. (This high prevalence in older women is due to the fact that they have high levels of both LDL- and HDL-cholesterol.) Additional information on the distributions of total and LDL-cholesterol levels in the population is given in Appendix I. This section addresses the CHD risk in different groups, with the implications for managing LDL-cholesterol.

RACE.—Race is not included in Table 4 because available evidence suggests that the clinical management of LDL-cholesterol should not differ according to race in the United States. (This report is not specifically directed at populations in other countries, but the guidelines would probably apply reasonably well to any country where CHD is endemic at similar levels to those in the United States.)

SEX.—Sex, on the other hand, should be considered as a risk factor, as described in Table 4, when determining the risk status of an individual patient. In women as in men, CHD is the major cause of death, and cholesterol levels are predictive of CHD. However, the rates of CHD are three to four times higher in men than in women in the middle decades of life and roughly two times higher in the elderly.[24,25] Hence, the absolute magnitude of the potential

Table 5.—US Prevalence of High Blood Cholesterol* by Age, Race, and Sex (Percent of Each Population)[23]				
	Men		Women	
Age, y	White	Black	White	Black
20-74	25.0	23.9	29.2	23.7
20-24	6.1	2.9	6.5	7.0
25-34	15.0	19.3	12.4	8.7
35-44	27.9	24.5	21.1	16.9
45-54	36.5	40.3	40.6	40.7
55-64	37.3	35.3	53.7	46.5
65-74	32.4	27.2	52.1	48.4

*Serum concentration of cholesterol ≥240 mg/dL.

benefit from lowering blood cholesterol in general, and the benefit/risk ratio of drug therapy in particular, is greater for men than for women. Thus, male sex is considered a risk factor in decisions about the cutpoints and goals of cholesterol-lowering treatment.

AGE.—Age is a complicated factor to consider. Beginning at 20 years of age, the mean total and LDL-cholesterol levels increase by about 40 mg/dL during the next two to three decades; in the elderly, the levels decline slightly (see Appendix I for age-specific data). Two major LDL-cholesterol cutpoints are recommended in this report: 160 mg/dL identifies the group with high-risk LDL-cholesterol, and (as discussed later in the section on drug treatment) 190 mg/dL identifies the group with "very-high-risk" LDL-cholesterol for whom consideration of drug therapy is warranted even in the absence of other risk factors. These cutpoints approximate the 75th and 90th percentiles for 35- to 60-year-old patients. Using these same cutpoints in younger patients will have the effect of designating a smaller proportion of the younger population as being in the high-risk categories.

The strategy recommended by the Cholesterol Consensus Conference for making clinical decisions about patients 20 to 39 years of age is to use cutpoints that correspond to the age-specific 75th and 90th percentile values (Appendix I). Using the Consensus Conference recommendations concerning the 75th percentile values, adults 20 to 29 years of age would be considered (in the terminology of the present report) to have high blood cholesterol for levels exceeding 200 mg/dL; those 30 to 39 years of age would be in this category if total cholesterol exceeded 220 mg/dL. Giving dietary treatment to the top 25% of the young adult population is probably desirable in order to prevent the development of atherosclerosis at an earlier stage in the disease. Recommending drug treatment to as large a group as the top 10% of young adults, however, is premature until additional evidence becomes available on the safety of using lipid-lowering drugs for many decades. There is, moreover, the important fact that age is a very strong risk factor, and therefore the absolute magnitude of the benefit (and the benefit/risk ratio) increases with age for the reasons given earlier.

Patients 60 years of age and above are another issue. There is little direct clinical trial evidence on whether elderly patients will benefit from intervention, and the strength of the association between LDL-cholesterol and CHD diminishes with age. However, LDL-cholesterol does continue to have some association with CHD, and the clinical trial evidence for the effectiveness of intervention after myocardial infarction suggests that lowering LDL-cholesterol is beneficial even in patients who already have

	Table 6.—Dietary Therapy of High Blood Cholesterol Level	
	Recommended Intake	
Nutrient	**Step-One Diet**	**Step-Two Diet**
Total fat	Less than 30% of total calories	Less than 30% of total calories
Saturated fatty acids	Less than 10% of total calories	Less than 7% of total calories
Polyunsaturated fatty acids	Up to 10% of total calories	Up to 10% of total calories
Monounsaturated fatty acids	10% to 15% of total calories	10% to 15% of total calories
Carbohydrates	50% to 60% of total calories	50% to 60% of total calories
Protein	10% to 20% of total calories	10% to 20% of total calories
Cholesterol	Less than 300 mg/d	Less than 200 mg/d
Total calories	To achieve and maintain desirable weight	To achieve and maintain desirable weight

advanced disease. Moreover, the fact that age is associated with a high risk of CHD in the later decades of life means that the absolute magnitude of the potential benefits of intervention remains substantial in the elderly.[25]

Summarizing the issue of sex and age, the recommendations and cutpoints in this report are meant to apply to all adults 20 years of age and above. There is room, however, for modifications based on the judgment of the physician and the preferences of the patient when dealing with individual patients, particularly young adults, the elderly, and women.

DIETARY TREATMENT
Cutpoints and Goals for Dietary Therapy

Patients with high-risk LDL-cholesterol levels (≥160 mg/dL), and those with borderline-high-risk LDL-cholesterol (130 to 159 mg/dL) who also have definite CHD or two other risk factors (Table 4), should enter a program of dietary therapy instituted by the physician. The *minimal* goals of therapy are as follows: (1) to lower LDL-cholesterol to below 160 mg/dL if the patient has neither definite CHD nor two other CHD risk factors (Table 4); or (2) to lower LDL-cholesterol to below 130 mg/dL if definite CHD or two other CHD risk factors (Table 4) are present. Ideally, dietary means should be used to attain even lower levels of LDL-cholesterol, if possible, to achieve a further reduction in CHD risk.

Although the goal of therapy is to lower the LDL-cholesterol concentration, measurement of serum total cholesterol can be used to monitor the response to diet. The principle is that LDL-cholesterol should be used for the definitive classification of patients and for decision making, but total cholesterol can be substituted for monitoring. For simplicity, a serum total cholesterol of 240 mg/dL corresponds roughly to an LDL-cholesterol of 160 mg/dL, while a total cholesterol of 200 mg/dL corresponds roughly to an LDL-cholesterol of 130 mg/dL. Thus, as a guide for monitoring, the minimal goals of therapy are: (1) to lower total cholesterol to below 240 mg/dL, if the patient has neither definite CHD nor two other CHD risk factors, or (2) to lower total cholesterol to below 200 mg/dL, if definite CHD or two other risk factors are present. It should be emphasized again that even lower levels of total cholesterol are desirable. The use of total cholesterol as a surrogate for LDL-cholesterol applies to patients with average levels of HDL-cholesterol without high total triglyceride levels. If the patient is found to have an abnormally high or low HDL-cholesterol or hypertriglyceridemia on initial classification, so that total cholesterol is not a good surrogate for LDL-cholesterol, it is appropriate to use LDL-cholesterol even in monitoring.

After the cholesterol response to diet has been obtained, LDL-cholesterol should again be measured in order to decide whether or not the goal of therapy has been achieved. In addition, levels of LDL-cholesterol should be employed for making a decision about drug therapy.

Overview and General Approach

Three dietary habits typically contribute significantly to elevated plasma cholesterol. First is a high intake of saturated fatty acids. The average intake is 13% to 15% of total calories, but many Americans consume 15% to 20% of their calories as saturated fatty acids. Second is a relatively high intake of cholesterol. Many patients with high-risk LDL-cholesterol levels exceed the current average intake of about 350 to 450 mg/d. Third is a high caloric intake that exceeds body requirements commonly causing obesity. The aim of dietary therapy is to reverse these excesses while maintaining and promoting good nutrition.

This document is directed at the high-risk patient, and its underlying theme is specific therapy for high blood cholesterol. Modification of the diet is an essential element in this therapy. The initial diet modifications recommended for patients in this report are very similar to the diet modifications recommended by the American Heart Association (Dallas) and other organizations for the public at large, as part of a population-based approach for lowering cholesterol. In the program described in this report, however, diet recommendations are provided to patients, in a medical treatment setting, in an intensive manner. Accordingly, the dietary intervention described here is referred to as "dietary treatment." It should be noted that the diets recommended in this report are consistent with good nutrition, and that their aim is to achieve healthy eating patterns. Physicians should emphasize to patients that the goal is not a temporary "diet," but a permanent change in eating behavior.

Diet modification should occur in two steps, which are outlined and compared in Table 6. These diets are designed to progressively reduce the intake of saturated fatty acids and cholesterol and eliminate excess total calories. The Step-One Diet should be prescribed by the physician and implemented by the physician and his or her immediate staff. This diet calls for an intake of total fat less than 30% of calories, saturated fatty acids less than 10% of calories, and cholesterol less than 300 mg/d. The patient's serum cholesterol level should be measured at four to six weeks and at three months after starting the Step-One Diet.

If the minimal goals of therapy are not achieved on this diet by three months, the patient should usually progress to the Step-Two Diet. Adoption of the Step-Two Diet would be facilitated by referral to a registered dietitian. This diet

Cholesterol Adult Treatment Panel Report

calls for a further reduction in saturated fatty acid intake to less than 7% of calories and cholesterol intake to less than 200 mg/d.

For many high-risk patients, the goals of cholesterol lowering can be achieved by dietary therapy alone. It is important that dietary therapy not be regarded as a failure prematurely. For most patients, dietary therapy should be continued for at least six months before adding drug therapy. Exceptions include patients with very-high LDL-cholesterol levels and other severe dyslipidemias (see Appendix II). If the desired goals of LDL-cholesterol lowering are met by diet modification alone, long-term monitoring is indicated. If reduction of LDL-cholesterol is not satisfactory, lipid-lowering drugs should be considered along with continued dietary intervention. (For detailed information about the effects of diet on serum lipids and lipoproteins and on CHD risk, including key studies and reviews, the reader should consult references 26 through 46.)

Recommended Diets

Step-One and Step-Two Diets—Nutrients and Rationale.—The recommended diets are presented in two steps—the Step-One and Step-Two Diets. The Step-One Diet calls for the reduction of the major and obvious sources of saturated fatty acids and cholesterol in the diet; for many patients this can be achieved without a radical alteration in dietary habits. The Step-Two Diet requires careful attention to the whole diet so as to reduce the intake of saturated fatty acids and cholesterol to a minimal level compatible with an acceptable and nutritious diet. Saturated fatty acids and cholesterol are not essential nutrients, and neither is required in the diet. The body can make these lipids in abundance, and they can be transported from one tissue to another to assure that any local shortage is supplied by lipids produced elsewhere in the body. The real need then is to reduce dietary saturated fatty acids and cholesterol to the levels required to achieve the goals of LDL-cholesterol lowering and still provide a diet that is nutritious and palatable. The fat-modified diets proposed in this report are designed to achieve these aims. The rationale for the recommended characteristics of the Step-One and Step-Two Diets can be described briefly.

A Nutritionally Balanced Diet.—A prerequisite for any therapeutic diet is that it be nutritionally adequate.[47] It must contain sufficient amounts of vitamins, minerals, and macronutrients to meet recommended allowances. The diet should contain a variety of foods. Fruits, vegetables, and legumes (peas and beans) are good sources of vitamin A, vitamin C, folic acid, fiber, and many minerals. Whole-grain and enriched breads, cereals, and other grain products contain B vitamins, protein, fiber, and some iron. Poultry and fish are good sources of protein. Meat products are rich in protein and contain iron in a form that is well absorbed; thus, meat can be included in a diet otherwise designed to lower serum cholesterol, although meat fat needs to be curtailed. The same is true of milk products; the nonfat portion of milk is rich in calcium and contains protein. While egg yolks are rich in cholesterol, egg whites contain protein and no cholesterol. Most nuts contain protein and fat, but their fat is largely unsaturated and thus does not raise the serum cholesterol level. Thus, while a serum-cholesterol-lowering diet requires modification of fat, the diet should be nutritious and palatable and include a variety of foods. The following considers the specific modifications that will be required.

Total Fat.—Total fat intake in both therapeutic diets should not exceed 30% of total calories. The purpose of decreasing total fat intake is twofold—to facilitate reduction of saturated fatty acid intake and to promote weight reduction in overweight patients by substituting foods of lower caloric density. Total fat in the current American diet averages approximately 35% to 40% of calories. Hence, for most high-risk patients, about one-fifth of their total fat now consumed must be eliminated. In the past, one approach to more intensive dietary therapy of high blood cholesterol (beyond the Step-One Diet) has been to reduce intake of total fat to 20% or less of calories, in parallel with progressive reductions in saturated fatty acids and cholesterol. However, very low fat intakes have low satiety value and often are not well accepted. Recent evidence indicates that a marked reduction in dietary fat is not required for satisfactory lowering of plasma LDL, provided that saturated fatty acids are reduced and the remaining fat is mainly unsaturated. In other words, a decrease in total fat to below 30% of calories may not be needed for the sole purpose of lowering the plasma cholesterol level. Nevertheless, a reduction in total fat to near 20% of calories will facilitate weight reduction and a decrease in saturated fatty acid intake for some patients. For these reasons, a further reduction of fat intake is not required in the Step-Two Diet, but neither is it excluded.

Saturated Fatty Acids.—In the Step-One Diet, saturated fatty acids should be decreased to less than 10% of calories. For most patients, saturated fatty acid intake will have to be reduced by about one-third to meet the requirements of the Step-One Diet, and another third for the Step-Two Diet. Several dietary fats are rich in saturated fatty acids. Animal fats that are high in saturated fatty acids include butter fat—contained in butter itself, whole milk, cream, ice cream, and cheese—beef fat, and pork fat. In addition, three plant oils—palm oil, palm kernel oil, and coconut oil—are especially rich in saturated fatty acids.

Polyunsaturated Fatty Acids.—When dietary saturated fatty acids are decreased, they can be replaced in part by polyunsaturated fatty acids. The polyunsaturates can be increased to 10% of calories, but they should not exceed this value. The current American diet contains about 7% of calories as polyunsaturated fatty acids, which should be a minimum value for the therapeutic diets. There are two major categories of polyunsaturated fatty acids, commonly referred to as omega-6 and omega-3. The major omega-6 fatty acid is linoleic acid, which has 18 carbon atoms and two double bonds. Substitution of linoleic acid for dietary saturated fatty acids results in a fall in the plasma cholesterol level. Although very high intakes of linoleic acid were once advocated for cholesterol lowering, lack of information about the consequences of long-term ingestion of large amounts of linoleic acid has led most investigators to recommend a ceiling of 10% of total calories. Several vegetable oils are rich in linoleic acid, including safflower oil, sunflower seed oil, soybean oil, and corn oil. Although polyunsaturated oils are high in linoleic acid and low in saturated fatty acids, they also are high in total calories (as are all fats and oils); consequently they can promote weight gain if consumed in large amounts.

The major sources of omega-3 fatty acids are the fish oils. Most omega-3 fatty acids in fish oil have very elongated carbon chains and are highly polyunsaturated. The major acids in this class are eicosapentaenoic acid (EPA) and docosahexaenoic acid (DHA). The omega-3 fatty acids have been found to lower triglyceride levels when given in high doses, but they are not necessarily the desired therapy for hypertriglyceridemia (Appendix II). There is little evidence that omega-3 fatty acids are useful for reducing LDL-cholesterol levels. Although it has been postulated by some that they will reduce the risk for CHD, this has not been established. Furthermore, it is not known whether long-term ingestion of these fatty acids will lead to undesirable side effects. The use of fish-oil capsules as a supplement in a therapeutic diet for high-risk cholesterol levels is not recommended here.

Consumption of omega-3 fatty acids should be differentiated from that of fish. Some fish are rich in omega-3 acids while others are not. Epidemiologic data suggest that frequent consumption of fish of any type, seemingly independent of omega-3 fatty acids, is associated with reduced CHD risk. Whether this is true or not, fish can serve as a useful substitute for meats that are richer in saturated fatty acids.

Monounsaturated Fatty Acids.—In both therapeutic diets, monounsaturated fatty acids, mainly oleic acid, should comprise 10% to 15% of total calories. Oleic acid is the major fatty acid found in olive oil, rapeseed (canola oil), and high-oleic forms of sunflower seed oil and safflower oil. For many years, oleic acid was considered to be "neutral" in its effect on plasma cholesterol, neither raising nor lowering the cholesterol level. However, recent evidence indicates that oleic acid may cause as much of a decrease in LDL-cholesterol levels as linoleic acid when either is substituted for saturated fatty acids in the diet. The current American diet contains 14% to 16% of calories as monounsaturated fatty acid. Much of it is consumed with animal fats, which are rich in saturated fatty acids. When animal fats are curtailed, a larger portion of monounsaturated fatty acids can come from vegetable oils.

Dietary Cholesterol.—Dietary cholesterol causes marked hypercholesterolemia and atherosclerosis in many laboratory animals, including nonhuman primates. Although high intakes of cholesterol in humans rarely cause striking rises in the plasma cholesterol level, controlled metabolic studies show that dietary cholesterol usually raises the plasma cholesterol level. The degree of rise varies from person to person. Overall, excess dietary cholesterol appears to contribute to the high LDL-cholesterol levels seen in high-risk patients and thus may add to CHD risk. Furthermore, concern about dietary cholesterol extends beyond its effects in raising the LDL-cholesterol level. Newly absorbed cholesterol enters the circulation with chylomicrons, which are degraded to cholesterol-rich chylomicron remnants; the latter may be atherogenic. Dietary cholesterol is not required for normal body function.

For practical purposes, a cholesterol intake of less than 300 mg/d is reasonable as part of the first step in dietary management of high-risk LDL-cholesterol. However, further restriction, as recommended in the Step-Two Diet, is justified for patients who do not achieve the goals of therapy on the Step-One Diet, despite adherence. Cholesterol in the diet comes from animal products. Particularly rich sources are egg yolk and organ meats (liver, sweetbreads, and brain). Some shellfish (eg, shrimp) also are moderately high in cholesterol, but not to the extent of egg yolk or organ meats. The flesh of all animals (beef, pork, lamb, chicken, fish) contains cholesterol; it is present in both muscle and fat, and both have approximately the same concentrations on a wet-weight basis. Dairy products containing butter fat also contribute cholesterol to the diet.

Protein.—The recommended intake of protein in both therapeutic diets is between 10% and 20% of calories. In laboratory animals, certain plant proteins have a cholesterol-lowering action relative to animal proteins. The same effect has not been established in humans. Thus, the type of protein in the therapeutic diets is not specified.

Carbohydrate.—Both recommended diets specify an intake of carbohydrates of 50% to 60% of calories. When dietary fat is reduced, it should be replaced by carbohydrate. Dietary carbohydrates include simple sugars (monosaccharides and disaccharides), complex digestible carbohydrates (starches), and complex indigestible carbohydrates (fiber). Complex carbohydrate should comprise more than half of digestible carbohydrates; this will help ensure ingestion of desirable quantities of vegetable products that contain vitamins, minerals, and fiber. In most people, when digestible carbohydrates are substituted for cholesterol-raising saturated fatty acids, the LDL-cholesterol level will fall to about the same extent as when oleic acid and linoleic acid are substituted in this manner. Very-high-carbohydrate diets can raise plasma triglycerides, but when fat intakes are in the vicinity of 30% of calories, this triglyceride response is minimal.

Total Calories.—Obesity is not only associated with elevated serum LDL-cholesterol levels, but is an independent risk factor for CHD. An important recommendation, therefore, is to reduce caloric intake to achieve weight reduction in overweight patients. Weight reduction will lower the LDL-cholesterol level in many people, as well as reduce plasma triglycerides and raise HDL-cholesterol levels. Some patients with high-risk LDL-cholesterol levels are extremely sensitive to caloric intake, and weight reduction and establishment of desirable body weight will completely correct their elevated LDL-cholesterol concentrations. The importance of caloric restriction in overweight, high-risk individuals cannot be overemphasized.

Weight reduction can be facilitated by exercise. Experience has shown that regular exercise will curb the appetite as well as burn off excess calories. It also will lower serum triglycerides and raise HDL-cholesterol levels, and, in some individuals, may lower the LDL-cholesterol level.

Fiber.—The indigestible carbohydrates and related polymers come under the category of dietary fiber. One type of fiber is insoluble, an example of which is the cellulose found in wheat bran. Insoluble fiber adds bulk to the stools and contributes to normal colon function. Some authorities believe that a relatively high intake of dietary fiber may help prevent diverticulosis and colon cancer, although this remains to be proven. Excessive intakes of insoluble fibers can be associated with gastrointestinal side effects and even interfere with absorption of vital nutrients such as calcium. Dietary fibers such as cellulose appear to have very little or no effect on blood cholesterol levels.

Another type of fiber is soluble in the intestine but not absorbed. This category includes pectins, certain gums, and psyllium. One of the gums is β-glucan, which is present in oat products and beans. High intake (eg, 15 to 25 g/d) of soluble fiber has been reported to lower the plasma cholesterol level by 5% to 15%. This high intake can produce gastrointestinal side effects, but prolonged usage frequently is associated with improved tolerance.

Alcohol.—The average intake of alcohol among Americans is approximately 5% of total calories, but this value varies widely among individuals. Although alcohol is not harmful when taken in moderation, a high consumption is known to have many adverse effects on health. Alcohol affects lipoprotein metabolism in several ways. It does not affect LDL-cholesterol concentrations, but it does increase triglyceride concentrations and HDL-cholesterol levels in many individuals. The mechanism for the rise in HDL-cholesterol is not known, nor is it known whether the higher level so produced imparts any protection against CHD. For patients who can consume moderate amounts of alcohol responsibly, its use can be allowed in the context of

Table 7.—Recommended Diet Modifications to Lower Blood Cholesterol		
	The Step-One Diet	
	Choose	**Decrease**
Fish, chicken, turkey, and lean meats	Fish, poultry without skin, lean cuts of beef, lamb, pork or veal, shellfish	Fatty cuts of beef, lamb, pork; spare ribs, organ meats, regular cold cuts, sausage, hot dogs, bacon, sardines, roe
Skim and low-fat milk, cheese, yogurt, and dairy substitutes	Skim or 1% fat milk (liquid, powdered, evaporated), buttermilk	Whole milk (4% fat): regular, evaporated, condensed; cream, half and half, 2% milk, imitation milk products, most nondairy creamers, whipped toppings
	Nonfat (0% fat) or low-fat yogurt	Whole-milk yogurt
	Low-fat cottage cheese (1% or 2% fat)	Whole-milk cottage cheese (4% fat)
	Low-fat cheeses, farmer or pot cheeses (all of these should be labeled no more than 2 to 6 g of fat per ounce)	All natural cheeses (eg, blue, roquefort, camembert, cheddar, Swiss), low-fat or "light" cream cheese, low-fat or "light" sour cream, cream cheeses, sour cream
	Sherbet, sorbet	Ice cream
Eggs	Egg whites (2 whites equal 1 whole egg in recipes), cholesterol-free egg substitutes	Egg yolks
Fruits and vegetables	Fresh, frozen, canned, or dried fruits and vegetables	Vegetables prepared in butter, cream, or other sauces
Breads and cereals	Homemade baked goods using unsaturated oils sparingly, angel food cake, low-fat crackers, low-fat cookies	Commercial baked goods: pies, cakes, doughnuts, croissants, pastries, muffins, biscuits, high-fat crackers, high-fat cookies
	Rice, pasta	Egg noodles
	Whole-grain breads and cereals (oatmeal, whole wheat, rye, bran, multigrain, etc)	Breads in which eggs are a major ingredient
Fats and oils	Baking cocoa	Chocolate
	Unsaturated vegetable oils: corn, olive, rapeseed (canola oil), safflower, sesame, soybean, sunflower	Butter, coconut oil, palm oil, palm kernel oil, lard, bacon fat
	Margarine or shortenings made from one of the unsaturated oils listed above, diet margarine	. . .
	Mayonnaise, salad dressings made with unsaturated oils listed above, low-fat dressings	Dressings made with egg yolk
	Seeds and nuts	Coconut

the above reservation. However, this report does not specifically recommend use of alcohol in the prevention of CHD.

Expected Responses to Dietary Therapy.—The degree of reduction of LDL-cholesterol levels that can be achieved by dietary therapy depends on the dietary habits of the patient before starting the diet and on the inherent responsiveness of the patient. In general, patients with high cholesterol levels show a greater absolute reduction in total and LDL-cholesterol concentrations than do individuals with relatively low cholesterol levels. Metabolic ward studies suggest that switching from the typical American diet to the Step-One Diet could reduce cholesterol levels on average by 30 to 40 mg/dL. Advancing to the Step-Two Diet can be expected to cause a further decline of approximately 15 mg/dL in cholesterol levels. Some individuals may demonstrate even greater reductions on the two diets, and others will have lesser responses. Most of the decrease in total blood cholesterol occurs in the LDL fraction.

Practical Approach to Dietary Therapy

Outline of Approach.—Once a patient is deemed at high risk, dietary therapy should begin in the physician's office. Diet is the cornerstone of treatment of high-risk cholesterol levels. The view that diet modification is impractical or doomed to failure for most patients is not justified. Many individuals have successfully modified their diets and have obtained a substantial reduction in cholesterol levels. Much of the problem of high cholesterol levels among Americans is due to dietary excesses, and diet modification is the rational approach to this problem for most people.

Role of the Physician.—The success of dietary therapy will depend to a large extent on the physician's attitudes, knowledge, and skills in motivating the patient and in organizing a team approach to dietary therapy. The physician can have a major impact on the patient's attitude toward diet modification. A positive attitude on the part of the physician is absolutely vital. The physician should describe to the patient his/her category of high blood cholesterol and should give an overview of the therapeutic plan. The role of diet, and possibly drugs, should be discussed. The physician will need to review the patient's dietary history. The patient should be questioned about current dietary habits with special attention to intake of foods rich in saturated fatty acids and cholesterol (eg, dairy fats—milk, butter, cheese, ice cream—frequency and choices of meat products, bakery goods, eggs, and organ meats). The need to modify eating behavior to achieve the goals of therapy should be indicated, and the plan for carrying out dietary treatment, as it involves other members of the team, can be described. Finally, the physician has a vital role to play in the monitoring of response, in reinforcement of the diet message, and in leadership of the therapeutic team. For assessing adherence to the diet, the physician can review the contents of Table 7 with the patient at follow-up visits.

Role of the Physician's Staff.—Another key component of the therapeutic team is the physician's staff. This may include registered nurses, registered physician's assistants, nurse clinicians, and other types of assistants. These individuals should receive appropriate training for their roles in patient management, which will include aiding in further dietary assessment and in dietary education and counseling. Nurses and other assistants can play key roles in patient education (eg, rationale for dietary change, selection of appropriate foods), in promoting behavioral changes, and in monitoring dietary changes. Various educational materials produced by the National Cholesterol Education Program and the American Heart Association can be used to assist in dietary education for patients. Referral to a registered dietitian can facilitate dietary instruction and monitoring of adherence, but if the physician's staff is appropriately trained, it can perform these functions for many patients.

Role of Registered Dietitians.—Registered dietitians (RDs) are educated in the science of nutrition and are professionally trained in dietary intervention. They must meet uniform standards for registration. The term "nutritionist" is used in a variety of ways. Some nutritionists are registered dietitians, but others may not be registered and may not have the clinical training in dietary counseling of a registered dietitian. Although such nutritionists may play a role in dietary education, referral to a registered dietitian is particularly valuable for more intensive dietary therapy, such as the Step-Two Diet, and evaluation of nutritional adequacy. Patients who have had difficulty in adhering or responding to the Step-One Diet also have much to gain from counseling by a registered dietitian. Patients who are not initially successful in the Step-One Diet may be referred to a dietitian for another Step-One Diet trial period before progressing to the Step-Two Diet. For some patients, based on the physician's judgment, referral to a registered dietitian may be appropriate from the outset of dietary therapy.

Dietitians can be identified through a local hospital as well as through state and district affiliates of the American Dietetic Association (208 S LaSalle St, Chicago, IL 60604). The American Dietetic Association maintains a roster of dietitians and responds to requests in writing for assistance in locating a registered dietitian in a given area. Dietitians with particular expertise in cholesterol management are available in most large medical centers where they are often part of a multidisciplinary lipid clinic team or cardiac rehabilitation team. The local affiliate of the American Heart Association may have a listing of dietitians who have particular interest and expertise in modifying the diet for purposes of cardiovascular risk reduction.

Schedule of Dietary Therapy.—Adherence to the prescribed diet is facilitated by monitoring the patient's response. The Step-One Diet should be employed for three months, and if the desired response is not obtained in spite of good diet adherence, the patient can progress to the Step-Two Diet for another three months. During this period, serum cholesterol levels should be monitored at regular intervals (described below). For most patients, dietary therapy to lower serum total and LDL-cholesterol

should be employed for at least six months before considering drugs. Exceptions to this approach are patients with severe elevations of serum cholesterol (Appendix II) and patients with definite CHD.

Recommended Dietary Patterns.—Most patients should be able to adopt and adhere to the Step-One Diet. Table 7 outlines ways to achieve the goals of dietary therapy, and a copy may be given to the patient along with additional educational materials. It should be emphasized to the patient that the recommended diet can be both tasty and nutritious, and that many choices of high-quality and acceptable foods are available in stores and restaurants.

A few general dietary changes underlie implementation of the Step-One Diet. To decrease intake of total fat, saturated fatty acids, and cholesterol, attention should be given to reducing foods containing butter fat—butter itself, cheese, ice cream, cream, whole (4%) milk, and even 2% milk. Only lean cuts of meat should be selected, visible fat should be trimmed away, and fat should be allowed to drain from meat after cooking. The skin of chicken should be removed, and fish should be substituted frequently for meat. Consumption of egg yolks and organ meats (liver, brain, sweetbreads) should be reduced. Shrimp, lobster, and other shellfish contain varying amounts of cholesterol, but are low in fat, and thus may be eaten occasionally. The vegetable oils rich in saturated fatty acids—coconut oil, palm kernel oil, and palm oil—are used in some commercial foods and food products; products that list these oils as ingredients on the label should generally be avoided.

Specific Food Subgroups.—Special attention should be given to certain common foods in the diet. This subsection provides specific recommendations:

MEATS.—Beef, pork, and lamb.—Use *lean* cuts of beef, pork, and lamb. Lean cuts of beef include extra-lean ground beef, sirloin tip, round steak, rump roast, arm roast or center-cut ham, loin chops, and tenderloin. Trim all fat off the outside of meats before cooking. It is not necessary to severely curtail the intake of red meat. Lean meat is rich in protein and contains a highly absorbable form of iron. Premenopausal women in particular should avoid severe reduction of lean red meat that would increase the risk for iron-deficiency anemia.

Processed meats.—Eat very little high-fat processed meats—bacon, bologna, salami, sausage, and hot dogs. Processed meats contain large quantities of "hidden" fat, and they are not rich in valuable nutrients.

Organ meats.—The organ meats—liver, sweetbreads, kidneys, and brain—are very rich in cholesterol, and they should be limited.

Chicken and turkey.—These are good sources of protein. The fat of poultry should be reduced by removal of skin and underlying fat layers. Chicken and turkey can be substituted for lean red meat in the diet, but they do not contain as much iron. Chicken and poultry should not be fried in fats rich in saturated fatty acids or covered with fat-rich sauces.

Fish.—Fish are a good source of protein. They contain cholesterol, but usually are low in saturated fatty acids. The preparation of fish is important. Like chicken and turkey, they should not be fried in saturated fats or covered with fat-rich sauces.

Shellfish.—Most shellfish contain less fat than meat and poultry. Their cholesterol content is variable (see Table 8). Some shellfish (eg, shrimp) are relatively high in cholesterol, but even these can be eaten occasionally within the recommended guidelines for cholesterol intake.

A reasonable approach to meat consumption is to limit intake of lean meat, chicken, turkey, and fish to six ounces

Table 8.—Cholesterol and Fat Content of Animal Products in Three-Ounce Portions (Cooked)		
Source	Cholesterol Content, mg/3 oz	Total Fat Content, g/3 oz
Red meats (lean)		
Beef	77	8.7
Lamb	78	8.8
Pork	79	11.1
Veal	128	4.7
Organ meats		
Liver	270	4.0
Pancreas (sweetbreads)	400	2.8
Kidney	329	2.9
Brains	1746	10.7
Heart	164	4.8
Poultry		
Chicken (without skin)		
Light	72	3.8
Dark	79	8.2
Turkey (without skin)		
Light	59	1.3
Dark	72	6.1
Fish		
Salmon	74	9.3
Tuna, light canned in water	55	0.7
Shellfish		
Abalone	90	0.8
Clams	57	1.7
Crab meat		
Alaskan King	45	1.3
Blue crab	85	1.5
Lobster	61	0.5
Oysters	93	4.2
Scallops	35	0.8
Shrimp	166	0.9

per day. The cholesterol and total fat content per three ounces (the recommended portion size) of various cooked meats are presented in Table 8.

DAIRY PRODUCTS.—Use skim milk or 1% milk instead of 2% or whole milk, which contains approximately 4% fat. Decrease natural and processed cheeses; substitute low-fat (2%) cottage cheese or synthetic cheeses produced from vegetable oils. Choose yogurt of the nonfat or low-fat (1% to 2%) type. Experiment with evaporated skim milk in recipes calling for heavy cream. Substitute low-fat yogurt or low-fat cottage cheese for sour cream in dips and salad dressings. Have at least two servings of very-low-fat dairy products, such as two glasses of skim (or 1%) milk, daily to help maintain calcium intake.

FATS AND OILS.—The general rule is to reduce intakes of fats and oils that are high in saturated fatty acids and cholesterol. Butter fat is high in both and should be curtailed as much as possible. Lard and beef fat are other blood cholesterol–raising animal fats. Vegetable fats do not contain cholesterol. However, certain vegetable fats— coconut oil, palm oil, and palm kernel oil—are very high in saturates and should be avoided; these are often used in bakery goods, processed foods, popcorn oils, and nondairy creamers. Labels on these foods should be read carefully to detect the presence of saturated vegetable oils.

Unsaturated vegetable oils and fats do not raise blood cholesterol, but they should be limited because they are high in calories. Generally, up to six to eight teaspoons a day is acceptable. Desirable liquid vegetable oils are corn oil, cottonseed oil, olive oil, rapeseed (canola) oil, safflower oil, soybean oil, and sunflower oil. Peanut oil is less desirable, but small amounts are acceptable. Margarine represents partially hydrogenated vegetable oil and is preferable to butter. Vegetable shortenings fall into the same category as margarine. Both contain quantities of *trans* fatty acids; these are not naturally occurring and should not be taken in excess. Mayonnaise and salad dressings often are made from unsaturated fats, but they too should be limited because of their high caloric content.

EGGS.—Eat no more than three egg yolks in a week on the Step-One Diet, and no more than one per week on the Step-Two Diet. Egg yolks often are hidden in cooked and processed foods. Egg whites contain no cholesterol, and they can be eaten often. Experiment with one to two egg whites instead of whole eggs in recipes, or use commercial egg substitutes that do not contain yolk.

FRUITS AND VEGETABLES.—It is advisable to feature fruits and vegetables as an important part of each meal. Both are rich in vitamins, fiber, and some minerals, and contribute to achieving the recommended allowances of these nutrients. Certain green and yellow vegetables may reduce the risk for cancer. Fruits (and even vegetables) can be used for snacks and desserts.

BREADS, CEREALS, PASTA, RICE, DRIED PEAS, AND BEANS.—These products are high in carbohydrate and protein and most are low in fat. Therefore, they can be increased in the diet as substitutes for fatty foods. However, they too contain calories and must not be eaten in excess. Cereals can be eaten as snacks as well as for breakfast. Dried peas and beans are good sources of protein. Combine large quantities of pasta, rice, legumes, and vegetables with smaller amounts of lean meat, fish or poultry to derive complete protein sources with less fat and calories.

NUTS.—Nuts tend to be high in fat, but the fat usually is unsaturated. The intake of nuts should thus be limited mainly to avoid excess calories. The same is largely true for peanut butter.

Other Eating Tips.—SNACKS.—Most candies should be limited as snacks; they tend to be rich in simple sugars and fats, and their caloric content outweighs their nutritional value. Some good choices in snacks are graham crackers, rye krisp, melba toast, soda crackers, bagels, English muffins, fruit, ready-to-eat cereals, and vegetables; these are preferable to snack crackers, french fries, and chips. Popcorn should be air popped or cooked in small amounts of liquid vegetable oil.

DESSERTS.—Eat fruits, low-fat fruit yogurt, and fruit ices instead of pastries, cake, and cookies. Also acceptable are sherbet, angel food cake, jello, frozen low-fat yogurt, and, occasionally, ice milk.

COOKING METHODS.—Choose those methods that use little or no fat. They include steaming, baking, broiling, grilling, or stir-frying in small amounts of fat. Foods can be cooked in the microwave or in a nonstick pan without added fat. Limit fried foods and avoid frying in saturated fat. Soups and stews should be chilled after cooking, and the congealed fat that forms on top after a few hours in the refrigerator should be skimmed off. When preparing meals avoid use of excess sodium, which can contribute to raising blood pressure in some people.

EATING AWAY FROM HOME.—Order entrees, potatoes, and vegetables without sauces or butter. When meat exceeds the size of a deck of cards (three to four ounces), the rest can be taken home for another meal. Choose

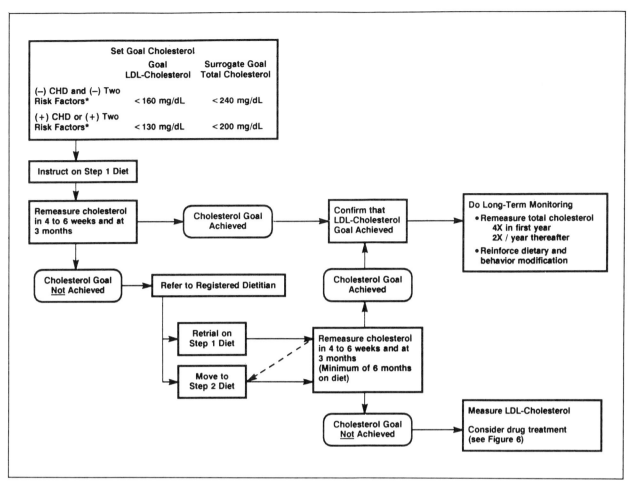

Fig 5.—Dietary treatment. Asterisk indicates one of which can be male sex
(Table 4); LDL, low density lipoprotein; CHD, coronary heart disease.

vegetable or fruit salads, and ask for salad dressings to be served on the side; use dressings sparingly. Limit high-fat toppings such as bacon, crumbled eggs, cheese, sunflower seeds, and olives, the latter two because they may be high in fat and salt. Ask for margarine instead of butter, and limit the amount of margarine used on bread and baked potatoes.

The physician who follows patients with high blood cholesterol frequently will be asked about specific food items. It may be helpful for the physician to have available a reference on food composition.[48,49]

Behavioral Modification.—Long-term adherence to the recommended diets can be achieved only through permanent modification of eating behavior. Several factors are required to achieve long-term success in adapting to a new diet. The rationale for diet change can be provided by the physician. Education of the patient in the principles of the fat-modified diet is the responsibility of the physician, the physician's immediate staff (eg, nurses), and, when utilized, a registered dietitian. The effectiveness of this approach will be facilitated by frequent communication among the different members of the team. Followup and monitoring by physicians is a key element in achieving the goals of LDL lowering on a long-term basis. Sometimes, permanent modification of eating behavior will require prolonged interaction with a registered dietitian. A brief summary of the process of dietary instruction and behavior modification as practiced by dietitians is provided in

Appendix III. This discussion may guide physicians in their own instructions to the patient.

An important adjunct to long-term change in eating behavior and life-style is a regular exercise program. Especially useful forms of exercise are activities that require movement of the body over distance, such as walking, stair climbing, running, cycling, and swimming. Improvements in cardiovascular fitness result from exercising regularly at moderate intensity for 15 to 30 minutes at least every other day. However, vigorous exercise must be carried out with caution in high-risk persons, and only with the advice of a physician and under the supervision of trained personnel.

Monitoring and Followup

Step-One Diet.—After starting the Step-One Diet, the serum total cholesterol level should be measured at four to six weeks and at three months (Fig 5). This will allow the patient enough time to adopt new eating habits and to respond to the dietary change. At the end of three months, the physician should assess the patient's adherence to the diet plan and response to dietary therapy. The response can be judged on the basis of the change in serum cholesterol level. If the response is satisfactory, ie, if the total cholesterol monitoring goal is met (<240 mg/dL without definite CHD or two other risk factors, <200 mg/dL with definite CHD or two other risk factors [Table 4]), then the LDL-cholesterol level should be measured in order to confirm that the LDL-cholesterol goal has been met. If the LDL goal is met, the phase of long-term monitoring can begin. If the response is not satisfactory, the patient should generally be referred to a registered dietitian and should progress to the Step-Two Diet or to another trial on the Step-One Diet. If this latter approach is selected, the patient should again be evaluated after four to six weeks and three months, with progression to the Step-Two Diet if the response is still not satisfactory.

Step-Two Diet.—On the Step-Two Diet, serum cholesterol levels should be measured after three to four weeks and three months of therapy. After three months of treatment with the Step-Two Diet, the physician should again assess the patient's adherence and response to the diet. It is important to document the extent of adherence to the therapeutic diet. If the desired goal for serum cholesterol–lowering has been attained, and a measurement of LDL-cholesterol level confirms that the LDL goal has been met, long-term monitoring can begin; if not, consideration should be given to drug therapy.

Diet Success: Long-term Monitoring.—The patient who has achieved the target goals for lowering of LDL-cholesterol by dietary therapy can be declared a diet success. Monitoring of total cholesterol should be carried out on a long-term basis. The fat-modified diet should be maintained indefinitely and the patient should be encouraged to adhere to the recommended eating pattern. Diet education should be continued and reinforced, by a registered dietitian if necessary. The patient should be counseled quarterly for the first year of long-term monitoring and twice yearly thereafter.

Total serum cholesterol should be measured prior to each visit, and the results should be used at the counseling session. For patients who have no lipoprotein abnormalities other than elevated LDL-cholesterol, monitoring at six-month intervals is appropriate. In such patients, the total cholesterol measurement, which can be made with a non-fasting blood sample and is less expensive than lipoprotein analysis, will provide a reasonable index of the LDL-cholesterol level. Many patients who previously have had high cholesterol levels on the typical American diet are "diet sensitive," which explains their originally high level. This means that continuous attention must be given to dietary adherence to avoid a "relapse" to high cholesterol concentrations. If the patient redevelops an elevated cholesterol level, the procedure outlined above for dietary therapy of elevated LDL-cholesterol may have to be reinstituted.

Inadequate Response to Diet.—A patient who fails to achieve the goals for lowering of total cholesterol (or LDL-cholesterol) by dietary therapy should be classified as having an inadequate response to diet. This does not necessarily mean diet failure, because a significant reduction in cholesterol levels may have occurred by diet modification. There are four categories of inadequate response to diet that can be distinguished.

1. Patients who have severe elevations of serum cholesterol often cannot achieve the goals of serum cholesterol lowering by diet, no matter how strict the diet. For these patients (Appendix II), it is not necessary to wait for six months of dietary therapy before adding drugs to the regimen.

2. Some patients with high LDL-cholesterol levels are biologically relatively resistant to LDL lowering by diet modification and will not achieve the cholesterol lowering goal despite good adherence to diet.

3. Others will adhere poorly to diet in spite of an intensive effort by the physician and counselors. After a few months it will be obvious that these patients will not adhere to dietary recommendations. Some physicians have the mistaken belief that most patients fall into this category, but this certainly is not true. A concerted effort by the physician, immediate staff, and registered dietitian should minimize the size of this group of patients.

4. For still other patients, a more prolonged period of dietary therapy may be justified. Up to a year, or even longer, may be required for a patient to learn to modify the diet by changing both the pattern of diet and eating habits. There may be a tendency for some physicians to employ drugs too soon instead of making the effort to change the patient's dietary habits. This tendency must be resisted. Adequate time should be allowed for the patient to attempt to modify the diet to achieve the desired goals of therapy.

Dietary Therapy for Special Groups

Severe Primary and Secondary Lipid Disorders.—Patients with severe primary hypercholesterolemia (eg, familial hypercholesterolemia) deserve maximal dietary therapy, ie, the Step-Two Diet. However, many of these patients will not respond adequately to diet and will require drug therapy (see Appendix II). Patients with severe primary hypertriglyceridemia should receive special attention to dietary management, which is described in more detail in Appendix II. The role of the diet in the treatment of low HDL-cholesterol and diabetic dyslipidemia likewise is discussed in Appendix II.

Elderly High-Risk Patients.—When considering dietary therapy for elderly patients classified as high risk, the value of diet modification for prevention of atherosclerotic disease must be balanced against the possibility of inadequate or inappropriate nutrition, which is often a problem in the elderly. The Step-One Diet seems prudent in elderly patients classified as high risk, but overly restrictive diets probably should be avoided. Intensive dietary therapy (eg, the Step-Two Diet) is not advisable in most elderly patients. Sound clinical judgment is required in making a decision about diet modification in older individuals classified as high risk, particularly because adequate intakes of calories and protein can be a major problem among the elderly.

Pregnant Women.—Elevations in cholesterol and triglyceride levels occur during pregnancy, with maximum levels in the third trimester. These increased levels are not generally clinically significant, but rare cases of hypertriglyceridemia and pancreatitis have been reported. Thus, some investigators recommend that serum triglyceride levels be measured at about the 28th week of gestation. Triglyceride levels generally return to baseline within six weeks postpartum, but elevations in LDL-cholesterol may occasionally persist for six to nine months. Such a response may represent a predisposition to elevated cholesterol. The approach to hyperlipidemic women who become pregnant is discussed in Appendix II.

Approach to Borderline–High Blood Cholesterol Group

Assessment of Risk.—Individuals with cholesterol levels in the range of 200 to 239 mg/dL are classified as having borderline–high blood cholesterol. Several studies indicate that cholesterol concentrations in the borderline-high range impart an increased CHD risk as compared with lower levels. However, while there is a progressive increase in risk as the blood cholesterol level rises from 200 to 240 mg/dL, the absolute risk does not rise sharply if no other risk factors are present (Table 3, "Background section"). For this reason, it is not necessary to enter most people with borderline–high blood cholesterol into active medical therapy. They nonetheless deserve to receive dietary information and cholesterol education as discussed below.

Special attention should be given to young adults with borderline–high blood cholesterol because they may be "tracking" toward the high-risk category later in life. In fact, many experts believe that young adults (20 to 39 years of age) with borderline–high blood cholesterol levels warrant full evaluation of serum lipoprotein fractions. This is an area where individualized clinical judgment is appropriate.

As with all patients, those with borderline–high blood cholesterol levels should be evaluated for other CHD risk factors and should be given preventive medical care for these factors if present. As indicated previously, patients in the borderline–high blood cholesterol group who have definite CHD or two other CHD risk factors (one of which can be male sex) should be managed in the same way as patients with high blood cholesterol levels.

Some experts believe that patients in the borderline–high blood cholesterol group who have one other major risk factor (eg, hypertension) also warrant lipoprotein measurements and possible dietary therapy. This is particularly so for young adults. Although this is not recommended here as a general approach for most patients with borderline–high blood cholesterol, it is clear that individualized clinical judgment and patient management is appropriate for this group.

Dietary Information and Patient Education.—For individuals with borderline–high blood cholesterol, intensive dietary therapy is not required. The population-based approach for lowering cholesterol levels in the entire community is expected, however, to have a significant impact on the diet and behavior of this group. Since these people are at increased risk for CHD, compared with individuals whose cholesterol levels are below 200 mg/dL, they should be made aware of the significance of their moderately increased risk and given information about how to modify the diet to lower the cholesterol level. The basic recommendation is for the patient to adopt an eating pattern similar to that of the Step-One Diet.

The same materials provided with the Step-One Diet might be made available to these patients by the physician and immediate staff, but intensive monitoring is not required. It should not be necessary to refer the patient to a registered dietitian, and the time devoted to patient instruction will be less than for the high-risk group. It is the physician's responsibility to inform the patient of his or her moderately increased risk, to advise changes in life-style and eating habits, to provide educational materials about diet, and to direct the individual to other sources of educational material. For instance, the local chapter of the American Heart Association usually stocks valuable materials containing dietary advice and practical approaches to diet modification. Sections of this report also can be copied for the patient.

Special attention should be given to dietary counseling of young adults with borderline–high blood cholesterol levels. They should be started on the Step-One Diet, but, in addition, they should be monitored for adherence and response more carefully than middle-aged patients in the same category. Young adults should be counseled on what to eat when away from home, and they should develop exercise habits that will be particularly useful as lifetime habits. Young adults who have an exceptionally high caloric intake because of a high level of exercise should be cautioned against excessive intake of saturated fatty acids,

cholesterol, and protein.

Reevaluation.—At the least, a follow-up measurement of the patient's cholesterol level should be made at one year and then at one- to two-year intervals. More frequent followup or measurements of lipoprotein fractions can be made at the discretion of the physician. Extra attention should be given to the followup of young adults with borderline–high blood cholesterol. Periodic determinations of serum cholesterol will indicate the physician's heightened and continuing concern; knowledge that the cholesterol level will be checked periodically should motivate the patient to adhere to the recommended diet; and these measurements will enable the physician to detect an increase in cholesterol level to the high blood cholesterol range, should it occur.

DRUG TREATMENT
When to Consider Drug Therapy/Treatment Goals

LDL-Cholesterol Levels for Initiation of Drug Therapy.—Patients whose LDL-cholesterol levels remain high despite adequate dietary therapy should be considered for drug treatment. At least six months of intensive dietary therapy and counseling should usually be carried out before initiating drug therapy. In individuals with severe elevations of LDL-cholesterol (>225 mg/dL) or with definite CHD, in whom dietary therapy alone is unlikely to be adequate or in whom the urgency of achieving substantial cholesterol lowering is greater, it may be appropriate to try dietary therapy alone for a period shorter than six months before considering drug therapy. A minimum of three months of dietary therapy is required to establish an adequate baseline for evaluating the efficacy of subsequent drug therapy. A registered dietitian, working with the physician to design an adequate treatment plan and assess dietary adherence, may enhance the effectiveness of dietary therapy sufficiently to obviate the need for drugs.

The LDL-cholesterol levels at which drug therapy should be considered after an adequate trial of dietary therapy alone are as follows:

(1) ≥190 mg/dL (very-high-risk LDL-cholesterol) in patients without definite CHD or two other CHD risk factors, one of which can be male sex (Table 4).

(2) ≥160 mg/dL (high-risk LDL-cholesterol) in patients with definite CHD or two other CHD risk factors (Table 4).

Clinical judgment is required when using these guidelines to make decisions about initiating drug therapy. All individuals with LDL-cholesterol levels ≥190 mg/dL are candidates for drug therapy, but the need is less pressing in older women. Men with LDL-cholesterol values between 160 and 190 mg/dL who have any other major risk factor generally should receive drug therapy. In women, however, a more conservative approach to drug therapy is appropriate, in view of the fact that the absolute risk of CHD is lower in women than in men. Thus, for women with LDL-cholesterol levels between 160 and 190 mg/dL, two other major risk factors or definite CHD should be present before initiating drug therapy. The distribution of LDL-cholesterol levels in the population is listed in Appendix I. It should be emphasized that maximum dietary therapy would significantly alter this distribution and decrease the percent of both men and women being considered for drug therapy.

Maximal efforts should be made in all patients to lower cholesterol levels and CHD risk by nonpharmacological approaches, such as diet, weight control, exercise, and other life-style modifications (eg, quitting smoking). This is especially important in patients who have not reached

Table 9.—Summary of the Major Drugs for Consideration*					
Drugs	Reduce CHD Risk	Long-term Safety	Maintaining Adherence	LDL-Cholesterol Lowering, %	Special Precautions
Cholestyramine, colestipol	Yes	Yes	Requires considerable education	15-30	Can alter absorption of other drugs, can increase triglyceride levels and should not be used in patients with hypertriglyceridemia
Nicotinic acid	Yes	Yes	Requires considerable education	15-30	Test for hyperuricemia, hyperglycemia, and liver function abnormalities
Lovastatin†	Not proven	Not established	Relatively easy	25-45	Monitor for liver function abnormalities, and possible lens opacities
Gemfibrozil‡	Not proven	Preliminary evidence	Relatively easy	5-15	May increase LDL-cholesterol in hypertriglyceridemic patients; should not be used in patients with gallbladder disease
Probucol	Not proven	Not established	Relatively easy	10-15	Lowers HDL-cholesterol; significance of this has not been established; prolongs QT interval

*CHD indicates coronary heart disease; LDL, low density lipoprotein; and HDL, high density lipoprotein.
†Recently approved by the Food and Drug Administration for marketing.
‡Not approved by the Food and Drug Administration for routine use in lowering cholesterol. The results of the Helsinki Heart Study should be available soon to define the effect on CHD risk and long-term safety.

their minimal LDL-cholesterol goal on dietary therapy alone, but who do not qualify for drug treatment according to the above guidelines. These patients include those without definite CHD or two other risk factors (see Table 4), whose LDL-cholesterol levels are in the range of 160 to 190 mg/dL, and those with definite CHD or two other risk factors, whose LDL-cholesterol levels are 130 to 160 mg/dL, on adequate dietary therapy. While drug therapy is not routinely recommended for such patients, consideration should be given to the use of low doses of bile acid sequestrants, especially in men. The sequestrants have a proven record of long-term safety. Moreover, many experts feel that patients with definite CHD should receive drug therapy if their minimal LDL-cholesterol goal (<130 mg/dL) has not been reached.

Low density lipoprotein–cholesterol is the best parameter to use in making the decision to use drugs and for monitoring the response to drug therapy (at least in the first few months). The decision to initiate drug treatment usually commits the patients to long-term therapy, for years or even for life. Since the number of potential patients who are candidates for prolonged administration of drugs is substantial, all decisions to initiate drug therapy must be made only after careful deliberation. Dietary therapy is clearly the safest treatment available. Hence, maximal efforts at dietary therapy should be made before initiating drug therapy, and should be continued even if drug therapy is needed. (For detailed information about the effects of drugs on serum lipids and lipoproteins and on CHD risk, including key studies and reviews, the reader should consult references 7, 10-13, and 50-60.)

Target Treatment Levels of LDL-Cholesterol.—The minimum goals of drug therapy are the same as those of dietary therapy, and are as follows:

(1) LDL-cholesterol <160 mg/dL in patients without definite CHD or two other CHD risk factors (one of which can be male sex, [Table 4]).

(2) LDL-cholesterol <130 mg/dL in patients with definite CHD or two other CHD risk factors (Table 4).

The LDL-cholesterol level that is necessary to promote substantial or maximal atherosclerotic regression has not been established, but some investigators believe that an LDL-cholesterol level as low as 100 mg/dL may be consid-

ered an ideal goal. Thus, it may be desirable to strive for an LDL-cholesterol level considerably below the minimal target goals of 160 mg/dL or 130 mg/dL, particularly in patients with definite CHD or with other major risk factors, once the decision to institute drug therapy has been made. There is no current evidence or opinion to suggest that further lowering of LDL-cholesterol below 100 mg/dL will produce significant additional benefit.

Selection and Use of Drugs

Overview and General Approach.—The major drugs for consideration include the following: bile acid sequestrants (cholestyramine, colestipol); nicotinic acid; HMG CoA reductase inhibitors (lovastatin); gemfibrozil; and probucol.

A brief summary of the major characteristics of these drugs is provided in Tables 9 and 10.

The drugs of first choice for patients without concurrent hypertriglyceridemia (triglyceride, <250 mg/dL) are the bile acid sequestrants and nicotinic acid. These drugs have been found to reduce CHD risk and to be generally safe in long-term use. They are effective in lowering LDL-cholesterol. Nicotinic acid is preferred for patients with concurrent hypertriglyceridemia (triglyceride, ≥250 mg/dL), because it lowers LDL-cholesterol without exacerbating the hypertriglyceridemia. The bile acid sequestrants can also effectively lower LDL-cholesterol in these patients, but their administration as single drug therapy will sometimes cause substantial increases in serum triglycerides.

Lovastatin is the first available drug in a new class, the HMG CoA reductase inhibitors. It is very effective in lowering LDL-cholesterol levels, produces modest reductions in triglyceride levels, and is easy to administer. The clinical use of lovastatin has been under study for only a few years, and its long-term safety and effects on CHD end points have not yet been established. It is, therefore, not classed as a drug of first choice in this report, and some caution is appropriate in its use.

Gemfibrozil and probucol are other available drugs that are also not classified as drugs of first choice. These drugs are generally not as effective in lowering LDL-cholesterol as are the bile acid sequestrants, nicotinic acid, or the

			Usual Time		
Drug	Starting Dose	Maximum Dose	and Frequency	Side Effects	Monitoring
Cholestyramine, colestipol	4 g twice daily, 5 g twice daily	24 g/d, 30 g/d	Twice daily, within an hour of major meals	Dose-dependent upper and lower gastrointestinal tract	Dosing schedules of coadministered drugs
Nicotinic acid	100-250 mg as single dose	3 g/d, rarely, doses up to 6 g are used	Three times a day with meals to minimize flushing	Flushing, upper gastrointestinal tract and hepatic	Uric acid, liver function, glucose
Lovastatin	20 mg once daily with evening meal	80 mg/d	Once (evening) or twice daily with meals	Gastrointestinal tract and hepatic, miscellaneous, including muscle pain	Liver function, creatine kinase, lens

Table 10.—Drugs Highly Effective in Lowering LDL-Cholesterol*

*LDL indicates low density lipoprotein.

HMG CoA reductase inhibitors. Moreover, these drugs have not been shown to reduce CHD risk and their safety for long-term use has not been established at this time. However, the results of a large clinical trial, the Helsinki Heart Study, evaluating the effects of gemfibrozil on CHD risk are expected soon.[59] If a clinically beneficial effect is seen, the recommended use of gemfibrozil will probably be expanded.

The cost of drugs may also warrant consideration. Cost should be viewed in relation to a drug's effectiveness and safety in cholesterol lowering. The following are the approximate yearly wholesale costs of drugs, derived from data in the 1986 Redbook; retail costs will be somewhat higher. Cholestyramine (Questran) at a daily dose of 16 g or colestipol (Colestid) at a daily dose of 20 g in bulk containers is $500 to $550; "generic" nicotinic acid at a daily dose of 3 g is $50, while Nico-Bid is $700; gemfibrozil (Lopid) at a daily dose of 1.2 g or probucol (Lorelco) at a daily dose of 1 g is approximately $375. Lovastatin is being marketed to the pharmacist at $1.25 per 20-mg tablet; at a dose of 40 mg/d, the yearly wholesale cost will be approximately $910.

Many patients with marked elevations of LDL-cholesterol will not be adequately controlled with single-drug therapy, and the use of combinations of drugs with synergistic mechanisms of action may be particularly effective in these patients. The mechanisms of action, clinical efficacy, and side effects of the drugs of first choice and the HMG CoA reductase inhibitors for the treatment of high-risk LDL-cholesterol levels are discussed in the following section. There then follows a more abbreviated discussion of the other drugs and of combination drug therapy.

Drugs of First Choice.—*Bile Acid Sequestrants: Cholestyramine and Colestipol.*—The major effect of the bile acid sequestrants is a lowering of the level of LDL-cholesterol. The sequestrants have the advantage that their use has been shown to reduce CHD risk in large-scale intervention trials and that long-term safety information is also available.[10,13] The sequestrants are not absorbed from the gastrointestinal tract and lack systemic toxicity. Thus, they are particularly suitable for treating younger patients, especially children and women considering pregnancy. The disadvantages of the sequestrants are related to the method of administration and the frequency of gastrointestinal side effects.

The primary action of the sequestrants, which are anion exchange resins, is to bind bile acids in the intestinal lumen; this interrupts the enterohepatic circulation of bile acids and leads to an increased hepatic synthesis of bile acids from cholesterol. Depletion of the hepatic pool of cholesterol results in an increase in LDL receptor activity in the liver. This in turn stimulates removal of LDL from plasma and lowers the concentration of LDL-cholesterol. Bile acid sequestrant therapy may increase hepatic VLDL production and thus increase the plasma concentration of triglycerides.

Cholestyramine and colestipol are both powders that must be mixed with water or fruit juice; they are taken in two (or, occasionally, three) divided doses with meals. The cholesterol-lowering effects of 4 g of cholestyramine are equivalent to those obtained with 5 g of colestipol. Decreases in LDL-cholesterol of 10% to 15% may be achieved with the initial suggested starting dosage schedule of 5 g of colestipol (or 4 g of cholestyramine) taken twice daily. In patients who do not respond adequately, the dose is increased gradually. Generally, the benefits of daily doses exceeding the equivalent of 16 g of cholestyramine are offset by poorer patient adherence and a greater incidence of gastrointestinal side effects. The response to therapy in individual patients is quite variable, but 15% to 30% reductions in the concentrations of LDL-cholesterol may be achieved with 16 to 24 g/d of cholestyramine or an equivalent dose of colestipol. The choice of one or the other of these drugs is dependent on individual patient preference based on taste and palatability. Cholestyramine is available in 9-g packets (each containing 4 g of cholestyramine and 5 g of orange-flavored filler) and in 378-g cans. Colestipol is available in 5-g packets and bottles containing 500 g, and there are no additives. The cost-per-unit dosage for cholestyramine is currently considerably less when it is purchased in bulk containers.

The bile acid sequestrants are contraindicated as single-drug therapy in patients with marked hypertriglyceridemia (triglyceride, >500 mg/dL) or patients with a history of severe constipation. The most common side effects associated with sequestrant therapy are gastrointestinal, and include constipation, bloating, epigastric fullness, nausea, and flatulence. Some suggestions for dealing with these side effects are provided in Appendix IV. These drugs are not absorbed, but they may interfere with the absorption of other anionic drugs if these are taken concurrently. It is generally advisable to take other medications at least one hour before or four hours after the bile acid sequestrants. The sequestrants can interfere with the absorption of digitoxin, warfarin, thyroxine, thiazide diuretics, beta blockers, and, potentially, many other drugs. Decreased absorption of fat-soluble vitamins and folic acid has been reported with prolonged high doses of the resins, primarily in patients with severe liver or small-bowel disease. Routine vitamin supplementation is not needed or recommended in adult patients. Biochemical side effects include a modest increase in plasma triglyceride concentrations in many patients and an occasional mild and usually transient increase in alkaline phosphatase and transaminase.

Nicotinic Acid.—The water-soluble B vitamin, nicotinic acid, has been used to lower plasma lipid levels for many years. Administration of nicotinic acid in the Coronary Drug Project was associated with a reduction in recurrent myocardial infarctions and in long-term total mortality.[11,53] Nicotinic acid lowers total and LDL-cholesterol and triglyceride levels and raises HDL-cholesterol levels. Decreases in total cholesterol levels of 25% may be observed. Nicotinic acid decreases the hepatic production of VLDL and, ultimately, the production of LDL-cholesterol. Nicotinamide is not effective in lowering LDL-cholesterol and cannot substitute for nicotinic acid.

Nicotinic acid is a very effective drug that requires considerable physician and patient education (Appendix IV). Although it has frequent side effects, these are generally reversible on reducing the dose or discontinuing the drug. Because of its proven efficacy and safety, the efforts required to use this agent are justified.

Nicotinic acid is the least costly of all the currently available agents. Side effects, especially flushing of the skin, often limit acceptance by patients. The flushing is prostaglandin mediated and can be significantly decreased by pretreatment with aspirin or nonsteroidal anti-inflammatory drugs. Tolerance to this flushing develops rapidly over several weeks. Flushing is greatly reduced by slowly increasing the dose of nicotinic acid and avoiding administration on an empty stomach. The use of sustained-release preparations will also reduce flushing, but the cost is considerably greater.[54] Flushing will return if doses are omitted from the prescribed schedule.

Nicotinic acid therapy is generally initiated with a single dose of 100 to 250 mg/d. This initial dose is usually given after dinner to minimize problems with flushing during normal daily activities. The frequency of dose and total daily dose is slowly increased every four to seven days until the first-level therapeutic dose of 1.5 to 2 g/d is reached. If the LDL-cholesterol is not lowered sufficiently, the dose should be increased to 3 g/d (1.0 g three times per day). In patients with marked elevations of plasma cholesterol, a higher daily dose up to 6 g/d is occasionally used.

Hyperuricemia and abnormalities in liver function studies are other common adverse effects, but are more likely with higher doses of nicotonic acid. Hyperglycemia and a number of gastrointestinal side effects occasionally occur. Liver function, blood glucose, and uric acid levels should be evaluated before beginning nicotinic acid and after reaching therapeutic dosage or increasing the dose level. The medication is supplied in 50-, 100-, and 500-mg tablets. The latter dosage is preferred for chronic therapy. Contraindications to nicotinic acid therapy include peptic ulcer, hepatic disease, and gouty arthritis or significant hyperuricemia.

New Drugs: Inhibitors of HMG CoA Reductase.—The discovery of specific competitive inhibitors of the rate-limiting enzyme in cholesterol biosynthesis (HMG CoA reductase) has opened up a new avenue of therapy for patients with primary hypercholesterolemia.[55,56] A number of drugs in this category are currently being evaluated including lovastatin, simvastatin, and pravastatin. Of these, lovastatin has been most extensively studied in humans and has recently been approved for marketing. Long-term safety information is limited or not available, and thus caution in its use is recommended. This is especially true for individuals who are not at high risk.

Although the effects of HMG CoA reductase inhibitors on CHD incidence have not yet been established, mean reductions in LDL-cholesterol of 25% to 45% have been noted in both familial and nonfamilial forms of hypercholesterolemia. The HMG CoA reductase inhibitors increase LDL receptor activity in the liver and increase the rate of receptor-mediated removal of LDL from plasma. Additionally, the production of LDL is also decreased. Patients are generally started on 20 mg of lovastatin once daily with the evening meal. The dose may be increased to 40 and then to 80 mg/d as a single evening dose or divided (twice a day) doses with meals. The cholesterol-lowering effects of lovastatin have persisted for the duration of the observed treatment periods up to two to four years.

Lovastatin at doses of 20 to 80 mg daily has been well tolerated. Reported side effects (often transient) to date have included changes in bowel function, headaches, nausea, fatigue, insomnia, skin rashes, and myositis (myalgia associated with markedly elevated creatine kinase [CPK] levels), which collectively have occurred in less than 5% of treated patients. Biochemical changes have included increases in transaminase and CPK levels. Approximately 1.9% of patients have developed persistent increases in transaminase levels of greater than three times normal after three to 16 months of therapy, requiring discontinuance of therapy. Careful monitoring of liver function studies is essential. Lovastatin does not impair steroid hormone production. There is a concern about the possibility that there may be effects on formation of lens opacities; although no effects have been detected to date in humans, this is still being investigated. Baseline and regular follow-up evaluation of the lens should be done.

If long-term safety can be satisfactorily established, these inhibitors of cholesterol biosynthesis will represent a major advance in the therapy of hypercholesterolemia. These agents are extremely effective in reducing LDL-cholesterol concentrations and, from the patient's point of view, are easy to take.

Other Drugs.—*Gemfibrozil.*—Gemfibrozil, a fibric acid derivative, is approved by the Food and Drug Administration primarily for triglyceride lowering to reduce the risk of pancreatitis, and not for routine use in lowering cholesterol to reduce the risk of CHD. It is sometimes used as single drug therapy in patients who do not tolerate the resins or nicotinic acid, and is occasionally used in combination with first-choice drugs (see the section on "Combined Drug Treatment"). The long-term safety and effects of gemfibrozil on CHD risk are still being evaluated in clinical trials. Preliminary evidence for long-term safety of gemfibrozil is available in the interim report of the Helsinki Heart Study.[59] This is a large, placebo-controlled study to evaluate the effect of this drug on CHD risk, and the results should be announced in the near future. If a clinically beneficial effect is demonstrated in this clinical trial, the recommended use of gemfibrozil will probably be expanded.

Gemfibrozil is primarily and highly effective in lowering triglycerides, and there is an associated increase in HDL-cholesterol. Because of the effect of this drug on HDL-cholesterol, the results of the Helsinki Heart Study may be of particular interest. To date, increases of HDL-cholesterol induced by treatment have not been conclusively shown to be associated with a decreased risk of CHD. A decrease in LDL-cholesterol of 10% to 15% may be seen in patients without elevated triglycerides treated with gemfibrozil. An increase in LDL-cholesterol may be seen in primary hypertriglyceridemia, and either increases or decreases in LDL-cholesterol may be seen in patients with elevated levels of both cholesterol and triglycerides. Gemfibrozil is well tolerated in most patients. The more common side effects include a variety of gastrointestinal symptoms, and occasional changes in hematologic parameters and liver function tests are noted. Gemfibrozil does potentiate the effects of oral anticoagulants and increases biliary lithogenicity. It is available as 300-mg capsules, and the usual dosage is 600 mg twice daily.*

Probucol.—Probucol therapy usually reduces LDL-cholesterol by about 8% to 15%, but there is also an associated reduction in HDL-cholesterol of up to 25%. There are no extensive, long-term clinical studies currently available for assessing probucol's safety or effect on CHD risk. Preliminary information indicates that probucol may inhibit the oxidation and tissue deposition of LDL. Probucol increases the rate of LDL catabolism, part of which may involve nonreceptor-mediated pathways.[57] The role of probucol in the treatment of patients with high LDL-cholesterol is uncertain because of concerns about the reduction in HDL-cholesterol, but xanthoma regression has also been reported as the HDL-cholesterol level decreases. Probucol is sometimes used as single drug therapy in patients who do not tolerate other drugs, and is occasionally used in combination with first-choice drugs (see the section on "Combined Drug Treatment").

Probucol is generally well tolerated, and side effects (including diarrhea, flatulence, abdominal pain, and nausea) occur in less than 5% of patients. Probucol causes prolongation of the QT interval, and the drug should be regarded as contraindicated in patients with electrocardiographic findings suggestive of ventricular irritability, with an initially prolonged QT interval, or taking other drugs that prolong the QT interval. Probucol is stored in adipose tissue, and blood levels fall slowly after therapy is discontinued. It is available in 250-mg tablets, and the usual dose is 500 mg twice daily.

Clofibrate.—Clofibrate, like gemfibrozil, is a fibric acid derivative. It is approved by the Food and Drug Administration primarily for triglyceride lowering to reduce the risk of pancreatitis, and not for routine use in lowering cholesterol to reduce the risk of CHD. Its effects on lipids and lipoproteins and its side effects are generally similar to those described above for gemfibrozil. Clofibrate is used less frequently than gemfibrozil, however, because of reports of long-term toxicity in clinical trials, particularly the World Health Organization Clofibrate Study.[58]

---

*Additional Note: The following statement was prepared by the Steering Committee of the Cholesterol Adult Treatment Panel (Drs Goodman, Cleeman, Brown, Grundy, Hulley, Hunninghake, and Rifkind) six weeks following the final approval of the report by the National Cholesterol Education Program Coordinating Committee:

Subsequent to the formal endorsement of this report by the National Cholesterol Education Program Coordinating Committee, the results of the Helsinki Heart Study were reported (Frick, MH, et al, *N Engl J Med* 1987;317:1237-1245). This randomized, double-blind five-year trial tested the clinical efficacy and safety of gemfibrozil, 600 mg twice daily, vs placebo in 4081 asymptomatic middle-aged men with elevated blood cholesterol levels. Gemfibrozil moderately reduced the serum levels of total and LDL-cholesterol, and also reduced triglycerides and increased HDL-cholesterol levels. The incidence of CHD was reduced by 34% in the drug-treated group (*P*<.02). This trial thus demonstrates the clinical efficacy and safety of gemfibrozil in reducing coronary risk in patients with high cholesterol levels. In view of these results, it would be reasonable for physicians to consider the use of gemfibrozil more readily when selecting drugs for patients with high cholesterol levels who meet the criteria for drug treatment. Gemfibrozil may be particularly useful, as an alternative to nicotinic acid, in patients with high-risk LDL-cholesterol levels who also have borderline hypertriglyceridemia (triglyceride levels, 250 to 500 mg/dL) and low HDL-cholesterol levels. More extensive review and evaluation of the results of the Helsinki Heart Study may further clarify the place of gemfibrozil in the treatment of patients with high blood cholesterol.

Miscellaneous Drugs.—These drugs are not recommended for general use.

Neomycin.—Neomycin is a nonabsorbable aminoglycoside antibiotic with cholesterol-lowering effects. Reductions in LDL-cholesterol levels of 20% to 25% have been reported. Side effects include diarrhea and abdominal cramps. Neomycin also has a potential to cause serious ototoxicity and nephrotoxicity. This drug is not approved by the Food and Drug Administration as a lipid-lowering agent, and its use should be considered investigational.

Dextrothyroxine.—Dextrothyroxine, the optical isomer of L-thyroxine, moderately lowers the concentrations of LDL-cholesterol, but does so at the expense of making the patient moderately hyperthyroid. Dextrothyroxine is approved by the Food and Drug Administration for use in selected young adults with primary hypercholesterolemia who are unable to take other effective lipid-lowering drugs. It is not recommended for use in this report because of the high incidence of adverse cardiovascular effects and hypermetabolic effects. Other available drugs have a more favorable benefit/risk ratio.

Investigational Drugs.—There is currently a flurry of activity in the development of new cholesterol-lowering agents. There are several new HMG CoA reductase inhibitors in various stages of development. Simvastatin and pravastatin are currently being extensively investigated in clinical trials. A number of newer fibric acid derivatives are available in Europe, and bezafibrate and fenofibrate have been fairly extensively evaluated in the United States. They appear to be more effective in lowering LDL-cholesterol than gemfibrozil or clofibrate.

Combined Drug Treatment.—If the response to single-drug therapy with one of the drugs of first choice is inadequate, combined drug therapy using two agents, preferably with synergistic mechanisms of action, should be considered to further lower LDL-cholesterol.[12,56,60] Experience with such drug combinations is somewhat limited, and it might be advisable to undertake such combination therapy in consultation with a lipid specialist. In patients without concurrent hypertriglyceridemia, the combination of a bile acid sequestrant with either nicotinic acid or lovastatin has the potential of lowering LDL-cholesterol by 45% to 60%. The addition of probucol or gemfibrozil to bile acid sequestrant therapy may occasionally be beneficial, but the efficacy of these combinations is significantly less than the abovementioned combinations. The combination of sequestrants and probucol may result in fewer gastrointestinal complaints.

For patients with both increased LDL-cholesterol levels and hypertriglyceridemia, nicotinic acid and lovastatin represent initial drugs of choice. Lovastatin and nicotinic acid can also be used in combination, or either of these two drugs can be combined with a bile acid sequestrant to obtain a possible additional 20% to 25% reduction in LDL-cholesterol. As yet, there is very little experience with the combination of lovastatin and nicotinic acid in terms of possible adverse effects such as hepatotoxicity. The addition of gemfibrozil to a bile acid sequestrant, lovastatin, or nicotinic acid will usually produce additional lowering of triglycerides, but the effect on change in LDL-cholesterol levels is quite variable. More experience is required with the combination of lovastatin and gemfibrozil to see if there is an increased risk of myositis.

Other Approaches.—Effective control of elevated levels of LDL-cholesterol will be attainable in the majority of patients using the primary drugs and drug combinations discussed above. Patients who do not achieve adequate cholesterol reduction after this type of therapy should be

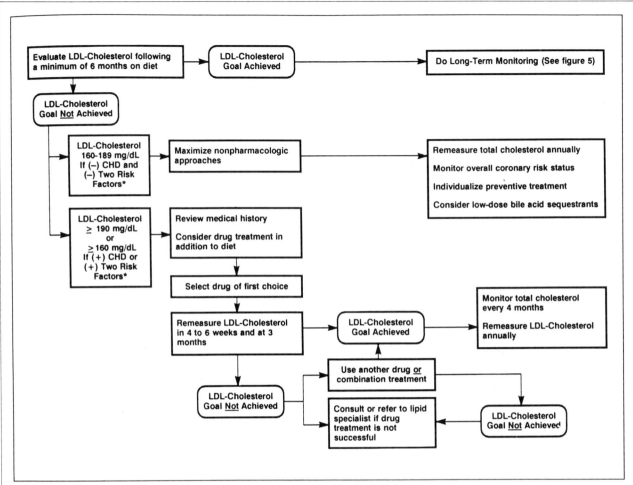

Fig 6.—Drug treatment. Asterisk indicates one of which can be male sex
(Table 4); LDL, low density lipoprotein; CHD, coronary heart disease.

referred to a specialist in lipid disorders. In addition to
investigational drugs or other drug combinations, other
approaches may be indicated. In patients with FH, plasmapheresis (either simple plasma exchange or plasma
exchange with some type of affinity chromatography) has
been used to selectively remove LDL from plasma. A
surgical procedure, partial ileal bypass, has occasionally
been used to lower LDL-cholesterol in heterozygous FH.
In homozygous FH, portacaval shunt and liver transplant
have been employed.

Monitoring and Followup of Patients

Drug therapy is usually not begun until patients have
had at least a six-month trial of dietary therapy. The
decision to begin drug therapy should be reviewed with
the patient along with the respective benefits and side
effects of the appropriate drugs.

It is important to have a minimum of two determinations
of lipoprotein levels during the last one to two months of
maximum dietary therapy, because the efficacy of drug
therapy needs to be judged against an accurately determined baseline. With good drug adherence, maximum
lowering of LDL-cholesterol is obtained within four weeks
of initating drug therapy. Thus, the first follow-up LDL-
cholesterol determination should be made four to six weeks
after initiating drug therapy. A second measurement

should be done at three months; a minimum of two
lipoprotein determinations is essential for evaluating drug
efficacy. The mean of these two determinations and a
careful assessment of drug adherence should be used to
initially judge the effectiveness of drug treatment. After
the response to drug therapy has been established and if
the response is adequate, then the patient should be seen
for a follow-up visit approximately every four months, in
order to monitor for side effects and assess the patient's
status and response to therapy. A lipoprotein profile (LDL-
cholesterol measurement) at yearly intervals will usually
be adequate; measurement of serum total cholesterol will
usually suffice for the interim visits (Fig 6). In the course
of long-term monitoring, if the total cholesterol or lipoprotein determination at a particular visit is out of keeping
with the patient's previous values, the determination should
be repeated to confirm the level.

The previously obtained laboratory work and medical
history and physical examination should be reviewed before
initiating drug therapy to see if any tests should be
repeated or whether additional tests are required. The
laboratory indications of adverse drug effects are generally
manifested by changes in blood count, or liver or kidney
function studies. These tests should definitely be repeated
within one to three months of initiation of drug therapy,
depending on the drug used, and at four- to 12-month

intervals thereafter. Additional testing may be required if abnormalities are noted, or if a high dose of drug is being used, or because of the known toxicity profile of a given drug (see previous discussion of major adverse effects for individual drugs). For example, more frequent transaminases are indicated when using lovastatin and more frequent uric acid and liver function determinations with higher doses of nicotinic acid.

The use of the bile acid sequestrants and nicotinic acid requires frequent observation or contact with the patient during the early stage of treatment. Clinic visits and/or telephone contact is usually indicated at least at monthly intervals for three to four months. Lovastatin requires continuing liver function and lens evaluation. Thus, there is a need for judgment regarding the frequency of visits and observation during the early phases of drug therapy. When the final drug regimen has been established, followup visits should continue at four-month intervals to promote adherence. Many of the routine patient contacts may not need direct physician involvement but may be handled instead by physician's assistants, nurses, pharmacists, or dietitians.

If the patient has had at least a 15% decrease in LDL-cholesterol and is tolerating the drug but has not achieved the minimal target goal for LDL-cholesterol, consideration should be given to adding another drug as discussed in the "Combined Drug Treatment" section. If the patient has not had a 15% decrease in LDL-cholesterol or is not tolerating the drug, the physician should either switch to another drug or proceed to combination therapy, if necessary. Consultation with a lipid specialist may be useful in the management of patients with persistently high LDL-cholesterol levels despite dietary and drug therapy.

Adherence to Drug Therapy

General Comments.—Drug therapy is likely to continue for a lifetime or for a very prolonged period of time. Hence, the patient must be well informed about the goals of drug treatment and the side effects of medication. The need for a long-term commitment must be emphasized. When dealing with the selection of bile acid sequestrants vs newer, "easier" drugs, safety must be emphasized. It is important to start with small doses of the drugs, especially when using sequestrants and nicotinic acid. The patient must have time to adapt to the drug regimen, and any difficulties must be remedied before proceeding to higher doses. Health professionals who are already involved in patient education would be a logical source of help for the patient who is having problems with side effects. The initial experience with a regimen is likely to predict long-term adherence.

The frequency of medication intake and its impact on life-style must be frankly discussed. The planned regimen should attempt to minimize changes in daily life-style. Reinforcement of adherence by periodic laboratory monitoring and reassurance is essential. There is also a need for patience, an adequate amount of time, and understanding on the part of the health professional. It must be emphasized to patients that the ultimate responsibility for management is theirs, and communication with the appropriate health professional is essential when problems arise. The importance of diet in addition to drugs must continue to be emphasized. Some practical suggestions concerning adherence are summarized in Appendix IV.

Patient Counseling/Assessment of Adherence.—The management of a risk factor like elevated serum cholesterol is multifactorial and in the ideal treatment setting would call on the expertise of a variety of professionals. Time and resources dictate a more prudent approach. Drug therapy for many patients can be successfully managed by the physician in his or her office along with the assistance of an office health professional who has skill and experience in teaching patients and some understanding of the side effects of drugs and approaches to their management. This person will generally be a nurse, or a nursing or physician's assistant. The community pharmacist is also a valuable resource for patient education. Additional educational efforts are usually required to ensure the successful utilization of the bile acid sequestrants and nicotinic acid, as compared with the other cholesterol-lowering drugs. There should be regular communication with the supervising physician, but many other health professionals can effectively educate the patient. A sensitive, caring individual who routinely sees the patient (constant caretaker model) and develops the patient's trust is often an important component of an effective adherence counseling program.

It is important that community health care providers utilize appropriate specialist consultation. Lipid specialists are available in most large metropolitan areas. Of major importance is the maintenance of continuing education in the cholesterol area, where knowledge is rapidly growing. Furthermore, consultation on an ongoing basis may be sought so that more difficult cases or situations can be reviewed and consultation obtained for planning treatment. If the target treatment goals for LDL-cholesterol are not achieved or if the patient is having considerable problems with side effects of medication, referral to a specialist in lipid disorders may be indicated. This is especially important if the patient has definite CHD, a genetic disorder with severe hypercholesterolemia, or other major risk factors. It is difficult to provide the best care possible through the use of a multidisciplinary team and also control the cost of treatment to the patient. Minimizing the number of office visits, limiting the number of direct care providers, and using the least costly provider with the broadest skills for routine care will help. Maximizing the response to dietary therapy will minimize the need for costly drug therapy. The use of standardized teaching materials that can be adapted to individual needs, and inexpensive followup between office visits (eg, telephone or postcard exchanges) may help patients successfully follow a regimen that has been tailored to their circumstances and that has every likelihood of effectively lowering their elevated cholesterol levels.

References

1. Consensus Development Conference: Lowering blood cholesterol to prevent heart disease. *JAMA* 1985;253:2080-2086.
2. Atherosclerosis Study Group: Optimal resources for primary prevention of atherosclerotic diseases. *Circulation* 1984;70:157A-205A.
3. Grundy SM: Cholesterol and coronary heart disease: A new era. *JAMA* 1986;256:2849-2858.
4. Hulley SB, Rhodes GG: The plasma lipoproteins as risk factors: Comparison of electrophoretic and ultracentrifugation results. *Metabolism* 1982;31:773-777.
5. Martin MJ, Hulley SB, Browner WS, et al: Serum cholesterol, blood pressure, and mortality: Implications from a cohort of 361 662 men. *Lancet* 1986;2:933-936.
6. Stamler J, Wentworth D, Neaton J: Is the relationship between serum cholesterol and risk of death from CHD continuous and graded? *JAMA* 1986;256:2823-2828.
7. Schaefer EJ, Levy RI: Pathogenesis and management of lipoprotein disorders. *N Engl J Med* 1985;312:1300-1310.
8. Brown NS, Goldstein JL: A receptor-mediated pathway for cholesterol homeostasis. *Science* 1986;232:34-47.
9. Ross R: The pathogenesis of atherosclerosis—an update. *N Engl J*

Med 1986;314:488-500.

10. Lipid Research Clinics Program: The Lipid Research Clinics Coronary Primary Prevention Trial results: I. Reduction in the incidence of coronary heart disease. *JAMA* 1984;251:351-364.

11. Canner PL, Berge KG, Wenger NK, et al: Fifteen-year mortality in Coronary Drug Project patients: Long-term benefit with niacin. *J Am Coll Cardiol* 1986;8:1245-1255.

12. Blankenhorn DM, Nessim SA, Johnson RL, et al: Beneficial effects of combined colestipol-niacin therapy on coronary atherosclerosis and coronary venous bypass grafts. *JAMA* 1987;257:3233-3240.

13. Lipid Research Clinics Program: The Lipid Research Clinics Coronary Primary Prevention Trial results: II. The relationship of reduction in incidence of coronary heart disease to cholesterol lowering. *JAMA* 1984;251:365-374.

14. Kannel WB, Neaton JD, Wentworth D, et al: Overall and CHD mortality rates in relation to major risk factors in 325 348 men screened for the MRFIT. *Am Heart J* 1986;112:825-836.

15. Study Group, European Atherosclerosis Society: Strategies for the prevention of coronary heart disease: A policy statement of the European Atherosclerosis Society. *Eur Heart J* 1987;8:77-88.

16. Jacobs D, Barrett-Conner E: Re-test reliability of plasma cholesterol and triglycerides: The Lipid Research Clinics Prevalence Study. *Am J Epidemiol* 1982;116:878-885.

17. Koke JD, Hawkins DL: Estimating baseline values of the variables of intervention in a clinical trial. *Contr Clin Trials* 1985;6:136-145.

18. Friedewald WT, Levy RI, Fredrickson DS: Estimation of the concentration of low-density lipoprotein cholesterol in plasma, without use of the preparative ultracentrifuge. *Clin Chem* 1972;18:499-502.

19. DeLong DM, DeLong ER, Wood PD, et al: A comparison of methods for the estimation of plasma low- and very-low-density lipoprotein cholesterol: The Lipid Research Clinics Prevalence Study. *JAMA* 1986;256:2372-2377.

20. Goldstein JL, Schrott HG, Hazzard WR, et al: Hyperlipidemia in coronary heart disease: II. Genetic analysis of lipid levels in 176 families and delineation of a new inherited disorder, combined hyperlipidemia. *J Clin Invest* 1973;52:1544-1568.

21. Castelli WP: The triglyceride issue: A view from Framingham. *Am Heart J* 1986;112:432-437.

22. Consensus Development Conference: Treatment of hypertriglyceridemia. *JAMA* 1984;251:1196-1200.

23. National Center for Health Statistics: Total serum cholesterol levels of adults 20 to 74 years of age: United States, 1976-1980, *Vital and Health Statistics*, Ser. II, No. 236. Dept Health and Human Services publication (PHS) 86-1686. Government Printing Office, May 1986.

24. Lerner DJ, Kanner WB: Patterns of coronary heart disease morbidity and mortality in the sexes: A 26-year follow-up of the Framingham population. *Am Heart J* 1986;111:383-390.

25. Feinlieb M, Gillum RF: CHD in the elderly: The magnitude of the problem in the US, in Wenger NK, Furberg CD, Pitt E (eds): *CHD in the Elderly.* New York, Elsevier, 1986, pp 29-59.

26. Grundy SM, Bilheimer D, Blackburn H, et al: Rationale of the diet-heart statement of the American Heart Association: Report of Nutrition Committee. *Circulation* 1982;65:839A-854A.

27. Stamler J: Population studies, in Levy RI, Rifkind BM, Dennis BH, et al (eds): *Nutrition, Lipids, and Coronary Diseases: A Global View.* New York, Raven Press, 1979, pp 25-88.

28. Hjermann I, Velve Byre K, Holme I, et al: Effect of diet and smoking intervention on the incidence of coronary heart disease. *Lancet* 1981;2:1303-1310.

29. Gotto AM Jr, Bierman EL, Connor WE, et al: Recommendations for treatment of hyperlipidemia in adults: A joint statement of the Nutrition Committee and the Council on Arteriosclerosis. *Circulation* 1984;69:1067A-1090A.

30. Keys A, Anderson JT, Grande F: Serum cholesterol response to changes in the diet. *Metabolism* 1965;14:747-787.

31. Hegsted DM, McGandy RB, Myers ML, et al: Quantitative effects of dietary fat on serum cholesterol in man. *Am J Clin Nutr* 1965;17:281-295.

32. Keys A, Grande F, Anderson JT: Bias and misrepresentation revisited: Perspective on saturated fat. *Am J Clin Nutr* 1974;27:188-212.

33. Keys A (ed): Coronary heart disease in seven countries. *Circulation* 1970;41(suppl 1):I-1-I-211.

34. Herold PM, Kinsella JE: Fish oil consumption and decreased risk of cardiovascular disease: A comparison of findings from animal and human feeding trials. *Am J Clin Nutr* 1986;43:566-598.

35. Mattson FH, Erickson BA, Kligman AM: Effect of dietary cholesterol on serum cholesterol in man. *Am J Clin Nutr* 1972;25:589-594.

36. Ginsberg H, Le NA, Mays C, et al: Lipoprotein metabolism in nonresponders to increased dietary cholesterol. *Arteriosclerosis* 1981;1:463-470.

37. Keys A: Serum cholesterol response to dietary cholesterol. *Am J Clin Nutr* 1984;40:351-359.

38. Schonfeld G, Patsch W, Rudell LL, et al: Effects of dietary cholesterol and fatty acids on plasma lipoproteins. *Am J Clin Invest* 1982;69:1072-1080.

39. Anderson LW, Story L, Sieling B, et al: Hypocholesterolemic effects of oat-bran or bean intake for hypercholesterolemic men. *Am J Clin Nutr*

1984;40:1146-1155.

40. Harlan WR, Hull AL, Schmouder RL, et al: Blood pressure and nutrition in adults: The National Health and Nutrition Examination Survey. *Am J Epidemiol* 1984;120:17-28.

41. Hennekens CH: Alcohol, in Kaplan NM, Stamler J (eds): *Prevention of Coronary Heart Disease.* Philadelphia, WB Saunders Co, 1983, pp 130-138.

42. Hubert HB, Feinlieb M, McNamara PM, et al: Obesity as an independent risk factor for cardiovascular disease: A 26-year follow-up of participants in the Framingham Heart Study. *Circulation* 1983;67:968-977.

43. Shekelle RB, Shryock AM, Paul O, et al: Diet, serum cholesterol, and death from coronary heart disease—The Western Electric Study. *N Engl J Med* 1981;304:65-70.

44. Kromhout D, Bosschieter EB, Coulander CdeL: The inverse reaction between fish consumption and 20-year mortality from coronary heart disease. *N Engl J Med* 1985;312:1205-1209.

45. American Heart Association: Dietary guidelines for healthy American adults: A statement for physicians and health professionals by the Nutrition Committee, American Heart Association. *Circulation* 1986;74:1465A-1468A.

46. Raab C, Tillotson JL (eds): *Heart to Heart: A Manual on Nutrition Counseling for the Reduction of Cardiovascular Disease Risk Factors.* National Institutes of Health Publication No. 83-1528.

47. US Dept Agriculture and Dept Health and Human Services: *Nutrition and Your Health: Dietary Guidelines for Americans.* ed 2. US Dept Agriculture Home and Garden Bulletin, No. 232, 1985.

48. Pennington J, Church H: *Bowes and Church's Food Values of Portions Commonly Used*, ed 14. Philadelphia, JB Lippincott, 1985.

49. US Dept Agriculture: Nutritive Value of Foods. US Dept Agriculture Home and Garden Bulletin, No. 72, 1986.

50. Brown WV, Goldberg IJ, Ginsberg HN: Treatment of common lipoprotein disorders. *Progr Cardiovasc Dis* 1984;27:1-21.

51. Hoeg JM, Gregg RE, Brewer HB Jr: An approach to the management of hypercholesterolemia. *JAMA* 1986;255:512-521.

52. Illingworth DR: Lipid-lowering drugs: An overview of indication and optimum therapeutic use. *Drugs* 1987;33:259-279.

53. Coronary Drug Project Research Group: Clofibrate and niacin in coronary heart disease. *JAMA* 1975;231:360-381.

54. Knopp RH, Ginsberg J, Albers JJ, et al: Contrasting effects of unmodified and time-released forms of niacin on lipoproteins in hyperlipidemic subjects: Clues to mechanism of action of niacin. *Metabolism* 1985;34:642-647.

55. Lovastatin Study Group II: Therapeutic response to lovastatin (mevinolin) in nonfamilial hypercholesterolemia: A multicenter trial. *JAMA* 1986;256:2829-2834.

56. Illingworth DR: Mevinolin (lovastatin) plus colestipol in therapy for severe heterozygous familial hypercholesterolemia. *Ann Intern Med* 1984;101:598-604.

57. Steinberg D: Studies on the mechanism of action of probucol. *Am J Cardiol* 1986;57:16H-21H.

58. Committee of Principal Investigators, World Health Organization Clofibrate Trial: A cooperative trial in the primary prevention of ischemic heart disease using clofibrate. *Br Heart J* 1978;40:1069-1118.

59. Helsinki Heart Study Ethical Committee: Safety as a factor in lipid-regulating primary prevention drug trials: The Helsinki Heart Study Interim Report: Royal Society of Medicine Services. *Int Congr Symp Senes* 1986;87:51-61.

60. Kane JP, Malloy MJ, Tun P, et al: Normalization of low-density lipoprotein levels in heterozygous familial hypercholesterolemia with a combined drug regimen. *N Engl J Med* 1981;304:251-258.

APPENDIXES

Appendix I

Table I-1.—Corresponding Levels of Lipids			
Cholesterol		Triglyceride	
mg/dL	mmol/L	mg/dL	mmol/L
35	0.9	250	2.8
130	3.4	400	4.5
160	4.1	500	5.6
190	4.9	1000	11.3
200	5.2	...	...
240	6.2	...	...

Table I-2.—Mean Serum Cholesterol Levels of Men and Women, SEM, Age-Adjusted Values, Selected Percentiles, Number of Examined Persons, and Estimated Population, by Race and Age: United States, 1978-1980

Race, Age, y	No. of Persons Examined	Estimated Population in Thousands	Mean	SEM	Percentile*								
					5th	10th	15th	25th	50th	75th	85th	90th	95th
Men													
All races†													
20-74	5604	63611	211	1.2	144	156	165	179	206	239	258	271	291
20-24	676	9331	180	1.7	129	136	145	155	176	202	215	227	246
25-34	1067	15895	199	1.5	141	152	159	172	194	220	240	254	275
35-44	745	11367	217	2.0	153	166	173	187	215	244	262	275	293
45-54	690	11114	227	1.8	159	176	182	197	223	255	271	283	303
55-64	1227	9607	229	1.8	164	176	184	198	225	254	277	288	307
65-74	1199	6297	221	1.8	153	167	175	191	217	249	265	279	301
White													
20-74	4883	55808	211	1.2	145	157	166	179	207	239	258	271	291
20-24	581	8052	180	1.8	131	138	146	155	176	202	216	229	244
25-34	901	13864	199	1.7	144	153	161	172	194	220	239	254	273
35-44	653	9808	217	1.8	153	166	173	187	214	244	260	272	291
45-54	617	9865	227	1.8	160	177	181	198	222	254	271	283	303
55-64	1086	8642	230	2.0	164	178	185	199	225	255	278	289	307
65-74	1045	5576	222	2.0	153	167	175	191	217	250	266	281	301
Black													
20-74	607	6102	208	2.5	133	146	156	171	200	238	260	273	301
20-24	79	1043	171	3.7†	...†	128	134	149	170	193	210	211	...†
25-34	139	1546	199	4.1†	129	136	144	163	192	226	248	259	301
35-44	70	1112	218	8.3†	...†	156	168	176	202	238	275	283	...†
45-54	62	1044	229	7.1†	...†	174	184	195	232	261	268	279	...†
55-64	129	801	223	4.8†	157	168	172	183	218	254	271	299	312
65-74	128	555	217	4.2	149	163	173	183	216	244	261	277	299
Age-adjusted values													
All races, 20-74	...	...	211	1.1	...	...	...	...	...	...	...	...	...
White, 20-74	...	...	211	1.1	...	...	...	...	...	...	...	...	...
Black, 20-74	...	...	209	2.5	...	...	...	...	...	...	...	...	...
Women													
All races†													
20-74	6260	69994	215	1.2	143	156	166	179	210	245	266	282	305
20-24	738	9994	184	1.9	132	140	145	157	180	204	216	230	250
25-34	1170	16856	192	1.4	135	145	154	164	188	215	233	243	263
35-44	844	12284	207	1.8	147	158	164	177	202	231	248	260	276
45-54	763	11918	232	2.2	164	178	188	199	228	257	275	290	306
55-64	1329	10743	249	2.0	180	193	203	215	242	277	299	314	336
65-74	1416	8198	246	1.6	173	189	198	214	241	274	295	309	327
White													
20-74	5418	60785	216	1.3	143	156	166	179	210	246	267	282	305
20-24	624	8408	184	2.1	133	140	147	159	181	204	215	230	249
25-34	1000	14494	192	1.5	135	145	153	164	188	215	235	244	261
35-44	726	10584	207	1.9	147	157	164	177	203	231	248	259	277
45-54	647	10369	232	2.6	166	179	188	199	228	257	274	290	308
55-64	1176	9601	249	1.7	180	193	203	215	244	277	298	312	330
65-74	1245	7329	246	1.7	174	190	199	214	242	275	296	309	328
Black													
20-74	729	7579	212	3.1	140	154	166	176	205	237	263	279	308
20-24	94	1304	185	4.9†	...†	136	144	156	178	204	220	237	...†
25-34	145	1953	191	4.1†	129	144	156	167	190	212	226	235	267
35-44	103	1415	206	4.5†	143	158	170	175	194	233	254	274	279
45-54	100	1215	230	7.2†	150	172	181	200	226	263	277	291	306
55-64	135	959	251	8.0†	178	185	198	211	233	280	318	336	345
65-74	152	733	243	4.2	173	189	198	211	237	269	290	308	323
Age-adjusted values													
All races, 20-74	...	...	215	1.2	...	...	...	...	...	...	...	...	...
White, 20-74	...	...	215	1.2	...	...	...	...	...	...	...	...	...
Black, 20-74	...	...	214	2.7	...	...	...	...	...	...	...	...	...

*Serum cholesterol values are given in milligrams per deciliter. To convert values to millimoles per liter, multiply by 0.02586. From National Center for Health Statistics.[23]

†Includes data for races not shown separately.

Table I-3.—Calculated Levels of Serum Low Density Lipoprotein (LDL) Cholesterol* for Persons† 20 to 74 Years of Age Fasting 12 Hours or More, by Sex and Age: Means and Selected Percentiles, United States, 1976-1980

Sex, Age, y	No. of Persons Examined	Estimated Population in Thousands	Mean	SD	Selected Percentiles									
					5th	10th	15th	25th	50th	75th	85th	90th	95th
Men													
20-74	1037	21 262	140	39	80	92	100	113	136	164	181	194	208
20-24	72	1852	109	36	...‡	70	74	88	104	129	149	154	...‡
25-34	174	5186	128	33	76	87	94	108	128	148	161	171	189
35-44	130	3866	145	40	81	96	105	116	138	176	192	203	206
45-54	106	3543	150	36	99	103	112	119	146	171	189	195	211
55-64	267	3943	148	39	84	101	108	118	147	171	191	206	217
65-74	288	2872	149	40	87	105	109	120	144	174	188	199	217
Women													
20-74	1246	27 102	141	43	81	91	98	110	136	164	186	199	220
20-24	105	3325	114	33	69	74	83	94	106	136	149	155	179
25-34	194	5517	121	33	72	83	90	98	116	139	154	166	187
35-44	166	4800	129	34	78	90	97	107	126	150	163	171	191
45-54	168	5155	157	45	94	104	116	125	156	184	200	213	226
55-64	282	4644	159	42	101	113	118	129	150	188	205	219	237
65-74	331	3661	162	44	98	109	122	135	158	186	207	226	245

*Serum LDL Cholesterol = Serum Total Cholesterol − HDL Cholesterol − (Triglycerides/5). Equation from Friedewald et al.[18] Persons with a serum triglyceride value greater than 400 mg/dL were excluded. From the National Center for Health Statistics: Division of Health Examination Statistics, unpublished data from the second National Health and Nutrition Examination Survey, 1976-1980.
†Includes other races in addition to black and white.
‡Sample size insufficient to produce statistically reliable results.

Table I-4.—Major Causes of Reduced Serum HDL-Cholesterol*

Cigarette smoking
Obesity
Lack of exercise
Androgenic and related steroids
   Androgens
   Progestational agents
   Anabolic steroids
β-Adrenergic blocking agents
Hypertriglyceridemia
Genetic factors
   Primary hypoalphalipoproteinemia

Appendix II. Special Patient and Population Groups

This section is provided to review for the practitioner the major forms of severe hypercholesterolemia, the problem of high plasma triglycerides, causes of reduced HDL-cholesterol, and manifestations of diabetic dyslipidemia. Its purpose is to assist the physician in management of these problems or help in identification of disorders that would be better treated by a specialist in this field. There are two reasons for referring a hyperlipidemic patient to a specialist. First, the dyslipidemia may be severe or complicated and beyond the experience of a given practitioner; and, second, the patient may require special testing that is beyond the capability of laboratories available to the physician. The latter may be particularly the case for rare or severe disorders of lipoprotein metabolism. In some instances, a precise etiologic diagnosis may be required for the correct treatment of a patient.

Severe Forms of Hypercholesterolemia

Familial Hypercholesterolemia.—This disorder is caused by a defect in the gene encoding for the LDL receptor such that the receptor is either absent or non-

functional. One gene for the LDL receptor normally is inherited from each parent. In the heterozygous form of FH, the patient has only one normal gene for LDL receptors, and LDL-cholesterol levels are approximately doubled, to levels exceeding 200 mg/dL. Heterozygous FH occurs approximately once in 500 people, and serum total cholesterol levels usually exceed 300 mg/dL; affected patients frequently have tendon xanthomas, corneal arcus, premature CHD, and a strong family history of hypercholesterolemia. Approximately 5% of patients with myocardial infarction before 60 years of age will have heterozygous FH. Affected men often develop CHD in their 30s or 40s, or even earlier; in women with FH, CHD often occurs in the 50s and 60s. Rarely, about once per million people, individuals inherit two abnormal genes for LDL receptors and hence are homozygous for FH. Their cholesterol levels range from 600 to 1000 mg/dL; they usually have planar and tuberous xanthomas of the hands, elbows, buttocks, and knees, as well as tendon xanthomas. Severe and often fatal coronary disease frequently develops in the teens.

Patients with heterozygous FH rarely respond adequately to dietary therapy alone. Certainly the Step-Two Diet will potentiate the action of specific cholesterol-lowering drugs, and affected patients should be encouraged to modify their diets to obtain maximal cholesterol lowering. Some patients with FH respond remarkably to diet, and the potential value of diet modification should not be overlooked. However, in most patients, it is not necessary to wait for six months of dietary therapy before beginning drug treatment. To obtain the goals of LDL lowering in patients with heterozygous FH, two drugs frequently are required. The combination of a bile acid sequestrant and nicotinic acid is a very potent available regimen. Recent evidence indicates that use of HMG CoA reductase inhibitors (eg, lovastatin) in combination with bile acid sequestrants will reduce LDL-cholesterol levels into the normal range in many people with heterozygous FH. In homozygous FH, more drastic means are required to lower LDL levels. These patients respond poorly to drugs, including reductase inhibitors, and more radical therapies have been tried, including portacaval shunt, liver transplantation, and direct removal of LDL by a modified form of plasmapheresis.

Familial Combined Hyperlipidemia.—Another form of primary hypercholesterolemia occurs in some individual members of families having FCHL. In FCHL, multiple lipoprotein phenotypes can occur in a single affected family. About one third of affected patients have increases in VLDL alone (type 4 hyperlipoproteinemia [HLP] pattern); another third have increases in LDL alone (type 2a HLP), while most others have elevations of VLDL plus LDL (type 2b HLP) or VLDL plus chylomicrons (type 5 HLP). Hyperapobetalipoproteinemia (increased LDL-apolipoprotein B [apo-B] with normal LDL-cholesterol) is another lipoprotein pattern commonly found in FCHL. The diagnosis of FCHL is made by testing of first-degree relatives and by finding multiple lipoprotein phenotypes in a single family. Patients with FCHL are at increased risk for CHD regardless of their lipoprotein phenotype. Familial hypercholesterolemia occurs in about 15% of patients with CHD before 60 years of age. The underlying metabolic defect in many families appears to be an overproduction of lipoproteins by the liver, and the resulting lipoprotein phenotype depends on how rapidly these excess lipoproteins are cleared from the circulation. For example, when rates of clearance of LDL are sluggish, the patient will develop an elevation of LDL-cholesterol.

Dietary therapy can play an important role in the treatment of primary hyperlipidemia due to overproduction of lipoproteins. Patients with FCHL may be extremely sensitive to even a few pounds of excess body weight, and reduction of weight to the desirable range sometimes will lower plasma lipid levels substantially. Further improvement in the lipoprotein pattern may be achieved by instituting a program of regular physical exercise. Restriction of dietary cholesterol and saturated fatty acids may further reduce LDL-cholesterol levels. In many patients with FCHL, however, drug therapy may be required to completely or adequately control plasma levels of lipoproteins. The drug of choice for FCHL is nicotinic acid, which interferes with the excessive formation of lipoproteins. For patients with FCHL who have elevated LDL with normal triglyceride levels and who cannot tolerate nicotinic acid, a bile acid binding resin or the new drug lovastatin can be used; these latter agents alone, however, may not be sufficient in patients with a concomitant elevation of plasma triglycerides, as will be discussed below in the "Hypertriglyceridemia" section.

Severe Primary Hypercholesterolemia.—About 1% of the adult population have cholesterol levels that are persistently over 300 mg/dL. A portion of individuals in this group will have heterozygous FH that is unrecognized, either because of a lack of tendon xanthomas or unavailability of first-degree relatives for testing. In others, a definite monogenic inheritance of elevated LDL-cholesterol cannot be demonstrated, and hence the term "polygenic" hypercholesterolemia has been used. While people in this category may merely represent the upper end of the spectrum of the population distribution of plasma cholesterol, they deserve special attention because of the severity of their hypercholesterolemia and their greatly heightened risk for CHD. Furthermore, patients of this category often have a diet-resistant form of hypercholesterolemia and must be managed with drugs. When it becomes obvious that patients of this type will not reach the goals of LDL lowering by dietary therapy alone, drug treatment can be instituted. Some patients may require a combination of drugs, as described above for FH, but others may respond adequately to a first-choice drug, or the new drug, lovastatin.

Familial Dysbetalipoproteinemia (Type 3 Hyperlipoproteinemia).—This is a relatively uncommon condition that occurs roughly in about one in 5000 persons in the United States, in which catabolism of remnants of VLDL and chylomicrons is delayed. The normal apo-E phenotype is E_3, while the phenotype of type 3 HLP is E_2. The basic abnormality lies in the primary structure of apolipoprotein E (apo-E). The structural alteration of apo-E prevents the normal binding of VLDL remnants to LDL receptors on liver and other cells. The accumulation of modified VLDL remnants (called beta-VLDL) accounts for the term *dysbetalipoproteinemia*. The VLDL in these patients have beta mobility on lipoprotein electrophoresis rather than the normal prebeta mobility. The disorder should be suspected when triglyceride levels are somewhat higher than cholesterol levels in the presence of striking cholesterol elevation. Patients with dysbetalipoproteinemia have an increased risk of premature CHD and peripheral vascular disease; they commonly are obese, glucose intolerant, hyperuricemic, and have tuboeruptive and palmar xanthomas. Despite hypercholesterolemia, the LDL-cholesterol rarely is increased in dysbetalipoproteinemia, and the increase in cholesterol levels occurs in the VLDL fraction; however, when LDL levels are calculated by equation, there will be an apparent increase in LDL-cholesterol. For this reason, in a patient with an elevation in both triglycerides and cholesterol, the physician should be alert to the possibility of dysbetalipoproteinemia, and appropriate testing should be done, including referral to a specialist if necessary.

If a patient with type 3 HLP is overweight, caloric restriction frequently reduces cholesterol levels to normal. If diabetes mellitus contributes to the hyperlipidemia, control of hyperglycemia will often be helpful, but may not eliminate the need to use specific lipid-lowering drugs. Clinical experience has shown that restriction of excess total calories, saturated fatty acids, and cholesterol in the diet will significantly reduce total cholesterol levels in many patients with familial dysbetalipoproteinemia. When hyperlipidemia persists in spite of maximal dietary therapy, drug therapy should be instituted. Nicotinic acid is the drug of choice for this disorder. The fibric acids (gemfibrozil and clofibrate) also have proven highly effective for reducing both cholesterol and triglycerides in dysbetalipoproteinemia. The bile acid sequestrants should not be used as single drug therapy in patients with type 3 HLP because these drugs will increase the cholesterol and triglyceride levels.

Hypertriglyceridemia

Definition.—The National Institutes of Health (NIH) Consensus Development Conference on Treatment of Hypertriglyceridemia defined definite hypertriglyceridemia as a fasting plasma triglyceride level exceeding 500 mg/dL.[22] This conference classified triglyceride levels in the range of 250 to 500 mg/dL as "borderline hypertriglyceridemia." The NIH Consensus Panel concluded: "There is little evidence that triglyceride levels below 250 mg/dL in the presence of normal cholesterol levels predict an increased risk of any disease. These levels (generally) can be considered normal." The present report generally follows the recommendations of this NIH Consensus Panel.

For most patients, triglyceride levels in the range of 250 to 750 mg/dL result mainly from increases in VLDL (type 4 HLP). When triglyceride levels are higher, the patient usually has elevations of both VLDL and chylomicrons (type 5 HLP). Very rarely patients have a congenital absence of lipoprotein lipase and have severe chylomicronemia (type 1 HLP).

Plasma Triglycerides and Disease.—The relationship between plasma triglyceride levels and cardiovascular disease is controversial. Although plasma triglyceride levels are positively associated with increased risk for cardiovascular disease in most population studies, in most they were not independently predictive for CHD after statistical adjustment for closely associated attributes such as total cholesterol, HDL-cholesterol, hypertension, cigarette smoking, and obesity. In the Framingham Heart Study, however, the plasma triglyceride level was found to be an independent predictor of CHD in women.[21] Even so, the plasma triglyceride level, rather than being a direct cause of atherosclerotic disease, probably reflects the presence of certain atherogenic lipoproteins. Certainly, many disease entities that elevate triglyceride levels, such as diabetes mellitus, nephrotic syndrome, and chronic renal disease, carry an increase in risk for CHD. Furthermore, some patients with FCHL have borderline hypertriglyceridemia and normal serum cholesterol levels and yet are still at increased risk for CHD. In these situations, the high triglyceride level may be a clue to the presence of other lipoprotein abnormalities that are more directly associated with CHD, such as low HDL-cholesterol, low apoprotein A-1, elevated apoprotein B, or atherogenic remnant lipoproteins that have not been well defined. When assessing the risk for CHD in a patient with borderline hypertriglyceridemia, reliance should be placed first on the standard cholesterol risk factors, viz, total cholesterol, LDL-cholesterol, and HDL-cholesterol. Beyond these, additional factors suggesting increased coronary risk in patients with hypertriglyceridemia are the presence in first-degree relatives of hypercholesterolemia, premature CHD, and, if the test is available, increased plasma levels of apo-B.

A link between plasma triglycerides and disease is most clearly evident in patients who have severe hypertriglyceridemia with chylomicronemia and eruptive xanthomata; these patients are prone to abdominal pain and/or pancreatitis, the latter occasionally being fatal. Severe elevations of chylomicrons directly induce pancreatitis, which can be prevented by triglyceride reduction.

Candidates for Specific Therapy.—Much of *borderline hypertriglyceridemia* seen in clinical practice is due to various exogenous or secondary factors raising the plasma triglyceride level. The most common is obesity. Others include excessive intake of alcohol, diabetes mellitus, hypothyroidism, chronic renal disease—uremia, nephrotic syndrome, maintenance dialysis, renal transplantation—liver disease, and, rarely, dysproteinemias. There are also a number of drugs that raise lipid levels as a significant side effect. These may primarily act on VLDL and raise triglyceride levels, rather than act on LDL. These include several drugs used to lower blood pressure (including the thiazide diuretics and β-adrenergic blocking agents), estrogenic hormones (including oral contraceptives), and retinoids. The clinician evaluating a patient's blood lipid levels should be aware of this phenomenon.

Borderline hypertriglyceridemia also can be one manifestation of certain familial hyperlipidemias. One such entity is FCHL, described above. Patients with FCHL have an increased risk for CHD regardless of their lipoprotein phenotype, including isolated borderline elevated plasma triglycerides. Because of heightened coronary risk, patients with FCHL deserve treatment with diet first, and, if necessary, with drugs. Furthermore, any patient with primary borderline hypertriglyceridemia who already has clinical manifestations of premature cardiovascular disease can be treated as if he or she has FCHL.

Borderline hypertriglyceridemia likewise can be a manifestation of another familial disorder called familial hypertriglyceridemia (FHTG). Most patients with FHTG appear to have a mild defect in lipolysis of triglyceride-rich lipoproteins combined with an overproduction of VLDL triglycerides. The VLDL are enriched in triglycerides, but the number of VLDL particles entering plasma apparently is not increased, and consequently LDL-cholesterol concentrations are not increased. Patients with FHTG seem to be at lesser risk for CHD than those with FCHL. In FHTG, there generally is a lack of elevated blood cholesterol, either in the patient or other family members, and affected members are less likely to have premature CHD. Caloric restriction and increased exercise can be strongly recommended for obese patients with FHTG, but drug therapy is generally not appropriate for this condition alone.

The NIH Consensus Panel based its definition of *definite hypertriglyceridemia* on the following considerations: "Fasting plasma triglyceride levels above 1,000 mg/dL carry a significant risk of pancreatitis. Based on this risk coupled with the large intraindividual variation in repeated triglyceride measurements, a triglyceride level greater than 500 mg/dL is considered to be abnormal, and warrants the label hypertriglyceridemia." Patients with definite hypertriglyceridemia also can have primary or secondary disorders of triglyceride metabolism, and, not infrequently, these two categories are present in a single patient.

Very high triglyceride levels (>1000 mg/dL) are due in large part to accumulation of chylomicrons. Rare genetic causes of severe chylomicronemia are congenital absence of lipoprotein lipase or apolipoprotein C-II, the latter being required for activation of lipoprotein lipase; these conditions usually become manifest first in childhood. Severe hypertriglyceridemia in adults sometimes is due to a primary disease (FHTG or FCHL) plus exacerbating secondary factors such as obesity, poorly controlled diabetes mellitus, excess use of alcohol, or drugs (eg, corticosteroids, estrogens, or β-adrenergic blocking agents). In such patients, both children and adults, immediate and long-term reduction of plasma triglycerides is mandatory to prevent recurrent abdominal pain and pancreatitis.

Dietary Therapy in Patients With Hypertriglyceridemia.—Changes in life-style (control of weight, increased physical activity, restriction of alcohol, and, in some cases, restriction of dietary fat) are the primary modes of therapy for hypertriglyceridemia. Patients with triglyceride levels in excess of 500 mg/dL, like those with high cholesterol levels, may benefit from counseling with a registered dietitian. Specific dietary approaches to the major forms of hypertriglyceridemia can be considered briefly.

For patients with severe hypertriglyceridemia and chylomicronemia, a very-low-fat diet (10% to 20% of total caloric intake as fat) should be instituted to prevent pancreatitis. The need to maintain this diet at all times must be emphasized. Some chylomicronemic patients are extremely sensitive to dietary fat and can develop pancreatitis from a single high-fat meal. In some patients, repeated bouts of pancreatitis will occur despite all attempts at dietary control, and drug therapy will be required.

In patients with borderline hypertriglyceridemia, emphasis should be on weight reduction and increasing physical activity. In this condition, very-low-fat, high-carbohydrate diets are not required and may actually accentuate hypertriglyceridemia. Therefore, it is not advisable to go beyond the Step-One Diet in reduction of fat intake. With secondary hypertriglyceridemias, one should treat the underlying disorder, but sometimes treatment can be facilitated by modifying the diet, usually by weight reduction and alcohol restriction.

Drug Therapy in Patients With Hypertriglyceridemia.—The NIH Consensus Panel reported: "drug therapy in hypertriglyceridemia should take a second place to modification of the diet. Drugs nevertheless may be required to avoid abdominal pain and pancreatitis in the presence of chylomicronemia. They also can be used to produce regression of xanthomata in patients of this kind or in those with familial dysbetalipoproteinemia. Drugs also may be employed in the attempt to retard atherogenesis in patients with genetic hyperlipidemias, such as FCHL or familial dysbetalipoproteinemia." The current report supports these recommendations.

For patients with marked hypertriglyceridemia, who do not respond adequately to modification of the diet, drug therapy can be justified to reduce the risk for acute pancreatitis. Nicotinic acid is the drug of choice here, but if this drug is not tolerated, many patients will respond sufficiently to a fibric acid (gemfibrozil or clofibrate) to eliminate the risk for pancreatitis. Bile acid binding resins are not appropriate for patients with hypertriglyceridemia.

The role of drugs in the treatment of borderline hypertriglyceridemia is controversial. Most patients in this category will have diet-induced hypertriglyceridemia and thus are not candidates for drug therapy. If a patient has the characteristics of FHTG, which does not carry an increased risk of CHD, the use of drugs is not warranted. On the other hand, if a hypertriglyceridemic patient has been shown to have FCHL, which imparts increased risk, lipid-lowering drug therapy is appropriate. Nicotinic acid is the drug of choice for FCHL, because it curtails the overproduction of lipoproteins that is characteristic of this disorder. An alternative approach is to reduce triglyceride levels with a fibric acid and to simultaneously lower LDL concentrations with either a bile acid binding resin or lovastatin. If a diagnosis of FCHL cannot be made by family testing, factors that suggest the presence of this disorder in individual patients include the presence of CHD, high blood cholesterol, high-risk LDL-cholesterol, reduced HDL-cholesterol, and a family history of CHD. Opinion is divided whether such patients are candidates for drug therapy. A conservative approach is to restrict the use of drugs to patients with high levels of total cholesterol and LDL-cholesterol. A more aggressive approach is to treat elevated triglycerides, high VLDL-cholesterol levels, and reduced HDL-cholesterol concentrations with nicotinic acid or a fibric acid; however, it must be emphasized that this latter approach has not been proven by controlled clinical trials to reduce the risk for CHD.

Reduced HDL-Cholesterol

In this document, a reduced serum level of HDL-cholesterol is defined as a concentration below 35 mg/dL. A reduced HDL-cholesterol level imparts an increased risk for CHD, and hence is classified as a major risk factor. As indicated in the text, the HDL-cholesterol concentration should be measured in all patients with high blood cholesterol levels, and in persons with borderline–high blood cholesterol levels and a high risk status (definite CHD or

two other major risk factors, one of which can be male sex). The presence of a reduced serum HDL-cholesterol is one factor favoring the use of drugs to treat high LDL-cholesterol concentrations.

The major causes of a reduced serum HDL-cholesterol level are listed in Appendix I, Table 4. Heavy cigarette smoking is a documented cause, and, in smokers, the reduction in HDL-cholesterol appears to be made worse by concomitant heavy use of coffee. Obesity is a major cause of reduced concentrations of HDL, and a closely related cause is a lack of physical activity. White men, but not necessarily black men, have lower HDL levels than women. Anabolic steroids and progestational agents decrease the HDL-cholesterol concentration. Among other drugs, the β-adrenergic blocking agents most consistently reduce the HDL level. Hypertriglyceridemia, even in mild forms, is frequently associated with significantly decreased levels of HDL-cholesterol, and, in some patients, elevated LDL-cholesterol is accompanied by a reduced concentration of HDL. Finally, poorly understood genetic factors account for a portion of cases of reduced HDL-cholesterol.

Although there have been no clinical trials demonstrating the benefit of raising HDL-cholesterol, the connection between reduced HDL-cholesterol and CHD risk justifies the attempt to raise HDL levels, particularly when this can be accomplished by hygienic means. Appropriate advice is to stop use of cigarettes in smokers, reduce body weight in the obese, increase exercise in the sedentary, and avoid use of anabolic steroids in athletes. For patients with a reduced HDL-cholesterol, avoiding the use of beta-blockers for treatment of hypertension may be prudent, although these drugs may be required for patients with definite CHD. One result of treating hyperlipidemia is that HDL-cholesterol concentrations frequently increase, which may be of added benefit.

Diabetic Dyslipidemia

Diabetes mellitus is a major risk factor for CHD, and, in accord with the recommendations of this report, the minimal goal of LDL lowering in diabetic men is to achieve a reduction of LDL-cholesterol to less than 130 mg/dL. For diabetic women, the minimal LDL-cholesterol goal is <160 mg/dL in the absence of CHD or another risk factor, or <130 mg/dL if definite CHD or another risk factor is present. Abnormal plasma lipid and lipoprotein levels frequently are seen in diabetics. Careful control of plasma glucose will reduce LDL levels, and HDL-cholesterol concentrations frequently will rise. Control of hyperglycemia is the key to improving the lipoprotein pattern in diabetics. The dietary therapy outlined for other high-risk patients with elevated LDL levels is recommended by many authorities for diabetic patients. Other investigators believe that intake of carbohydrates should not exceed 40% to 45% of total calories; if this latter approach is accepted, the intake of saturated fatty acids and cholesterol still should be curtailed, as recommended for other patients at high risk.

The most obvious lipoprotein abnormality in patients with noninsulin-dependent diabetes mellitus (NIDDM) is hypertriglyceridemia. In occasional, poorly controlled diabetics, severe chylomicronemia can develop, and risk for acute pancreatitis is high. In these unusual patients, intake of fat must be severely restricted, at least temporarily, to prevent further synthesis of chylomicrons; furthermore, adequate doses of insulin are needed to restore normal activity of lipoprotein lipase. The milder forms of hypertriglyceridemia that occur in many diabetics are the result of poor control of hyperglycemia, and their triglycerides can be reduced by improved glucose control. If hypertriglyceridemia persists despite good control of plasma glucose levels, the patient may have an underlying familial form of hyperlipidemia.

Pregnant Women With Preexisting Lipid Disorders

Generally, the dietary therapy previously prescribed for the lipid disorder should be continued during pregnancy. If dietary therapy is very restrictive, careful consideration should be given to assuring adequate nutrient intake. Drug therapy should be discontinued during pregnancy, since the effect of lipid-lowering drugs on the fetus has not been carefully studied. Women with a prior history of hypertriglyceridemia should be monitored carefully; triglyceride levels above 1000 mg/dL are associated with an increased risk of pancreatitis. Consultation with a lipid specialist may be indicated for patients with severe forms of hyperlipidemia.

Appendix III. Intensive Dietary Instruction and Behavior Modification

In a majority of patients with high-risk LDL-cholesterol levels, the Step-One Diet should prove sufficient to reach the goals of dietary therapy. For most patients, it should not be necessary to refer to a dietitian. A dietitian can, however, be helpful even for these patients. For a minority of patients, more intensive dietary therapy will be needed, and referral to a registered dietitian will be important in order to effectively implement therapy. The dietitian can play a vital role in education of the patient in the process of dietary change, and the dietitian will be especially valuable for instruction of the patient in the Step-Two Diet. In this Appendix, the general approach to intensive dietary therapy under the supervision of a registered dietitian is outlined. The purpose of this section is to provide the physician and immediate staff with information about the techniques employed by many dietitians for institution and maintenance of intensive dietary therapy (including the Step-Two Diet). If the physician and staff are thoroughly familiar with the principles of dietary therapy, as outlined in this Appendix, this understanding will facilitate their interaction with the dietitian and will increase the chances of success in achieving the goal of therapy by diet modification alone. The usual steps employed by the dietitian are the following.

Assessment of Nutritional Status and Eating Habits.—A thorough assessment of the patient's dietary history and current eating habits is useful in implementation of dietary change. This assessment will include the recording of the patient's current weight and weights at significant ages. The dietitian will estimate percentage of desirable body weight, and, in some cases, the percentage of body fat, to determine whether the patient needs to lose weight. A detailed description of current eating habits will be obtained. Examples of the types of information that are obtained include the following: (1) What times of the day does the patient usually eat? (2) Are some meals routinely skipped? (3) At what time does the patient eat his/her largest meal? (4) Where are meals typically prepared (eg, in a restaurant, work cafeteria, fast-food restaurant, deli, at home, or in the homes of others)? (5) Are meals eaten at home prepared from packaged foods or fresh from the market? (6) Which are favorite foods and what foods are disliked? and (7) What foods will be most difficult to increase or decrease? Furthermore, the dietitian will attempt to assess the patient's general state of knowledge of nutrition and its relation to high cholesterol levels, educational level, motivation, attitudes toward diet, and structure of social support.

Initial Instructions for Diet Modification.—The dietitian will describe for the patient an overall plan for diet modification. The connection between dietary habits and blood cholesterol level will be emphasized, and particular emphasis will be given to reducing the consumption of saturated fatty acids and cholesterol, and to reducing excess body weight. The dietitian may review the contents of Table 7 with the patient and will give particular attention to foods that are unusually rich in saturated fatty acids and cholesterol. A few individuals may be taught to compute a daily record of food intake that delineates specific foods, where they are prepared, and their quantity. To learn to record quantities of different foods will require specific instruction for using measuring cups, spoons, and a food scale. The dietitian may feel that certain patients will benefit by keeping a food record for about three days as an educational exercise.

In this initial instructional process, the dietitian likely will review the patient's daily routine both during the week and on weekends, and will assist the patient in identifying life-style factors that might interfere with adherence. The patient will be urged to actively participate in discussion and may be given the option of evaluating several eating plans before deciding on a final diet plan. It will be pointed out to the patient that he/she may find certain foods to be unappealing at first, but over a period of time, new preferences in taste will develop.

Particular attention will be given to the sources of fat in the diet, especially fat that is "hidden" in foods such as bakery goods, cheeses, and processed meats. Suggestions will be made on how to select appropriate snack foods and prepared foods. The patient may be taught the principle of "controlled cheating," ie, how to plan and adjust for occasional episodes off the diet without becoming discouraged and discontinuing the diet altogether. Instruction will be given on how to change the type of milk used, how to reduce meat portion size, how to substitute egg whites for whole eggs in baking, and how to use margarines and oils in the place of fats rich in saturated fatty acids. The dietitian probably will attempt to involve other individuals of significance (eg, parents, spouse, and children) in dietary instructions.

Institution of Fat-Modified Diets.—Patients usually are started on a diet that corresponds as closely as possible to their normal eating habits. For example, if the patient always skips breakfast, he/she will not be requested to eat breakfast at the outset. If the patient always eats lunch in the cafeteria at work, he/she will be taught to make reasonable food choices rather than starting to bring lunch from home. Specific goals for eating habits will be set to allow progress toward the attainment of the composition of the Step-One Diet. Only after this first step has been attained will the dietitian attempt to progress to the Step-Two Diet.

Although the objective of the Step-One Diet is less than 10% of calories as saturated fatty acids, it usually is difficult for the average person to estimate whether the target is being met. A realistic approach will provide specific recommendations about diet change, such as reducing meat portion size to four ounces, or substituting a tuna sandwich for a cheese sandwich two days a week. It usually is necessary to implement the specific goals in a graduated fashion, rather than all at once. This will prevent the patient from being overwhelmed, will allow him/her sufficient time for adjustment, and will engender a feeling of success and not failure. Some patients will be asked to self-monitor eating behaviors related to their eating-habit goals on a regular basis during the initiation phase. The dietitian may need to review these records periodically to detect problem areas. Finally, a schedule for follow-up visits with the dietitian often is employed to ensure adoption of and adherence to the new diet.

Strategy for Behavior Modification.—Involvement of the patient in developing appropriate behavior strategies is crucial for successful dietary change and long-term adherence to the recommended diet. For the obese patient, techniques of behavior modification have been moderately successful for achieving weight reduction, and they may be instituted for overweight patients. Further, the dietitian may modify these techniques to train patients to alter the diet composition. These techniques focus on unconscious eating habits, compulsive behavior, binge eating, lack of resistance to social pressures for eating cholesterol-raising foods, use of eating to relieve anxiety and depression, and lack of will power or self-control. The dietitian can explore all of these areas with the patient and guide him/her in overcoming these eating problems. Patients will be given the opportunity to "talk through" their eating problems and to "brainstorm" new ways to improve their eating behavior.

Monitoring and Reinforcement.—Progress in achieving the specified dietary goals will be monitored by both the patient and the diet counselor. It is helpful for the physician to provide information on response in cholesterol levels as a guide to success in diet modification. Self-monitoring tools that are designed to meet the needs of the patient may be utilized. For example, three-day food records often are an effective monitoring tool. These records provide an estimate of adherence and can help to identify any real or potential problems. These records also can enable the patient to become more aware of the diet and related behaviors, assist in analysis of progress in dietary change, and provide reinforcement of new behavior.

A schedule of regular follow-up visits is helpful to achieve adherence to the diet. There is a tendency for adherence to drift downward with time, and this often can be avoided by periodic visits with the dietitian. It will be especially important to give supportive followup and assistance during periods of life change or stress (eg, marriage or divorce, loss of loved ones, job change); renewed self-monitoring during these periods may be especially helpful. Occasional meetings with other family members can help to reinforce adherence to diet modification. A constant review of the basics will be needed to offset distortions of information resulting from misunderstandings or erroneous messages picked up from the media or other sources.

Individuals are increasingly making use of personal computers for activities at home. Software programs are now available, or will become available, for analyzing food records, for providing nutrient analysis, and for support of changes in eating patterns. These programs are available for both the lay public and for professionals at several levels of complexity. Their use for modification of the diet for individuals seems to hold great potential.

Role of the Patient and Family in Dietary Therapy.— Although intakes of saturated fatty acids and cholesterol have declined in the United States, most of our population continues to consume a diet that contributes to undesirably high cholesterol levels. The current social environment often does not provide easy access to appropriate food choices nor does it sufficiently reinforce diet modification. It is thus helpful to incorporate a social support element in nutrition education and dietary counseling. Inclusion of family and spouses in intervention sessions will significantly increase the chances of success of dietary strategies to lower cholesterol. Worksite and group strategies may be particularly successful when they integrate dietary change into the social context. New interactive methods have advantages over traditional didactic methods for providing information and reinforcement.

Appendix IV. Practical Suggestions to Improve Drug Adherence

Pre-Initiation Assessment.—In addition to selection of a drug based on its efficacy, an attempt should be made to select a drug that the patient is likely to tolerate. The patient should participate in this discussion and can be given the option of evaluating several drugs before deciding upon the final treatment plan. A few examples of the type of preliminary deliberation might include the following:

Sequestrants.—Good choice for young, motivated, and safety-conscious individuals. May not be a good choice for the patient who has significant constipation, existing hemorrhoids, recurrent symptoms of peptic ulcer or hiatus hernia; has a history of taking multiple drugs; or travels extensively.

Nicotinic Acid.—Good choice where cost is a major consideration, a tablet is preferred, or long-term effects on CHD or safety are desired. The drug may not be tolerated in the postmenopausal woman with flushing, or in the patient with angina pectoris or extensive coronary disease.

Lovastatin.—Good choice for the patient receiving multiple medications, with extensive disease, or severe forms of hypercholesteremia. The patient may have concerns about the lack of long-term safety information.

There are no absolute predictors of adherence, but one should be prepared to offer special assistance to patients with conditions frequently associated with reduced adherence. These include the following: current life changes, eg, marital status change, job or housing change, and so on; current or past history of psychological distress; smokers; lack of social support; erratic or irregular schedules; and recurring physiological complaints, particularly those that might be exacerbated by any side effects of the medication.

Pre-Initiation Education (This Is Particularly Important With the Bile Acid Sequestrants and Nicotinic Acid).—*Sequestrants.*—Demonstrate preparation of medication. Discuss how volume of fluid may affect palatability and large volumes may increase the sense of fullness. Rapid ingestion may cause air swallowing. If water is unsatisfactory, an unsweetened juice (avoid calories) may improve palatability. A heavy or pulpy juice may minimize complaints relative to consistency. Fluid and fiber intake (the latter may also produce some additional cholesterol lowering effect) should be increased to alleviate constipation. Laxatives should not be used, but stool softeners may be indicated occasionally.

Nicotinic acid.—Discuss flushing, its expected duration, development of tolerance, and the need to avoid taking medication on an empty stomach. Flushing may be diminished initially by pretreatment with an inhibitor of prostaglandin synthesis or use of a variety of sustained-release preparations such as Nico-Bid. Note that the cost of the sustained-release preparations is much greater than that of the usual nicotinic acid tablets.

Identify the most likely side effects and ways the patient has handled such symptoms in the past. Identify ways the patient can manage these side effects should they occur. It is important to reinforce the patient's capability to manage these symptoms if they do occur.

Review the patient's daily routine both during the week and on weekends. Help the patient to identify life-style factors that might interfere with adherence, and to identify ways in which the regimen or the daily routine could be adjusted to enhance adherence.

Teach the patient how to maintain a daily record of medication intake as well as how to use that record to identify factors, if any, which contribute to missed medication doses or to self-adjustments to the medication dosage.

Teach the patient about cholesterol-adherence relationships. In particular, stress the variability that exists in measured cholesterol values due to both laboratory and biological factors (eg, measurement methods, laboratory variation, seasonal variability, weight change, dietary intake, and stress).

Initiation of Treatment.—Tailor drug regimen to patient characteristics rather than asking for life-style changes in addition to those already prescribed.

Establish a regular follow-up schedule that will allow for the early identification and remediation of any problems. If possible, supplement the regular visit schedule with between-visit telephone checks until the regimen is solidly in place.

Gradually build up to the prescribed dose to minimize the occurrence of side effects and to allow the patient to adjust to the regimen.

Introduce self-monitoring and review these records at follow-up appointments until the patient is consistently adhering to the medication regimen at full dosage. Assist with any adherence difficulties promptly.

Ongoing Maintenance of Adherence.—Provide regular feedback to the patient regarding his or her cholesterol level so that the patient is aware of the treatment's success, and thus, the importance of adherence.

Involve spouses or other family members in the patient's therapy. Social support has a strong influence on long-term adherence.

Request that the patient periodically self-monitor adherence to the medication regimen. Use these records to evaluate the patient's adherence and to identify any difficulties the patient may be experiencing.

Maintain regularly scheduled followup with the patient, with active pursuit after missed appointments. Regular supervision is an important factor in maintaining adherence.

Give prompt attention to any changes in treatment response or in adherence.

Increase attention and the frequency of follow-up visits or telephone contact during periods of life stress or life change to minimize the adherence problems that are likely to ensue.

Encourage self-monitoring during periods of stress or life change to help the patient maintain awareness of the medication regimen and to identify problems that may be arising.

Teach the patient to solve problems. The ability to manage everyday therapy problems helps remove barriers to effective treatment.

INDEX

ACKNOWLEDGEMENTS

The publishers would like to acknowledge the help given to them by the Library of the Royal Society of Medicine.

The papers listed below are reproduced by permission of their respective copyright holders.

Academic Press Inc. (London) Ltd
European Heart Journal
Paper 34

Acta Medica Scandinavica
Paper 3

The American College of Physicians
Papers 7, 13

American College of Cardiology
Journal of the American College of Cardiology
Paper 30

The American Heart Association Inc.
Circulation
Papers 12, 18

Copyright – American Medical Association
Journal of the American Medical Association
Papers 9, 26, 27, 29, 31, 32

Copyright – American Medical Association
Archives of Internal Medicine
Paper 35

The American Society of Biological Chemists
Paper 4

Copyright – American Society for Clinical Investigation
Journal of Clinical Investigation
Papers 15, 16, 17, 19

The Biochemical Society
Paper 11

British Medical Journal
Paper 24

The C.V. Mosby Company
Paper 28

Federation of European Biochemical Societies
Papers 21, 22

J.L. Goldstein
Paper 14

The Lancet Ltd
Papers 6, 20, 25

R.W. Mahley
Paper 23

New England Journal of Medicine
Papers 10, 33

The Reuben H. Donnelley Corporation
Paper 8

Charles C. Thomas
Paper 5